Register Now for O to Your Book:

SPRINGER PUBLISHING COMPANY
CONNECT™

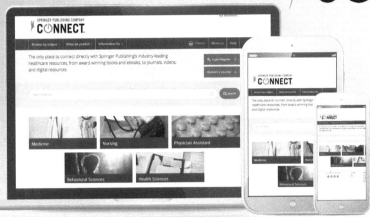

Your print purchase of *Neurocritical Care Board Review, Second Edition*, **includes online access to the contents of your book**—increasing accessibility, portability, and searchability!

Access today at:

http://connect.springerpub.com/content/book/978-0-8261-2382-4
or scan the QR code at the right with your smartphone and enter the access code below.

P9JA3D8H

Scan here for quick access.

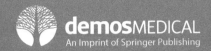

demosMEDICAL
An Imprint of Springer Publishing

View all our products at springerpub.com/demosmedical

Neurocritical Care Board Review

Questions and Answers

Second Edition

Editors

Asma Zakaria, MD
Neurointensivist
Division of Medical Critical Care Services
Inova Fairfax Hospital;
Assistant Professor
Department of Medicine
Virginia Commonwealth University
Falls Church, Virginia

Pouya Tahsili-Fahadan, MD
Neurointensivist
Division of Medical Critical Care Services
Inova Fairfax Hospital;
Assistant Professor
Department of Medicine
Virginia Commonwealth University
Falls Church, Virginia;
Adjunct Assistant Professor
Department of Neurology
Johns Hopkins University
Baltimore, Maryland

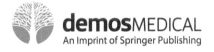
demosMEDICAL
An Imprint of Springer Publishing

Visit our website at www.Springerpub.com

ISBN: 9780826123596
ebook ISBN: 9780826123824

Acquisitions Editor: Beth Barry
Compositor: diacriTech

Medicine is an ever-changing science. Research and clinical experience are continually expanding our knowledge, in particular our understanding of proper treatment and drug therapy. The authors, editors, and publisher have made every effort to ensure that all information in this book is in accordance with the state of knowledge at the time of production of the book. Nevertheless, the authors, editors, and publisher are not responsible for errors or omissions or for any consequences from application of the information in this book and make no warranty, expressed or implied, with respect to the contents of the publication. Every reader should examine carefully the package inserts accompanying each drug and should carefully check whether the dosage schedules mentioned therein or the contraindications stated by the manufacturer differ from the statements made in this book. Such examination is particularly important with drugs that are either rarely used or have been newly released on the market.

Library of Congress Cataloging-in-Publication Data

Names: Zakaria, Asma, editor. | Tahsili-Fahadan, Pouya editor.
Title: Neurocritical care board review : questions and answers / edited by
    Asma Zakaria and Pouya Tahsili-Fahadan.
Description: Second edition. | New York : Demos Medical Publishing, an
    imprint of Springer Publishing Company, LLC., [2019] | Includes
    bibliographical references and index.
Identifiers: LCCN 2018039932 | ISBN 9780826123596
Subjects: | MESH: Nervous System Diseases–therapy | Critical Care |
    Examination Questions
Classification: LCC RC346 | NLM WL 18.2 | DDC 616.8/0428076–dc23 LC record available at
https://lccn.loc.gov/2018039932

Printed in the United States of America.

20 21 22 / 5 4 3

To Mimi and Ayza, who sacrificed their mama time for this project.
To Bülent, for teaching me patience and picking up the slack where I faltered.
To my parents for always being there.
AZ

To my wife, Noushin, who has accepted me as I am. I promise to cook for you
forever!
To my children, Jasmine and Darius.
To my mother and my father, Sharareh and Dr. Hossein Tahsili Fahadan.
PTF

Contents

PART II. GENERAL CRITICAL CARE: PATHOLOGY, PATHOPHYSIOLOGY, AND THERAPY

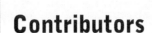

Contributors

Sasha D. Adams, MD, FACS   Associate Professor, Acute Care Surgery, McGovern Medical School, University of Texas Health Science Center at Houston, Houston, Texas

Lily Agrawal, MD   Professor of Medicine, Endocrinology Section, VA Hospital, Hines, Illinois

Nasiya Ahmed, MD   Assistant Professor, Department of Internal Medicine, Division of Geriatric and Palliative Medicine, University of Texas Health Science Center at Houston, Houston, Texas

Amy R. Alger, MD, FACS   Assistant Professor, Trauma and Critical Care Surgery, Department of Surgery, Duke University Medical Center, Durham, North Carolina

Teresa A. Allison, PharmD, BCPS, BCCCP   Clinical Pharmacy Specialist, Neurosciences, Memorial Hermann –Texas Medical Center, Department of Pharmacy, Houston, Texas

Laith Altaweel, MD   Neurointensivist, Division of Medical Critical Care Services, Inova Fairfax Hospital, Falls Church, Virginia

Réza Behrouz, DO, FAAN   Associate Professor, Division of Cerebrovascular Diseases, Department of Neurology, School of Medicine, University of Texas Health Science Center at San Antonio, San Antonio, Texas

Suur Biliciler, MD   Associate Professor, Neurology, McGovern Medical School, University of Texas Health Science Center at Houston, Houston, Texas

Nori L. Bradley, MD, MSc, FRCSC   Intensivist, Department of Critical Care Medicine, Medical Director, Organ Donation, Royal Columbian Hospital, New Westminster, British Columbia, Canada

Shivika Chandra, MD   Department of Neurology, University of Texas Health Science Center at Houston, Houston, Texas

Mehul Desai, MD   Associate Director of Adult ECMO, Medical Critical Care Services, Inova Heart and Vascular Institute, Fairfax, Virginia

Mary Ann Emanuele, MD   Professor of Medicine, Loyola University Medical Center, Endocrinology Division, Maywood, Illinois

Nicholas Emanuele, MD   Professor of Medicine, Loyola University Medical Center and Chief, Endocrinology Section, VA Hospital, Hines, Illinois

Yoshua Esquenazi, MD   Assistant Professor, Department of Neurosurgery, McGovern Medical School, University of Texas Health Science Center at Houston, Houston, Texas

Howard J. Fan, MD   Neurointensivist, Dignity Health Neuroscience Institute of Northern California, Mercy San Juan Hospital, Carmichael, California

Salia Farrokh, PharmD, BCPS, BCCCP   Clinical Pharmacy Specialist, Neuro Intensive Care, Johns Hopkins Hospital, Baltimore, Maryland

Matthew Flaherty, MD   Neurointensivist, Neurocritical Care, Stroke of Arizona, Phoenix, Arizona

Elissa K. Fory, MD   Neurologist, Bloomfield Hills, Michigan

Elizabeth Franco, PharmD   ICU/ED Clinical Pharmacy Specialist, CHI St Luke's Health –The Woodlands Hospital, Woodlands, Texas

Corey E. Goldsmith, MD   Assistant Professor of Neurology, Department of Neurology, Baylor College of Medicine, Houston, Texas

Aaron M. Goodman, MD   Assistant Professor of Medicine, Department of Medicine, Division of Blood and Marrow Transplantation, Moores Cancer Center, University of California San Diego, La Jolla, California

Hiba A. Haider, MD   Assistant Professor of Neurology, Division of Epilepsy, Emory University School of Medicine, Atlanta, Georgia

Giridhar P. Kalamangalam, MD, DPhil   Associate Professor, Department of Neurology, University of Florida, Gainesville, Florida

Aditya Kasarabada, MD, MPH, FCCP   Critical Care Attending, Medical Critical Care Services, Inova Fairfax Medical Campus, Falls Church, Virginia

Anand Kaul, MD   Resident, Department of Neurosurgery, Temple University, Philadelphia, Pennsylvania

Keith Kerr, MD   Chief Resident Physician, Department of Neurosurgery, McGovern Medical School, University of Texas Health Science Center at Houston, Houston, Texas

Daphne H. Knicely, MD   Assistant Professor of Medicine, Associate Director for Nephrology Fellowship Program, Division of Nephrology, Johns Hopkins University School of Medicine, Baltimore, Maryland

Doris Kung, DO   Assistant Professor, Neurology, Baylor College of Medicine, Houston, Texas

Justin Kwan, MD   Associate Professor, Neurology, Department of Neurology, Temple University, Lewis Katz School of Medicine, Philadelphia, Pennsylvania

Asad Latif, MD, MPH   Assistant Professor, Department of Anesthesiology and Critical Care Medicine, Division of Adult Critical Care Medicine, Johns Hopkins University School of Medicine, Baltimore, Maryland

Monica Lee, PharmD, BCCCP   Emergency Department Clinical Pharmacy Specialist, Houston Methodist West Hospital, Houston, Texas

Carolina B. Maciel, MD   Assistant Professor, Department of Neurology, University of Florida, Gainesville, Florida

Alaleh Mazhari, DO, FACE   Associate Professor of Medicine, Loyola University Medical Center, Endocrinology Division, Maywood, Illinois

Farah Meah, DO   Assistant Professor of Medicine, Endocrinology Section, VA Hospital, Hines, Illinois

Flavia Nelson, MD   Associate Professor of Neurology, Director, Multiple Sclerosis Division, University of Minnesota Twin Cities, Department of Neurology, Minneapolis, Minnesota

Anh Nguyen, MD   Neurointensivist, Houston Methodist Neurological Institute, Houston, Texas

Soo J. Park, MD   Hematology/Oncology Fellow, Department of Medicine, Division of Hematology-Oncology, Moores Cancer Center, University of California San Diego, La Jolla, California

Carlos Perez, MD   Child Neurology Fellow, Department of Pediatrics, Division of Child and Adolescent Neurology, University of Texas Health Science Center at Houston, Houston, Texas

Cecile L. Phan, MD   Clinical Associate Professor, Division of Neurology, Department of Medicine, Faculty of Medicine and Dentistry, University of Alberta, Edmonton, Alberta, Canada

Subhashini Ramesh, MD   Neurointensivist, Division of Medical Critical Care Services, Inova Fairfax Hospital, Falls Church, Virginia

Rohini Samudralwar, MD   Assistant Professor, Department of Neurology, McGovern Medical School, University of Texas Health Science Center at Houston, Houston, Texas

Scott R. Shepard, MD   Assistant Professor, Department of Neurosurgery, University of Texas Health Science Center at Houston, Houston, Texas

Brett Simpson, MD   Resident Physician, Department of Neurosurgery, McGovern Medical School, University of Texas Health Science Center at Houston, Houston, Texas

Philip M. Sommer, MD   Clinical Instructor, Department of Anesthesiology, Perioperative Care, and Pain Medicine, New York University Langone Health, New York, New York

Pouya Tahsili-Fahadan, MD   Neurointensivist, Division of Medical Critical Services, Inova Fairfax Hospital; Assistant Professor, Department of Medicine, Virginia Commonwealth University, Falls Church, Virginia; Adjunct Assistant Professor, Department of Neurology, Johns Hopkins University, Baltimore, Maryland

Nitin Tandon, MD   Professor, Department of Neurosurgery, McGovern Medical School, University of Texas Health Science Center; Director, Epilepsy Surgery Program, Texas Epilepsy Neural Technologies and NeuroInformatics Institute, Houston, Texas

Sumeska Thavarajah, MD   Assistant Professor of Medicine, Clinic Director for the Bayview Nephrology Clinic, Division of Nephrology, Johns Hopkins University School of Medicine, Baltimore, Maryland

Mithila Vullaganti, MD   Assistant Professor, Neurology, Department of Neurology, Tufts Medical Center, Boston, Massachusetts

Jing Wang, PhD   Physician Assistant, Division of Medical Critical Care Services, Inova Fairfax Hospital, Falls Church, Virginia

Grant M. Warmouth, MD   Staff Neurophysiologist, American Neuromonitoring Associates, St. Louis, Missouri

George W. Williams, MD   Associate Professor, Departments of Anesthesiology and Neurosurgery, Division of Neurocritical Care, University of Texas Health Science Center at Houston, Houston, Texas

Bülent Yapicilar, MD   Neurosurgeon, Nova Neuroscience, Vienna, Virginia

Asma Zakaria, MD   Neurointensivist, Division of Medical Critical Care Services, Inova Fairfax Hospital; Assistant Professor, Department of Medicine, Virginia Commonwealth University, Falls Church, Virginia

Preface

Since its recognition as a subspecialty in 2005, the neurocritical care community has significantly grown. An increasing number of hospitals across the United States provide subspecialized neurocritical care, and fellowship-trained neurointensivists are in demand more than ever. The first neurocritical care board examination was administered in 2007 by the United Council for Neurologic Subspecialties (UCNS) to assess competency in all aspects of neurocritical care. *Neurocritical Care Board Review, First Edition: Questions and Answers* was the first neurocritical care board review book and was warmly welcomed by both practicing and future neurointensivists. So far, almost 70 programs have received accreditation for fellowship training in neurocritical care, and more than 1,300 providers from different backgrounds and disciplines, including emergency medicine, general and vascular neurology, pediatrics, internal medicine, intensive care, and anesthesiology, as well as vascular and trauma surgeons and neurosurgeons have been certified as neurocritical care diplomats.

Recent advances in neurocritical care and requirements for board preparation demanded a new edition. *Neurocritical Care Board Review, Second Edition: Questions and Answers* underwent complete and thorough revision to reflect the reviews and comments from the first edition and feedback from our colleagues across different specialties and institutions. In keeping with the original intent of this book, we approached physicians from various medical and surgical specialties to author chapters based on the board curriculum, frequently encountered challenges or consults, and what they believed to be an appropriate level of understanding that an intensivist should have on a given topic. The chapters are named and arranged in a similar format to the board curriculum to allow for easy review and organization when studying for the boards. The question-and-answer (Q&A) format kept in the second edition allows the reader to perform thorough self-assessment prior to taking the exam. Several new questions have been added to each chapter. The answers are detailed and cover the majority of the board syllabus with updated references for additional reading. Recent advances in acute treatment of ischemic stroke and general critical care have revolutionized the field, and we have tried to incorporate these findings into this edition.

Neurocritical Care Board Review, Second Edition: Questions and Answers is intended to be a comprehensive study guide and self-assessment tool for candidates sitting for both initial certification and recertification in neurocritical care. In addition, trainees taking the surgical or medicine critical care boards will also find it useful as it covers the neurocritical care component of their board curriculums. *Neurocritical Care Board Review, Second Edition: Questions and Answers* is an easy-to-read, concise yet comprehensive, and portable learning resource not only for board preparation, but also for medical students, residents, and fellows rotating in the neurocritical care unit. Nurses, advance practice providers, and non-neurointensivist physicians who participate in the care of neurocritical care patients will also find this book to be an easy guide to the management of many frequently encountered issues, with case examples and imaging to further guide their education.

In June 2018, the American Board of Medical Specialties (ABMS) adopted a new subspecialty certification in neurocritical care involving the American Board of Psychiatry and Neurology (ABPN), American Board of Anesthesia (ABA), American Board of Emergency Medicine (ABEM), and American Board of Neurosurgery (ABNS). While the UCNS "recertification" and "initial certification" examinations are scheduled to be held in December 2018 and 2019, respectively, the new neurocritical care subspecialty offered by ABMS will allow for "uniformity in the training and skill sets of neurointensivists through ACGME-accredited fellowship training." We encourage all candidates to visit www.abms.org, www.neurocriticalcare.org, and www.ucns.org to peruse eligibility criteria as well as information regarding examination registration, format, and content.

Assembling this book has been a labor of love for us, and we hope that the readers of this book will also enjoy it and learn from it. All credit goes to our co-authors and colleagues, as well as our mentors, especially Drs. Diringer, Geocadin, and Powner. For those of you taking the Neurocritical Care Boards, we hope it serves its purpose of being a quick and easy self-assessment tool, reference, and guide. Good luck and we would love to hear your feedback!

Asma Zakaria, MD
Pouya Tahsili-Fahadan, MD
Inova Fairfax Hospital
Falls Church, Virginia

Neurologic Disease States: Pathology, Pathophysiology, and Therapy

1

CNS Ischemia and Hemorrhage

■ QUESTIONS

1. A 58-year-old man with long-standing hypertension has acute onset of right hemiplegia and aphasia 6 hours prior to his arrival in the ED. He is obtunded, with a dense left gaze deviation, and the left pupil is 6 mm and poorly reactive to light, while the right is 4 mm and reacts to light. The patient vomits and is subsequently intubated and then taken to CT scan, where he is found to have a large left hemisphere hypodensity with mass effect and uncal herniation. Of the following steps, which is most proven to lead to a good outcome?

   A. Osmotherapy with 23.4% saline
   B. Increase respiratory rate (RR) to 24
   C. Decompressive hemicraniectomy
   D. Administer intravenous (IV) alteplase
   E. Elevate head of bed to 30°

2. A 68-year-old man presents with acute onset left hemiparesis and headache. His symptoms started approximately 2.5 hours prior to arrival to the ED. His blood pressure (BP) on presentation was 218/110 mmHg. An emergent CT of the head shows an 18-mL intracerebral hemorrhage. His International Normalized Ratio (INR) is 1.0 and his platelet count is 112 cells/μL. Which of the following is true in his case?

   A. Lowering of systolic BP is associated with a better functional recovery
   B. Hemostatic medications (such as recombinant factor VII) mitigate hemorrhage volume growth and therefore improve outcomes
   C. Due to his thrombocytopenia, platelet transfusion is indicated
   D. All of the above are true

3. A 78-year-old man with hypertension, tobacco use, and hyperlipidemia presents with an episode of transient aphasia lasting 30 minutes and difficulty with right arm coordination. He is examined 1 hour later and found with no deficits. An MRI shows no acute stroke. Carotid duplex suggests 70% to 90% stenosis of the proximal left internal carotid artery at the bulb. He has no history of coronary artery disease (CAD), and his ECG is normal. The best option for stroke prevention in this patient is:

   A. High-dose statin therapy
   B. Aspirin
   C. Carotid stenting
   D. Carotid endarterectomy

4. A 54-year-old man with hypertension and hyperlipidemia experiences acute right hemiparesis and aphasia. He was last seen normal approximately 5 hours ago by his wife. In the ED, his blood pressure (BP) is 184/98 mmHg. His National Institutes of Health Stroke Scale (NIHSS) is 18. A noncontrasted CT shows no abnormal hypodensity, but a "dense middle cerebral artery (MCA) sign" on the left. His International Normalized Ratio (INR) is 0.9 and his platelet count is 225 cells/μL. What is the best next step in his care?

   A. Administer intravenous (IV) alteplase as soon as possible
   B. Prepare for endovascular treatment of left MCA occlusion
   C. Obtain a CT perfusion scan to assess for viable tissue
   D. Lower his systolic pressure to less than 140 mmHg immediately

5. A 21-year-old woman presents with brief right facial sensory loss and mild right upper extremity incoordination. Her symptoms resolve without any residual deficit. The MRI shows no infarct, but the magnetic resonance angiography (MRA) suggests high-grade right-middle cerebral artery stenosis. An angiogram confirms the stenosis and reveals extensive hypertrophy and collateralization in the lenticulostriate vessels. Her blood pressure (BP) is 135/65, and her lipid profile reveals a total cholesterol of 236 and a low-density lipoprotein of 112. The best option for subsequent management of this patient is:

   A. High-dose statin therapy
   B. Aspirin
   C. Endovascular stenting of the right-middle cerebral artery (MCA)
   D. Surgical bypass of the right MCA

6. A 72-year-old woman with a history of coronary artery disease (CAD) presents with acute onset of left hemiparesis, which started 2 hours ago. In the ED, her blood pressure (BP) is 184/98 mmHg. Noncontrasted CT of the head shows a 15-mL right basal ganglia intracerebral hemorrhage (ICH). Upon reviewing her medications list, the nurse notices that she is on aspirin 325 mg on a daily basis. The patient confirms this. Which one of the following is true is her case?

   A. Since she has been on an antiplatelet agent, platelet transfusion is indicated
   B. Since she has been on an antiplatelet agent, administration of DDAVP is indicated
   C. Platelet transfusion will have no benefit on outcomes in this patient
   D. Platelet transfusion will act as an antidote to aspirin and reverse its effect

7. An 85-year-old woman with mild dementia but no significant vascular disease presents to the ED within 1 hour of abrupt onset of nausea and altered mental status. Her blood pressure (BP) is 135/76, heart rate (HR) 104, respiratory rate (RR) 16, and temperature 36.8°C. Her exam is notable for dense left hemineglect. Her motor exam is limited by her neglect but appears normal. A CT scan of the brain shows a 4-cm right parietal intracerebral hemorrhage (ICH). Which of the following treatments could significantly worsen her outcome?

   A. Placement of an intraventricular catheter to measure intracranial pressure (ICP)
   B. Surgical evacuation of the hematoma within 4 hours
   C. Prophylactic seizure therapy with levetiracetam
   D. Early nutrition support with tube feeds

8. A 45-year-old man with poorly controlled hypertension presents with new onset ataxia and dysarthria with a systolic blood pressure (BP) of 225/115. A noncontrast head CT shows a 4-cm right cerebellar hemisphere hemorrhage with compression of the fourth ventricle and dilation of the lateral and third ventricles. The next best step in management is:

   A. Target mean arterial pressure (MAP) of less than 100 mmHg with labetalol push and nicardipine drip
   B. Insert intraventricular drain and normalize intracranial pressure (ICP)

C. Surgical evacuation of the cerebellar hematoma

D. Perform a cerebral angiogram to evaluate for aneurysm

9. A 35-year-old man with poorly controlled hypertension presents to the ED with acute dysarthria. His initial blood pressure (BP) is 175/110. A noncontrast head CT shows a 1-cm pontine hemorrhage. He is placed on a nicardipine drip, but before his BP responds, he becomes obtunded and a follow-up CT shows significant hematoma expansion to involve 3 cm of the mid pons. He is intubated and moved to the ICU with a Glasgow Coma Scale (GCS) score of 6. Upon arrival to the ICU, the nursing staff comments that this patient has a poor prognosis and asks you to discuss do-not-resuscitate (DNR) status with the family. The most appropriate next step is to:

A. Explain to the family that the patient will likely not survive to a functional status and they should consider no cardiopulmonary resuscitation (CPR) if he worsens overnight

B. Call an ethics consult to evaluate elements of the case for futility of care

C. Notify the family of the severity of the injury, but strongly urge them to allow CPR and full code status for the next 24 hours

D. Notify the case manager that the patient will likely need long-term care, and plan for early tracheotomy and a gastrostomy tube

10. A 60-year-old woman has a severe headache followed by left hemiplegia. She is brought to the ED and a noncontrast head CT shows a 15-mL right thalamic hemorrhage with intraventricular extension, including within the third and fourth ventricles. Her blood pressure (BP) is 187/100, heart rate (HR) is 20, respiratory rate (RR) is 20, and temperature is 37.2°C. She is awake and cooperative but is slowly becoming more lethargic. Her BP is cautiously lowered with labetalol to a mean arterial pressure (MAP) of 120 mmHg. She has an intraventricular drain placed that allows intracranial pressure (ICP) monitoring and cerebrospinal fluid (CSF) drainage. Which of the following therapies has been shown to reduce disability in this patient?

A. Intraventricular tissue plasminogen activator (tPA)

B. Intraventricular recombinant factor VII

C. Active aspiration of the intraventricular blood

D. None of the above

11. A 23-year-old woman is postpartum day 2 from a normal vaginal delivery for which she received an epidural anesthetic, which was a "wet tap" with spinal leak. She is scheduled to be discharged home but has a lingering headache and mild nausea, which has been attributed to a spinal headache. She then has a generalized seizure and becomes difficult to arouse. Her sclera are injected. She is intubated and taken for noncontrast CT, which shows diffuse cerebral edema with multiple dilated vessels in the vertex. There are two small cortical hemorrhages, one 1 cm in the left frontal region, and the other 6 mm in the right parietal region. What is the likely diagnosis?

A. Ruptured arteriovenous malformation (AVM)

B. Ruptured left middle cerebral artery (MCA) aneurysm

C. Cerebral venous thrombosis

D. Brainstem infarction

12. For the same patient, what is the best initial management?

A. Heparin drip

B. Interventional thrombolysis

C. Mannitol

D. Hemicraniectomy

13. A 45-year-old woman is an unrestrained passenger in a motor vehicle accident where she sustains a blow to the right side of her head. Other than a brief loss of consciousness and head pain, she has no deficits. She has a negative noncontrast head CT in an ED after the event and is discharged home. Over the next several weeks, she notices diplopia, tearing, chemosis, conjunctival injection, and a pulsating sensation of the left eye, prompting further evaluation. Upon seeing her in your office, the most useful diagnostic test is:

    A. Brain MRI with contrast
    B. Cerebral angiogram
    C. Optic nerve sheath ultrasound
    D. Formal visual field assessment

14. A 24-year-old woman who has given birth to a healthy infant 2 weeks ago presents with headache and personality change per her husband. Symptoms began the last evening and progressed. She states that her blood pressure (BP) was poorly controlled during and after pregnancy and she is currently on labetalol 200 mg twice daily. This regimen was started after she was hospitalized for 2 days 1 week ago with a diagnosis of preeclampsia. She has been experiencing "migraine" headaches since the birth of her child and has been using her usual sumatriptan frequently. On exam, her BP is 188/112 mmHg. She is alert and fully oriented, but complains of a severe frontal headache. A CT of the head shows a 20-mL right frontal intracerebral hemorrhage (ICH) and subarachnoid blood in the right Sylvian fissure. What is the best course of action in her case?

    A. Start heparin immediately for cerebral venous thrombosis
    B. Lower BP and obtain CT angiography
    C. Administer subcutaneous sumatriptan to control the headache and obtain CT angiography
    D. Start an antiepileptic medication and magnesium

15. A 26-year-old nurse has frequent nausea and vomiting during pregnancy. After an episode of vomiting, she becomes aphasic and has difficulty moving her right arm. She is brought to the ED, where her symptoms begin to improve, but on exam, she remains impaired in language fluency and has a right-arm drift. Initial CT is normal, but subsequent MRI shows an infarction in the left insula and precentral gyrus. She undergoes magnetic resonance angiogram (MRA) of the neck, which shows a 6-cm dissection of the carotid artery originating from the carotid bulb. The lumen is reduced in diameter to approximately 70%. She has been improving with no further symptoms. The best treatment at this point is:

    A. Endovascular stenting
    B. Aspirin
    C. Warfarin
    D. Endarterectomy

16. Which of the following statements regarding blood pressure (BP) management in stroke patients is true?

    A. There is significant class-specific evidence for the superiority of calcium channel blockers in stroke patients over other BP–reducing medications
    B. Stopping BP medications in hospitalized acute stroke patients leads to worse outcomes
    C. Careful BP lowering in the hospital was demonstrated to lead to better outcomes in the Scandinavian Candesartan Acute Stroke Trial (SCAST)
    D. Two-drug therapy is indicated as an initial strategy in patients with an observed BP of 160/100

17. A 93-year-old man presents with acute onset left hemiparesis and hemineglect. Symptoms started 40 minutes ago and have not changed. His blood pressure (BP) is 178/88 mmHg. CT of the head is unremarkable. He has a history of atrial fibrillation and takes warfarin. His International Normalized Ratio (INR) in the ED is 1.6. His wife states that he had a stroke 4 months ago. Which one of the following is true in this patient?

    A. Intravenous (IV) tissue plasminogen activator (tPA) is contraindicated due to his advanced age
    B. IV tPA is contraindicated due to his elevated INR
    C. IV tPA is not contraindicated in this patient
    D. IV tPA is contraindicated due to a recent stroke

18. A 60-year-old woman with hypertension but no prior stroke or other cerebrovascular disorders presents to the hospital via emergency medical service (EMS) after being found down by her son. Her son had dinner with her the evening before and she said goodnight to him around 11 p.m. He saw her walking normally from her bedroom at 8 a.m., but they did not talk. At 10 a.m., she called him at work and was difficult to understand so he came home and found her on the floor. It is now 11:30 a.m. Her blood pressure (BP) is 175/100, heart rate (HR) is 74 and regular, and temperature is 36.9°C. The patient has a right gaze with dense left hemiplegia. CT of the brain shows blurring of the gray–white junction in the right middle cerebral artery (MCA) territory, but no definite hypodensity. Her National Institutes of Health (NIH) Stroke Scale is calculated to be 22. The right MCA is hyperdense. Is this patient a candidate for thrombolysis?

    A. No, her last-known normal was the prior evening, which is outside the tissue plasminogen activator (tPA) window
    B. No, her last-known normal was 8 a.m., which is outside the approved 3-hour window for tPA
    C. Yes, her time of onset was 10 a.m., which is within the approved 3-hour window for tPA
    D. Yes, her last-known normal was 8 a.m., which is within the 4.5-hour window for tPA

19. A 76-year-old woman with a history of atrial fibrillation presents with sudden onset of left hemiparesis and hemineglect. The CT shows a 33-mL right parietal intracerebral hemorrhage (ICH). She is taking dabigatran. The last dose of this medication was 4 hours ago. What is the best treatment for this patient in view of anticoagulation-related ICH?

    A. Fresh frozen plasma
    B. Prothrombin complex concentrate
    C. Idarucizumab
    D. Intravenous vitamin K

20. An 89-year-old woman who lives alone has acute onset of left hemiparesis and dysarthria. She is brought to the ED, receives intravenous (IV) tissue plasminogen activator (tPA), and improves to her baseline despite evidence of a 3-cm infarction in the right insula on MRI. The MRI otherwise shows age-appropriate atrophy without a significant amount of white matter disease. During her evaluation, she is found to be in atrial fibrillation. What regimen should be recommended for secondary stroke prevention?

    A. Aspirin
    B. Aspirin plus clopidogrel
    C. Warfarin
    D. Amiodarone without anticoagulation

21. In which scenario is anticonvulsant therapy recommended?

    A. Prophylaxis in ischemic stroke patients with large cortical infarctions
    B. Prophylaxis in hemorrhagic lobar stroke patients with significant edema
    C. Prophylaxis in ischemic stroke patients, posthemicraniectomy
    D. Ischemic stroke patients who have an isolated, brief seizure 2 weeks after initial stroke

22. A 31-year-old woman with no significant medical problems experienced a severe headache while jogging. She went to the ED and was alert but had a severe, throbbing headache and no focal neurologic symptoms. Her blood pressure (BP) was 173/105, and noncontrast head CT was normal. She went home from the ED, and the following day, she experienced aphasia while speaking to a friend on the phone. She returned to the ED, where her symptoms resolved, but a repeat CT scan showed a small, distal, right parietal convexity subarachnoid hemorrhage (SAH). Lumbar puncture (LP) was normal with no inflammation. Cerebral angiography showed no aneurysm or arteriovenous malformation (AVM), but multiple areas of vasoconstriction. She was treated with fluids, and an extensive autoimmune workup was negative. On follow-up imaging 3 months later, one would expect to find:

    A. Complete resolution of the vasoconstriction
    B. Mycotic aneurysms
    C. Hypertrophy of the lenticulostriates
    D. Diffuse white matter disease

23. A 49-year-old woman with no significant past medical history is staying at a hotel on a business trip abroad when she has acute onset of dysarthria and left-sided weakness with sensory loss. She is found to have a moderate-sized right-middle cerebral artery (MCA) infarction on MRI, but no sign of large vessel disease. Her hypercoagulable workup is negative, ECG and telemetry are normal, and transthoracic echocardiogram is normal, but transesophageal echocardiogram shows a right-to-left shunt across a patent foramen ovale during the Valsalva maneuver. The patient is very interested in "fixing the problem" and would like to have the patent foramen ovale (PFO) closed. The most appropriate next step in management is:

    A. Refer the patient to a cardiologist for PFO closure
    B. Start combination of aspirin and clopidogrel
    C. Start anticoagulation immediately
    D. Obtain lower extremity venous Doppler

24. A 73-year-old woman with hyperlipidemia and hypertension experiences a 30-minute episode of dysarthria and right-side weakness. She comes to the ED and is fully recovered. Her initial blood pressure (BP) is 163/102. CT is normal, and ECG shows normal sinus rhythm. What is her ABCD2 score, and should she be admitted to the hospital?

    A. 3, no admission required
    B. 4, no admission required
    C. 4, admission required
    D. 5, admission required

25. A 69-year-old man has chest pain and is found to have an aortic dissection requiring emergent surgical repair. Postoperatively, he is noted to be paraplegic. Which of the following strategies is worthwhile in this patient?

    A. Reduction of mean arterial pressure (MAP) to target less than 100 mmHg
    B. Placement of a lumbar drain
    C. Avoid bypass methods during surgery for distal reperfusion
    D. Prolong ICU sedation to avoid oxygen consumption

■ ANSWERS

1. **The answer is C.** Hemicraniectomy is a life-saving remedy in the setting of massive hemispheric infarct. The results of the HAMLET–DESTINY–DECIMAL pooled analysis of hemicraniectomy versus medical management provide strong evidence for this therapy. A total of 93 patients were included in the pooled analysis. More patients in the decompressive surgery group than in the control group had a modified Rankin Score (mRS) less than or equal to 4 (75% vs. 24%; pooled absolute risk reduction 51%), an mRS 3 (43% vs. 21%; 23%), and survived (78% vs. 29%; 50%); with numbers needed to treat of two for survival with mRS 4, four for survival with mRS 3, and two for survival irrespective of functional outcome. In this scenario, the patient is an ideal candidate for surgery based on his age and the early nature of the edema. Osmotherapy is an important temporizing measure to reduce edema for 2 to 6 hours, but it is not the best answer as it is not a therapy that has been subjected to a large, randomized trial to show better outcomes in the absence of definitive management. Similarly, raising the head of the bed or increasing the respiratory rate will produce a decrease in intracranial pressure (ICP) but will not be expected to provide sufficient benefit to lead to a better outcome. Intra-arterial thrombolysis would be poorly tolerated in a patient with a large hypodensity on CT and signs of herniation. It would most likely worsen the patient's outcome based on analysis of the PROACT II trial.

   Anderson CS, Heeley E, Huang Y, et al. INTERACT2 Investigators. Rapid blood-pressure lowering in patients with acute intracerebral hemorrhage. *N Engl J Med*. 2013;368(25):2355-2365. doi:10.1056/NEJMoa1214609

   Vahedi K, Hofmeijer J, Juettler E, et al. Early decompressive surgery in malignant infarction of the middle cerebral artery: a pooled analysis of three randomized control trials. *Lancet Neurol*. 2007;6(3):215-222. doi:10.1016/S1474-4422(07)70036-4

2. **The answer is A.** The Intensive Blood Pressure Reduction in Acute Cerebral Hemorrhage (INTERACT 2) trial showed significantly better functional recovery on an ordinal analysis of scores on the modified Rankin scale (odds ratio for greater disability, 0.87; 95% confidence interval, 0.77 to 1.00; $p = .04$). In ATACH-2 trial, risk of death or disability at 3 months did not differ between intensive (goal 110–139 mmHg) versus standard (goal 140–179 mmHg) systolic blood pressure lowering within 4.5 hours of symptom onset. B is incorrect since the Factor Seven for Acute Hemorrhagic Stroke (FAST) trial showed that although hemostatic therapy with recombinant activated factor VII reduced hematoma growth in patients with acute intracerebral hemorrhage (ICH), it did not improve survival or functional outcomes. C is incorrect because platelet count of 110 cells/μL does not meet the criteria for severe thrombocytopenia, for which platelet transfusion is indicated base on the American Heart Association guidelines.

   Hemphill JC 3rd, Greenberg SM, Anderson CS, et al. Guidelines for the management of spontaneous intracerebral hemorrhage: a guideline for healthcare professionals from the American Heart Association/American Stroke Association. *Stroke*. 2015;46(7):2032-2060. doi:10.1161/STR.0000000000000069

   Mayer SA, Brun NC, Begtrup K, et al. Efficacy and safety of recombinant activated factor VII for acute intracerebral hemorrhage. *N Engl J Med*. 2008;358(20):2127-2137. doi:10.1056/NEJMoa0707534

   Qureshi AI, Palesch YY, Barsan WG, et al. Intensive blood-pressure lowering in patients with acute cerebral hemorrhage. *N Engl J Med*. 2016;375(11):1033-1043.doi:10.1056/NEJMoa1603460

3. **The answer is D.** This patient has suffered a transient ischemia attack (TIA) of the left hemisphere. The high-grade (>70%) stenosis found in the ipsilateral carotid artery (ICA) places this patient at approximately 26% risk of stroke in 2 years, according to the North American Symptomatic Carotid Endarterectomy Trial (NASCET). The addition of aspirin or statin therapy is appropriate, but they are not sufficient to exclude revascularization, which remains the best option and offers the most relative risk reduction of the choices provided (65% for endarterectomy vs. approximately 20% for aspirin and approximately 30%–35% for statins). Carotid stenting and endarterectomy are comparable methods to achieve revascularization, and choosing the right option depends on the patient's comorbidities. In a patient with a high risk of perioperative myocardial infarction, stenting would be preferable. This

patient has no such risk from the information given. Furthermore, in the Carotid Revascularization Endarterectomy versus Stenting Trial (CREST), patients older than 70 years had less risk of stroke with endarterectomy than stenting. In this case, endarterectomy is the best option. Considerations such as location of the plaque, risk of cranial nerve palsies, and cosmetic scarring should be kept in mind, but in this case, the lesion is easily accessible with surgery.

Brott TG, Hobson RW 2nd, Howard G, et al. Stenting versus endarterectomy for treatment of carotid-artery stenosis. *N Engl J Med.* 2010;363(1):11-23. doi:10.1056/NEJMoa0912321

4. **The answer is B.** IV alteplase is not indicated as he is outside of the window for this medication. He is still within the 6 hours window of endovascular intervention. Based on the severity of his deficit and a left "dense MCA sign" that correlated with his symptoms, we know that the culprit lesion is a left MCA occlusion. In the interest of time—since only 1 hour is left to closure of endovascular window—CT perfusion will be of little benefit. Lowering of BP is not indicated in this particular scenario. D is incorrect; there is no such target for ischemic stroke.

Powers WJ, Derdeyn CP, Biller J, et al. 2015 American Heart Association American Stroke Association focused update of the 2013 guidelines for the early management of patients with acute ischemic stroke regarding endovascular treatment: a guideline for healthcare professionals from the American Heart Association American Stroke Association. *Stroke.* 2015;46(10):3020-3035. doi:10.1161/STR.0000000000000074

5. **The answer is D.** This patient presents with classic angiographic findings of Moyamoya disease. Statin therapy has no proven role in Moyamoya disease and based on this patient's age, it is highly unlikely that the angiographic results represent atherosclerosis. Aspirin therapy is a reasonable consideration but should not be carried out in the long term without surgical management because of the risk of the hypertrophied vessels rupturing and causing a basal ganglia hemorrhage. Endovascular stenting is contraindicated and results in rapid restenosis. Surgical management with superficial temporal artery bypass to the MCA (also called extracranial–intracranial (EC–IC bypass) is effective and associated with a lower risk of ischemia and hemorrhage.

Smith ER, Scott RM. Surgical management of moyamoya syndrome. *Skull Base.* 2005;15(1):15-26. doi:10.1055/s-2005-868160

6. **The answer is C.** The Platelet Transfusion in Cerebral Haemorrhage (PATCH) trial was a randomized, open-label, phase 3 trial that showed platelet transfusion seems inferior to standard care for people taking antiplatelet therapy before ICH. In fact, participants who received platelet transfusion had more serious adverse events during their hospital stay than those who were not transfused. DDAVP has not shown to be of benefit in patients with ICH and antiplatelet use prior to that.

Baharoglu MI, Cordonnier C, Al-Shahi Salman R, et al. Platelet transfusion versus standard care after acute stroke due to spontaneous cerebral haemorrhage associated with antiplatelet therapy (PATCH): a randomised, open-label, phase 3 trial. *Lancet.* 2016;387(10038):2605-2613. doi:10.1016/S0140-6736(16)30392-0

7. **The answer is B.** The Surgical Trial in Intracerebal Hemorrhage (STICH) trial showed no benefit to surgical evacuation of ICH and subsequent trials of early evacuation showed worse outcomes. In particular, this patient is likely to have cerebral amyloid angiopathy, and surgery carries a significant risk of adjacent tissue hemorrhage. Although surgery remains controversial in most cases, isolated craniectomy without hematoma evacuation would be worthwhile to consider in a patient with impending herniation from supratentorial ICH. There is no evidence that prophylactic seizure therapy improves outcomes, although in the case of levetiracetam, there is also no evidence of worsening outcomes. Early nutritional support has been shown to improve outcomes. An intraventricular catheter for monitoring ICP is indicated if the Glasgow Coma Scale score (GCS) is less than 8 and has not been observed to worsen outcomes.

Mendelow AD, Gregson BA, Fernandes HM, et al. Early surgery versus initial conservative treatment in patients with spontaneous supratentorial intracerebral haematomas in the International Surgical Trial in Intracerebral Haemorrhage (STICH): a randomised trial. *Lancet.* 2005;365(9457):387-397. doi:10.1016/S0140-6736(05)70233-6

Morgenstern LB, Demchuk AM, Kim DH, et al. Rebleeding leads to poor outcome in ultra-early craniotomy for intracerebral hemorrhage. *Neurology.* 2001;56(10):1294-1299. doi:10.1212/WNL.56.10.1294

Naidech AM, Garg RK, Liebling S, et al. Anticonvulsant use and outcomes after intracerebral hemorrhage. *Stroke.* 2009;40(12):3810-3815. doi:10.1161/STROKEAHA.109.559948

8. **The answer is C.** According to the guidelines of the American Heart Association, patients with cerebellar hemorrhage who are deteriorating neurologically or who have brainstem compression and/or hydrocephalus from ventricular obstruction should undergo surgical removal of the hemorrhage as soon as possible, and that initial treatment of these patients with ventricular drainage rather than surgical evacuation is not recommended. Cerebral angiogram is a worthwhile diagnostic test, but it should be performed after the craniectomy.

Hemphill JC 3rd, Greenberg SM, Anderson CS, et al. Guidelines for the management of spontaneous intracerebral hemorrhage: a guideline for healthcare professionals from the American Heart Association American Stroke Association. *Stroke.* 2015;46(7):2032-2060. doi:10.1161/STR.0000000000000069

9. **The answer is C.** This patient has a potentially devastating hemorrhage in a region of the brain that could lead to permanent disability. Nonetheless, based on his intracerebral hemorrhage (ICH) score, his 30-day mortality risk is only 26%. The use of DNR orders in the ICU varies significantly by institution. In a meta-analysis of ICU prognosis, factors such as gender, GCS, ICH volume, intraventricular hemorrhage (IVH), age, midline shift, uncal herniation, cisternal effacement, location of the hemorrhage, and glucose level were all considered as prognostic factors, but DNR status was the only variable that significantly predicted mortality. Furthermore, in this study DNR orders were implemented and care withdrawn on average at 2 days. This suggests that DNR orders worsen patient outcome, especially when implemented early. It is important to involve family members in the decision-making process, but unless a patient has a preexisting DNR order or long-standing, well-known wishes to not receive aggressive care, DNR orders should be postponed for at least 24 hours.

Becker KJ, Baxter AB, Cohen WA, et al. Withdrawal of support in intracerebral hemorrhage may lead to self-fulfilling prophecies. *Neurology.* 2001;56(6):766-772. doi:10.1212/WNL.56.6.766

10. **The answer is D.** Clot Lysis Evaluation of Accelerated Resolution of Intraventricular Hemorrhage III (CLEAR III) was a randomized, double-blinded, placebo-controlled, multiregional trial that showed that in patients with intraventricular hemorrhage (IVH) and a routine extraventricular drain, irrigation with alteplase did not substantially improve functional outcomes at the modified Rankin Score (mRS) 3 cutoff compared with irrigation with saline. Answers B and C are unrealistic.

Hanley DF, Lane K, McBee N, et al. Thrombolytic removal of intraventricular haemorrhage in treatment of severe stroke: results of the randomised, multicentre, multiregion, placebo-controlled CLEAR III trial. *Lancet.* 2017;389(10069):603-611. doi:10.1016/S0140-6736(16)32410-2

11. **The answer is C.** Cerebral venous thrombosis is a difficult diagnosis to make based on non-contrast head CT and requires a high degree of suspicion. A contrast-enhanced CT will often reveal the thrombosis more readily, and if suspected, this is a rare indication for contrast-enhanced CT in acute stroke. The CT findings include dilated cortical veins, cortical subarachnoid blood, and dense-appearing cerebral sinuses. With contrast, the dense sinus sign becomes the so-called empty delta sign and is present in about one third of cases. CT remains normal in many cases. A number of patients who lack typical vascular risk factors are at risk for venous thrombosis, such as pregnant women; patients with

hematological, oncological, and autoimmune diseases; and patients with head trauma or recent intrathecal or spinal procedures. The findings of scleral injection make venous insufficiency very likely. Ruptured AVM or aneurysm would be expected to produce more obvious signs of subarachnoid blood in a patient who deteriorates rapidly and is preceded with a much more severe headache. A brainstem infarction should not produce cortical hemorrhages.

Hacein-Bey L, Varelas PN, Ulmer JL, et al. Imaging of cerebrovascular disease in pregnancy and the puerperium. *AJR Am J Roentgenol.* 2016;206(1):26-38. doi:10.2214/AJR.15.15059

12. **The answer is A.** In most patients with cerebral venous thrombosis, there is an excellent response to heparin infusion. This treatment should be continued even in the presence of small cortical bleeds. Bleeding in cerebral venous thrombosis is caused by high venous pressure, and thus adequate anticoagulation is necessary to manage the underlying problem. The other treatments listed are reasonable considerations in a patient who does not respond to intravenous (IV) heparin. Osmotherapy can cause dehydration and venous constriction and worsen the thrombotic situation, but it has a role when attempts at reducing intracranial pressure (ICP) have failed or are not available, including lumbar drainage, acetazolamide, and optic nerve fenestration. Hemicraniectomy should be considered when all other options at relieving ICP have failed and herniation is a concern.

Ferro JM, Canhão P. Cerebral venous sinus thrombosis: update on diagnosis and management. *Curr Cardiol Rep.* 2014;16(9):523. doi:10.1007/s11886-014-0523-2

13. **The answer is B.** The presentation is typical of a carotid–cavernous fistula. This abnormal communication between the carotid artery and the cavernous sinus often arises from trauma, but can occur spontaneously, and should be suspected in any patient with unexplained chemosis, especially if it involves any degree of ophthalmoplegia. The contents of the cavernous sinus include cranial nerves III and IV, which are compressed by the enlarging fistula and cause ophthalmoplegia. Treatment is typically endovascular occlusion of the fistula.

Ellis JA, Goldstein H, Connolly ES Jr, et al. Carotid-cavernous fistulas. *Neurosurg Focus.* 2012;32(5):E9. doi:10.3171/2012.2.FOCUS1223

14. **The answer is B.** Cerebral venous thrombosis is a possibility, but given the sequence of events such as a history of poorly controlled BP and postpartum overuse of triptans, the most likely diagnosis is postpartum angiopathy (PPA). The most common presentation of PPA is cerebral hemorrhage. Lowering the BP carefully and obtaining a CT angiogram will provide details on the underlying cause of the patient's hemorrhage. A is wrong because one should not start heparin indiscriminately until an unequivocal diagnosis of cerebral venous thrombosis is made. The other two choices are incorrect. Administration of triptans in the face of elevated and history of uncontrolled BP is contraindicated. Choice D is not a valid answer.

Fugte JE, Ameriso SF, Ortiz G, et al. Variable presentations of postpartum angiopathy. *Stroke.* 2012;43(3):670-676. doi:10.1161/STROKEAHA.111.639575

15. **The answer is B.** In the Cervical Artery Dissection in Stroke Study (CADISS), a randomized, end-point blinded study of 250 patients showed no difference in efficacy of antiplatelet and anticoagulant drugs at preventing stroke and death in patients with symptomatic carotid and vertebral artery dissection. In this pregnant woman, warfarin would not be desirable because of teratogenicity. Surgical options for management of dissection exist, but are quite rare and typically reserved for ligation when endovascular and medical management are not possible. Endovascular repair has become more frequent, and while prospective data for its efficacy and safety are lacking, it is commonly used when a patient does not respond to initial medical management or has intracranial extension of the dissection, neither of which are present in this scenario.

CADISS trial investigators, Markus HS, Hayter E, et al. Antiplatelet treatment compared with anti-coagulation treatment for cervical artery dissection (CADISS): a randomised trial. *Lancet Neurol.* 2015;14(4):361-367. doi:10.1016/S1474-4422(15)70018-9

16. **The answer is D.** Two-drug therapy is indicated as an initial strategy in patients with an observed BP of 160/100. According to the Joint National Committee (JNC) 7 guidelines, patients with BP greater than 160 systolic or greater than 100 diastolic are considered stage 2 hypertension, and initial therapy with two-drug classes is recommended. BP goals and strategies remain controversial, and increasing evidence suggests there is little to be gained by either permissive hypertension or modest lowering of BP acutely. In the SCAST, careful blood pressure lowering had no effect on outcome, and in the Continue or Stop post-Stroke Antihypertensives Collaborative Study (COSSACS) trial, neither continuing nor stopping BP medications in hospitalized stroke patients had an effect on outcomes. There is good evidence for secondary stroke prevention with a number of classes of antihypertensive medications. While calcium channel blockers are a reasonable strategy, there is no reason to choose this class over thiazide diuretics, angiotensin converting enzyme (ACE) inhibitors, or angiotensin receptor blockers. Thiazide diuretics, remain the first line of recommendation in JNC 7.

Robinson TG, Potter JF, Ford GA, et al. Effects of antihypertensive treatment after acute stroke in the Continue or Stop Post-Stroke Antihypertensives Collaborative Study (COSSACS): a prospective, randomised, open, blinded-endpoint trial. *Lancet Neurol.* 2010;9(8):767-775. doi:10.1016/S1474-4422(10)70163-0

Sandset EC, Bath PM, Boysen G, et al. The angiotensin-receptor blocker candesartan for treatment of acute stroke (SCAST): a randomised, placebo-controlled, double-blind trial. *Lancet.* 2011;377(9767):741-750. doi:10.1016/S0140-6736(11)60104-9

17. **The answer is C.** IV tPA is not contraindicated in this patient. Age is not an exclusionary factor for administration of IV tPA, so long as the patient is 18 and older. His International Normalized Ratio (INR) is 1.7; he would exclude if his INR was greater than 1.7. His stroke was more than 3 months ago.

Powers WJ, Rabinstein AA, Ackerson T, et al. 2018 guidelines for the early management of patients with acute ischemic stroke. A guideline for healthcare professionals from the American Heart Association/American Stroke Association. *Stroke.* 2018;49(3):e46-e110. doi:10.1161/STR.0000000000000158

18. **The answer is D.** Determining eligibility for thrombolysis depends on establishing a "last known well" time in most cases, unless the stroke onset is directly observed. The 10 a.m. phone call cannot be used as a last known normal since the patient was not observed between 8 a.m. and 10 a.m. to be well. Nonetheless, the clinician should use all available information to make this determination and consider each scenario in the context of both history and imaging. The CT suggests an acute stroke, so it is reasonable to assume that the stroke is only a few hours old. Furthermore, the son's report of his mother walking at 8 a.m. is sufficient to establish that she was well at 8 a.m. even though she did not speak. If a patient has isolated aphasia or dysarthria, this might not be enough information, but in a patient with an obvious MCA infarction, it is safe to assume that she would not have been able to walk normally if this stroke was in evolution at 8 a.m. Finally, the window for thrombolysis has been expanded to 4.5 hours based on the European Cooperative Acute Stroke Study III (ECASS III) trial. Patients older than 80 years, those with NIH Stroke Scale score greater than 25, and those with diabetes and prior stroke were excluded in this trial. This patient has none of these exclusions, so she qualifies for the extended time window.

Hacke W, Kaste M, Bluhmki E, et al. Thrombolysis with alteplase 3 to 4.5 hours after acute ischemic stroke. *N Engl J Med.* 2008;359(13):1317-1329. doi:10.1056/NEJMoa0804656

19. **The answer is C.** The patient has suffered ICH due to dabigatran. This drug is not reversed by vitamin K, and fresh frozen plasma and prothrombin complex concentrate are unlikely to be effective. The only proven treatment for hemorrhage due to dabigatran is the monoclonal antibody fragment idarucizumab, which binds dabigatran with an affinity that is 350 times higher than that observed for thrombin. In a prospective cohort study of 90 patients, idarucizumab completely reversed the anticoagulant effect of dabigatran within minutes.

Pollack CV Jr, Reilly PA, Eikelboom J, et al. Idarucizumab for dabigatran reversal. *N Engl J Med.* August 6, 2015;373(6):511-520. doi:10.1056/NEJMoa1502000

20. **The answer is C.** Although the risk of major intracranial hemorrhage (ICH) increases with advanced age, the risk of ischemic stroke from atrial fibrillation increases as well and remains significantly greater than the risk of ICH. A prospective trial of 973 patients older than 75 years assigned to warfarin versus aspirin for atrial fibrillation found that ischemic strokes were more than twice as common in the aspirin group (44 events vs. 21 in warfarin group), but that major bleeds were equivalent (three in the warfarin group and four in the aspirin group). Warfarin in this population produced a 52% relative risk reduction in ischemic stroke with no significant increase in risk of major hemorrhage. The combination of aspirin plus clopidogrel for stroke prevention produced a modest improvement in ischemic stroke in the Atrial Fibrillation Clopidogrel Trial with Irbesartan for Prevention of Vascular Events (ACTIVE-A) trial, but a similar increase in bleeding risk equating to no net benefit.

Connolly SJ, Pogue J, Hart RG, et al. Effect of clopidogrel added to aspirin in patients with atrial fibrillation. *N Engl J Med.* 2009;360(20):2066-2078. doi:10.1056/NEJMoa0901301
Mant J, Hobbs FD, Fletcher K, et al. Warfarin versus aspirin for stroke prevention in an elderly community population with atrial fibrillation (the Birmingham Atrial Fibrillation Treatment of the Aged Study, BAFTA): a randomised controlled trial. *Lancet.* 2007;370(9586):493-503. doi:10.1016/S0140-6736(07)61233-1

21. **The answer is D.** There is no data to support the use of prophylactic anticonvulsants in stroke patients. Furthermore, even in patients who are at an elevated risk of poststroke seizure, such as the scenarios listed in choices A to C, there is no evidence that preventing seizure improves outcomes. In ischemic stroke patients, current guidelines support the use of anticonvulsants only if a patient has a clinically definite seizure. It is reasonable to use anticonvulsants for a period of time and consider gradual discontinuation once the patient has become seizure free.

Powers WJ, Rabinstein AA, Ackerson T, et al. 2018 guidelines for the early management of patients with acute ischemic stroke. A guideline for healthcare professionals from the American Heart Association/American Stroke Association. Stroke. 2018;49(3):e46-e110. doi:10.1161/STR.0000000000000158

22. **The answer is A.** The patient most likely has reversible cerebral vasoconstriction syndrome (RCVS). This is an underdiagnosed entity that causes thunderclap headache and can easily be mistaken for primary central nervous system (CNS) angiitis and delayed cerebral ischemia from SAH. It is also known as "pseudovasculitis" because the findings on angiography so closely mimic vasculitis. RCVS is associated with a number of drugs, as well as exertion, pregnancy, and other headache types. A number of treatments have been used, but none are well established by trial data. The disease is self-limited but can be complicated by seizure and cerebral ischemia in up to 20% of patients. The clinical picture is not consistent with endocarditis, so mycotic aneurysms would be unlikely. The hypertrophy of lenticulostriates is a result of Moyamoya disease, which affects only the proximal vessels, whereas this patient had diffuse disease on initial imaging. While white matter infarctions are possible, they are rare, and often limited only to a single region, not diffuse.

Sattar A, Manousakis G, Jensen MB. Systematic review of reversible cerebral vasoconstriction syndrome. *Expert Rev Cardiovasc Ther.* 2010;8(10):1417-1421. doi:10.1586/erc.10.124

23. **The answer is D.** This patient has a cryptogenic stroke. PFO is more prevalent in patients with cryptogenic stroke than in the general population, but based on the results of the CLOSURE study, there is no benefit to PFO closure with the device used in that trial. Results of two recent trials, patent foramen oval closure or anticoagulation vs. antiplatelets after stroke (CLOSE) and patent foramen oval closure or antiplatelet therapy for cryptogenic stroke (REDUCE), show that in patients with recent stroke and PFO with an associated atrial septal aneurysm or moderate to large aunt, PFO closure in addition to antiplatelet is superior to antiplatelet one with an increased risk of peri-procedural complications including, atrial fibrillation. However, before any medical or surgical decision is made, lower extremity Doppler or magnetic resonance venography (MRV) is necessary to rule out deep vein thrombosis (DVT) as a source of paradoxical embolus. In the absence of a lower extremity DVT, anticoagulation is not indicated. There is no evidence that dual antiplatelet therapy is superior to monotherapy in patients with PFO without evidence of lower extremity DVT.

Mas J-L, Derumeaux G, Guillon B, et al. Patent foramen oval closure or anticoagulation vs. anti platelets after stroke. *N Engl J Med*. 2017;377(11):1011-1021. doi:10/1056/NEJMoa1705915

Messé SR, Gronseth G, Kent DM, et al. Practice advisory: recurrent stroke with patent foramen ovale (update of practice parameter): report of the Guideline Development, Dissemination, and Implementation Subcommittee of the American Academy of Neurology. *Neurology*. 2016;87(8):815-821. doi:10.1212/WNL.0000000000002961

Sondergaard L, Kasner S, Rhodes J, et al. Patent foramen oval closure or antiplatelet therapy for cryptogenic stroke. *N Engl J Med*. 2017;377(11):1033-1042. doi:10/1056/NEJMoa1707404

24. **The answer is D.** The ABCD2 system is a method for determining 2-, 7-, 30-, and 90-day stroke risk. Hospitals, EDs, and insurers are using it as a guide for decisions on admission versus outpatient evaluation. "A" stands for age: a patient gets one point for age greater than or equal to 60. "B" stands for blood pressure (BP): a patient gets one point if either the systolic BP is greater than or equal to 140 mmHg, or the diastolic BP is greater than or equal to 90 mmHg. "C" stands for clinical criteria: a patient gets one point for isolated speech impairment without weakness, and two points for unilateral weakness. "D" stands for diabetes: a patient gets one point if he or she is diabetic. The second "D" stands for duration: a patient gets one point for an episode of 10 to 59 minutes, and two points for an episode greater than or equal to 60 minutes. This patient scores a five, based on the description. Although different organizations use various cutoffs for decision making, a score of four or five results in a 2-day stroke risk of 4.1%, which justifies hospital admission.

Johnston SC, Rothwell PM, Nguyen-Huynh MN, et al. Validation and refinement of scores to predict very early stroke risk after transient ischaemic attack. *Lancet*. 2007;369(9558):283-292. doi:10.1016/S0140-6736(07)60150-0

25. **The answer is B.** Spinal cord infarction remains a poorly studied condition, but among the available strategies, two are worthwhile based on data from case series. First, the placement of a lumbar drain reduces intrathecal pressures and allows for increased cord perfusion. MAP should not be lowered for the same reason. Second, the use of distal bypass during surgery to restore cord perfusion in segments disrupted by grafting seems to improve outcomes. This strategy is likely best accomplished by monitoring somatosensory evoked potentials (SSEPs) during aortic repair and opting for bypass when the SSEPs show poor signal transmission. Prolonging ICU sedation may lead to other complications such as critical illness polyneuropathy (CIP) or myonecrosis and is not supported by any data.

Romi F, Naess H. Spinal cord infarction in clinical neurology: a review of characteristics and long-term prognosis in comparison to cerebral infarction. *Eur Neurol*. 2016;76(3-4):95-98. doi:10.1159/000446700

2 Subarachnoid Hemorrhage and Vascular Malformations

BÜLENT YAPICILAR AND ASMA ZAKARIA

▤ QUESTIONS

1. A 40-year-old female presents to the ED complaining of severe headache and new vision changes in her right eye. She is anxious because her mother died of a brain hemorrhage. Her past medical history is significant for nephrectomy 2 years ago, lupus, and poorly controlled hypertension. She has been smoking one pack of cigarettes per day for the past 20 years and is a heavy drinker. Her exam is unremarkable except her right eye is blind with a dilated pupil and ptosis. What is the next step in the management of this patient after reviewing this initial CT scan?

   A. Get a CT with contrast
   B. Get a cerebral angiogram
   C. Spinal tap
   D. Ophthalmology consult
   E. Magnetic resonance venogram (MRV)

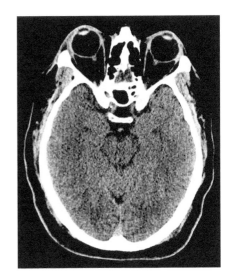

2. The spinal tap is done, and the cerebrospinal fluid (CSF) shows xanthochromia. The patient undergoes a cerebral angiogram and a right posterior communicating aneurysm is clipped. Two days after surgery, the patient becomes less responsive but without focal deficits. What do you suspect?

   A. Seizure
   B. Stroke
   C. Hydrocephalus
   D. Vasospasm
   E. Subdural hematoma (SDH)

3. The patient is more awake after an external ventricular drain (EVD) is placed; however, a few hours later she becomes lethargic with anisocoria and right hemiparesis. What is the cause of the neurological change?

   A. Seizure
   B. Vasospasm
   C. Subdural hematoma
   D. Stroke
   E. Hyponatremia

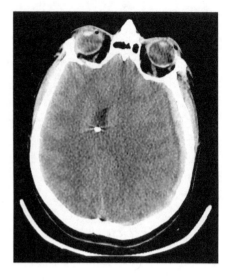

4. What is **not** a risk factor for having a subarachnoid hemorrhage (SAH) in this patient?

   A. Smoking
   B. Family history
   C. Hypertension
   D. Systemic lupus erythematosus (SLE)
   E. Alcohol

5. A 65-year-old male presents to the ED with headache and lethargy. His wife states that he has had a bad headache for the past 5 days. A CT scan shows acute subarachnoid hemorrhage (SAH). An external ventricular drain is placed, and an anterior communicating aneurysm is coiled. Two days after the procedure, the patient's sodium drops to 126 and he has a left prona-tor drift. What is the cause for his neurologic change?

   A. Seizure
   B. Vasospasm
   C. Rebleeding
   D. Stroke
   E. Hyponatremia

6. A cerebral angiogram with angioplasty is done and the patient improves. Over the next couple of days, the patient should be closely monitored for all of the following signs of vasospasm, **except:**

   A. Abulia
   B. Motor deficit
   C. Aphasia
   D. Headaches
   E. Hyporeflexia

7. The risk for developing vasospasm is greatest with:

   A. Intracerebral hematoma
   B. Intraventricular hematoma and posterior fossa subarachnoid blood
   C. Subarachnoid blood less than 1 mm thickness
   D. Subarachnoid blood more than 1 mm thickness
   E. Perimesencephalic subarachnoid blood

8. The gold standard for diagnosing cerebral vasospasm is:

   A. Transcranial duplex (TCD)
   B. CT perfusion (CTP) scan
   C. CT angiogram (CTA)
   D. Cerebral angiogram
   E. MRI diffusion

9. Which of the following cardiac findings is **not** associated with subarachnoid hemorrhage (SAH)?

   A. Elevated troponin
   B. Short QT interval
   C. Elevated B-type natriuretic peptide (BNP)
   D. Sinus bradycardia
   E. Left ventricular (LV) dysfunction

10. Risk factors for rebleeding of an aneurysm include all of the following, **except**:

    A. Size of aneurysm
    B. Hunt and Hess grade at admission
    C. Fisher grade at admission
    D. Seizure at ictus
    E. Systolic Blood Pressure (SBP) greater than 160 mmHg

11. Which of the following drugs is preferred for controlling hypertension in subarachnoid hemorrhage (SAH)?

    A. Nicardipine
    B. Esmolol
    C. Labetalol
    D. Sodium nitroprusside
    E. Enalapril

12. Subarachnoid hemorrhage (SAH) can typically present with all of the following, **except**:

    A. Inferior nasal quadrantanopsia
    B. Hemiparesis
    C. Exophthalmos
    D. Horner's syndrome
    E. Third nerve palsy with pupillary sparing

13. According to the International Subarachnoid Aneurysm Trial (ISAT), all of the following are true, **except**:

    A. Anterior circulation aneurysms less than 7 mm have a 0% risk of rupture
    B. The risk for epilepsy was lower in the endovascular group
    C. Higher rebleeding rate was seen in the endovascular group
    D. Higher aneurysm occlusion rate was seen in the surgical group
    E. There was a reduction in risk of death or dependency in the endovascular group

14. All of the following are true regarding neurogenic pulmonary edema, **except**:

    A. Increases the incidence of cerebral vasospasm
    B. Can mimic congestive heart failure
    C. Results in PaO2/FiO2 less than 200

D. Can be seen within minutes of initial insult

E. Should be treated with an alpha-agonist

15. All of the following are true regarding hyponatremia in subarachnoid hemorrhage (SAH), **except**:

A. Hyponatremia is the most common electrolyte imbalance in SAH

B. Hyponatremia is not associated with a higher risk of vasospasm and poor prognosis

C. Urine osmolality (UOsm) and urine sodium (UNa) levels can be used to distinguish cerebral salt wasting (CSW) and Syndrome of Inappropriate Antidiuretic Hormone (SIADH)

D. Hyponatremia in SAH is hypotonic hyponatremia

E. It usually occurs between day 3 and day 14 after rupture

16. The correct transducer position in monitoring cerebral perfusion pressure (CPP) with an elevated head position is:

A. Arterial line and intracranial pressure (ICP) monitor transducers at the level of the heart

B. Arterial line and ICP monitor transducers at the level of the foramen of Monro

C. Arterial line transducer at the level of the heart and ICP monitor transducer at the level of the foramen of Monro

D. No difference as long as the arterial line and ICP monitor transducers are at the same level

E. ICP monitor transducer should always be above the arterial line transducer

17. Which of the following vasopressors is used as a first-line agent to augment blood pressure in cerebral vasospasm?

A. Phenylephrine

B. Epinephrine

C. Dopamine

D. Dobutamine

E. Vasopressin

18. What is the strongest prognostic indicator for poor outcome in subarachnoid hemorrhage (SAH)?

A. Initial clinical grade

B. Aneurysm rerupture

C. Older age

D. Global cerebral edema on initial CT scan

E. Fever

19. All of the following are true regarding the use of nimodipine in the management of subarachnoid hemorrhage (SAH), **except**:

A. Nimodipine is an L-type calcium channel blocker

B. It has been shown to improve neurological outcome

C. It can cause hypotension

D. It improves cerebral vasospasm

E. There is no difference in clinical efficacy between intravenous (IV) and enteral nimodipine use

20. All of the following regarding continuous EEG (cEEG) monitoring in subarachnoid hemorrhage (SAH) are true, **except**:

A. cEEG changes can be seen at the onset of vasospasm

B. Intracortical recording has less artifact compared to scalp recording

C. Alpha–delta ratio (ADR) correlates better than mean amplitude for predicting vasospasm

D. cEEG can detect ischemia in the absence of infarction

E. cEEG monitoring is particularly useful in poor-grade patients

21. A patient presents with the CT scan shown. Which is the correct answer regarding this condition?

A. Cerebral angiogram should always be done
B. Will never rebleed
C. Does not cause vasospasm
D. Needs long-term follow-up
E. Has a rehemorrhage rate of 4% in the first 24 hours

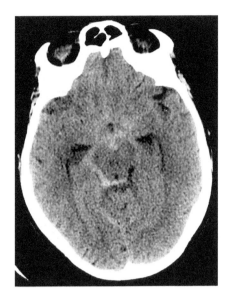

22. Which of the following is true regarding Transcranial Doppler (TCD) ultrasound in cerebral vasospasm?

A. Lindegaard ratio greater than 3 correlates with severe spasm
B. TCD has good sensitivity in identifying patients with vasospasm
C. It is a screening tool to assess peripheral vasculature
D. It is most accurate for detecting spasm in the middle cerebral artery (MCA)
E. It can detect vasospasm only in the anterior circulation

23. A 27-year-old male presents with a subarachnoid hemorrhage (SAH). He is awake and alert with no focal neurologic findings. A cerebral angiogram is performed and the resulting image is shown here. What is the next step in the management of this patient?

A. No intervention because the A Randomized Trial of Unruptured Brain Arteriovenous Malformation (ARUBA) study showed superiority of observation over intervention
B. Arterio-venous malformation (AVM) embolization will also indirectly obliterate the aneurysm in a delayed fashion
C. The patient should get the AVM and aneurysm treated in a delayed fashion
D. Treat only the aneurysm at this admission
E. Radiosurgery can be utilized for the management of this patient

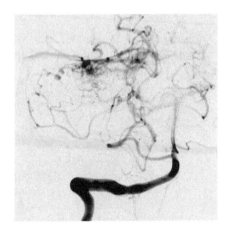

24. A 67-year-old patient with atrial fibrillation on warfarin presents with a dense left hemiparesis. The patient was last known well 5 hours ago and has a National Institutes of Health (NIH) stroke scale of 10. Current International Normalized Ratio (INR) is 1.8. What should be the next step in managing this patient?

    A. Intravenous (IV) tissue plasminogen activator (tPA) stat
    B. Transfuse fresh-frozen plasma (FFP) to correct elevated INR
    C. Activate pathway for mechanical thrombectomy
    D. Heparin drip with partial thromboplastin time (PTT) goal 60 to 90
    E. Hemicraniectomy for right middle cerebral artery (MCA) stroke

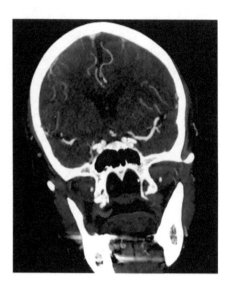

25. A 46-year-old patient with a cerebral aneurysm and a sister who died of a ruptured cerebral aneurysm is worried about her children having the same problem. She asks you about screening and treatment?

    A. She should not worry about her children having the same problem
    B. Her children should undergo a cerebral angiogram to rule out an aneurysm
    C. CT angiogram of the brain once is enough for screening
    D. The children should get long-term screening using magnetic resonance angiography (MRA)
    E. Her children with aneurysm should be treated the same as the general population

26. A 56-year-old male presents with this angiogram. Which of the following statements is **incorrect**:

    A. Patients who undergo treatment with embolization have lower rebleeding rates than clipping
    B. Patients who undergo coiling of their aneurysm have a higher recurrence rate
    C. Clipping the aneurysm has a higher mortality rate than embolization
    D. Ruptured aneurysms have a higher recanalization rate after coiling
    E. Larger aneurysms have a higher recanalization rate after coiling

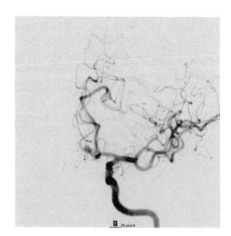

27. A 16-year-old patient with history of sickle cell disease (SCD) and multiple strokes in the past presents to the emergency room with headaches. Imaging is concerning for moyamoya syndrome (MMS). What is the best treatment for this patient?

    A. Anticoagulation
    B. Cerebral bypass surgery
    C. Blood transfusions for patients with decreased Transcranial Doppler (TCD) velocities
    D. Exchange transfusion to hemoglobin S (HbS) target less than 30%
    E. Hyperventilation to decrease intracerebral pressure

■ ANSWERS

1. **The answer is C.** CT can detect greater than 95% of subarachnoid hemorrhages (SAHs) within 24 hours and 98% within 12 hours after rupture. Blood appears as high-density signal in the cisterns. A CT can look falsely negative, as in this case, if the volume of blood is very small, if the bleeding occurred several days prior, or if the hematocrit is extremely low. The next step in managing this patient is to perform a lumbar puncture to rule out blood in the cerebrospinal fluid (CSF) space. The presence of xanthochromia is helpful in distinguishing true SAH from a traumatic tap. According to the guidelines, spectroscopy is the recommended method of analysis and should be done on the final bottle. An increased bilirubin and oxyhemoglobin level is suggestive of SAH while a negative value practically rules it out. Xanthochromia can be detected if the patient presents greater than 4 hours after ictus. If less than 4 hours, the less reliable method of counting red blood cells (RBCs) in the CSF and comparing the clearance between bottles 1 and 4 may be employed. In a comparative study, the non-SAH group had a clearance rate of 70% and an RBC count in bottle 4 of less than 500, while patients with SAH cleared only 30% of their red cells with an RBC count anywhere between 900 and 2 million in bottle 4. The patient has ptosis from a third nerve palsy, suggesting a posterior communicating artery (PComm) aneurysm, in addition to blindness secondary to a concurrent vitreous hemorrhage (Terson's syndrome). An MRV is indicated if there is concern for a venous sinus thrombosis.

Beetham R. Recommendations for CSF analysis in subarachnoid haemorrhage. *J Neurol Neurosurg Psychiatr*. 2004;75(4):528. doi:10.1136/jnnp.2003.023176

Diringer MN. Management of aneurysmal subarachnoid hemorrhage. *Crit Care Med*. 2009;37(2): 432-440. doi:10.1097/CCM.0b013e318195865a

Gorchynski J, Oman J, Newton T. Interpretation of traumatic lumbar punctures in the setting of possible subarachnoid hemorrhage: who can be safely discharged? *Cal J Emerg Med*. 2007; 8(1):3-7.

Tormey W, O'Shea P, Brennan P. National guidelines for analysis of cerebrospinal fluid for bilirubin in suspected subarachnoid haemorrhage. *Ann Clin Biochem*. 2012;49(pt 1):102-103. doi: 10.1258/acb.2011.011123

2. **The answer is C.** The patient is likely developing early hydrocephalus, which occurs in 20% to 30% of cases within the first 48 hours. Delayed hydrocephalus (up to several weeks) develops in one-fourth of surviving patients and is associated with older age, female gender, and intraventricular blood. There is no difference between patients treated by clipping or coiling. Poor clinical grade is the best predictor for the occurrence of hydrocephalus. It is not typical for vasospasm (or stroke) to develop within 2 days. Vasospasm can be seen as early as day 3, reaching a maximum incidence on days 6 to 8, and rarely as late as day 15 and beyond. An SDH should present earlier and usually with a focal deficit like hemiparesis or dilated pupil. Seizure is always a possibility in this patient population and should be ruled out if the CT scan does not confirm hydrocephalus.

Germanwala AV, Huang J, Tamargo RJ. Hydrocephalus after aneurysmal subarachnoid hemorrhage. *Neurosurg Clin N Am*. 2010;21(2):263-270. doi:10.1016/j.nec.2009.10.013

3. **The answer is C.** The patient has a rapid clinical change after the placement of a ventricular drain. The clinical presentation is highly suggestive of an acute hemorrhage caused by the drain placement.

Maniker AH, Vaynman AY, Karimi RJ, et al. Hemorrhagic complications of external ventricular drainage. *Neurosurgery*. 2006;59(4 suppl 2):ONS419-424; discussion ONS424. doi: 10.1227/01.NEU.0000222817.99752.E6

4. **The answer is D.** Risk factors that have clearly been associated with an increased risk of aneurysmal SAH (aSAH) include hypertension, smoking, alcohol abuse, and a family history (at least one first-degree relative) of aSAH.

Connolly ES Jr, Rabinstein AA, Carhuapoma JR, et al. Guidelines for the management of aneurysmal subarachnoid hemorrhage: a guideline for healthcare professionals from the American Heart Association/American Stroke Association. *Stroke*. 2012;43(6):1711-1737. doi:10.1161/STR.0b013e3182587839

5. **The answer is B.** The patient has signs and symptoms consistent with cerebral vasospasm as apparent on the following angiogram:

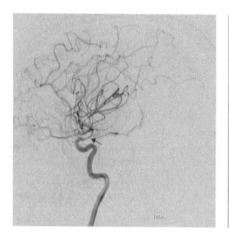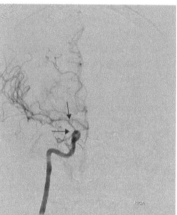

Cerebral Vasospasm on Angiography

Cerebral vasospasm usually occurs between days 3 to 15 postictus. In some patients, it may persist beyond day 15. Clinical vasospasm must be differentiated from radiographic vasospasm. Although angiographic vasospasm is observed in up to 70% of patients, only 30% of these patients become clinically symptomatic, supporting the idea that additional factors play a role in the development of delayed cerebral ischemia (DCI). DCI is a clinical diagnosis of a new neurologic deficit in the setting of SAH. Cerebral vasospasm can cause DCI; however, not every patient with DCI has vasospasm and vice versa. Nimodipine is the only drug available to reduce long-term poor outcomes (level 1 evidence). The CONSCIOUS 1 and 2 studies showed a reduction in cerebral vasospasm with the use of endothelin 1 antagonist; however, this did not translate into improved outcomes. The pathophysiology of DCI seems to be multifactorial at this time. Patients with SAH are at risk for DCI at any time within the first 21 days. Triple-H therapy has been widely used for the treatment of cerebral vasospasm; however, recent studies question the benefit of hemodilution and hypervolemia. In patients refractory to medical management, endovascular therapy has been utilized. The problem is the transient effect of the intervention. Statins have also been used to treat cerebral vasospasm, possibly exerting their beneficial effects by decreasing glutamate-mediated excitotoxicity and moderation of the inflammatory response by upregulating cytokines and increasing nitric oxide (NO) levels. A recent meta-analysis of existing data showed that statins, despite attenuating the incidence of cerebral vasospasm, did not reduce DCI or mortality. DCI has been the target of vigorous research (lumbar cerebrospinal fluid [CSF] drainage, endothelin 1 antagonists [CONSCIOUS 1–3], intravenous [IV] magnesium, Nicardipine pellets placed intraoperatively, and intrathecal thrombolytics and calcium channel blockers) but unfortunately none of the proposed interventions have shown an improvement in clinical outcomes to date.

Kramer AH, Fletcher JJ. Locally-administered intrathecal thrombolytics following aneurysmal subarachnoid hemorrhage: a systematic review and meta-analysis. *Neurocrit Care*. 2011;14(3):489-499. doi:10.1007/s12028-010-9429-z

Muroi C, Seule M, Mishima K, et al. Novel treatments for vasospasm after subarachnoid hemorrhage. *Curr Opin Crit Care*. 2012;18(2):119-126. doi:10.1097/MCC.0b013e32835075ae

Rabinstein AA, Lanzino G, Wijdicks EF. Multidisciplinary management and emerging therapeutic strategies in aneurysmal subarachnoid haemorrhage. *Lancet Neurol.* 2010;9(5):504-519. doi:10.1016/S1474-4422(10)70087-9

Schubert GA, Seiz M, Hegewald AA, et al. Hypoperfusion in the acute phase of subarachnoid hemorrhage. *Acta Neurochir.* 2011;110(1):35-39. doi:10.1007/978-3-7091-0353-1_6

Shen J, Huang KY, Zhu Y, et al. Effect of statin treatment on vasospasm-related morbidity and functional outcome in patients with aneurysmal subarachnoid hemorrhage: a systematic review and meta-analysis. *J Neurosurg.* 2016;127(2):291-301. doi:10.3171/2016.5.JNS152900

Tseng MY. Summary of evidence on immediate statins therapy following aneurysmal subarachnoid hemorrhage. *Neurocrit Care.* 2011;15(2):298-301. doi:10.1007/s12028-011-9596-6

Washington CW, Zipfel GJ. Detection and monitoring of vasospasm and delayed cerebral ischemia: a review and assessment of the literature. *Neurocrit Care.* 2011;15(2):312-317. doi:10.1007/s12028-011-9594-8

Weir B, Grace M, Hansen J, et al. Time course of vasospasm in man. *J Neurosurg.* 1978;48(2):173-178. doi:10.3171/jns.1978.48.2.0173

6. **The answer is E.** All of the other options have been observed in patients with cerebral vasospasm. Abulia and lower extremity motor deficits are seen in vasospasm involving the anterior cerebral artery. Aphasia and motor deficit involving upper and lower extremity is seen with middle cerebral artery (MCA) spasm. An increased tone is often suggestive of vasospasm. Hyporeflexia is not usually a finding in cerebral vasospasm.

Keyrouz SG, Diringer MN. Clinical review: prevention and therapy of vasospasm in subarachnoid hemorrhage. *Crit Care.* 2007;11(4):220. doi:10.1186/cc5958

7. **The answer is D.** The relationship between CT imaging of subarachnoid blood and the risk of vasospasm was first published by Miller Fisher in 1980 and is since used as the Fisher classification. Twenty-three of 24 patients with localized clot or blood greater than 1 mm in thickness developed severe spasm and one patient, moderate vasospasm. Intraventricular or intracerebral hematoma had no effect on vasospasm. Of the five patients in this group, three had no vasospasm and two had mild spasm. One patient had subarachnoid blood in the posterior fossa. Subarachnoid blood can be seen in a grade 4 hemorrhage as described by Fisher; however, it cannot be a significant amount.

Fisher CM, Kistler JP, Davis JM. Relation of cerebral vasospasm to subarachnoid hemorrhage visualized by computerized tomographic scanning. *Neurosurgery.* 1980;6(1):1-9. doi:10.1227/00006123-198001000-00001

8. **The answer is D.** Cerebral angiography is the gold standard for diagnosing cerebral vasospasm. It is the best imaging study to evaluate large and small vessel disease and to initiate treatment at the same time. It is invasive and has a 1% complication rate. Therefore, alternative imaging tools are used more often. TCD is a good noninvasive monitoring tool with high specificity, particularly for the middle cerebral artery (MCA). However, it has low sensitivity and negative predictive value and is very operator dependent. CTA is a very promising tool if beam artifact and processing limitations can be overcome. CTA tends to overestimate the degree of spasm compared to conventional angiogram and is less accurate for distal vasospasm. A recent meta-analysis using data from 10 studies showed 80% sensitivity and 93% specificity for cerebral vasospasm. CTP is of particular interest since we understand that angiographic vasospasm is only one of multiple factors contributing to delayed cerebral ischemia. Measuring cerebral blood flow might provide more comprehensive information. Early CTP showed a significant difference in cerebral blood flow, mean transit time, and cerebral blood volume in patients who developed symptomatic vasospasm. Late CTP had a specificity of 91% and sensitivity of 95% compared to conventional angiogram. Early CTP may help in predicting vasospasm and late CTP findings correlate highly with the development of cerebral vasospasm and delayed cerebral ischemia.

Greenberg ED, Gold R, Reichman M, et al. Diagnostic accuracy of CT angiography and CT perfusion for cerebral vasospasm: a meta-analysis. *Am J Neuroradiol*. 2010;31(10):1853-1860. doi:10.3174/ajnr.A2246

Washington CW, Zipfel GJ. Detection and monitoring of vasospasm and delayed cerebral ischemia: a review and assessment of the literature. *Neurocrit Care*. 2011;15(2):312-317. doi:10.1007/s12028-011-9594-8

Wintermark M, Dillon WP, Smith WS, et al. Visual grading system for vasospasm based on perfusion CT imaging: comparisons with conventional angiography and quantitative perfusion CT. *Cerebrovasc Dis*. 2008;26(2):163-170. doi:10.1159/000139664

9. **The answer is B.** SAH is associated with many systemic complications, including cardiac dysfunction and failure (stunned, neurogenic, or Takotsubo cardiomyopathy). It is believed that increased intracranial pressure causes hypothalamic injury and excessive release of catecholamines. Classic changes after elevated levels of catecholamines are myocardial contraction band necrosis causing LV dysfunction and a rise in troponin and BNP levels. Troponin is 100% sensitive in detecting LV dysfunction after SAH compared to MB isoenzyme of creatine kinase (CKMB), and reaches peak levels at day 1 to decay thereafter. Peak troponin and BNP levels have predictive value and are associated with higher mortality after SAH. Higher admission Hunt and Hess grade, intraventricular hemorrhage, loss of consciousness at ictus, and abnormal admission ECG changes are predictive of a higher troponin level. In 50% to 100% of cases, a variety of ECG changes, along with arrhythmias, can be found after SAH. These changes are transient and include ST elevation and depression, QT prolongation (but not shortening), peaked or inverted T waves, large U waves, peaked P, and pathological Q waves. Clinically important cardiac arrhythmias, most often atrial fibrillation and flutter but also sinus bradycardia, are associated with poor outcomes, and can be seen in 4% of cases. An interesting phenomenon encountered in SAH is the apical ballooning syndrome, also known as Takotsubo cardiomyopathy. Regional wall motion abnormalities (RWMA) involving the apex with sparing of the base produces an LV dysfunction with a ventriculogram resembling a Japanese octopus trapping pot. The motion defect can cause an apical LV thrombus with fatal outcome.

Frontera JA, Parra A, Shimbo D, et al. Cardiac arrhythmias after subarachnoid hemorrhage: risk factors and impact on outcome. *Cerebrovasc Dis*. 2008;26(1):71-78. doi:10.1159/000135711

Lee VH, Oh JK, Mulvagh SL, et al. Mechanisms in neurogenic stress cardiomyopathy after aneurysmal subarachnoid hemorrhage. *Neurocrit Care*. 2006;5(3):243-249. doi:10.1385/NCC:5:3:243

Mayer SA, LiMandri G, Sherman D, et al. Electrocardiographic markers of abnormal left ventricular wall motion in acute subarachnoid hemorrhage. *J Neurosurg*. 1995;83(5):889-896. doi:10.3171/jns.1995.83.5.0889

Naidech AM, Kreiter KT, Janjua N, et al. Cardiac troponin elevation, cardiovascular morbidity, and outcome after subarachnoid hemorrhage. *Circulation*. 2005;112(18):2851-2856. doi:10.1161/CIRCULATIONAHA.105.533620

Tung PP, Olmsted E, Kopelnik A, et al. Plasma B-type natriuretic peptide levels are associated with early cardiac dysfunction after subarachnoid hemorrhage. *Stroke*. 2005;36(7):1567-1569. doi:10.1161/01.STR.0000170699.59783.d6

10. **The answer is E.** Rebleeding of an aneurysm has devastating consequences and is associated with higher mortality. Most studies show that the rerupture risk is highest in the first 24 hours and particularly within the first 6 hours after the ictus. The traditional rebleeding rate based on the International Cooperative Aneurysm Study is 4%, but the actual rebleeding rate is likely much higher since the 4% refers to the population that reaches a tertiary care center and excludes patients in the field or in community EDs. Ohkuma et al. reported a 13% prehospitalization rate of rebleeding. Aneurysm size greater than 1 cm along with poor initial neurological presentation and seizure at onset were risk factors for rebleeding. Controversy still exists regarding hypertension as a risk factor versus a consequence of rebleeding. The 2012 American Heart Association (AHA) guidelines recommend an SBP less than 160 preoperatively to balance the risk of rebleeding with maintaining cerebral perfusion pressure (level 2A). Along with early intervention (open or endovascular), antifibrinolytic therapy has been used to prevent rebleeding (AHA level 2B evidence).

Connolly ES Jr, Rabinstein AA, Carhuapoma JR, et al. Guidelines for the management of aneurysmal subarachnoid hemorrhage: a guideline for healthcare professionals from the American Heart Association/American Stroke Association. *Stroke.* 2012;43(6):1711-1737. doi:10.1161/STR.0b013e3182587839

Guo LM, Zhou HY, Xu JW, et al. Risk factors related to aneurysmal rebleeding. *World Neurosurg.* 2011;76(3-4):292-298; discussion 253. doi.10.1016/j.wneu.2011.03.025

Hillman J, Fridriksson S, Nilsson O, et al. Immediate administration of tranexamic acid and reduced incidence of early rebleeding after aneurysmal subarachnoid hemorrhage: a prospective randomized study. *J Neurosurg.* 2002;97(4):771-778. doi:10.3171/jns.2002.97.4.0771

Kassell NF, Torner JC. Aneurysmal rebleeding: a preliminary report from the Cooperative Aneurysm Study. *Neurosurgery.* 1983;13(5):479-481. doi:10.1227/00006123-198311000-00001

Leipzig TJ, Redelman K, Horner TG. Reducing the risk of rebleeding before early aneurysm surgery: a possible role for antifibrinolytic therapy. *J Neurosurg.* 1997;86(2):220-225. doi:10.3171/jns.1997.86.2.0220

Lord AS, Fernandez L, Schmidt JM, et al. Effect of rebleeding on the course and incidence of vasospasm after subarachnoid hemorrhage. *Neurology.* 2012;78(1):31-37. doi:10.1212/WNL.0b013e31823ed0a4

Naidech AM, Janjua N, Kreiter KT, et al. Predictors and impact of aneurysm rebleeding after subarachnoid hemorrhage. *Arch Neurol.* 2005;62(3):410-416. doi:10.1001/archneur.62.3.410

Ohkuma H, Tsurutani H, Suzuki S. Incidence and significance of early aneurysmal rebleeding before neurosurgical or neurological management. *Stroke.* 2001;32(5):1176-1180. doi:10.1161/01.STR.32.5.1176

Steiger HJ, Medele R, Brückmann H, et al. Interdisciplinary management results in 100 patients with ruptured and unruptured posterior circulation aneurysms. *Acta Neurochir (Wien).* 1999;141(4):359-366; discussion 366. doi:10.1016/S0090-3019(02)00717-6

11. **The answer is A.** The American Heart Association (AHA) guidelines recommend controlling hypertension using esmolol, labetalol, or nicardipine due to their short-acting nature and safety profile. In a retrospective study, nicardipine was superior in controlling hypertension compared to labetolol. In addition, the blood pressure responded more rapidly to nicardipine. Hypotension also occurred more often in the labetolol group: 9% versus 3%. Nicardipine, a pure vasodilator (L-type calcium channel) should also be used for patients with chronic obstructive pulmonary disease (COPD), congestive heart failure, or a history of bronchospasm. Esmolol and labetalol should be used if tachycardia needs to be treated along with hypertension. Nitroprusside should be avoided because of its ability to dilate intracerebral venous and arterial vasculature and raise intracranial pressure (ICP). It has an unreliable dose–response profile, tends to cause rebound hypertension, and can cause cyanide toxicity. Enalapril is not suitable for emergency treatment because of its long duration (6–12 hours) and delayed onset (15–30 minutes) of action.

Rose JC, Mayer SA. Optimizing blood pressure in neurological emergencies. *Neurocrit Care.* 2004;1(3):287-299. doi:10.1385/NCC:1:3:287

Woloszyn AV, McAllen KJ, Figueroa BE, et al. Retrospective evaluation of nicardipine versus labetalol for blood pressure control in aneurysmal subarachnoid hemorrhage. *Neurocrit Care.* 2012;16(3):376-380. doi:10.1007/s12028-012-9700-6

12. **The answer is E.** Third nerve palsy can occur with a posterior communicating artery (PComm) aneurysm but usually involves the pupil. Pupillary involvement is almost pathognomonic for aneurysms, particularly if they are greater than or equal to 5 mm. Cases of pupillary sparing have been reported; however, this is the exception. The third nerve lies in the subarachnoid space close to the PComm, and the pupillary fibers lie on the dorsomedial surface, making them more vulnerable to compression from aneurysms. In contrast, ischemic causes for third nerve palsies affect the central fibers, sparing the pupil. Middle cerebral artery (MCA) aneurysms can present with temporal lobe seizures or hemiparesis, even if they are unruptured, due to mass effect. Carotid artery aneurysms, particularly of the ophthalmic segment, but also anterior communicating and cavernous sinus aneurysms, can present with various visual field deficits such as bitemporal hemianopsia, homonymous hemianopsia, and quadrantanopsia. Ophthalmic aneurysms present initially with an inferior nasal field cut because of the pressure on the overlying falciform ligament. Horner's syndrome

can occur with a cavernous segment aneurysm of the carotid artery compressing the postganglionic sympathetic pathway, while exophthalmus may be a symptom of a carotid cavernous fistula after aneurysm rupture into the cavernous sinus. Posterior circulation aneurysms can present with Weber's syndrome and other brainstem compression syndromes as well as third, sixth, and lower cranial nerve palsies. Unruptured anterior communicating artery aneurysms can present with dementia, abulia, or pituitary dysfunction from mass effect.

Arle JE, Abrahams JM, Zager EL, et al. Pupil-sparing third nerve palsy with preoperative improvement from a posterior communicating artery aneurysm. *Surg Neurol.* 2002;57(6):423-426; discussion 426. doi:10.1016/S0090-3019(02)00717-6

Batjer HH. *Cerebrovascular Disease*. Philadelphia, PA: Lippincott Williams & Wilkins; 1997.

Rucker CW. The causes of paralysis of the third, fourth and sixth cranial nerves. *Am J Ophthalmol.* 1966;61(5 pt 2):1293-1298. doi:10.1016/0002-9394(66)90258-3

Trobe JD, Glaser JS, Post JD. Meningiomas and aneurysms of the cavernous sinus: neuro-ophthalmologic features. *Arch Ophthalmol.* 1978;96(3):457-467. doi:10.1001/archopht.1978.03910050233009

13. **The answer is A.** The rupture risk of an aneurysm according to size and location was published in the International Study of Unruptured Intracranial Aneurysms (ISUIA). The study enrolled and found that smaller aneurysms located in the anterior circulation had a lower rupture risk compared to larger aneurysms and aneurysms located in the posterior circulation. All the other answers are correct.

Molyneux AJ, Kerr RS, Yu LM, et al. International subarachnoid aneurysm trial (ISAT) of neurosurgical clipping versus endovascular coiling in 2143 patients with ruptured intracranial aneurysms: a randomised comparison of effects on survival, dependency, seizures, rebleeding, subgroups, and aneurysm occlusion. *Lancet.* 2005;366(9488):809-817. doi:10.1016/S0140-6736(05)67214-5

Wiebers DO, Whisnant JP, Huston J 3rd, et al. Unruptured intracranial aneurysms: natural history, clinical outcome, and risks of surgical and endovascular treatment. *Lancet.* 2003;362(9378):103-110. doi:10.1016/S0140-6736(03)13860-3

14. **The answer is E.** Neurogenic pulmonary edema is a fairly common pulmonary complication and can be seen with any type of brain injury. The pathogenesis involves overactivation of the sympathetic nervous system. Two theories exist, and both probably play a role in the pathogenesis: the blast theory and the permeability theory. The sympathetic surge causes capillary leakage regardless of the systemic blood pressure. Edema is caused by damage to capillary endothelium, which contains both alpha- and beta-adrenergic receptors. According to the blast theory, the systemic blood pressure surge shifts blood from the systemic circulation to the low-pressure pulmonary circulation, causing barotrauma to the capillary endothelium, damaging the alveolar membrane, and resulting in pulmonary edema. This can be seen within minutes, and symptoms often resolve after 24 to 48 hours unless there are persistently high intracranial pressures (ICPs) and ongoing central nervous system (CNS) injury. Centrally distributed, bilateral infiltrates are seen on x-ray, associated with frothy blood-tinged sputum. The therapy is mainly supportive using mechanical ventilation as well as alpha-antagonists like phentolamine, or beta-stimulating catecholamines to treat adrenergic-induced systemic vascular and pulmonary hypertension. Alternatively, some reports suggest dobutamine or dopamine to improve cardiac contractility. High positive end-expiratory pressure (PEEP) should be used with caution in the setting of elevated ICP. Several studies have shown that the incidence of cerebral vasospasm is increased with neurogenic pulmonary edema, and some studies have shown a higher mortality rate. These results are probably due to a higher initial Hunt and Hess grade and less aggressive hemodynamic resuscitation and hypertensive treatment of these patients due to aggravation of cardiac or respiratory failure with hypervolemic or euvolemic therapy.

Davison DL, Terek M, Chawla LS. Neurogenic pulmonary edema. *Crit Care.* 2012;16(2):212. doi:10.1186/cc11226

Friedman JA, Pichelmann MA, Piepgras DG, et al. Pulmonary complications of aneurysmal subarachnoid hemorrhage. *Neurosurgery.* 2003;52(5):1025-1031; discussion 1031. doi:10.1227/01.NEU.0000058222.59289.F1

Lakkireddigari SK, Durga P, Nayak M, et al. Preoperative neurogenic pulmonary edema: a dilemma for decision making. *J Anaesthesiol Clin Pharmacol*. 2012;28(2):232-234. doi:10.4103/0970-9185.94905

Muroi C, Keller M, Pangalu A, et al. Neurogenic pulmonary edema in patients with subarachnoid hemorrhage. *J Neurosurg Anesthesiol*. 2008;20(3):188-192. doi:10.1097/ANA.0b013e3181778156

15. **The answer is C.** Hyponatremia is the most common electrolyte imbalance seen in SAH, occurring in 30% to 50% of SAH patients, and usually presents 3 to 14 days after aneurysm rupture. It can be seen more frequently with blood in the third ventricle, suprasellar cistern and with anterior communication artery (AComm) aneurysm rupture. It can present as headache, nausea, vomiting, anorexia, and lethargy, and, if untreated, these patients may rapidly develop cerebral edema and experience seizures and brain herniation. The differential diagnosis is broad and includes hormonal disorders (e.g., thyroid, cardiac, medications, and volume-related problems). It may be caused by either cerebral salt wasting (CSW) or Syndrome of Inappropriate Antidiuretic Hormone Secretion (SIADH) in SAH patients; however, prospective data showing decreased plasma volume and increased natriuretic peptide in SAH with hyponatremia favors CSW as the underlying cause. The pathogenesis of the former is still unknown, but it is believed to be caused by elevated natriuretic peptides mediated by the sympathetic system. Both cause hypotonic hyponatremia with elevated urine osmolality greater than 200 mOsm/kg and urine Na greater than 25 mOsm/kg. The fluid balance in CSW is negative, and resuscitation is necessary. SIADH is associated with expanded intravascular volume and fluid restriction is the treatment. In the setting of SAH and vasospasm this is dangerous and this management is discouraged in practice. The use of mineralocorticoids has been shown to ameliorate hyponatremia. Fludrocortisone, because of its greater mineralocorticoid profile, is the preferred form. The recommended rate of correction varies between 8 and 12 mmol/L in 24 hours. There is no conclusive data that shows that hyponatremia influences prognosis in SAH patients. In a prospective study with 298 patients, *hypernatremia* was independently associated with poor outcome at 3 months. This study, contrary to older literature, did not show an association of hyponatremia with vasospasm or poor outcome. The likely explanation is that in the past, patients were treated with fluid restriction.

Diringer MN, Bleck TP, Claude Hemphill J 3rd, et al. Critical care management of patients following aneurysmal subarachnoid hemorrhage: recommendations from the Neurocritical Care Society's Multidisciplinary Consensus Conference. *Neurocrit Care*. 2011;15(2):211-240. doi:10.1007/s12028-011-9605-9

Hasan D, Wijdicks EF, Vermeulen M. Hyponatremia is associated with cerebral ischemia in patients with aneurysmal subarachnoid hemorrhage. *Ann Neurol*. 1990;27(1):106-108. doi:10.1002/ana.410270118

Qureshi AI, Suri MF, Sung GY, et al. Prognostic significance of hypernatremia and hyponatremia among patients with aneurysmal subarachnoid hemorrhage. *Neurosurgery*. 2002;50(4):749-755; discussion 755. doi:10.1097/00006123-200204000-00012

Rabinstein AA, Wijdicks EF. Hyponatremia in critically ill neurological patients. *Neurologist*. 2003;9(6):290-300. doi:10.1097/01.nrl.0000095258.07720.89

16. **The answer is B.** Incorrect placement and calibration of the arterial line transducer may overestimate CPP by greater than 25%. According to a study, the arterial line transducer was at the ear level in only 10% of ICUs. When the patient's head is elevated by 30°, both transducers must be placed at the foramen of Monro for most accurate monitoring.

Nates JL, Niggemeyer LE, Anderson MB, et al. Cerebral perfusion pressure monitoring alert! *Crit Care Med*. 1997;25(5):895-896. doi:10.1097/00003246-199705000-00033

17. **The answer is A.** Phenylephrine is the drug preferred to elevate blood pressure in cerebral vasospasm, although it should be used with caution in patients with coronary artery disease, glaucoma, and thyroid disease. It is an alpha-agonist elevating the blood pressure by vasoconstriction and may cause some degree of reflex bradycardia. Phenylephrine has essentially no beta-adrenergic receptor activity at clinically used intravenous doses. It has an immediate

onset of action and the effect lasts for 20 to 40 minutes. Epinephrine is an alpha-1 and beta-1 agonist, causes tachycardia, and should be used for patients with bradycardia or where blood pressure and cardiac output need to be augmented. Dopamine and dobutamine can also activate beta-1 receptors, causing tachycardia. Dopamine in high doses is used in similar situations as norepinephrine. Dobutamine is preferred when the blood pressure is already elevated and cardiac output is low. It is not a strong vasopressor, because its beta-2 action causes vasodilation counteracting its beta-1 action, but it does have positive inotropic and chronotropic effects. Vasopressin causes vasoconstriction through AVPR1 receptor activity and has been shown to be effective in the management of refractory hypertensive therapy in conjunction with other vasopressors. It should be used with caution given its association with vasospasm and cerebral edema in animal models.

Dóczi T, László FA, Szerdahelyi P, et al. Involvement of vasopressin in brain edema formation: further evidence obtained from the Brattleboro diabetes insipidus rat with experimental sub-arachnoid hemorrhage. *Neurosurgery.* 1984;14(4):436-441. doi:10.1227/00006123-198404000-00008

Miller JA, Dacey RG Jr, Diringer MN. Safety of hypertensive hypervolemic therapy with phenyle-phrine in the treatment of delayed ischemic deficits after subarachnoid hemorrhage. *Stroke.* 1995;26(12):2260-2266. doi:10.1161/01.STR.26.12.2260

Muehlschlegel S, Dunser MW, Gabrielli A, et al. Arginine vasopressin as a supplementary vaso-pressor in refractory hypertensive, hypervolemic, hemodilutional therapy in subarachnoid hemorrhage. *Neurocrit Care.* 2007;6(1):3-10. doi:10.1385/NCC:6:1:3

Rose JC, Mayer SA. Optimizing blood pressure in neurological emergencies. *Neurocrit Care.* 2004;1(3):287-299. doi:10.1385/NCC:1:3:287

Trandafir CC, Nishihashi T, Wang A, et al. Participation of vasopressin in the development of cere-bral vasospasm in a rat model of subarachnoid haemorrhage. *Clin Exp Pharmacol Physiol.* 2004;31(4):261-266. doi:10.1111/j.1440-1681.2004.03986.x

18. **The answer is A.** According to the American Stroke Association (ASA)/American Heart Association (AHA) guidelines for the management of aneurysmal subarachnoid hemorrhage, the severity of clinical presentation is the strongest prognostic indicator for SAH (Class 1 evidence). Additional predictors for poor outcome are rebleeding, older age, preex-isting severe illness, hyperglycemia, fever, cerebral edema, symptomatic vasospasm, intra-ventricular or intracerebral hematoma, and cerebral infarction.

Connolly ES Jr, Rabinstein AA, Carhuapoma JR, et al. Guidelines for the management of aneurysmal subarachnoid hemorrhage: a guideline for healthcare professionals from the American Heart Association/American Stroke Association. *Stroke.* 2012;43(6):1711-1737. doi:10.1161/STR.0b013e3182587839

19. **The answer is D.** Nimodipine is an L-type calcium channel blocker and is the only med-ication that has been shown to improve outcome in SAH. Although the exact mechanism of this observation is not known, it does not appear to be through alleviation of cere-bral vasospasm. Proposed hypotheses include blocking calcium-dependent excitotoxicity, antiplatelet aggregation activity, and dilation of lepto-meningeal or small dural collaterals not seen on angiogram. Adverse effects have also been described, like hypotension, increased intracranial pressure (ICP), and decreased brain tissue oxygenation. The use of IV nimodipine did not show any benefit compared to the enteral route.

Dumont AS, Tjoumakaris SI, Jabbour PM, et al. Intravenous versus enteral nimodipine in aneurys-mal subarachnoid hemorrhage: is there an advantage? *World Neurosurg.* 2012;78(1-2):48-49. doi:10.1016/j.wneu.2012.05.001

Soppi V, Karamanakos PN, Koivisto T, et al. A randomized outcome study of enteral versus intra-venous nimodipine in 171 patients after acute aneurysmal subarachnoid hemorrhage. *World Neurosurg.* 2012;78(1-2):101-109. doi:10.1016/j.wneu.2011.09.030

Stiefel MF, Heuer GG, Abrahams JM, et al. The effect of nimodipine on cerebral oxygenation in patients with poor-grade subarachnoid hemorrhage. *J Neurosurg.* 2004;101(4):594-599. doi:10.3171/jns.2004.101.4.0594

20. **The answer is A.** The use of cEEG to detect reversible ischemic changes was first applied in the 1970s in carotid surgeries. Different parameters have since been investigated that corre-late best with ischemic changes. An alpha–delta ratio is practical and correlates with delayed

cerebral ischemia (DCI) and vasospasm. Changes can be seen up to 3 days prior, which allows for timely therapeutic interventions and is particularly beneficial in poor-grade patients with no clinical examination to follow. cEEG monitoring in these patients is also beneficial to detect nonconvulsive seizures (NCS), which can be seen in nearly 20% of patients after SAH. Intracortical recording seems to be more accurate in predicting vasospasm, is less prone to artifact, has better signal-to-noise ratio, and can be used for automated detection. Loss of faster frequencies can be seen when cerebral blood flow (CBF) level decreases to 25 to 35 mL/g/min. As the CBF decreases further toward infarction threshold (10–12 mL/g/min), the cEEG becomes silent and the damage becomes irreversible.

Claassen J, Mayer SA, Kowalski RG, et al. Detection of electrographic seizures with continuous EEG monitoring in critically ill patients. *Neurology*. 2004;62(10):1743-1748. doi:10.1212/01.WNL.0000125184.88797.62

Foreman B, Claassen J. Quantitative EEG for the detection of brain ischemia. *Crit Care*. 2012;16(2):216. doi:10.1186/cc11230

Stuart RM, Waziri A, Weintraub D, et al. Intracortical EEG for the detection of vasospasm in patients with poor-grade subarachnoid hemorrhage. *Neurocrit Care*. 2010;13(3):355-358. doi:10.1007/s12028-010-9414-6

21. **The answer is A.** Perimesencephalic subarachnoid hemorrhage (SAH) accounts for approximately 10% of patients with SAH. Despite extensive workup, the bleeding source remains unknown in these patients. Hypothesized causes include venous anomaly, ruptured perforating artery, and capillary telangiectasia. By definition, the bleeding is anterior to the midbrain with or without extension to the ambient cistern or basal part of the Sylvian cistern with incomplete filling of the interhemispheric fissure. Recognizing the correct bleeding pattern is important because non-perimesencephalic SAH with a negative angiogram has a more significant clinical course. Patients with perimesencephalic SAH usually have a good clinical grade at presentation. They can develop vasospasm with studies showing up to a 16% incidence. These patients therefore need admission to the ICU and a workup like any other SAH. The clinical course, however, is much more benign and the ICU stay much shorter. Only one case report exists describing a patient with a recurrent hemorrhage. All patients with perimesencephalic SAH should undergo at least one cerebral angiogram at admission. CT angiogram (CTA) or MR angiogram (MRA) is not recommended as an initial study. Controversy exists regarding a follow-up angiogram because of the low yield, and some authors do not recommend it. The patient does not need to be followed long term as good data exist suggesting an asymptomatic course.

Gross BA, Lin N, Frerichs KU, et al. Vasospasm after spontaneous angiographically negative subarachnoid hemorrhage. *Acta Neurochir (Wien)*. 2012;154(7):1127-1133. doi:10.1007/s00701-012-1383-4

Kim YW, Lawson MF, Hoh BL. Nonaneurysmal subarachnoid hemorrhage: an update. *Curr Atheroscler Rep*. 2012;14(4):328-334. doi:10.1007/s11883-012-0256-x

22. **The answer is D.** The MCA is the most reliable vessel for accurately detecting vasospasm with TCD. Posterior circulation vasculature can also be measured, but less accurately than the anterior circulation. Lindegaard ratio is the ratio between MCA and extracranial internal carotid artery (ICA) velocities, and a value greater than 6 correlates with severe cerebral vasospasm. Transcranial duplex studies have poor sensitivity. Nearly 40% of patients who develop delayed cerebral ischemia failed to reach the velocity threshold of 120 cm/sec. It is not useful for screening peripheral vasculature.

Carrera E, Schmidt JM, Oddo M, et al. Transcranial Doppler for predicting delayed cerebral ischemia after subarachnoid hemorrhage. *Neurosurgery*. 2009;65(2):316-323; discussion 323. doi:10.1227/01.NEU.0000349209.69973.88

23. **The answer is D:** This patient presented with a ruptured aneurysm associated with an AVM. Aneurysms are found in 2.7% to 58% of AVMs and may have an increased risk for rupture and rerupture. This wide range is reflective of the different classifications available, as well as the diagnostic tools used in the studies. Aneurysm classification into intranidal, extranidal,

and arterial (prenidal) or venous (postnidal) is important because of the different rupture potential. The reported rupture risk is up to 9.8% but there remains controversy over which location—intranidal versus prenidal—poses a higher risk. Aneurysms unrelated to the AVM exhibit a similar rupture risk to aneurysms in the general population and should be treated accordingly.

The source of the hemorrhage is sometimes difficult to determine. If the patient presents with SAH alone, the bleeding is likely aneurysmal. If concomitant intracranial hemorrhage (ICH) is present, it becomes more difficult to elucidate the source and the relationship between the ICH epicenter and the AVM or aneurysm should be mapped. Once the source is identified as the aneurysm, as in this patient, expedited treatment should be initiated. If an aneurysmal source can be ruled out, the AVM rupture is usually treated in a delayed fashion. Aneurysms can obliterate once the AVM has been treated successfully due to change in flow dynamics. However, waiting for this is not advisable in the setting of a ruptured aneurysm.

Management of unruptured AVMs has become more controversial since the ARUBA trial. This randomized trial for unruptured AVM randomized 226 patients into observation or intervention arms and was stopped early by the National Institutes of Health (NIH) because of the superiority of the observation group. The trial has incited a lot of controversy, and among the criticism was the short mean follow-up time of 33 months. The data is now being analyzed according to the different treatment modalities and AVM characteristics. Spetzler Martin grade 1 and 2 AVMs have a 95% success rate with surgery. Radiosurgery is not an option in this patient's AVM as it will not address the ruptured aneurysm.

Flores BC, Klinger DR, Rickert KL, et al. Management of intracranial aneurysms associated with arteriovenous malformations. *Neurosurg Focus*. 2014;37:E11. doi:10.3171/2014.6.FOCUS14165

Platz J, Berkefeld J, Singer OC, et al. Frequency, risk of hemorrhage and treatment considerations for cerebral arteriovenous malformations with associated aneurysms. *Acta Neurochir (Wien)*. 2014;156:2025-2034. doi:10.1007/s00701-014-2225-3

Redekop G, TerBrugge K, Montanera W, et al. Arterial aneurysms associated with cerebral arteriovenous malformations: classification, incidence, and risk of hemorrhage. *J Neurosurg*. 1998;89:539-546. doi:10.3171/jns.1998.89.4.0539

Salomon R, Sander Connolly E. Arteriovenous malformations of the brain. *N Engl J Med*. 2017;376:1859-1866. doi:10.1056/NEJMra1607407

24. **The answer is C.** This patient's angiogram shows an occlusion of the right middle cerebral artery (MCA). He is in the time window for endovascular thrombectomy. Since 2015, five randomized controlled trials have shown improvement in functional outcome at 90 days after mechanical thrombectomy for patients with large vessel occlusion. Patients underwent thrombectomy up to 12 hours after onset of symptoms, if imaging studies showed good collateral circulation or a small core infarction (Escape). The newer DAWN trial pushes this window to up to 24 hours after symptom onset if imaging is favorable. Prior to any intervention the patient should undergo noncontrast CT imaging to determine the Alberta stroke program early CT (ASPECT) score and rule out a large core infarct or intracerebral hemorrhage. This patient is out of the IV tPA window and there is no role for heparin here. The patient's need for a hemicraniectomy cannot be determined based on an angiogram.

Berkhemer OA, Fransen PS, Beumer D, et al. A randomized trial of intraarterial treatment for acute ischemic stroke. *N Engl J Med*. 2015;372:11-20. doi:10.1056/NEJMoa1411587

Campbell BC, Mitchell PJ, Kleinig TJ, et al. Endovascular therapy for ischemic stroke with perfusion-imaging selection. *N Engl J Med*. 2015;372(11):1009-1018. doi:10.1056/NEJMoa1414792

Goyal M, Demchuk AM, Menon BK, et al. Randomized assessment of rapid endovascular treatment of ischemic stroke. *N Engl J Med*. 2015;372(11):1019-1030. doi:10.1056/NEJMoa1414905

Jovin TG, Chamorro A, de Miguel MA, et al. Thrombectomy within 8 hours after symptom onset in ischemic stroke. *N Engl J Med*. 2015;372(24):2296-2306. doi:10.1056/NEJMoa1503780

Nogueira RG, Jadhav AP, Haussen DC, et al. Thrombectomy 6 to 24 hours after stroke with a mismatch between deficit and infarct. *N Engl J Med.* 2018;378(1):11-21. doi: 10.1056/NEJMoa1706442

Saver, JL, Goyal M, Bonafe A, et al. Stent-retriever thrombectomy after intravenous t-PA vs. t-PA alone in stroke. *N Engl J Med.* 2015;372(24):2285-2295. doi:10.1056/NEJMoa1415061

25. **The answer is D.** Individuals with two first-degree relatives with a ruptured aneurysm should undergo screening because of increased lifelong risk of subarachnoid hemorrhage (SAH) and aneurysm formation, according to the European Stroke Organization and the American Heart Association. Several chromosomes have been implicated in aneurysm formation (specifically chromosomes 4, 8, and 9). In addition, it appears the risk is higher in smokers, suggesting that environmental factors and genetic predisposition exert their effect in concert. The Familial Intracranial Aneurysm study revealed a 21% incidence of aneurysms among first-degree relatives who underwent imaging. Further, a 17-fold increase in rupture rate of intracranial aneurysms has been demonstrated in individuals with a family history, compared to individuals with sporadic aneurysms. Even in family members with initially negative studies, continued surveillance using Magnetic Resonance Angiography (MRA; to limit radiation exposure) should be performed given the high rate de novo aneurysm formation.

Bor AS, Rinkel GJ, van Norden J, et al. Long-term, serial screening for intracranial aneurysms in individuals with a family history of aneurysmal subarachnoid haemorrhage: a cohort study. *Lancet Neurol.* 2014;13(4):385-392. doi:10.1016/S1474-4422(14)70021-3

Broderick JP, Brown RD Jr, Sauerbeck L, et al. Greater rupture risk for familial as compared to sporadic unruptured intracranial aneurysms. *Stroke.* 2009;40(6):1952-1957. doi: 10.1161/STROKEAHA.108.542571

Brown RD Jr, Broderick JP. Unruptured intracranial aneurysms: epidemiology, natural history, management options, and familial screening. *Lancet Neurol.* 2014;13(4):393-404. doi:10.1016/S1474-4422(14)70015-8

Brown RD Jr, Huston J, Hornung R, et al. Screening for brain aneurysm in the Familial Intracranial Aneurysm study: frequency and predictors of lesion detection. *J Neurosurg.* 2008;108(6):1132-1138. doi: 10.3171/JNS/2008/108/6/1132

Connoly ES Jr, Rabinstein AA. Guidelines for the management of hemorrhage: a guideline for healthcare professionals from the American Heart Association/Stroke Association. *Stroke.* 2012;43:1711-1737. doi:10.1161/STR.0b013e3182587839

Steiner T, Juvela S. European Stroke Organization guidelines for the management of intracranial aneurysms and subarachnoid hemorrhage. *Cerebrovascular Dis.* 2013;35(2):95-112. doi:10.1159/000346087

26. **The answer is A.** Whether an aneurysm should be clipped or coiled has changed significantly since the landmark International Subarachnoid Aneurysm Trial (ISAT) publication in 2002. Since then, the long-term results of the UK cohort have been published which showed that the risk for rebleeding and recurrence remains higher in the endovascular group. Patients in the coiled group were more likely to be alive (83% vs. 79%) and independent (mRS 0–2 at 10 years, 82% vs. 78%) compared to the clipped group. More striking results were seen in the Barrow Ruptured Aneurysm Trial (BRAT), which had a 6-year follow-up. Although there were no significant differences in the poor outcomes (mRS >2) between the coiling and clipping groups, the rate of re-treatment and complete aneurysm obliteration after 6 years strongly favored clipping. It is still too early to use the term "cure" after 10 years for a disease that can recur and have fatal outcomes with rebleeding. The Cerebral Aneurysm Rerupture After Treatment (CARAT) study revealed a 58% mortality among early postprocedure reruptures with a trend toward higher rates with coiling patients. Beyond that, rerupture is rare with both modalities. With the emergence of newer technologies, including flow diversion, this problem may become less of an issue in the future. Coiling remains a valid long-term alternative to clipping.

CARAT Investigators. Rates of delayed rebleeding from intracranial aneurysms are low after surgical and endovascular treatment. *Stroke.* 2006;37(6):1437-1442. doi:10.1161/01.STR.0000221331.01830.ce

Jeon, JP, Cho YD, Rhim JK, et al. Fate of coiled aneurysms with minor recanalization at 6 months: rate of progression to further recanalization and related risk factors. *Am J Neuroradiol.* 2016;37(8):1490-1495. doi:10.3174/ajnr.A4763

Johnston SC, Dowd CF, Higashida RT, et al. Predictors of rehemorrhage after treatment of ruptured intracranial aneurysms: the Cerebral Aneurysm Rerupture After Treatment study. *Stroke.* 2008;39(1):120-125. doi:10.1161/STROKEAHA.107.495747

Molyneux AJ, Birks, Clarke A, et al. The durability of endovascular coiling versus neurosurgical clipping of ruptured cerebral aneurysms: 18-year follow-up of the UK cohort of the International Subarachnoid Aneurysm Trial. *Lancet.* 2015;385:691-697. doi:10.1016/S0140-6736(14)60975-2

Molyneux AJ, Kerr RS. International subarachnoid aneurysm trial (ISAT) of neurosurgical clipping versus endovascular coiling in 2143 patients with ruptured intracranial aneurysms: a randomized trial. *Lancet.* 2002;360:1267-1274. doi:10.1016/S0140-6736(02)11314-6

Spetzler RF, Zabramski JM, McDougall CG, et al. Analysis of saccular aneurysms in the Barrow Ruptured Aneurysm Trial. *J Neurosurg.* 2017;128(1):120-125. doi:10.3171/2016.9.JNS161301

27. **The answer is B.** Patients with SCD have a 330 times higher risk of stroke compared to the general population. Forty percent of SCD patients will have moyamoya-like vessels thought to be due to chronic sickle cell occlusion of the vaso vasorum. SCD, when combined with MMS, has double the risk for recurrent vascular events. Therefore early detection and treatment is important. Medical management or anticoagulation is insufficient for patients having SCD and MMS. Patient with elevated Transcranial Doppler velocities (usually >200 cm/sec) should be treated with exchange transfusions to a target HbS level of 30% to 50%. Hyperventilation would increase the risk for stroke because of the vasospasm risk. The best long-term therapy for these patients is direct or indirect cerebral bypass surgery, which reduces the stroke rate six-fold.

Dobson SR, Holden KR, Nietert PJ, et al. Moyamoya syndrome in childhood sickle cell disease: a predictive factor for recurrent cerebrovascular events. *Blood.* 2002;99(9):3144-3150. doi: 10.1182/blood.V99.9.3144

Smith ER, McClain CD, Heeney M, et al. Pial synangiosis in patients with moyamoya syndrome and sickle cell anemia: perioperative management and surgical outcome. *Neurosurg Focus.* 2009;26(4):E10. doi:10.3171/2009.01.FOCUS08307

Yang, W, Porras JL, Takemoto CM, et al. Effectiveness of surgical revascularization for stroke prevention in pediatric patients with sickle cell disease and moyamoya syndrome. *J Neurosurg Pediatr.* 2017;20(3):232-238. doi:10.3171/2017.1.PEDS16576

3

Neurotrauma

ANAND KAUL AND SCOTT R. SHEPARD

▪ QUESTIONS

1. Indications for craniotomy for acute epidural hematoma (EDH) include all of the following **except**:

   A. Pupillary anisocoria
   B. Midline shift greater than 5 mm
   C. Hematoma volume greater than 30 cm^3
   D. Lack of a lucid interval
   E. Clot thickness greater than 15 mm

2. The lesion seen on the scan at right is most consistent with:

   A. Cerebellar contusion
   B. Cerebellar intracerebellar hematoma
   C. Posterior fossa subdural hematoma (SDH)
   D. Posterior fossa epidural hematoma (EDH)

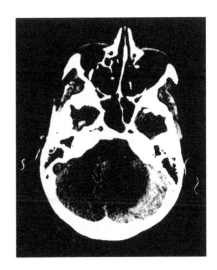

3. The primary effect of mannitol in the treatment of elevated intracranial pressure (ICP) is:

   A. Osmotic fluid removal from the brain
   B. Rheologic effects to change the shape of red blood cells and decrease blood viscosity
   C. Free radical sequestration
   D. Decrease in the cerebral metabolic rate

4. A 43-year-old is admitted to the ICU following a fall down a flight of stairs. She reports brief loss of consciousness following the fall. CT scan of the head demonstrates a small inferior frontal pole contusion. Initially she complained of pain in her neck and numbness in her arms bilaterally. By the next morning she noted her arms felt weak, describing them to be heavy

and numb all over. She has right greater than left as well as distal greater than proximal weakness in her upper extremities. Her lateral C spine x-ray and CT C spine facet view are seen as follows:

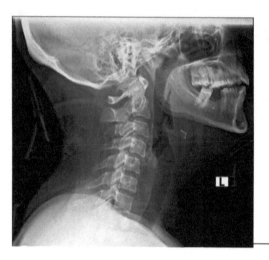
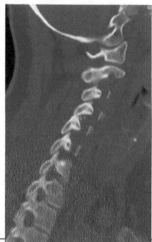

Which of following aspects of this patient's Subaxial Injury Classification (SLIC) score are true?

A. There is translational morphology to spinal deformity without disruption of the discoligamentous complex with incomplete spinal cord injury which will not require operative intervention for fixation.

B. There is no abnormality of spinal morphology, discoligamentous complex likely to be intact although there is evidence of incomplete spinal cord injury. Will likely be stable without operative intervention.

C. There is likely to be translational morphology of spinal deformity with disruption of the discoligamentous complex and incomplete spinal cord injury necessitating operative intervention.

D. There is a burst fracture morphology indeterminate injury to disco ligamentous complex and incomplete spinal cord injury that will be sufficiently managed with external fixation.

5. What is true about the type and stability of injury demonstrated by the imaging studies in Question 4?

A. Chance fracture, stable
B. Burst fracture, unstable
C. Jefferson fracture, unstable
D. Hangman's fracture, unstable
E. Perched facet, unstable

6. All of the following statements regarding the older patients with acute subdural hematomas (SDHs) are true **except**:

A. It is possible to predict death and low Glasgow Coma Scale (GCS) scores in older patients undergoing surgery for acute SDH on the basis of the admission eye-opening score of the GCS

B. Patients age 18 to 30 years with acute SDH undergoing surgery have a 25% overall mortality, whereas patients older than 50 years with acute SDH undergoing surgery have a 75% mortality rate

   C. Several multivariate analyses have failed to demonstrate age as an independent predictor of outcome in older patients undergoing craniotomy for acute SDH

   D. In one study, 17 of 23 comatose patients with acute SDH older than 65 died, while the rest remained in a persistent vegetative state

7. Which of these statements regarding basilar skull fractures is **not** true?

   A. Basilar skull fractures occur in 7% to 16% of all patients with skull fractures

   B. These fractures are often indicated by the presence of pneumocephalus on head CT in the absence of open cranial vault fractures

   C. Prophylactic antibiotics have been demonstrated to reduce the risk of meningitis

   D. These skull fractures are frequently accompanied by periorbital ecchymoses (raccoon's eyes) or postauricular ecchymoses (Battle's sign)

   E. These fractures rarely require surgical intervention

8. Which of the following statements regarding posttraumatic cerebrospinal fluid (CSF) fistulae is true?

   A. CSF otorrhea is more likely to resolve spontaneously than CSF rhinorrhea

   B. Posttraumatic CSF fistulae occur in 50% of all patients with basilar skull fractures

   C. Less than one third resolve spontaneously

   D. Meningitis occurs in less than 3%

   E. Most posttraumatic CSF fistulae are not evident for 3 to 6 days after injury

9. Hypertonic saline has been demonstrated to:

   A. Increase cerebral blood flow more than mannitol on an equimolar basis

   B. Decrease intracranial pressure (ICP) more than mannitol on an equimolar basis

   C. Have a shorter duration of action than mannitol

   D. Have a greater risk of nephrotoxicity than mannitol

10. Which of the following is not a risk factor for blunt cerebrovascular injury?

   A. Displaced midface fracture (LeFort II or LeFort III)

   B. Basilar skull fracture with carotid canal involvement

   C. C7-T1 jumped facets and subluxation with spinal cord transection

   D. Closed head injury with diffuse axonal injury (DAI) and Glasgow Coma Scale (GCS) less than 6

   E. Near hanging with anoxia

11. Use of corticosteroids in the treatment of acute spinal cord injury in adults has been demonstrated to:

   A. Dramatically increase motor function in patients 6 months after the injury

   B. Increase the risk of systemic complications, including wound infections, sepsis, and pneumonia

   C. Decrease the risk of systemic complications following acute spinal cord injury

   D. Demonstrate benefit to patients if administration is initiated between 24 and 72 hours following acute spinal cord injury

12. A 21-year-old man is involved in a high-speed motor vehicle accident in which he strikes a telephone pole, resulting in an extended loss of consciousness. On arrival at the ICU, he is noted to have a Glasgow Coma Scale (GCS) of 5T, with a motor score of 4 and intact brainstem reflexes. He is intubated with the vital signs of temperature of 98.3°F, heart rate (HR) 68 beats/min, regular, mean arterial pressure (MAP) 90 mmHg, and oxygen saturation of 99% with fraction of inspired oxygen (FiO$_2$) of 40%. Urine drug screen is negative, and there is no detectable alcohol in his serum sample. Referring to his CT scan, the most likely diagnosis is:

    A. Traumatic encephalopathy
    B. Acute subdural hematoma (SDH)
    C. Brainstem contusion
    D. Diffuse axonal injury (DAI)
    E. Nonconvulsive status epileptic

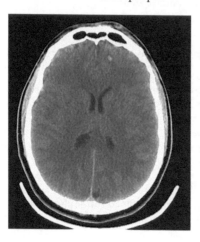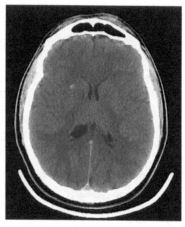

13. The Rescue intracranial pressure (ICP) study is a recently published randomized trial of decompressive hemicranictomy versus further medical management in the treatment of uncontrolled ICP in traumatic brain injury (TBI) patients after failure of initial medical therapy. All of the following are true statements about the results of this study except:

    A. The death rate in the surgical group was 26.9% and the mortality rate in the medical group was 48.9%
    B. The adverse event rate was 16.3% in the surgical group and 9.2% in the medical group
    C. There was no significant difference in favorable outcomes between the medical and surgical groups at 6 months; however, at 12 months, the surgical group demonstrated a statistically significant improvement in the rate of favorable outcomes
    D. The surgical and medical groups had an approximately equivalent rate of patients in the moderate recovery and good recovery categories
    E. The surgical group had a statistically significant increase in the incidence of favorable outcomes at 6-month follow-up and an increase in the ICU length-of-stay compared with the medical group

14. Risk factors for increase in the size of traumatic cerebral contusions/hemorrhages include:

    A. Male sex
    B. Age older than 60 years
    C. Elevation of partial thromboplastin time (PTT)
    D. Deterioration of Glasgow Coma Scale (GCS) after resuscitation
    E. All of the above

15. Which of these statements regarding prophylactic hypothermia in traumatic brain injury (TBI) is true?

    A. Prophylactic hypothermia has been clearly demonstrated to benefit outcome from acute TBI in children.
    B. Prophylactic hypothermia has a complication rate similar to other brain injury treatments in normothermic patients.
    C. Prophylactic hypothermia decreases mortality, but does not improve outcome in adults with acute TBI.
    D. Prophylactic hypothermia does not improve mortality or outcome in the treatment of adults and children with TBI.

16. Prophylactic anticonvulsants in the setting of traumatic brain injury (TBI) have been demonstrated to:

    A. Decrease the incidence of early posttraumatic seizures
    B. Decrease the incidence of both early and late posttraumatic seizures
    C. Not alter the incidence of posttraumatic seizures but reduce the severity of posttraumatic seizures
    D. Decrease the incidence of late posttraumatic seizures

17. Which of the following statements is true regarding the role of decompressive hemicraniectomy in the treatment of the patient with traumatic brain injury (TBI)?

    A. Randomized prospective trials have shown that decompressive hemicraniectomy decreases mortality and improves outcomes
    B. Decompressive hemicraniectomy may be effective in treating refractory intracranial pressure (ICP)
    C. Decompressive hemicraniectomy has no role in the treatment of increased ICP in the patient with TBI and should only be used to treat the malignant middle cerebral artery (MCA) syndrome
    D. Decompressive hemicraniectomy should never be performed in patients younger than 18 years

18. Which of the following statements regarding posttraumatic vasospasm (PTV) is not true?

    A. Contrary to nimodipine use in aneurysmal subarachnoid patients, nimodipine has been demonstrated to decrease the rate of radiographic vasospasm in traumatic brain injury (TBI) patients.
    B. Young age, lower admission Glasgow Coma Scale (GCS), and presence of traumatic subarachnoid hemorrhage (SAH) are risk factors for the development of PTV.
    C. The duration of PTV, 3 days to 3 weeks, is similar to the duration of vasospasm in aneurysmal subarachnoid patients.
    D. Incidence of PTV reported in the literature ranges from 35.6% to 61%.
    E. Two phases of PTV have been described, an early phase and a late phase.

19. Indications for intracranial pressure (ICP) monitoring include all of the following **except**:

    A. Severe alcohol withdrawal in the traumatic brain injury (TBI) patient
    B. Glasgow Coma Scale (GCS) score 3 to 8 with an abnormal CT scan
    C. Normal head CT scan with any two of these features: age older than 40 years, unilateral or bilateral motor posturing, and systolic blood pressure (SBP) <90
    D. Patients with abnormal head CT scans with GCS greater than 8 who are undergoing prolonged general anesthesia or pharmacologic muscle relaxants and will not have a neurologic examination that may be assessed

20. Treatments designed to decrease intracranial pressure (ICP) should begin when:

    A. ICP increases 10 mmHg from the pressure when the ICP monitor was placed
    B. There is a presence of any midline shift on the head CT
    C. ICP reaches a threshold of between 15 and 20 mmHg
    D. ICP reaches a threshold of between 20 and 25 mmHg

21. Ventriculostomy infections have been demonstrated to:

    A. Increase with the duration of use, and infection rates increase substantially after 7 days
    B. Occur in less than 3% of patients
    C. Occur less commonly in patients with intraventricular hemorrhage (IVH)
    D. Significantly decrease with routine catheter exchange every 5 days

22. Which of the following is true regarding prophylaxis against venous thromboembolic events (VTE) in traumatic brain injury (TBI) patients?

    A. The Brain Trauma Foundation Guidelines (2016) recommend specific agents and timing for VTE prophylaxis in TBI patients.
    B. Enoxaparin has been demonstrated to be superior to both unfractionated heparin and dalteparin in VTE prevention in TBI patients
    C. The incidence of VTE in TBI patients not treated with chemoprophylaxis against VTE is between 2% and 5%
    D. TBI patients with worsening of their hemorrhage between the first and second postinjury head CT scans have a 13-fold increased risk of continued hemorrhage progression when treated with enoxaparin for prophylaxis against VTE

23. A 35-year-old man is 3-week status post-decompressive hemicraniectomy when he develops a new contralateral left upper-extremity monoparesis over several days. He is afebrile with a normal white count and denies any new trauma. Extensive laboratory evaluation is within normal limits. EEG demonstrates expected slowing over the affected hemisphere and does not reveal any evidence of seizure. There has not been any clinical evidence of seizure. Referring to this repeat CT scan, the most likely diagnosis is:

    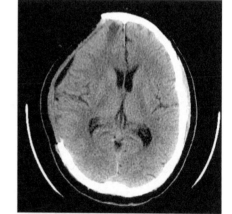

    A. Postictal paralysis
    B. Hydrocephalus
    C. Conversion disorder
    D. "Syndrome of the trephined"

24. Which of the following statements regarding barbiturate-induced coma is true?

    A. Has been demonstrated to be beneficial in improving patient outcome from severe traumatic injury when used in a prophylactic fashion
    B. Is less effective than mannitol in lowering increased intracranial pressure (ICP)
    C. Rarely induces systemic hypotension when infused at target rates
    D. Causes an unacceptable increase in core body temperature

25. Which of the following is **not** true regarding the complications associated with ventriculostomy placement?

A. The risk of all hemorrhage after ventriculostomy placement is 7%
B. The risk of clinically significant hemorrhage after ventriculostomy placement is approximately 1%
C. The risk of hemorrhage increases significantly in patients whose International Normalized Ratio (INR) is between 1.4 and 1.6 compared with patients whose INR is between 1.2 and 1.4
D. In children, ventriculostomy insertion is associated with a three-fold higher risk of hemorrhage compared with intraparenchymal monitor placement

▪ ANSWERS

1. **The answer is D.** The indications for surgery for an acute EDH include the following: hematoma size greater than 30 cm³, clot thickness greater than 15 mm, midline shift greater than 5 mm, and pupillary anisocoria in the presence of an EDH not due to other factors such as ocular trauma. The lucid interval occurs in less than 20% of patients with EDH and is not a factor in the decision for surgery in patients with EDH. Patients with EDH in whom the hematoma is less than 30 cm³, the clot is less than 15 mm in diameter, there is less than 5 mm of midline shift, and whose Glasgow Coma Scale (GCS) is greater than 8 can be managed conservatively; however, they must be monitored very closely and undergo early repeat CT scan. Peres' review of the literature demonstrated that in initially nonoperative acute epidural hematomas 82/471 patients (17.4%) required delayed craniotomy for evacuation due to progression of hemorrhage. Endovascular management with arterial embolization in nonoperative acute EDH has been demonstrated to be safe and a potentially effective means of treating some types of blunt vascular injuries and avoiding the need for craniotomy.

   Bullock MR, Chesnut R, Ghajar J, et al. Surgical management of acute epidural hematomas. *Neurosurgery*. 2006;58(3 suppl):S7-S15; discussion Si-Siv. doi:10.1227/01.neu.0000210363.91172.a8

   Peres CM, Caldas JM, Puglia P, et al. Endovascular management of acute epidural hematomas: clinical experience with 80 cases. *J Neurosurg*. 2018;128(4):1044-1050. doi:10.3171/2016.11.JNS161398

2. **The answer is C.** This lesion is a posterior fossa SDH. Posterior fossa hematomas are uncommon in traumatic brain injury (TBI), and occur in less than 3% of TBI patients. The most common posterior fossa hematoma seen in the setting of trauma is an EDH, accounting for less than 10% of all EDHs. Posterior fossa SDHs are even less common and account for only 0.5% to 2.5% of all SDHs, whereas posterior fossa intraparenchymal hematomas account for only 1.7% of all traumatic intraparenchymal hematomas. Although trauma-related posterior fossa hemorrhages are uncommon, they pose a particular hazard for patients because of the limited size of the posterior fossa and the tendency for these patients to rapidly deteriorate.

   Bullock MR, Chesnut R, Ghajar J, et al. Surgical management of posterior fossa mass lesions. *Neurosurgery*. 2006;58(3 suppl):S47-S55; discussion Si. doi:10.1227/01.neu.0000210366.36914.38

3. **The answer is B.** The primary mechanism of mannitol's effect on ICP is through its ability to decrease blood viscosity by altering the shape of the red blood cells (rheologic effect) and is not through its osmotic effects. This change in viscosity improves cerebral blood flow, especially at the level of the microcirculation, resulting in a decrease in ICP. The rheologic effects of mannitol occur within minutes of mannitol administration, whereas the osmotic effects of mannitol are not apparent for 15 to 30 minutes after administration. Mannitol is also a free radical scavenger. Mannitol does not directly affect the cerebral metabolic rate.

   Bratton SL, Chesnut RM, Ghajar J, et al. Guidelines for the management of severe traumatic brain injury. II. Hyperosmolar therapy. *J Neurotrauma*. 2007;24(suppl 1):S14-S20. doi:10.1089/neu.2007.9994

4. **The answer is C.** The SLIC scale takes into account the mechanism of injury as well as the integrity of the discoligamentous complex and overall neurological status as predictors of injury severity. It sheds light on prognosis and has been helpful in accurately determining treatment course of action in regard to nonoperative and operative management of subaxial cervical spine injury. By SLIC classification, this patient's injury was scored as follows: injury morphology—translational, 4 points; discoligamentous complex—disrupted, 2 points; neurological status—incomplete cord injury, 3 points. Her total SLIC score was 9, indicating a need for operative treatment.

   Bullock MR, Chesnut R, Ghajar J, et al. Surgical management of acute epidural hematomas. *Neurosurgery*. 2006;58(3 suppl):S7-S15; discussion Si. doi:10.1227/01.neu.0000210363.91172.a8

   Bullock MR, Chesnut R, Ghajar J, et al. Surgical management of posterior fossa mass lesions. *Neurosurgery*. 2006;58(3 suppl):S47-S55; discussion Si. doi:10.1227/01.neu.0000210366.36914.38

Patel AA, Hurlbert RJ, Bono CM, et al. Classification and surgical decision making in acute subaxial cervical spine trauma. *Spine.* 2010;35:S228-S234. doi:10.1097/BRS.0b013e3181f330ae

Vaccaro AR, Hulbert RJ, Patel AA, et al. Spine Trauma Study Group. The subaxial cervical spine injury classification system: a novel approach to recognize the importance of morphology, neurology, and integrity of the disco-ligamentous complex. *Spine.* 2007;32:2365-2374. doi: 10.1097/BRS.0b013e3181557b92

5. **The answer is E.** The inferior articulating facet joint is fractured and is now in a "perched" position on the superior articulating facet of C5. The facet joint is considered a major stabilizer of cervical motion in multiple dimensions within the cervical spine. Disruption of the facet joint can cause significant linear/rotational translation of the facets and subaxial spine which can damage nerve roots and/or the spinal cord itself. The mechanism of the injury deals with hyperextension usually combined with lateral bending and/or rotation. Facet fractures comprise up to 6.7% of all types of cervical spine fractures. A systematic review by Kepler et al. reviewed 11 different studies with a total of 368 patients that had either bilateral or unilateral isolated cervical facet fractures and determined that operative management yielded better clinical outcomes that nonoperative management in regard to maintenance of reduction. Aarabi et al. analyzed a cohort of 25 patients and determined that even in patients with nondisplaced unilateral subaxial facet fractures, those treated with operative management had a lower failure rate.

Aarabi B, Mirvis S, Shanmuganathan K, et al. Comparative effectiveness of surgical versus nonoperative management of unilateral, nondisplaced, subaxial cervical spine facet fractures without evidence of spinal cord injury. *J Neurosurg: Spine.* 2014;20(3):270-277. doi: 10.3171/2013.11.spine13733

Bratton SL, Chestnut RM, Ghajar J, et al. Guidelines for the management of severe traumatic brain injury. II. Hyperosmolar therapy. *J Neurotrauma.* 2007;24(suppl 1):S14-S20. doi: 10.1089/neu.2007.9994

Hadley MN, Fitzpatrick BC, Sonntag VK, et al. Facet fracture-dislocation injuries of the cervical spine. *Neurosurgery.* 1992;30:661-666. doi:10.1016/s0196-0644(05)81775-5

Kepler CK, Vaccaro AR, Chen E, et al. Treatment of isolated cervical facet fractures: a systematic review. *J Neurosurg: Spine.* 2016;24(2):347-354. doi:10.3171/2015.6.spine141260

6. **The answer is A.** Although there is a relationship between poor outcome and age as well as poor outcome and low GCS, it is not possible to predict death based on advanced age and poor presentation GCS. In a study by Kotwica and Brzezinski, a statistically significant difference in outcome at 3 months was demonstrated between younger patients and older patients. Patients aged 18 to 30 had a mortality rate of 25%, and patients older than 50 years with an acute SDH had a mortality rate of 75%. Although many studies have demonstrated a relationship between age and outcome in patients with acute SDH, several multivariate analyses have not demonstrated such a relationship.

Bullock MR, Chesnut R, Ghajar J, et al. Surgical management of acute subdural hematomas. *Neurosurgery.* 2006;58(3 suppl):S16-S24; discussion Si. doi:10.1227/01.neu.0000210364.29290.c9

Howard MA 3rd, Gross AS, Dacey RG Jr, et al. Acute subdural hematomas: an age-dependent clinical entity. *J Neurosurg.* 1989;71(6):858-863. doi:10.3171/jns.1989.71.6.0858

Kotwica Z, Brzezinski J. Acute subdural haematoma in adults: an analysis of outcome in comatose patients. *Acta Neurochir (Wien).* 1993;121(3-4):95-99. doi:10.1007/bf01809257

7. **The answer is C.** Although the use of prophylactic antibiotics in basilar skull fractures is a common practice, it has not been demonstrated to decrease the risk of meningitis in these patients. Five randomized controlled trials failed to demonstrate that there was a reduction in the frequency of meningitis, mortality from all causes, and meningitis-related mortality in patients receiving prophylactic antibiotics for skull base fractures compared with those who did not receive prophylactic antibiotics. Current data do not support the use of prophylactic antibiotics in patients with closed basilar skull fractures. This includes patients with evidence of cerebrospinal fluid (CSF) leakage. Basilar skull fractures occur in up to one-sixth of patients with skull fractures and rarely require surgical intervention. Pneumocephalus on CT scan is often an indicator of a basilar skull fracture, especially in the absence of a cranial vault fracture

in proximity to the region of pneumocephalus. Periorbital ecchymoses (raccoon's eyes) or postauricular ecchymoses (Battle's sign) are common indicators of skull base fractures.

Ratilal BO, Costa J, Sampaio C, et al. Antibiotic prophylaxis for preventing meningitis in patients with basilar skull fractures. *Cochrane Database Syst Rev.* 2011;8:CD004884. doi: 10.1002/14651858.cd004884.pub3

8. **The answer is A.** Posttraumatic CSF leakage is a common problem in the traumatic brain injury (TBI) patient and occurs in 12% to 30% of patients with basilar skull fractures. The fractures most commonly associated with CSF leakage are frontal or ethmoid sinus fractures and longitudinal temporal bone fractures. Sixty percent of traumatic CSF leaks present within 48 hours of injury, and approximately 70% spontaneously resolve within 48 hours. CSF otorrhea has a higher spontaneous resolution rate than CSF rhinorrhea. Some patients develop posttraumatic CSF leakage months to years after a TBI. Meningitis occurs in between 7% and 30% of all patients who develop a posttraumatic CSF leak, with *Streptococcus pneumoniae* being the most frequently isolated pathogen.

Friedman JA, Ebersold MJ, Quast LM. Persistent posttraumatic cerebrospinal fluid leakage. *Neurosurg Focus.* 2000;9(1):e1. doi:10.3171/foc.2000.9.1.1

9. **The answer is B.** Hypertonic saline and mannitol are both effective in lowering ICP. In the study by Battison et al., nine patients received two treatments each of 200 mL of 20% mannitol and 100 mL of 7.5% saline, with 6% dextran-70 solution (HSD) in a random order. Median ICP reductions were greater using hypertonic saline solution versus mannitol infusion, with the mean ICP reduction of 13 mmHg for hypertonic saline versus 7.5 mmHg reduction with mannitol. In another study, by Vialet et al., 20 patients were assigned treatment with either 20% mannitol or 7.5% hypertonic saline solution in a random order, each given at a dose of 2 mL/kg. The frequency and duration of recurrent elevated ICP episodes were higher in patients treated with mannitol than in those treated with hypertonic saline.

Battison C, Andrews PJ, Graham C, et al. Randomized, controlled trial on the effect of a 20% mannitol solution and a 7.5% saline/6% dextran solution on increased intracranial pressure after brain injury. *Crit Care Med.* 2005;33(1):196-202; discussion 257. doi: 10.1097/01.ccm.0000150269.65485.a6

Munar F, Ferrer AM, de Nadal M, et al. Cerebral hemodynamic effects of 7.2% hypertonic saline in patients with head injury and raised intracranial pressure. *J Neurotrauma.* 2000;17(1):41-51. doi: 10.1089/neu.2000.17.41

Vialet R, Albanèse J, Thomachot L, et al. Isovolume hypertonic solutes (sodium chloride or mannitol) in the treatment of refractory posttraumatic intracranial hypertension: 2 mL/kg 7.5% saline is more effective than 2 mL/kg 20% mannitol. *Crit Care Med.* 2003;31(6):1683-1687. doi: 10.1097/01.ccm.0000063268.91710.df

10. **The answer is C.** There are two widely used guidelines for screening patients with blunt trauma for cerebrovascular injury: the Denver criteria and the Memphis criteria. According to the Denver criteria, the following are the risk factors for blunt cerebrovascular injury: LeForte II or III fracture pattern, cervical spine fracture or subluxation, basilar skull fracture with the involvement of the carotid canal, diffuse axonal injury with GCS less than 6, and near hanging with anoxic brain injury. The Memphis criteria list the following as risk factors for blunt cerebrovascular injury: cervical spine fracture, LeFort II or LeForte III facial fracture, basilar skull fracture with the involvement of the carotid canal, Horner's syndrome, neurologic deficit not explained by imaging studies, and neck soft-tissue injury (seat belt sign, hematoma, or hanging). A fracture/dislocation at C7-T1 is generally not considered a risk factor for vertebral artery injury because the vertebral arteries enter the foramen transversarium at the level of C6 in 90% of patients and enter at the C7 level in the remaining 10%. Therefore a subluxation at C7-T1 is unlikely to result in a vertebral artery injury in the absence of other risk factors for cerebrovascular injury.

Arthurs ZM, Starnes BW. Blunt carotid and vertebral artery injuries. *Injury.* 2008;39(11):1232-1241. doi:10.1016/j.injury.2008.02.042

Biffl WL, Moore EE, Offner PJ, et al. Optimizing screening for blunt cerebrovascular injuries. *Am J Surg*. 1999;178(6):517-521. doi:10.1016/s0002-9610(99)00245-7

Bromberg WJ, Collier BC, Diebel LN, et al. Blunt cerebrovascular injury practice management guidelines: the Eastern Association for the Surgery of Trauma. *J Trauma*. 2010;68(2):471-477. doi:10.1097/TA.0b013e3181cb43da

11. **The answer is B.** The use of ultra-high-dose corticosteroids following acute, nonpenetrating spinal cord injury has not been demonstrated to significantly improve the outcomes in spinal cord injury patients in three separate randomized controlled clinical trials, the National Acute Spinal Cord Injury Study (NASCIS). The most recent of these studies, NASCIS 3, examined megadose methylprednisolone (initial bolus 30 mg/kg, then 5.4 mg/kg infusion) for 24 or 48 hours in acute nonpenetrating spinal cord injury. There was no statistically significant improvement in outcome or motor scores in the original analysis. In NASCIS 3, mortality from respiratory morbidity was six times higher in the 48-hour group. There was a two-fold increase in the incidence of severe pneumonia and a four-fold increase in the incidence of severe sepsis in the 48-hour group compared with the 24-hour group. This was not statistically significant as the NASCIS 3 study was underpowered for this analysis. In NASCIS 2, there was a two-fold increase in wound infections in the steroid group, and in NASCIS 1, there was a four-fold increase in wound infection rates in the steroid group. The NASCIS studies are part of a significant controversy and have undergone extensive post hoc analyses that point to some benefit in specific subgroups of patients. This post hoc analysis was used to justify treatment of spinal cord-injured patients with high-dose steroids. Nearly all of the major spine and trauma organizations now have position statements stating that the use of steroids in acute spinal cord injury is not indicated.

Bracken MB, Shepard MJ, Collins WF, et al. A randomized, controlled trial of methylprednisolone or naloxone in the treatment of acute spinal-cord injury. Results of the Second National Acute Spinal Cord Injury Study. *N Engl J Med*. 1990;322(20):1405-1411. doi:10.1056/NEJM199005173222001

Bracken MB, Shepard MJ, Holford TR, et al. Administration of methylprednisolone for 24 or 48 hours or tirilazad mesylate for 48 hours in the treatment of acute spinal cord injury. Results of the Third National Acute Spinal Cord Injury Randomized Controlled Trial. National Acute Spinal Cord Injury Study. *JAMA*. 1997;277(20):1597-1604. doi:10.1001/jama.277.20.1597

Hurlbert RJ. The role of steroids in acute spinal cord injury: an evidence-based analysis. *Spine*. 2001;26(24S):S39-S46. doi:10.1097/00007632-200112151-00009

12. **The answer is D.** The most likely diagnosis is DAI. The most common cause of depressed consciousness in the traumatic brain injury (TBI) patient without metabolic or pharmacologic alterations and without elevated intracranial pressure (ICP) or large structural brain injury is DAI. Some authors believe that the term "diffuse axonal injury" in and of itself is a misnomer, as it is technically a more discrete localized axonal injury caused by shear injury that occurs most frequently when the brain accelerates or decelerates at a high speed with arc-type vectors through the axons. This leads to axonal disruption and neuronal dysfunction and often results in severe neurologic impairment with minimal evidence of injury on CT scan. Recovery from DAI is very variable and, at this time, there is no algorithm that can accurately predict the outcomes.

Meythaler JM, Peduzzi JD, Eleftheriou E, et al. Current concepts: diffuse axonal injury–associated traumatic brain injury. *Arch Phys Med Rehabil*. 2001;82(10):1461-1471. doi:10.1053/apmr.2001.25137

13. **The answer is E.** The Rescue ICP demonstrated a decreased length of stay in the ICU for the surgical group, not an increased length of stay. At the 6-month follow-up, the surgical group had a higher rate of favorable outcomes (42.8%) versus the medical group (34.6%), but this was not a statistically significant difference. In the study, favorable outcomes were defined as scores of 4 to 8 on the Extended Glasgow Outcome Scale (GOS-E). At 12-month follow-up, the surgical group had a favorable outcome rate of 45.4% and the medical group had a favorable outcome rate of 32.4%. This difference was statistically significant.

Hutchinson PJ, Kolias AG, Timofeev IS, et al. Trial of decompressive craniectomy for traumatic intracranial hypertension. *NEJM*. 2016;375:1119-1130. doi:10.1177/1751143716685246

14. **The answer is E.** All are risk factors for the progression of traumatic cerebral contusions in acute head injury. Early progressive hemorrhage occurs in almost half of acutely head-injured patients who undergo a CT scan within 2 hours of injury. It is most common in cerebral contusions, and it is associated with intracranial pressure (ICP) elevations. The factors listed—male sex, age older than 60 years, early deterioration of GCS after initial resuscitation, and elevated PTT—appear to be the key determinants of hemorrhage progression. Although it is not possible to predict which patients will demonstrate clinically significant progression of their cerebral contusions and there is no definitive guideline for the timing of follow-up CT scans in patients with cerebral contusions, it is important to understand who is at the highest risk for such progression and to obtain early repeat CT scans.

Chang EF, Meeker M, Holland MC. Acute traumatic intraparenchymal hemorrhage: risk factors for progression in the early post-injury period. *Neurosurgery*. 2006;58(4):647-656; discussion 647. doi:10.1227/01.neu.0000197101.68538.e6
Oertel M, Kelly DF, McArthur D, et al. Progressive hemorrhage after head trauma: predictors and consequences of the evolving injury. *J Neurosurg*. 2002;96(1):109-116. doi:10.3171/jns.2002.96.1.0109

15. **The answer is D.** Induced hypothermia is one of the most investigated treatments in TBI. Although some smaller studies have attributed some benefit to prophylactic hypothermia in the treatment of TBI, several large randomized studies have failed to demonstrate any benefit of prophylactic hypothermia on mortality in children or adults with TBI. In pooled data of some randomized controlled trials of hypothermia in adults, there is a tendency toward better Glasgow Outcome Scale scores in the hypothermia group. Individual randomized trials have failed to demonstrate this benefit, and thus there is not a definitive improvement in the outcome in TBI patients treated with prophylactic hypothermia. Several meta-analyses by the Cochrane Injuries Group have failed to demonstrate that hypothermia is a beneficial treatment for TBI. The guidelines for the management of severe TBI state that prophylactic hypothermia is an option for the treatment of TBI; however, it is not a Class I or Class II intervention. Hypothermia remains an option for the treatment of patients with refractory intracranial hypertension following maximal medical therapy.

Alderson P, Gadkary C, Signorini DF. Therapeutic hypothermia for head injury. *Cochrane Database Syst Rev*. 2004;4:CD001048. doi:10.1002/14651858.cd001048.pub2
Bratton SL, Chestnut RM, Ghajar J, et al. Guidelines for the management of severe traumatic brain injury. II. Hyperosmolar therapy. *J Neurotrauma*. 2007;24(suppl 1):S14-S20. doi:10.1089/neu.2007.9994
Clifton GL, Miller ER, Choi SC, et al. Lack of effect of induction of hypothermia after acute brain injury. *N Engl J Med*. 2001;344(8):556-563. doi:10.1056/nejm200102083440114
Hutchison JS, Ward RE, Lacroix J, et al. Hypothermia therapy after traumatic brain injury in children. *N Engl J Med*. 2008;358(23):2447-2456. doi:10.1056/NEJMoa0706930

16. **The answer is A.** Posttraumatic seizures are a significant problem in the TBI patient, occurring in between 4% and 25% of adults and in as many as one third of children with TBI. Posttraumatic seizures may be divided into three groups: immediate seizures (occurring <24 hours after injury), early seizures (occurring less than a week after injury), and late seizures (occurring more than 7 days after injury). Prophylactic anticonvulsants in the setting of TBI have been demonstrated to decrease the risk of early posttraumatic seizures. In the landmark study by Temkin et al., phenytoin was demonstrated, in a randomized double-blind study, to decrease the risk of early posttraumatic seizures from 14.2% to 3.6%. Unfortunately, treatment with phenytoin beyond a week did not decrease the rate of late posttraumatic seizures.

Khan AA, Banerjee A. The role of prophylactic anticonvulsants in moderate to severe head injury. *Int J Emerg Med*. 2010;3(3):187-191. doi:10.1007/s12245-010-0180-1
Temkin NR, Dikmen SS, Wilensky AJ, et al. A randomized, double-blind study of phenytoin for the prevention of post-traumatic seizures. *N Engl J Med*. 1990;323(8):497-502. doi:10.1056/NEJM199008233230801

17. **The answer is B.** The routine use of decompressive hemicraniectomy to improve the outcome in adults with severe TBI and refractory ICP elevation is not supported by any randomized clinical trials. For the pediatric population, decompressive hemicraniectomy reduces the risk of death and unfavorable outcome in one small pilot study in which there were limiting issues. This treatment may be justified in patients younger than 18 years when medical treatment has failed to control ICP. In the adult population, the results of nonrandomized trials and controlled trials with historical controls suggest that decompressive hemicraniectomy is a useful option when sustained and maximal medical treatment has failed to control ICP. In the recently published decompressive craniectomy (DECRA) in diffuse traumatic brain injury study from Australia, the following conclusion was published: "In adults with severe diffuse traumatic brain injury and refractory intracranial hypertension, early bifrontotemporoparietal decompressive craniectomy decreased intracranial pressure and the length of stay in the ICU but was associated with more unfavorable outcomes." This study provides data that the use of up-front, early decompressive hemicraniectomy does not improve outcome in TBI. While DECRA does not address the utility of decompressive hemicraniectomy in treating patients with elevated ICP refractory to maximal medical therapy, Rescue ICP demonstrated a reduction in mortality and increased survival with severe disability in this patient population. Decompressive hemicraniectomy remains a useful option in the treatment of these patients.

Cooper DJ, Rosenfeld JV, Murray L, et al. Decompressive craniectomy in diffuse traumatic brain injury. *N Engl J Med.* 2011;364(16):1493-1502. doi:10.1056/NEJMx110081

Hutchinson PJ, Kolias AG, Timofeev IS, et al. Trial of decompressive craniectomy for traumatic intracranial hypertension. *NEJM.* 2016;375:1119-1130. doi:10.1056/NEJMoa1605215

Taylor A, Butt W, Rosenfeld J, et al. A randomized trial of very early decompressive craniectomy in children with traumatic brain injury and sustained intracranial hypertension. *Childs Nerv Syst.* 2001;17(3):154-162. doi:10.1007/s003810000410

18. **The answer is A.** Nimodipine has not been demonstrated to decrease the rate of angiographic vasospasm in PTV, although there was a trend toward decreased risk of death and severe disability in a Cochrane database review of calcium channel blockers in acute TBI patients. PTV has been shown to have two phases, an acute phase occurring before 24 hours, which is independent of the presence of SAH, and a late phase occurring, 48 to 72 hours after injury, that is correlated with the presence of traumatic SAH. Risk factors for PTV are young age, lower admission GCS, and presence of traumatic SAH. PTV has been reported to occur in between 35.6% and 61% of TBI patients. Symptomatic PTV can be difficult to diagnose in TBI patients as they often have limited neurologic exams.

Perrein A, Petry L, Reis L, et al. Cerebral vasospasm after traumatic brain injury: an update. *Minerva Anestesiol.* 2015;81:1219-1228.

19. **The answer is A.** Alcohol withdrawal itself is not a reason for placement of an ICP monitor. The Guidelines for the Management of TBI, published by the Brain Trauma Foundation, review this subject extensively and provide a consensus statement that there is strong level II evidence to support the use of ICP monitoring in patients with severe TBI. There is also level III evidence that any patients who have any two out of three features—age older than 40 years, unilateral or bilateral motor posturing, SBP <90—should have an ICP monitor placed. ICP monitor placement should also be considered for any trauma patient with an abnormal head CT who will not have a neurologic examination that may be assessed on a frequent basis because of prolonged general anesthesia or extended use of skeletal muscle relaxants. These guidelines are not restrictive, and ICP monitoring can be used for any patient about whom there is a concern for elevated ICP due to radiographic or clinical features.

Bratton SL, Chestnut RM, Ghajar J, et al. Guidelines for the management of severe traumatic brain injury. XV. Steroids. *J Neurotrauma.* 2007;24(suppl 1):S91-S95. doi:10.1089/neu.2007.9981

20. **The answer is D.** This is one of the most debated topics in neurosurgery and neurocritical care. There is a study by Eisenberg et al., which is the only prospective, double-blind, placebo-controlled study, demonstrating improvements in outcome for lowering ICP. In this study, a threshold of 25 was used. The consensus position in the guidelines for the management of severe traumatic brain injury (TBI) is that ICP-lowering treatments should be initiated at an ICP threshold of 20 to 25 mmHg. This is considered a level II recommendation on the basis of available evidence. It should be noted that occasional patients may herniate at ICPs less than 25 mmHg, especially when mass lesions greater than 20 mL are present in the cerebellum or temporal lobe. In addition, the ICP at which patients begin to experience deleterious effects is different for each patient, and some patients will not experience the deleterious effects until their ICP is greater than 25 mmHg, especially if their cerebral perfusion is maintained in an acceptable range.

Bratton SL, Chestnut RM, Ghajar J, et al. Guidelines for the management of severe traumatic brain injury. XV. Steroids. *J Neurotrauma*. 2007;24(suppl 1):S91-S95. doi:10.1089/neu.2007.9981

Eisenberg HM, Frankowski RF, Contant CF, et al. High-dose barbiturate control of elevated intracranial pressure in patients with severe head injury. *J Neurosurg*. 1988;69(1):15-23. doi:10.3171/jns.1988.69.1.0015

21. **The answer is A.** Infection rates after ventriculostomy placement are one of the most heavily studied and controversial issues in neurocritical care and neurosurgery. The published infection rates range from less than 1% to 45%. Most studies report between a 5% and 23% infection rate, depending on the criteria used to define infections and the statistical methodology used. The key issue is that ventriculostomy infections are a significant problem and increase patient risk and cost significantly. Several factors are well established with respect to ventriculostomy infections. They increase significantly after a catheter has been in place for more than 7 days, and they are significantly increased in patients with IVH. Routine catheter exchange after 5 to 7 days, a common practice, does not appear to decrease the infection rate.

Beer R, Lackner P, Pfausler B, et al. Nosocomial ventriculitis and meningitis in neurocritical care patients. *J Neurol*. 2008;255(11):1617-1624. doi:10.1007/s00415-008-0059-8

Harrop JS, Sharan AD, Ratliff J, et al. Impact of a standardized protocol and antibiotic-impregnated catheters on ventriculostomy infection rates in cerebrovascular patients. *Neurosurgery*. 2010;67(1):187-191; discussion 191. doi:10.1227/01.NEU.0000370247

Hoefnagel D, Dammers R, Ter Laak-Poort MP, et al. Risk factors for infections related to external ventricular drainage. *Acta Neurochir (Wien)*. 2008;150(3):209-214; discussion 214. doi: 10.1007/s00701-007-1458-9

Holloway KL, Barnes T, Choi S, et al. Ventriculostomy infections: the effect of monitoring duration and catheter exchange in 584 patients. *J Neurosurg*. 1996;85(3):419-424. doi: 10.3171/jns.1996.85.3.0419

22. **The answer is D.** In the study by Levy et al., TBI patients with increase of their hemorrhage between the first and second postinjury head CT scans have a 13-fold increased risk of continued hemorrhage progression when treated with enoxaparin for prophylaxis against VTE. The Brain Trauma Foundation Guidelines (2016) do not recommend a specific agent for deep vein thrombosis (DVT) prophylaxis in TBI patients and do not provide guidance for the timing of initiation of VTE prophylaxis in TBI patients. The incidence of VTE in TBI patients not treated with chemoprophylaxis against VTE in the literature has been reported in the range of 6% and 20% of TBI patients. Enoxaparin has not been demonstrated to be superior to either unfractionated heparin or dalteparin in VTE prevention in TBI patients.

Arnold JD, Bart BW, Baker DE, et al. Unfractionated heparin three times per day versus enoxaparin in the prevention of deep venous thrombosis in trauma patients. *Am Surg*. 2010;76(6):567-570.

Levy A, Slaottolo R, Bar-Or R, et al. Pharmocaologic thromboprophylaxis is a risk factor for hemorrhage progression in a subset of patients with traumatic brain injury. *J Trauma*. 2010;68:886-894. doi:10.1097/TA.0b013e3181d27dd5

Shen X, Dutcher SK, Plamer J, et al. A systematic review of the benefits of anticoagulation following traumatic brain injury. *J Head Trauma Rehabil*. 2015;30(4):829-837. doi: 10.1097/HTR.0000000000000077

Tykocki T, Guzek K. Anticoagulation therapy in traumatic brain injury. *World Neurosurg*. 2016;89:497-504. doi:10.1016/j.wneu.2016.01.063

23. **The answer is D.** This patient is experiencing the "syndrome of the trephined." This is an uncommon and poorly understood phenomenon of the delayed onset of a neurological deficit after decompressive craniectomy. It can range from a mild neurologic deficit to severe hemispheric dysfunction and alteration in consciousness. There are many theories as to its etiology; however, there is no proven mechanism. It is frequently reversed by cranioplasty, although there often is a delay in improvement of symptoms. Given the lack of clinical or radiographic evidence of seizure, it is unlikely that this patient has a postictal paralysis. Although hydrocephalus is a common sequela of traumatic brain injury (TBI), this patient does not have hydrocephalus. Conversion disorder is an unlikely diagnosis in a patient with a serious head injury.

Akins PT, Guppy KH. Sinking skin flaps, paradoxical herniation, and external brain tamponade: a review of decompressive craniectomy management. *Neurocrit Care*. 2008;9(2):269-276. doi: 10.1007/s12028-007-9033-z

Stiver SI, Wintermark M, Manley GT. Reversible monoparesis following decompressive hemicraniectomy for traumatic brain injury. *J Neurosurg*. 2008;109(2):245-254. doi: 10.3171/JNS/2008/109/8/0245

24. **The answer is B.** Mannitol is more effective in lowering ICP than pentobarbital. In the study by Schwartz et al., 59 patients were treated in a prospective, randomized comparison of pentobarbital and mannitol for the treatment of elevated ICP following traumatic brain injury (TBI). In both patients with and without significant intracranial hematomas, mannitol was more effective than pentobarbital in decreasing and controlling ICP. In a prospective randomized study by Ward et al., prophylactic use of barbiturate coma failed to provide any improvement in outcome compared with the control group. Furthermore, barbiturate use caused clinically significant hypotensive episodes in half of the patients. In the Cochrane review of barbiturate coma, approximately one in four patients developed clinically significant hypotensive episodes. Hypotension is a major risk factor for poor outcome in TBI patients. Barbiturates cause a decrease in core body temperature, not an increase in temperature.

Lee MW, Deppe SA, Sipperly ME, et al. The efficacy of barbiturate coma in the management of uncontrolled intracranial hypertension following neurosurgical trauma. *J Neurotrauma*. 1994;11(3):325-331. doi:10.1089/neu.1994.11.325

Roberts I. Barbiturates for acute traumatic brain injury. *Cochrane Database Syst Rev*. 2000;2:CD000033. doi:10.1002/14651858.CD000033

Schwartz ML, Tator CH, Rowed DW, et al. The University of Toronto head injury treatment study: a prospective, randomized comparison of pentobarbital and mannitol. *Can J Neurol Sci*. 1984;11(4):434-440. doi:10.1017/s0317167100045960

Ward JD, Becker DP, Miller JD, et al. Failure of prophylactic barbiturate coma in the treatment of severe head injury. *J Neurosurg*. 1985;62(3):383-388. doi:10.3171/jns.1985.62.3.0383

25. **The answer is C.** In a recent study, Bauer et al. demonstrated that there is no difference in the risk of hemorrhage after ventriculostomy insertion in patients with an INR between 1.2 and 1.6 compared with patients whose INR was less than 1.2. The risk of hemorrhage after ventriculostomy placement in a large meta-analysis by Bauer et al. was reported as 7.0% from pooled data of studies with more than 25 patients, with most of the studies reporting a rate between 4.5% and 9.4%. The same study reported a clinically significant hemorrhage rate of 0.8%, with most studies reporting a rate between 0.2% and 1.4%. In a study by Anderson et al., the rate of any type of hemorrhage after ventriculostomy insertion in children was 17.6% compared with a 6.5% risk of hemorrhage after intraparenchymal monitor placement.

Anderson RC, Kan P, Klimo P, et al. Complications of intracranial pressure monitoring in children with head trauma. *J Neurosurg*. 2004;101(1 suppl):53-58. doi:10.3171/ped.2004.101.2.0053

Bauer DF, McGwin G Jr, Melton SM, et al. The relationship between INR and development of hemorrhage with placement of ventriculostomy. *J Trauma*. 2011;70(5):1112-1117. doi: 10.1097/TA.0b013e3181e7c2ae

Bauer DF, Razdan SN, Bartolucci AA, et al. Meta-analysis of hemorrhagic complications from ventriculostomy placement by neurosurgeons. *Neurosurgery*. 2011;69(2):255-260. doi: 10.1227/NEU.0b013e31821a45ba

4 Seizures and Epilepsy

GRANT M. WARMOUTH, CAROLINA B. MACIEL,
AND GIRIDHAR P. KALAMANGALAM

QUESTIONS

1. A 63-year-old right-handed man is brought to the ED approximately 5 hours after the acute onset of right-sided facial droop, right arm weakness, and "halting speech." According to his wife, the patient was cursing at the football game on television, when he started to stutter, make guttural noises, and then seemingly stared blankly and did not respond to her. She noticed that his right arm was shaking rhythmically. Soon thereafter, the shaking stopped and the patient started to make semi-purposeful movements (reaching for objects with his left hand) but still appeared "dazed." The patient has never had a prior stroke or head trauma, has never had any surgeries, has had no medical procedures done this year, and has had no recent complaints. His serum glucose is 130 mg/dL, sodium is 137 mEq/L, magnesium is 1.7 mEq/L, his platelets are $220 \times 10^3/\mu$L, blood alcohol level is undetectable, and urine toxicology is negative. His blood pressure is 160/89 mmHg (with similar readings obtained by emergency medical service [EMS] in the field). The initial head CT is unremarkable. During your interview in the ED, you observe the patient halt purposeful movements and stare blankly, and you witness subtle shaking of the right arm for about 20 seconds. His nurse tells you that he has seemed "spaced out" and sleepy during his brief period in the ED. The next most appropriate step is:

   A. Give the patient tissue plasminogen activator (tPA) per standard protocol and arrange for him to be admitted to the neuro-ICU for monitoring
   B. Do a lumbar puncture and send cerebrospinal fluid (CSF) for white blood cell (WBC) count, red blood cell (RBC) count, glucose, protein, herpes simplex virus-1 (HSV-1) polymerase chain reaction (PCR), HSV-2 PCR, and Gram stain
   C. Load the patient with phenytoin and arrange for continuous EEG (cEEG) monitoring in the neuro-ICU
   D. Do an urgent MRI to evaluate for acute cerebral infarction
   E. None of the above

2. A patient has just been admitted to your ICU who presented to the ED with status epilepticus (SE) and no further history. Seizures were reported as generalized convulsions, per emergency medical services (EMS) and ED staff. The patient's vitals are temperature 38.0°C, heart rate (HR) 99 bpm, blood pressure (BP) 140/77 mmHg, respiratory rate (RR) 14 breaths per minute, and SpO2 97% on 2 L nasal cannula. There are two peripheral intravenous (IV) lines in place. Lab tests show no electrolyte abnormalities, normal blood urea nitrogen and creatinine, normal liver function tests, and glucose of 135 mg/dL; the urine toxicology screen results are pending. The patient received a total of 8 mg of lorazepam IV in the ED and was loaded with fosphenytoin at 20 mg/kg IV (at 150 mg/min). Owing to continued brief seizure activity, a subsequent dose of fosphenytoin 10 mg/kg was administered; this fosphenytoin finished infusing about 3 minutes ago. The patient now begins to assume tonic posturing and then proceeds over the next 20 seconds to generalized clonic activity. You have ordered lorazepam 2 mg IV × 1 STAT. You plan to proceed with which of the following medications?

A. Fosphenytoin 20 mg/kg IV
B. Thiamine 100 mg IV
C. Midazolam 0.4 mg/kg IM
D. Intubate the patient and start a propofol infusion
E. None of the above

3. A 23-year-old male patient is known to have juvenile absence epilepsy. He takes lamotrigine as an outpatient. He is admitted to the neuro-ICU with subacute onset of confusion. Continuous EEG (cEEG) monitoring shows irregular generalized spike and wave activity at 3.0 Hz to 3.5 Hz waxing and waning throughout the entirety of the first 20 minutes the patient is monitored. At this point, the patient is correctly diagnosed as being in absence status epilepticus (SE). Which of the following medications should be avoided?

A. Lorazepam
B. Diazepam
C. Phenytoin
D. Keppra
E. Valproic acid

4. An adult patient is unresponsive and has absent brainstem reflexes. A standardized apnea test was not able to be successfully completed because of refractory hypoxemia. The patient had an episode of ventricular fibrillation (following a cervical spine discectomy) with a prolonged 40-minute course of cardiopulmonary resuscitation (CPR). A CT scan of the head done 18 hours later showed diffuse loss of the gray–white matter junction. It is now 48 hours after the cardiac arrest. A routine bedside EEG is ordered, and a sample is shown as follows. The entire 20-minute EEG appeared consistent with this sample. This EEG:

A. Is not consistent with the clinical diagnosis of brain death because of preserved EEG activity
B. Is consistent with the clinical diagnosis of brain death (but it is not sufficient as a confirmatory test for brain death, as the duration was only 20 minutes and less than 16 EEG channels were used)
C. Shows generalized approximately 1-Hz spikes, consistent with seizure
D. Is a finding typically seen with anesthetic doses of propofol
E. None of the above

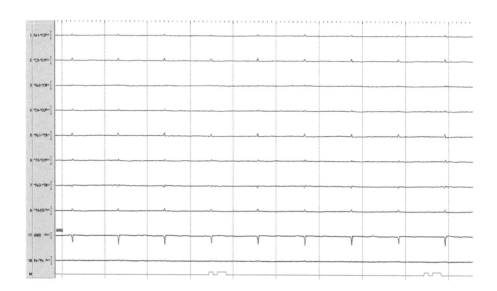

5. Relevant special requirements for a brain death EEG protocol include

 A. The EEG gain should be recorded and interpreted at a gain of no less than 2 μV/mm
 B. The EEG should show at least 30 minutes of interpretable data
 C. During the EEG, the technician should test EEG reactivity to external stimuli, especially noxious excitations
 D. Following resuscitation from circulatory arrest, at least 8 hours should pass from the onset of coma until the EEG examination
 E. All of the above

6. An adult patient meets all the clinical diagnostic criteria for brain death. An EEG is done as per brain death standard protocol, which shows electrocerebral inactivity (ECI). Approximately what percentage of clinically brain-dead patients show this EEG pattern?

 A. 90%
 B. 80%
 C. 50%
 D. 25%
 E. Less than 10%

7. A 29-year-old woman with Takayasu's arteritis presented to the ED 6 hours after the onset of lethargy and somnolence. In the ED, she was unresponsive and had sluggish pupillary responses, bilateral oculomotor palsies, quadriparesis, and weak flexor responses to noxious stimuli in all the four limbs. An MRI revealed bilateral midbrain infarctions. She was admitted to the neuro-ICU, and an EEG within the first 24 hours is shown as follows. During the EEG, the patient was not responsive to noxious stimuli in all four limbs or to loud auditory stimuli. What type of pattern does this EEG show, and what are the implications for recovery?

 A. Spindle coma, generally a favorable prognosis for recovering consciousness
 B. Spindle coma, generally a very poor prognosis for recovering consciousness
 C. Stage II sleep, excellent neurologic recovery
 D. Alpha coma, excellent neurologic recovery
 E. None of the above

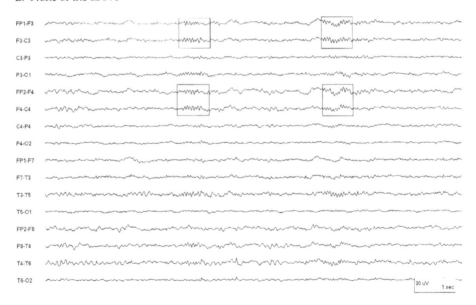

Source: Courtesy of Hirsch LJ, Brenner RP. *Atlas of EEG in Critical Care*. West Sussex, UK: Wiley-Blackwell, 2010: Figure 2.29, p. 78.

8. A 62-year-old man with hypertension and diabetes is admitted to the ICU after an asystolic cardiac arrest. The time period from cardiac arrest to initiation of cardiopulmonary resuscitation (CPR) is unknown. CPR was performed for 35 minutes before a sustained sinus rhythm was acquired. Approximately 24 hours after admission, the patient remains unresponsive to all noxious stimuli and is on no paralytic or sedative medications. During the EEG, the patient is not responsive to noxious stimuli in all four limbs or to loud auditory stimuli. The EEG shows the following pattern, which remained unchanged following external stimulation. What type of pattern does this EEG show, and what are its implications?

A. Beta coma, often associated with good prognosis for meaningful neurologic recovery
B. Delta–theta coma, often associated with poor prognosis for meaningful neurologic recovery
C. Spindle coma, often associated with good prognosis for meaningful neurologic recovery
D. Alpha coma, often associated with poor prognosis for meaningful neurologic recovery
E. None of the above

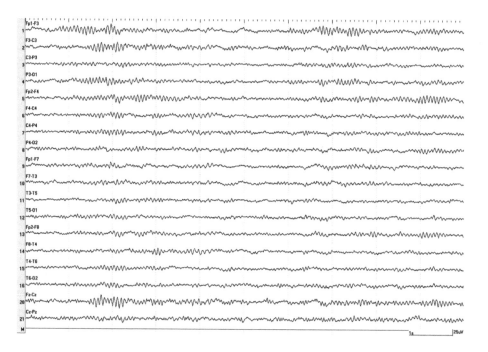

9. The causes of a diffuse encephalopathy are multiple and diverse. In general, the EEG findings seen in a diffuse encephalopathy are typically nonspecific for etiology, but there is a typical progression of nonspecific EEG findings that correlate with worsening encephalopathy. Which of the following EEG patterns are most consistent with a mild diffuse encephalopathy?

A. A generalized diffuse burst-suppression (BS) pattern
B. Generalized rhythmic delta activity (GRDA) seen upon a background of diffuse delta–theta activity
C. On a 48-hour recording, no variability in EEG pattern. No normal sleep activity or state changes are seen
D. Slowing of the posterior dominant rhythm ("alpha-rhythm") to a poorly sustained, reactive 7 Hz. There are fragmentary runs of generalized 4- to 5-Hz theta activity
E. None of the above

10. A 53-year-old woman presented with a 5-day history of fevers (102°F), headache, confusion, and bizarre behavior. Examination is remarkable for slowing of mentation, and the patient appears hypomanic. Following is an EEG done upon admission. What is the abnormal pattern shown on this EEG, and is it related to the patient's current presentation?

    A. Frequent left temporal spikes; not related to current presentation. Patient likely has a long history of localization-related epilepsy

    B. Lateralized periodic discharges (LPDs) in the left temporal region; not related to current presentation. LPDs are often seen in chronic disorders, and the patient has an acute illness

    C. Frequent left temporal spikes; likely related to current presentation. Patient likely has an acute illness, leading to exacerbation of an underlying epileptic focus in the left temporal lobe

    D. LPDs in the left temporal region; due to current acute illness. LPDs are a manifestation of acute cerebral injury

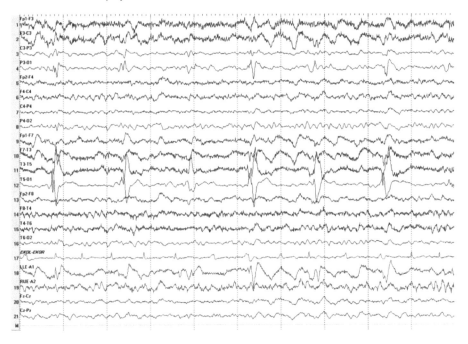

11. The following EEG could be seen in which of these clinical settings?

    A. After appropriate treatment for convulsive status epilepticus (SE)
    B. Lithium toxicity
    C. Creutzfeldt–Jakob disease
    D. Baclofen toxicity
    E. All of the above

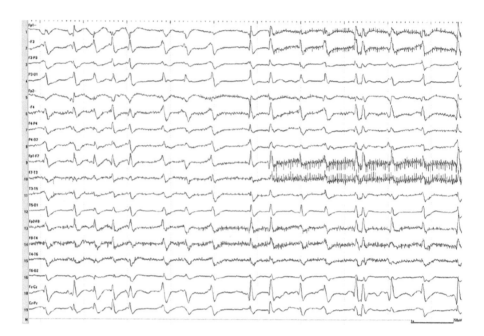

12. A 55-year-old man with cirrhosis is admitted to the neuro-ICU with a 3-day history of fluc-tuating mental status. Per history, there have been periods of alert, confused interactivity alternating with periods of somnolence. Complex partial seizures with postictal confusion, nonconvulsive status epilepticus (NCSE), and metabolic encephalopathy are on the differen-tial. An EEG is done (shown later). What are these EEG complexes?

A. Lateralized periodic discharges (LPDs)
B. Generalized rhythmic delta activity (GRDA), frontally predominant
C. Spike-slow wave complexes
D. Generalized periodic discharges (GPDs) with triphasic morphology
E. None of the above

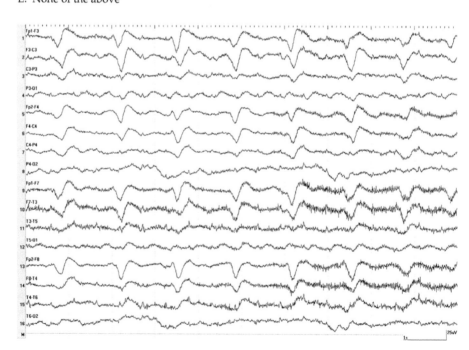

13. A 25-year-old man sustained right frontal head injury in an automobile accident. The patient has been in the neuro-ICU for 24 hours, and he is being monitored with continuous EEG (cEEG). The following finding was seen on a routine EEG. No clinical changes were seen in the patient during the cEEG. What does this EEG show?

   A. Nonconvulsive focal right frontal–temporal seizure
   B. Right frontal–temporal breach rhythm
   C. Mu rhythm (benign normal variant)
   D. Electrode artifact at F4

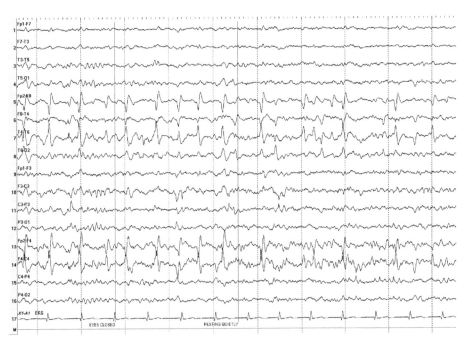

14. A 45-year-old man suffered cardiac arrest and remains comatose for 3 days after resuscitation. He is normothermic, is on no sedative or paralytic medications, and shows preserved pupillary reflexes, weak corneal reflexes, and no motor response. The patient has not had myoclonic status epilepticus (MSE). Median nerve somatosensory-evoked potential (SSEP) testing is done 24 to 72 hours following rewarming. Which of the following findings on SSEP testing 1 to 3 days after cardiac arrest or postrewarming is predictive of a poor neurologic outcome?

   A. Bilaterally absent N9 potentials
   B. Bilaterally absent N13 responses
   C. Bilaterally absent N20 responses
   D. SSEPs have not been established as useful for predicting neurologic outcome in this clinical setting
   E. Bilaterally prolonged N20 latencies

15. The following EEG pattern is commonly seen in comatose patients. This pattern is associated with which of these clinical settings?

   A. Hypothermia
   B. Hyperthermia
   C. Untreated convulsive status epilepticus (SE)
   D. Untreated nonconvulsive SE (NCSE)
   E. Creutzfeldt–Jakob disease

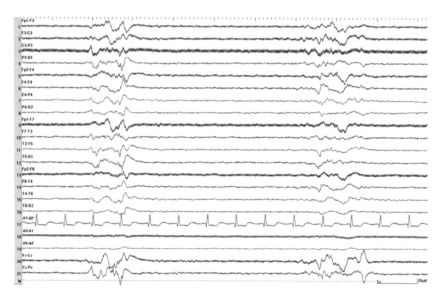

16. A 61-year-old woman is undergoing left carotid endarterectomy (CEA). EEG is monitored continuously during the procedure. The baseline EEG shows symmetric hemispheric amplitudes and EEG frequencies. Three minutes after cross clamping of the left internal carotid artery, the EEG appears as follows. Based on these findings, the surgeon should be advised of which of the following?

   A. The patient has experienced a new left middle cerebral artery (MCA) distribution infarct; proceed with the surgery without further intervention
   B. The surgery is progressing as expected; there are no surprising findings on EEG, as left hemispheric amplitude decrement is anticipated after left carotid cross clamping
   C. The patient is having a seizure; lorazepam should be administered
   D. There is marked and significant new amplitude decrement over the left hemisphere, and arterial shunting should be done to prevent irreversible ischemia to the left cerebral hemisphere

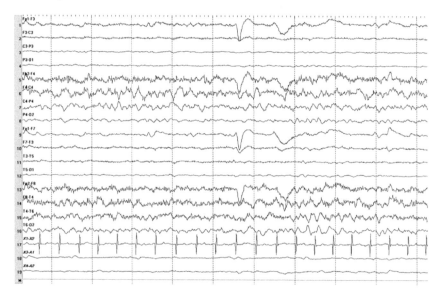

17. Nonconvulsive status epilepticus (NCSE) in the ICU setting is

   A. Associated with no significant morbidity or mortality beyond that typically seen with a generalized tonic–clonic seizure lasting 2 minutes
   B. Associated with high mortality (>50%) regardless of NCSE duration
   C. Associated with low mortality (<10%) regardless of NCSE duration
   D. Associated with higher morbidity and mortality with longer NCSE duration
   E. None of the above

18. A 87-year-old woman on Coumadin for stroke prophylaxis in the setting of a mechanical aortic valve presents with mild right hemiparesis, fluctuation in word-finding difficulties, and headache. A noncontrast CT of the head demonstrates a left convexity subdural hemorrhage measuring 1.5 cm with 0.5-mm midline shift. A continuous EEG (cEEG) is ordered and demonstrated as follows. Which of the following is true regarding this EEG?

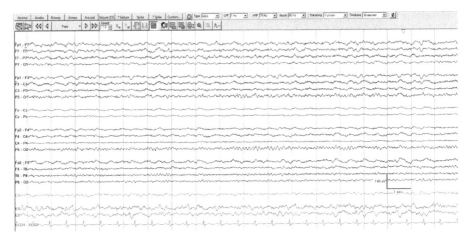

   A. Focal slowing, attenuation of faster frequencies, and lower amplitudes in the left hemisphere, frontotemporally maximal
   B. Intermittent left frontal sharp waves
   C. Left frontal lateralized periodic discharges (LPDs)
   D. Seizure originating from the left frontal region
   E. Bifrontal right greater than left slowing

19. Which of the following clinical scenarios would be appropriate for continuous EEG (cEEG) monitoring in the ICU?

   A. A patient with fluctuating mental status and concern for nonconvulsive status epilepticus (NCSE)
   B. A patient presenting with convulsive status epilepticus (SE), now somnolent after appropriate treatment in the ED
   C. A patient with acute subarachnoid hemorrhage (SAH)
   D. A patient with a large acute right hemisphere intracerebral hemorrhage (ICH)
   E. All of the above

20. A 35-year-old man without any past medical history was an unhelmeted rider involved in a motorcycle collision. He is intubated in the field, and brought emergently to the emergency room (ER) where the exam is notable for sluggish pupillary reactivity and extensor posturing. An intracranial pressure (ICP) monitor is placed, measuring an ICP of 40 cm H_2O. A CT of the head demonstrates bifrontal contusions and global cerebral edema. Neurosurgery

decides against surgical management of this traumatic brain injury (TBI). After maximization of osmotic therapy, you decide to use barbiturate coma to optimize medical therapy. Which of the following is correct regarding pentobarbital?

A. Barbiturates can lower ICP by reducing cerebral metabolic activity, and should be titrated to burst suppression (BS) on EEG

B. Barbiturates are strong inducers of CYP 450, leading to faster clearance of drugs that undergo hepatic metabolism

C. Pentobarbital and intravenous (IV) phenobarbital formulations contain polyethylene glycol (PG), and can lead to severe anion gap metabolic acidosis at high doses

D. Hypotension and ileus are common side effects of pentobarbital infusion

E. All of the above

21. A 65-year-old woman with a history of hypertension presents after being found down. She had complained of sudden onset of headache just prior to collapsing and arrives to the ED intubated, spontaneously moving the right side and weakly withdrawing to noxious stimulation on the left. CT of the head reveals thick diffuse subarachnoid hemorrhage (SAH). CT angiogram shows a right anterior communicating artery aneurysm. The patient undergoes coiling of the aneurysm without complications. She is extubated on the following day but remains confused and exhibits fluctuating left leg weakness. She is connected to continuous EEG (cEEG) for evaluation of nonconvulsive seizures and for ischemia detection by quantitative EEG (qEEG). An 8-hour Alpha:Delta Ratio (ADR) trend with delamination of parasagittal leads demonstrated by the black box, and a snapshot of the raw EEG are shown as follows. Which of the following is correct about electroencephalographic signs of cerebral hypoperfusion?

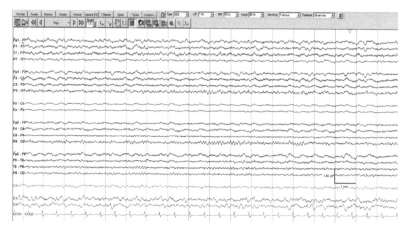

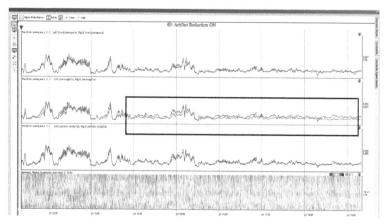

A. The most reliable trend for ischemia detection is the global Asymmetry Index Spectrogram between hemispheres

B. An asymmetry with lower values of ADR in the parasagittal leads on the right is suggestive of decreased perfusion and ongoing ischemia in the ipsilateral anterior cerebral artery distribution

C. Hyperexcitable patterns lying on the ictal–interictal continuum are not associated with the development of delayed cerebral ischemia in poor-grade aneurysmal SAH

D. An asymmetry with lower values of ADR in the frontotemporal leads on the left is suggestive of decreased perfusion and ongoing ischemia in the contralateral middle cerebral artery distribution

E. All of the above

22. Cortical spreading depolarizations (CSDs) have been implicated in the pathophysiology of migraines. More recently, with the use of electrocorticography and multimodal monitoring, CSDs have been associated with secondary brain injury in which of the following diseases?

A. Aneurysmal subarachnoid hemorrhage (SAH)
B. Traumatic brain injury (TBI)
C. Acute ischemic stroke
D. Intracerebral hemorrhage (ICH)
E. All of the above

23. A 75-year-old woman with coronary artery disease (CAD) on dual antiplatelet therapy, end-stage renal disease on hemodialysis, and type 1 diabetes mellitus (DM) is found unresponsive at home after she did not show up for dinner plans with friends. One of the friends listens to her home voicemail learns that she missed two hemodialysis appointments that week. On arrival to the ED, she is hypertensive to 180/120 mmHg and comatose, with intermittent spontaneous bilateral extensor posturing. A CT scan of the head is unremarkable. A lumbar puncture is deferred due to dual antiplatelet and she is started on cefepime, vancomycin, and acyclovir. Her EEG is demonstrated as follows. Regarding hyperexcitable patterns with triphasic morphology, which is correct?

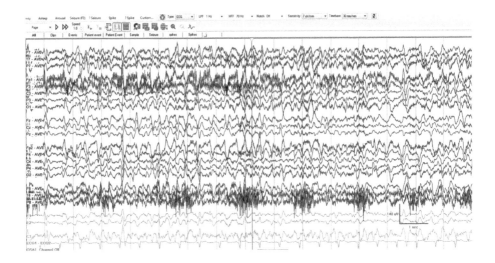

A. Triphasic morphology by definition represents hepatic failure and STAT lactulose should be given regardless of blood ammonia levels
B. Patients being monitored on continuous EEG (cEEG) who exhibit epileptiform findings with triphasic morphology have the same risk of developing seizures as any other generalized periodic discharges (GPDs)
C. Triphasic waves can only be seen in metabolic disorders such as renal and hepatic failure
D. Hyperexcitable findings with triphasic morphology do not respond to benzodiazepine or nonsedating antiseizure medications
E. All of the above

24. A previously healthy 23-year-old woman is transferred to your neuro-ICU from an outside hospital for a second opinion regarding her catatonia prior to undergoing electroconvulsive therapy per psychiatry recommendations. She was admitted 5 weeks ago to the psychiatric ward with bizarre behavior and paranoia, and progressed to this nonverbal catatonic state despite aggressive pharmacologic management with benzodiazepines and antipsychotics. On exam, she is profoundly dysautonomic with heart rate (HR) ranging from 55 to 120 bpm, normotensive, afebrile, sweating profusely, and does not regard, track, or follow any commands. You note that she has orofacial and hand dyskinetic movements. An EEG demonstrates extreme delta brush (EDB). Regarding this patient's condition, which of the following is correct?

A. The clinical and EEG findings are suggestive of anti-N-methyl-D-aspartate (NMDA) receptor encephalitis. A lumbar puncture (LP) should be pursued to test for the presence of receptor-specific antibodies
B. EDB is pathognomonic of anti-NMDA receptor encephalitis and no further workup is necessary
C. Seizures are rare in anti-NMDA receptor encephalitis and when they occur do not warrant pharmacologic treatment
D. Anti-NMDA receptor encephalitis is seen as a paraneoplastic syndrome due to small-cell lung cancer and a CT of the chest is the next recommended test in the workup of this patient
E. All of the above

25. A 24-year-old man was admitted to the hospital following a witnessed first-time generalized tonic–clonic seizure while standing in line at a restaurant. According to the family, he was experiencing forgetfulness and difficult maintaining concentration during the preceding weeks. In the ED, he is drowsy but otherwise is completely back to baseline. An MRI of the brain demonstrates a partially calcified left frontotemporal mass measuring 3.5×2.0 cm without abnormal enhancement. Following surgery he is noted to have fluctuation in the mental status and is connected to continuous EEG (cEEG), which demonstrates stimulus-induced left frontotemporal periodic discharges with associated rhythmic delta activity (demonstrated as follows). Which of the following are correct regarding lateralized periodic discharges (LPDs)?

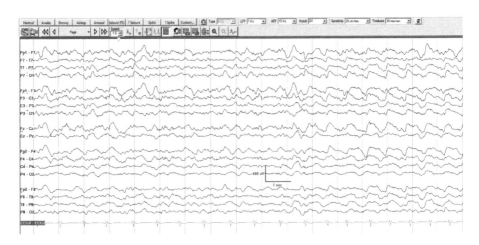

A. LPDs are not considered a hyperexcitable pattern as they are not associated with an increased seizure risk, thus cEEG may be discontinued
B. Hyperexcitable patterns such as LPDs and lateralized rhythmic delta activity (LRDA) are associated with approximately 60% risk of developing electrographic seizures within 48 hours of monitoring
C. LPDs are a specific electrographic finding of brain tumors
D. When LPDs occur in lockstep with clonic jerks, they correspond to the electrographic signature of a clinical seizure and are called ictal LPDs
E. B and D are correct

26. A 49-year-old man suffered a ventricular fibrillation cardiac arrest and is status postpercutaneous coronary intervention and therapeutic hypothermia. His course has been complicated by shock liver and acute renal insufficiency. At 72 hours after complete rewarming and discontinuation of sedatives and neuromuscular blockade, he remains comatose. He has preserved pupillary reflex and corneal reflexes, but has no motor response to noxious stimulation. A CT scan of the head obtained at 48 hours postcardiac arrest is unrevealing. Median nerve somatosensory-evoked potential (SSEP) performed during rewarming demonstrates prolonged right N20 latency, and absent N20 peak on the left. He has been monitored on continuous EEG (cEEG), which did not demonstrate epileptiform discharges and has improved background continuity (decreased suppression percentage). Today's EEG following a bedside stimulation protocol is shown as follows. Regarding the use of EEG for prognostication of hypoxic–ischemic encephalopathy, which of the following are correct?

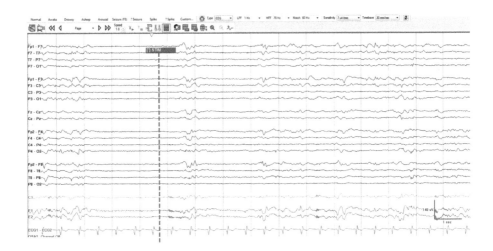

A. EEG is a validated neuroprognostic tool and is currently recommended with high level of evidence by American Academy of Neurology, American Heart Association, and European Society of Intensive Care Medicine guidelines

B. The presence of epileptiform discharges at any time during cEEG of cardiac arrest survivors predicts poor outcomes with a positive predictive value of 100%

C. Preserved reactivity, defined as any reproducible change in continuity, amplitude, or frequency of background, is the most traditionally used EEG criterion for neuroprognostication in hypoxic–ischemic encephalopathy

D. Malignant EEG patterns such as unreactive background to external stimuli and burst suppression at any time are predictive of poor outcomes with a positive predictive value of 100%

E. All of the above

27. You are called to see a 57-year-old man with depression and alcoholic cirrhosis who was admitted to the medical ICU after being found down with empty bottles of extra-strength acetaminophen 2 days prior. He has been treated with N-acetylcysteine. He had been stuporous with preserved brainstem reflexes until this morning, when 40 minutes into his first session of emergent hemodialysis for severe hyperammonemia (ammonia of 474 μmol/L) he developed bilateral midriasis with unreactive pupils and spontaneous extensor posturing. A continuous EEG (cEEG) was ordered to capture the stereotypic posturing and is shown later (raw EEG and comprehensive 2-hour trend with rhythmicity spectrogram, color density power spectra, relative asymmetry spectrogram, amplitude EEG, and suppression panels). His laboratory studies are notable for marked transaminitis (aspartate transaminase [AST]/ alanine transaminase [ALT] 3,827/11,800 U/L), International Normalized Ratio (INR) 2.16, and sodium 139 mmol/L. In this clinical context, what is the next step in the management for this patient?

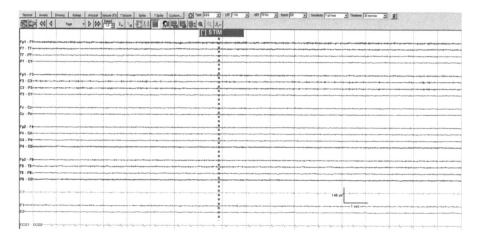

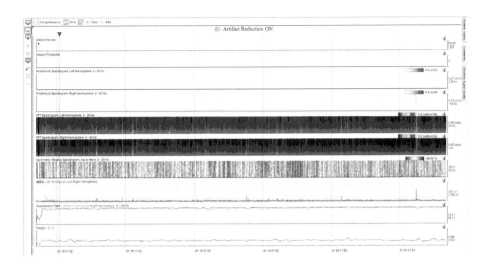

A. 0.1 mg/kg of lorazepam STAT as this patient is in nonconvulsive status epilepticus (NCSE)
B. Midazolam 0.2 mg/kg intravenous (IV) bolus as this patient is in NCSE
C. MRI of the brain with and without gadolinium
D. Arrange for an apnea test and brain-death assessment
E. Stop hemodialysis, obtain STAT CT for the head

28. An 87-year-old woman on Coumadin for stroke prophylaxis in the setting of a mechanical aortic valve presents with mild right hemiparesis and spells of speech arrest lasting for 2 minutes. A noncontrast CT of the head demonstrates a left convexity subdural hemorrhage measuring 0.5 cm without midline shift. A 20-minute EEG is obtained and demonstrated lateral rhythmic delta activity (LRDA) shown as follows. Which of the following is true regarding this patient?

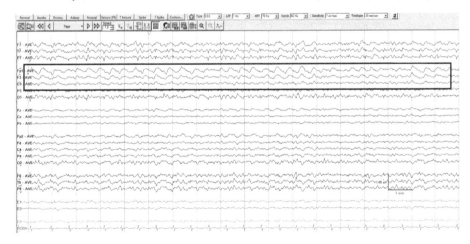

A. Midazolam 0.2 mg/kg intravenous (IV) bolus should be given STAT as this patient is at high risk for nonconvulsive status epilepticus (NCSE).
B. When present in the temporal region (temporal intermittent rhythmic delta activity [TIRDA]), LRDA is a benign variant and is not associated with an increased seizure risk.
C. Patients with lateralized periodic discharges (LPDs) but not LRDA on EEG have an increased seizure risk.
D. This patient should be maintained on continuous EEG (cEEG) for additional 24 to 48 hours due to a high seizure risk.
E. All of the above

29. A 52-year-old man with hypertension and hepatitis C suffers a pulseless electrical activity cardiac arrest during an esophagoduodenoscopy that was complicated by esophageal perforation. Return of spontaneous circulation (ROSC) was obtained at 15 minutes. Therapeutic hypothermia (TH) was not employed. You are called to see the patient. Upon arrival to the surgical ICU he remains comatose and is noted to have myoclonic activity of face and trunk with any stimulation. There is transient improvement with 2 mg intravenous (IV) lorazepam. He is connected to the EEG and diagnosed with myoclonic status epilepticus (MSE) as jerks are in lockstep with epileptiform activity on EEG (shown later). Regarding this case of postanoxic myoclonic status, which of the following is true?

A. Goals of care discussions need to occur immediately as postanoxic myoclonic status is associated with no chance for meaningful recovery.
B. This patient should undergo aggressive treatment of MSE as his EEG has favorable features.
C. Myoclonic status is particularly sensitive to phenytoin and lamotrigine, and these are the drugs of choice in this case.
D. This clinical vignette describes a case of Lance Adams syndrome, which is not associated with a poor long-term prognosis.
E. None of the above

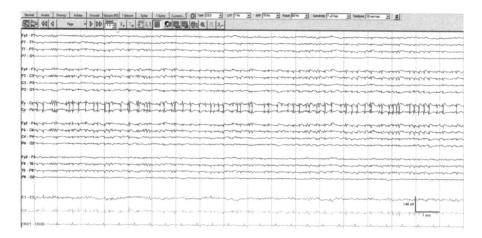

■ ANSWERS

1. **The answer is C.** This patient presents with a likely acute left middle cerebral artery stroke complicated by recurrent acute symptomatic seizures as, according to the history, hemiparesis preceded the witnessed rhythmic arm jerking. This patient meets criteria for status epilepticus (SE) given the frequent occurrence of seizures without the return to mentation baseline in between events. Historically, SE was considered persistent or repetitive seizure activity lasting at least 30 minutes without recovery of consciousness between events. However, the urgent nature of this condition and the critical importance of timely diagnosis and treatment inspired the revised definition of SE that is now widely accepted as any seizure lasting for ≥5 minutes, or ≥2 discrete seizures between which there is incomplete recovery of level of consciousness. This patient appears to be having repetitive complex partial seizures (dazed, staring, right-hand movements) and although he is not unconscious or comatose, he has not recovered to his baseline level of consciousness. This patient's SE should be treated emergently and should be the first priority of the possible answers. The first tier in the treatment of ongoing seizures is appropriately dosed benzodiazepine administration, which are often underdosed. This patient should be loaded with adequately dosed antiseizure medication (second-line agents) such as fosphenytoin/phenytoin at 20 mg/kg, or valproic acid at 20 to 40 mg/kg, or phenobarbital 20 mg/kg as they are all comparatively effective. Additionally, this patient should be admitted to the neuro-ICU, and have cEEG monitoring for nonconvulsive and clinically silent ongoing seizure activity. The differential for an acute confusional state (and seizures) does include cerebral infections such as encephalitis (answer B). However, the clinical history here is suggestive of an acute cerebral infarction with complex partial seizures. An argument could also be made for simply new onset of complex partial SE with Todd's paralysis; however, the weakness preceding any seizure-like activity makes it less likely. Seizures in acute ischemic stroke are reported in less than 10% of cases and, when they occur, are associated with delay in systemic reperfusion treatments (door-to-needle times). Nonetheless, this patient is outside the window for tPA administration (answer A). Of note, the patient remains eligible for endovascular rescue therapy. An MRI should be obtained to confirm acute infarction, but this would not be the next most appropriate step (answer E). The history is rather abrupt for encephalitis, but HSV encephalitis should be considered if the MRI were to show typical T2 and fluid-attenuated inversion recovery (FLAIR) hyperintensities in the temporal lobes (or if the MRI did not show an acute infarction as suspected). The most common cause of SE is a prior history of epilepsy, but approximately half of SE occurs in patients without prior history of seizures. In these patients, the most common cause is stroke, accounting for about 20%.

Alme KN, Engelsen BA, Naik M, et al. Identifying patients at risk of acute symptomatic seizure after ischemic stroke. *Acta Neurol Scand.* 2017;136:265-271. doi:10.1111/ane.12721. Available at: http://www.ncbi.nlm.nih.gov/pubmed/28025821.

Alvarez V, Rossetti AO, Papavasileiou V, et al. Acute seizures in acute ischemic stroke: does thrombolysis have a role to play? *J Neurol.* 2013;260:55-61. doi:10.1111/ane.12721. Available at: http://www.ncbi.nlm.nih.gov/pubmed/22743792.

Brophy GM, Bell R, Claassen J, et al. Guidelines for the evaluation and management of status epilepticus. *Neurocrit Care.* 2012;17:3-23. doi:10.1007/s12028-012-9695-z. Available at: http://www.ncbi.nlm.nih.gov/pubmed/22528274.

Glauser T, Shinnar S, Gloss D, et al. Evidence-based guideline: treatment of convulsive status epilepticus in children and adults: report of the Guideline Committee of the American Epilepsy Society. *Epilepsy Curr.* 2016;16:48-61. doi:10.5698/1535-7597-16.1.48. Available at: http://www.ncbi.nlm.nih.gov/pubmed/26900382.

Guidelines for epidemiologic studies on epilepsy. Commission on Epidemiology and Prognosis, International League Against Epilepsy. *Epilepsia.* 1993;34:592-596 http://www.ncbi.nlm.nih.gov/pubmed/8330566.

Hirsch LJ, Gaspard N. Status epilepticus. *Continuum (Minneap Minn).* 2013;19:767-794. doi:10.1212/01.CON.0000431395.16229.5a. Available at: http://www.ncbi.nlm.nih.gov/pubmed/8330566.

Kamal N, Sheng S, Xian Y, et al. Delays in door-to-needle times and their impact on treatment time and outcomes in get with the guidelines-stroke. *Stroke.* 2017;48:946-954. doi:10.1161/STROKEAHA.116.015712. Available at: http://www.ncbi .nlm.nih.gov/pubmed/28228574.

Treiman DM, Meyers PD, Walton NY, et al. A comparison of four treatments for generalized convulsive status epilepticus. Veterans Affairs Status Epilepticus Cooperative Study Group. *N Engl J Med.* 1998;339:792-798. doi:10.1056/NEJM199809173391202. Available at: http://www.ncbi.nlm.nih.gov/pubmed/9738086.

2. **The answer is D.** The management of SE can be complicated. The treating physician has two concurrent goals in the management of SE: one is to stop all seizure activity as quickly as possible, and the other is to determine an etiology for the SE. There are different published treatment protocols for SE, which tend to vary only in minor details. All protocols begin with basic life support, sending labs to look for an etiology for the SE, and the administration of thiamine 100 mg IV and 50 mL of 50% dextrose IV unless an adequate glucose level is known. (Note that this patient's glucose was normal, and in clinical practice, a glucose level can be established rapidly with a finger stick). As a tier one, appropriately dose benzodiazepine (e.g., lorazepam 4 mg IV with possibility of repeating to a maximum of 0.1 mg/kg or midazolam 10 mg IV/IM/buccal/IN) is the first-line treatment. As a second line, appropriately dosed fosphenytoin 20 mg/kg, valproic acid 40 mg/kg, or phenobarbital 20 mg/kg are commonly used; however, there are several other intravenous therapeutic options without a head-to-head comparison available in the literature at present. If seizures persist, now called refractory SE, intravenous continuous infusions are needed. Propofol (loading 10 mg/kg maximum, infusion 20–200 mcg/kg/min) and midazolam (loading 0.2 mg/kg IV and not 0.4 mg/kg IM as displayed in answer C; infusion 0.1–2.9 mg/kg/hr) are the most commonly used agents; however, several other options including pentobarbital and ketamine are also acceptable. Complete references to level of evidence and options can be found in the Neurocritical Care Society and American Epilepsy Society guidelines. Whenever loading with fosphenytoin or phenytoin it is important to maintain hemodynamic monitoring, as these drugs are associated with arrhythmias and hypotension due to their effect on sodium ion channels. Moreover, phenytoin has zero-order kinetics and an additional 20 mg/kg after a total administered dose of 30 mg/kg already given in this patient may lead to toxicity as levels increase nonlinearly. Prior to rebolusing phenytoin, it is important to obtain levels and correct to serum albumin, as this is a heavily protein-bound drug. There are several ways to calculate loading and adjusted maintenance dosing of phenytoin based on the volume of distribution of this drug (0.5–1 L/kg; 0.8 L/kg is most commonly used). A commonly used formula for a reloading dose is (target phenytoin total level − current corrected total phenytoin level) × (dosing weight × 0.8). The actual body weight in kilograms should be used in the majority of circumstances, and in obese patients a correction for the weight is as follows: ideal body weight + 1.33 × (actual body weight − ideal body weight) to a maximum of 100 kg. A similar formula can be used for valproic acid by changing the volume of distribution to 0.4 L/kg (range 0.1 – 0.4 L/kg).

Abernethy DR, Greenblatt DJ. Phenytoin disposition in obesity. Determination of loading dose. *Arch Neurol.* 1985;42:468-471. http://www.ncbi.nlm.nih.gov/pubmed/3994563.

Bergen DC. Pharmacokinetics of phenytoin: reminders and discoveries. *Epilepsy Curr.* 2009;9:102-104. doi:10.1111/j.1535-7511.2009.01307.x. Available at: http://www.ncbi.nlm.nih .gov/pubmed/PMC2728486.

Brophy GM, Bell R, Claassen J, et al. Guidelines for the evaluation and management of status epilepticus. *Neurocrit Care* 2012;17:3-23. doi:10.1007/s12028-012-9695-z. Available at: http://www.ncbi.nlm.nih.gov/pubmed/22528274.

Glauser T, Shinnar S, Gloss D, et al. Evidence-based guideline: treatment of convulsive status epilepticus in children and adults: report of the guideline Committee of the American Epilepsy Society. *Epilepsy Curr.* 2016;16:48-61. doi:10.5698/1535-7597. Available at: 16.1.48.http://www.ncbi.nlm.nih.gov/pubmed/23739110.

Zaccara G, Messori A, Moroni F. Clinical pharmacokinetics of valproic acid– 1988. *Clin Pharmacokinet.* 1988;15:367-389.doi:10.2165/00003088-198815060-00002. Available at: http://www.ncbi.nlm.nih.gov/pubmed/28228574.

3. **The answer is C.** The cEEG shows irregular generalized spike and wave, or polyspike and wave activity at approximately 3.0 to 3.5 Hz (consistent with absence SE). There are several medications known to exacerbate absence seizures. These include phenytoin, carbamazepine, oxcarbazepine, and tiagabine. Therefore, the patient should not be given phenytoin. This is a caveat to the treatment of SE. If a patient is known to have childhood or juvenile absence epilepsy, then the treatment regimen protocol should exclude phenytoin. The most appropriate initial drugs in the setting of absence SE are benzodiazepines, such as lorazepam, midazolam, or diazepam, to break the seizure. It would then be most appropriate to load valproic acid to reach a rapid serum therapeutic range. In the clinical scenario outlined in this question, it is also appropriate to check serum lamotrigine levels to see whether the patient is subtherapeutic on this outpatient medication, as medication noncompliance could be the cause of the absence SE.

Hirsch LJ, Gaspard N. Status epilepticus. *Continuum (Minneap Minn)*. 2013;19:767-794. doi:10.1212/01.CON.0000431395.16229.5a. Available at: http://www.ncbi.nlm.nih.gov/pubmed/8330566.

4. **The answer is B.** The EEG shows electrocerebral inactivity (ECI) and diffuse ECG artifact. The EEG is flat except for the prominent ECG artifact. Note that all the apparent cerebral activity is always time linked with ECG QRS complex, and this is how ECG artifact is confirmed in the EEG. The electric field produced by the heart can be recorded from the scalp, and it is commonly seen on the EEG of ECI recordings. Note that two of the established criteria for a brain death protocol EEG are duration of at least 30 minutes and the use of a minimum of 16 EEG channels.

Stecker MM, Sabau D, Sullivan L, et al. American Clinical Neurophysiology Society guideline 6: Minimum technical standards for EEG recording in suspected cerebral death. *J Clin Neurophysiol*. 2016;33:324-327. doi:10.1097/WNP.0000000000000322. Available at: http://www.ncbi.nlm.nih.gov/pubmed/27482789.

5. **The answer is E.** All of the answers are correct. These are the relevant special considerations that must be followed for a brain death protocol EEG. In particular, note that the EEG must be interpreted at a gain of 2 μV/mm. (Typically, adult EEGs are interpreted at gains of 7–10 μV/mm.) With lower gain settings, the EEG waveforms appear larger. Thus, this setting of 2 μV/mm will essentially magnify any present electrocerebral activity, and this is necessary before concluding that an EEG shows complete electrocerebral inactivity (ECI). Also note that typical routine hospital and outpatient EEGs are 20 minutes in duration. For a brain death protocol, a minimum of 30 minutes of interpretable recording should be obtained.

Stecker MM, Sabau D, Sullivan L, et al. American Clinical Neurophysiology Society guideline 6: Minimum technical standards for EEG recording in suspected cerebral death. *J Clin Neurophysiol*. 2016;33:324-327. doi:10.1097/WNP.0000000000000322. Available at: http://www.ncbi.nlm.nih.gov/pubmed/27482789.

6. **The answer is A.** When thinking about EEG patterns seen in the setting of clinical brain death, the most common pattern seen is ECI. However, it is important to note that this finding is not diagnostic of brain death (which is a clinical definition). The ECI pattern is seen in about 96.5% of adult patients and 89% children fulfilling clinical criteria for brain death. If there is concern about the reliability of ECI findings due to technical or other reasons, the EEG may be repeated in 6 hours for adults and at least 24 hours in children.

Stecker MM, Sabau D, Sullivan L, et al. American Clinical Neurophysiology Society guideline 6: Minimum technical standards for EEG recording in suspected cerebral death. *J Clin Neurophysiol*. 2016;33:324-327. doi:10.1097/WNP.0000000000000322. Available at: http://www.ncbi.nlm.nih.gov/pubmed/27482789.

7. **The answer is A.** The figure shows a background of mixed 4- to 7-Hz theta activity with prominent 12- to 16-Hz spindle activity, consistent with spindle coma. Spindles are typically one of the hallmarks of stage II sleep. However, spindle coma and stage II sleep are distinguished by clinical context; patients are arousable from stage II sleep with gentle to noxious stimuli or with auditory stimuli, whereas those in spindle coma remain unresponsive. Most

commonly, spindle coma is seen in patients with high mesencephalic (midbrain) lesions, as in this case. However, spindle coma can also be seen with posttraumatic and postencephalitic encephalopathies. This EEG pattern is, in general, a harbinger of a favorable prognosis for some meaningful neurologic recovery (but definitely not necessarily an indicator of complete recovery or a speedy recovery).

Ikeda A, Klem G, Luders H. *Metabolic, Infectious, and Hereditary Encephalopathies*. 3rd ed. Philadelphia, PA: Lippincott Williams & Wilkins; 2003.

8. **The answer is D.** The EEG shows prominent monotonous diffuse alpha activity representing alpha coma, which has been traditionally associated with a poor prognosis. Nonetheless, alpha coma is a descriptive electrographic term representing a heterogeneous group of patients and a diverse category of etiologies including diffuse brain insults after cardiopulmonary arrest, patients with brainstem lesions at or just caudal to the pontomesencephalic junction, and patients with various toxic or metabolic abnormalities, including barbiturate overdose and hyperglycemic, hyperosmolar coma. Knowing the etiology and other electrographic features, such as the presence of background reactivity to external stimulation, is crucial to assess the prognostic significance of this EEG finding. This patient had an unreactive recording and most likely will have an unfavorable prognosis.

Austin EJ, Wilkus RJ, Longstreth WT Jr. Etiology and prognosis of alpha coma. *Neurology*. 1988;38:773-777.doi:10.1212/wnl.38.5.773. Available at: http://www.ncbi .nlm.nih.gov/pubmed/3362375.

Kaplan PW, Genoud D, Ho TW, et al. Etiology, neurologic correlations, and prognosis in alpha coma. *Clin Neurophysiol*. 1999;110:205-213doi:10.1016/s1388-2457(98)00046-7. Available at: http://www.ncbi.nlm.nih.gov/pubmed/10210610.

Westmoreland BF, Klass DW, Sharbrough FW, et al. Alpha-coma. Electroencephalographic, clinical, pathologic, and etiologic correlations. *Arch Neurol*. 1975;32:713-718. doi:10.1001/archneur.1975.00490530035001. Available at:http://www.ncbi.nlm.nih.gov/ pubmed/1180739.

9. **The answer is D.** A discussion of the myriad of causes of diffuse encephalopathies is beyond the scope of this chapter. However, regardless of underlying etiology, the EEG often follows a typical progression as an encephalopathy progresses from "mild" to "severe." The earliest changes are often a mild slowing of the occipital dominant rhythm (alpha rhythm) in wakefulness into the theta range; diffuse fragmentary or more sustained theta and delta activity can also be seen. As encephalopathy worsens, the alpha rhythm and normal faster activities (alpha and frontal beta) will be lost, and diffuse theta and delta activity become more prominent and sustained. Normal sleep architecture can also be lost (K-complexes and spindles). With worsening, periods of diffuse amplitude attenuation and GRDA, often frontally predominant, can be seen; the normal EEG variability and state transitions are lost. The EEG becomes unreactive to external stimuli (pain). As encephalopathy worsens still, the EEG will reach a diffuse burst suppression pattern and ultimately will reach electrocerebral inactivity (ECI).

Hirsch LJ, Brenner RP. *Atlas of EEG in Critical Care*. West Sussex, UK: Wiley-Blackwell; 2010.

10. **The answer is D.** The EEG clearly shows LPDs (formerly known as periodic lateralized epileptiform discharges [PLEDs]) in the left temporal lobe. These are not just frequent left temporal spikes, given their recurrence in nearly regular intervals (periodicity) for over six cycles. LPDs typically recur every 1 to 2 seconds (as seen in this EEG) and consist of a spike or sharp wave (may be polyphasic), which may be followed by a slow wave. Acute structural lesions are the most common cause of LPDs, often ischemic or hemorrhagic strokes, but any acute or chronic cerebral injury that could result in seizures can generate LPDs. Herpes simplex virus (HSV) encephalitis is commonly considered when LPDs are seen in the appropriate clinical context (as in this case), since most patients with HSV encephalitis will develop LPDs. In summary, LPDs should be considered a marker of acute cerebral injury, and these discharges are a transient finding, diminishing over days to weeks. LPDs are associated with

seizures in approximately 60% to 70% of patients. Moreover, LPDs may also occur in patients without acute brain injuries, and their occurrence is associated with alteration of consciousness and worse outcomes at discharge.

Hirsch LJ, Brenner RP. *Atlas of EEG in Critical Care*. West Sussex, UK: Wiley-Blackwell; 2010.

Hirsch LJ, LaRoche SM, Gaspard N, et al. American Clinical Neurophysiology Society's standardized critical care EEG terminology: 2012 version. *J Clin Neurophysiol.* 2013;30: 1-27. doi:10.1097/WNP.0b013e3182784729. Available at: http://www.ncbi.nlm.nih. gov/pubmed/23377439.

Garcia-Morales I, Garcia MT, Galan-Davila L, et al. Periodic lateralized epileptiform discharges: etiology, clinical aspects, seizures, and evolution in 130 patients. *J Clin Neurophysiol.* 2002;19:172-177. doi:10.1097/00004691-200203000-00009. Available at: http://www. ncbi.nlm.nih.gov/pubmed/11997729.

Sainju RK, Manganas LN, Gilmore EJ, et al. Clinical correlates and prognostic significance of lateralized periodic discharges in patients without acute or progressive brain injury: a case-control study. *J Clin Neurophysiol.* 2015;32:495-500. doi: 10.1097/WNP.0000000000000206. Available at: http://www.ncbi.nlm.nih.gov/pubmed/26200591.

11. **The answer is E.** The EEG shows generalized periodic discharges (GPDs, formerly known as generalized periodic epileptiform discharges [GPEDs]). GPDs are bilateral, bisynchronous, and symmetric discharges occurring at nearly regular intervals for over six cycles and are considered a nonspecific finding that is commonly seen in the ICU in a variety of clinical settings. These include postanoxic coma, metabolic disorders, Creutzfeldt–Jakob disease, and Hashimoto encephalopathy. Medication toxicity can also result in this EEG pattern, most notably with lithium toxicity (but can also be seen with baclofen and cefepime). GPDs (unlike lateralized periodic discharges [LPDs]) are associated with seizures in approximately 20% to 30% of cases, regardless of triphasic morphology of discharges.

Foreman B, Claassen J, Abou Khaled K, et al. Generalized periodic discharges in the critically ill: a case-control study of 200 patients. *Neurology.* 2012;79:1951-1960. doi:10.1212/WNL.0b013e3182735cd7. Available at: http://www.ncbi.nlm.nih.gov/ pubmed/23035068 Accessed August 15, 2017.

Foreman B, Mahulikar A, Tadi P, et al. Generalized periodic discharges and 'triphasic waves': a blinded evaluation of inter-rater agreement and clinical significance. *Clin Neurophysiol.* 2016;127:1073-1080. doi:0.1016/j.clinph.2015.07.018. Available at: http:// www.ncbi.nlm.nih.gov/pubmed/26294138 Accessed August 15, 2017.

Hirsch LJ, LaRoche SM, Gaspard N, et al. American Clinical Neurophysiology Society's standardized critical care EEG terminology: 2012 version. *J Clin Neurophysiol.* 2013;30: 1-27. doi:10.1097/WNP.0b013e3182784729. Available at: http://www.ncbi.nlm.nih.gov/ pubmed/23377439.

12. **The answer is D.** The EEG shows GPDs with a triphasic morphology. Classically, the discharge is characterized by three phases, as displayed in this case. Note the initial negative (upward) component of the complex, with subsequent larger amplitude positive (downward) deflection, and with a final negative component; hence the former "triphasic waves" term. However, according to the American Clinical Neurophysiology Society nomenclature, a discharge with a triphasic morphology may have two phases with each phase longer than the previous, and the positive phase of highest amplitude. In this example, note the frontal predominance, as this is commonly seen in discharges with triphasic morphology. These discharges are classically seen in hepatic encephalopathy. However, they can also be seen in any toxic/metabolic encephalopathy and in acute brain injury, and should not be considered diagnostic of hepatic encephalopathy. Typically, they occur at 0.5 to 1.5 Hz and may wax and wane in morphology and persistence throughout the recording. GPDs are associated with seizures in approximately 20% to 30% of cases, regardless of the triphasic morphology of discharges.

Foreman B, Claassen J, Abou Khaled K, et al. Generalized periodic discharges in the critically ill: a case-control study of 200 patients. *Neurology.* 2012;79:1951-1960. doi:10.1212/WNL.0b013e3182735cd7. Available at: http://www.ncbi.nlm.nih.gov/ pubmed/23035068 Accessed August 15, 2017.

Foreman B, Mahulikar A, Tadi P, et al. Generalized periodic discharges and 'triphasic waves': a blinded evaluation of inter-rater agreement and clinical significance. *Clin*

Neurophysiol. 2016;127:1073-1080. doi: 10.1016/j.clinph.2015.07.018. Available at: http://www.ncbi.nlm.nih.gov/pubmed/26294138, Accessed August 15, 2017.

Hirsch LJ, LaRoche SM, Gaspard N, et al. American Clinical Neurophysiology Society's standardized critical care EEG terminology: 2012 version. *J Clin Neurophysiol.* 2013;30: 1-27. doi:10.1097/WNP.0b013e3182784729. Available at: http://www.ncbi.nlm.nih.gov/pubmed/23377439.

Kaplan PW, Sutter R. Affair with triphasic waves—their striking presence, mysterious significance, and cryptic origins: what are they? *J Clin Neurophysiol.* 2015;32: 401-405. doi:10.1097/WNP.0000000000000151. Available at: http://www.ncbi.nlm.nih.gov/pubmed/26426768.

Sutter R, Stevens RD, Kaplan PW. Clinical and imaging correlates of EEG patterns in hospitalized patients with encephalopathy. *J Neurol.* 2013;260:1087-1098. doi:10.1007/s00415-012-6766-1. Available at: http://www.ncbi.nlm.nih.gov/pubmed/23196336.

Sutter R, Stevens RD, Kaplan PW. Significance of triphasic waves in patients with acute encephalopathy: a nine-year cohort study. *Clin Neurophysiol.* 2013;124:1952-1958. doi: 10.1016/j.clinph.2013.03.031. Available at: http://www.ncbi.nlm.nih.gov/pubmed/23684126.

13. **The answer is A.** This EEG shows a typical nonconvulsive seizure as seen in the ICU setting. The electrographic criteria for seizure activity include clear evolution in frequency, morphology, or location of an ongoing cEEG pattern. This particular EEG shows the evolution of approximately 2-Hz right frontal–temporal spikes into 1-Hz spikes on the second half of the EEG. The following 10 to 30 seconds of acquired EEG would be expected to show resolution of the spikes, with possible right frontal–temporal delta–theta slowing. Thus, this finding is an electrographic seizure (labeled as nonconvulsive based on the clinical history provided). A breach rhythm is from a skull defect (such as craniotomy or burr hole), which results in an increase in voltage and more sharp morphology in the underlying EEG. Faster frequencies are more accentuated with breach than slower frequencies. Mu rhythm is a benign, normal variant typically seen in healthy individuals in the ambulatory setting, consisting of 7- to 11-Hz arciform waveforms over the central head regions. This normal variant is attenuated with movement or thought of movement of the contralateral hand. The EEG abnormalities seen are not limited to the F4 electrode.

Hirsch LJ, LaRoche SM, Gaspard N, et al. American Clinical Neurophysiology Society's standardized critical care EEG terminology: 2012 version. *J Clin Neurophysiol.* 2013;30: 1-27. doi: 10.1097/WNP.0b013e3182784729. Available at: http://www.ncbi.nlm.nih.gov/pubmed/23377439.

Westmoreland B.Electroencephalography: Adult, normal and benign variants. In Clinical Neurophysiology, 3rd Ed , 2009. (Eds: Daube JR & Rubin DI). New York. Oxford University Press.

14. **The answer is C.** According to the international guidelines in neuro-prognostication post–cardiac arrest, the bilateral absence of the N20 component of the median nerve SSEP 1 to 3 days or later after cardiac arrest or complete rewarming accurately predicts a poor outcome. The N9 (Erb's point) waveform reflects peripheral nerve activity propagating through the brachial plexus and would be expected to remain present. The N13 waveform reflects activity in the dorsal horns of the spinal cord, and this would also be expected to remain present. The N20 waveform reflects activity in the thalamocortical radiations/sensory cortex (some debate remains to the exact generator).

ACNS. Guideline 9D: g on short-latency somatosensory evoked potentials. *J Clin Neurophysiol.* 2006;23:168-179. doi:10.1097/00004691-200604000-00013. Available at: http://www.ncbi.nlm.nih.gov/pubmed/16612233.

Callaway CW, Donnino MW, Fink EL, et al. Part 8: post-cardiac arrest care: 2015 American Heart Association guidelines update for cardiopulmonary resuscitation and emergency cardiovascular care. *Circulation.* 2015;132:S465-82. doi:10.1161/CIR.0000000000000262. Available at: http://www.ncbi.nlm.nih.gov/pubmed/26472996.

Sandroni C, Cariou A, Cavallaro F, et al. Prognostication in comatose survivors of cardiac arrest: an advisory statement from the European Resuscitation Council and the European Society of Intensive Care Medicine. *Intensive Care Med.* 2014;40:1816-1831. doi:10.1007/s00134-014-3470-x. Available at: http://www.ncbi.nlm.nih.gov/pubmed/25398304.

Wijdicks EF, Hijdra A, Young GB, et al. Practice parameter: prediction of outcome in comatose survivors after cardiopulmonary resuscitation (an evidence-based review): report of the Quality Standards Subcommittee of the American Academy of Neurology. *Neurology*. 2006;67:203-210. doi: 10.1212/01.wnl.0000227183.21314.cd. Available at: http://www.ncbi.nlm.nih.gov/pubmed/16864809.

15. **The answer is A.** This EEG pattern is known as a burst-suppression (BS) pattern, and it is seen only in the clinical context of coma. BS is an alternating pattern. It consists of bursts of bilaterally synchronous (usually), widespread mixed-frequency activity, which may have intermixed spikes or sharp waves. These bursts alternate with periods of globally absent EEG activity (or low-voltage delta–theta activity) totaling 50% to 90% of recording. When suppression percentage is between 10% and 49%, the recording is said to be discontinuous. BS is commonly seen after a severe insult to the brain, most commonly hypoxic or anoxic insult (in which case it carries a poor prognosis). BS can also be seen with reversible causes of coma, such as hypothermia; drug intoxication (e.g., benzodiazepines, barbiturates, high doses of narcotics); and after the administration of anesthetics (e.g., propofol, benzodiazepines, barbiturates, ketamine, sevoflurane, isoflurane). During the treatment of SE, the goal is often to achieve seizure suppression, but in some cases, a BS pattern is pursued with the use of anesthetics. There is still debate in the scientific community as to which goal should be pursued with the use of anesthetics, as emerging evidence suggests that increased suppression does not necessarily translate into a higher likelihood of a subsequent successful wean of anesthetic therapy; however, the characteristics of the bursts do. Note that Creutzfeldt–Jakob disease results in the appearance of generalized periodic discharges (GPDs) and not BS.

Hirsch LJ, LaRoche SM, Gaspard N, et al. American Clinical Neurophysiology Society's standardized critical care EEG terminology: 2012 version. *J Clin Neurophysiol*. 2013;30: 1-27. doi:10.1097/WNP.0b013e3182784729. Available at: http://www.ncbi.nlm.nih. gov/pubmed/23377439.

Johnson EL, Martinez NC, Ritzl EK. EEG characteristics of successful burst suppression for refractory status epilepticus. *Neurocritical Care*. 2016;25:407-414. doi:10.1007/s12028-016-0294-2. Available at: http://www.ncbi.nlm.nih.gov/pubmed/27406818.

Rossetti AO, Tovar Quiroga DF, Juan E, et al. Electroencephalography predicts poor and good outcomes after cardiac arrest: a two-center study. *Crit Care Med*. 2017;45;e674-e682. doi:10.1097/CCM.0000000000002337. Available at: http://www.ncbi.nlm.nih.gov/ pubmed/28406812.

Thompson SA, Hantus S. Highly epileptiform bursts are associated with seizure recurrence. *J Clin Neurophysiol*. 2016;33:66-71. doi:10.1097/WNP.0000000000000232. Available at: http://www.ncbi.nlm.nih.gov/pubmed/26844972.

Westmoreland B. Adult EEG: Abnormal nonepileptiform activity. In Clinical Neurophysiology, 3rd Ed , 2009. (Eds: Daube JR & Rubin DI). New York. Oxford University Press.

16. **The answer is D.** During CEA surgery, it is common to monitor EEG and median nerve and posterior tibial nerve somatosensory-evoked potential (SSEP). The EEG is sensitive for detecting new cortical ischemia and assesses large areas of the cerebral cortex. New cortical ischemia is seen as ipsilateral slowing or amplitude attenuation/decrement, or both. The normal mean cerebral blood flow (CBF) is approximately 50 mL/100 g/min. Mild hypoperfusion down to approximately 22 mL/100 g/min typically is well tolerated without EEG changes. When CBF falls below this 22 mL/100 g/min threshold, the EEG will show slowing or amplitude attenuation, or both. A further decrease to 7 to 15 mL/100 g/min will result in suppression of EEG activity. Perfusion below 12 to 15 mL/100 g/min will result in neural damage. In most patients, there will be adequate collateral flow (via the circle of Willis) to prevent cerebral ischemia when one internal carotid artery is clamped. However, in about 20% of patients, carotid clamping results in significant cerebral ischemia with an associated high risk of acute cerebral infarction. The changes seen in this EEG are indicative of new left cerebral hemispheric hypoperfusion and ischemia. The surgeon should be alerted to this and to the fact that carotid artery bypass shunting is needed.

Sepkuty JP Gutierrez S. Carotid surgery. In A Practical Approach to Neurophysiologic Intraoperative Monitoring, 2008 (Ed: Husain AM). New York: Demos.

17. **The answer is D.** The EEG criteria for NCSE historically lacked consensus, as it depends on clinical context (e.g., age, history of epileptic encephalopathy or not, and in boundary syndromes such as coma with epileptiform changes but not quite meeting criteria for unequivocal status epilepticus) in addition to the EEG findings. The Salzburg Consensus Criteria are well accepted and propose different definitions according to the presence or absence of epileptic encephalopathy. NCSE *in patients without known epileptic encephalopathy* is diagnosed when epileptic discharges sustain greater than 2.5 Hz; or ≤2.5 Hz or rhythmic delta/theta activity (>0.5 Hz) *and* one of the following: subtle clinical ictal phenomena during the EEG pattern (clinical correlate), typical spatiotemporal evolution, or clinical/EEG improvement following intravenous (IV) antiseizure medications. *For patients with known epileptic encephalopathy,* NCSE represents increased prominence from baseline of the same features listed for those without epileptic encephalopathy, so long as they are accompanied by an observable change in the clinical state of the patient or there is clinical/EEG improvement following IV antiseizure medications. Note that these criteria are broad, relying significantly on the clinical aspect for a more tailored EEG interpretation. In NCSE, seizure duration tends to be the best predictor of mortality. A study of NCSE in the ICU setting demonstrated that if seizure duration was less than 10 hours, 60% of patients returned home and 10% died. However, if NCSE duration was greater than 20 hours, none returned home and 85% died. Thus, rapid recognition and treatment of NCSE in the ICU has important implications for clinical outcome.

Beniczky S, Hirsch LJ, Kaplan PW, et al. Unified EEG terminology and criteria for nonconvulsive status epilepticus. *Epilepsia.* 2013;54(suppl 6):28-29. doi:10.1111/epi.12270. Available at: http://www.ncbi.nlm.nih.gov/pubmed/24001066.

Sutter R, Kaplan PW. Electroencephalographic criteria for nonconvulsive status epilepticus: synopsis and comprehensive survey. *Epilepsia.* 2012;53(suppl 3):1-51. doi:10.1111/j.1528-1167.2012.03593.x. Available at: http://www.ncbi.nlm.nih.gov/pubmed/22862158.

Young GB, Jordan KG, Doig GS. An assessment of nonconvulsive seizures in the intensive care unit using continuous EEG monitoring: an investigation of variables associated with mortality. *Neurology.* 1996;47:83-89. doi:10.1212/WNL.47.1.83. Available at: http://www.ncbi.nlm.nih.gov/pubmed/8710130.

18. **The answer is A.** Subdural (and epidural) hematomas can be associated with all of the EEG patterns mentioned in the answers, but the epoch displayed captures focal slowing and attenuation ipsilateral to the lesion, which is the correct answer. Focal slowing and amplitude attenuation are caused by underlying cortical malfunction and increased distance between the brain and recording electrodes. Blood is irritating to the cerebral cortex, so focal sharp waves or spikes, LPDs, and seizures may be seen with any area of cerebral hemorrhage affecting the cortex.

Hirsch LJ, Brenner RP. *Atlas of EEG in Critical Care.* West Sussex, UK: Wiley-Blackwell; 2010.

19. **The answer is E.** The rationale for cEEG monitoring in the ICU is founded on the following attributes: (a) EEG is tightly linked to cerebral metabolism; (b) EEG is sensitive to ischemia and hypoxia; (c) EEG detects neuronal dysfunction at a reversible stage; (d) EEG detects neuronal damage or recovery, while clinical examination may not; (e) EEG is the best method to detect epileptiform activity, including NCSE; (f) cEEG provides dynamic information that routine bedside EEG cannot; and (g) EEG provides useful information about localization. Thus, cEEG has utility in many clinical ICU settings, including acute cerebral ischemia, ICH, uncontrolled seizures (including SE and concern for NCSE), coma, intracranial infections, and head trauma. Beyond its obvious role for assessing epileptiform activity and seizures, cEEG is a valuable tool for assessing ischemia in aneurysmal SAH, focal ischemia, and early detection of increased intracranial pressures. cEEG is also useful for monitoring anesthetic and drug effects (commonly described as the depth of anesthesia) and for monitoring periodic patterns that may be of prognostic value or indicate a higher risk for seizures (i.e., lateralized periodic discharges [LPDs] or generalized periodic discharges [GPDs]).

Herman ST, Abend NS, Bleck TP, et al. Consensus statement on continuous EEG in critically ill adults and children, part I: indications. *J Clin Neurophysiol.* 2015;32: 87-95.

doi:10.1097/WNP.0000000000000166. Available at: http://www.ncbi.nlm.nih.gov/pubmed/25626778.

20. **The answer is E.** Pentobarbital is an effective antiseizure medication used in refractory status epilepticus and can be used in refractory intracranial hypertension as it reduces the cerebral metabolic activity. It is important to be aware of the significant acute adverse effects of this therapy. Pentobarbital and IV formulations of phenobarbital contain high concentrations of PG, which is the vehicle commonly used in IV formulations of drugs (e.g., lorazepam). Approximately 55% of PG undergoes metabolism with the final product being lactate, which in high concentrations may lead to metabolic anion gap acidosis. Whenever used with the intent to reduce cerebral metabolism and flow in traumatic injuries and ICP crisis, barbiturate coma must be monitored with continuous EEG (cEEG) and infusions titrated to burst suppression. Pentobarbital is a strong inducer of several cytochrome P-450 subclasses, which leads to significant drug interactions. Decreased gut motility and hypotension are common serious side effects of this therapy.

Miller MA, Forni A, Yogaratnam D. Propylene glycol-induced lactic acidosis in a patient receiving continuous infusion pentobarbital. *Ann Pharmacother*. 2008;42:1502-1506. doi: 10.1345/aph.1L186. Available at: http://www.ncbi.nlm.nih.gov/pubmed/18698010.

Roberts I, Sydenham E. Barbiturates for acute traumatic brain injury. *Cochrane Database Syst Rev*. 2012;12:CD000033. doi:10.1002/14651858.CD000033.pub2. Available at: http://www.ncbi.nlm.nih.gov/pubmed/23235573.

21. **The answer is B.** The American Clinical Neurophysiology Society recommends cEEG for the detection of nonconvulsive seizures in critically ill patients and suggests that cEEG can be useful for the detection of ischemia in aneurysmal SAH. Early detection of tissue at risk for ischemia is crucial in order to optimize perfusion and improve outcomes. EEG provides high temporal resolution and is extremely sensitive to changes in cerebral blood flow. It can be particularly useful in patients with high clinical grades (Hunt and Hess IV–V) as the exam is very poor and insensitive to detect changes in perfusion; and in patients with high radiologic grade (modified Fisher 3, thick cisternal blood) as they are at higher risk for ischemic complications. qEEG allows for an objective trend during the monitoring period. The most commonly used qEEG parameter for ischemia monitoring is the ADR that is reported based on vascular distributions: middle cerebral artery, anterior cerebral artery, and posterior cerebral artery. Percent alpha variability is also a useful qEEG parameter. Additionally, the emergence of new focal asymmetries with attenuation of faster frequencies or slowing of background, or even emergence of interictal discharges, on raw EEG are all important findings that may suggest ischemia in aSAH. Hyperexcitable patterns lying on the ictal interictal continuum are associated with the development of delayed cerebral ischemia in poor-grade aSAH. In the presented case, clear right frontocentral slowing is seen in the raw EEG and correlated with delamination of ADR trends in the parasagittal panel (black box, left hemisphere represented in blue, right hemisphere represented in red) suggesting ipsilateral anterior cerebral artery (ACA) ischemia. This asymmetry between left and right is also displayed in the global Asymmetry Index Spectrogram where frequencies of 3 to 5 Hz are more prevalent on the right and faster frequencies more prevalent on the left (predominance of red and blue hues by frequency band, respectively); however, asymmetry spectrogram is not the most sensitive or reliable trend, as it is susceptible to artifact and provides a global outline of frequency bands between hemispheres, thus lacking spatial specificity.

Claassen J, Mayer SA, Hirsch LJ. Continuous EEG monitoring in patients with subarachnoid hemorrhage. *J Clin Neurophysiol*. 2005;22:92-98. doi:10.1097/01.WNP.0000145006.02048.3A. Available at: http://www.ncbi.nlm.nih.gov/pubmed/15805808.

Herman ST, Abend NS, Bleck TP, et al. Consensus statement on continuous EEG in critically ill adults and children, part I: indications. *J Clin Neurophysiol*. 2015;32:87-95. doi:10.1097/WNP.0000000000000166. Available at: http://www.ncbi.nlm.nih.gov/pubmed/25626778.

Kim JA, Rosenthal ES, Biswal S, et al. Epileptiform abnormalities predict delayed cerebral ischemia in subarachnoid hemorrhage. *Clin Neurophysiol*. 2017;128:1091-1099. doi:

10.1016/j.clinph.2017.01.016. Available at: http://www.ncbi.nlm.nih.gov/pubmed/28258936.

Labar DR, Fisch BJ, Pedley TA, et al. Quantitative EEG monitoring for patients with subarachnoid hemorrhage. *Electroencephalogr Clin Neurophysiol*. 1991;78:325-332. doi:10.1016/0013-4694(91)90094-K. Available at: http://www.ncbi.nlm.nih.gov/pubmed/1711451.

Muniz CF, Shenoy AV, O'Connor KL, et al. Clinical development and implementation of an institutional guideline for prospective EEG monitoring and reporting of delayed cerebral ischemia. *Journal of Clinical Neurophysiology: official publication of the American Electroencephalographic Society*. 2016;33:217-26. doi:10.1097/WNP.0000000000000281. Available at: http://www.ncbi.nlm.nih.gov/pubmed/27258445.

Vespa PM, Nuwer MR, Juhasz C, et al. Early detection of vasospasm after acute subarachnoid hemorrhage using continuous EEG ICU monitoring. *Electroencephalogr Clin Neurophysiol*. 1997;103:607-615. doi:10.1016/S0013-4694(97)00071-0. Available at: http://www.ncbi.nlm.nih.gov/pubmed/9546487.

22. **The answer is E.** CSDs are waves of sudden and near-complete disruption of cellular ionic homeostasis that are slowly propagating across contiguous cortex and not respective vascular distributions. CSDs can be triggered by focal ischemia and have been implicated in secondary brain injury in TBI, ICH, acute ischemic stroke, and SAH. Delayed cerebral ischemia in SAH can occur from vasospasm or electrophysiologic cerebral dysfunction and inverse neurovascular coupling. Inverse coupling describes severe hypoperfusion in response to CSD and has been implicated in the remote ischemic events after SAH.

Dreier JP, Fabricius M, Ayata C, et al. Recording, analysis, and interpretation of spreading depolarizations in neurointensive care: review and recommendations of the COSBID research group. *J Cereb Blood Flow Metab*. 2016;37:1595-1625. doi:10.1177/0271678X16654496. Available at: http://www.ncbi.nlm.nih.gov/pubmed/27317657.

Dreier JP, Major S, Manning A, et al. Cortical spreading ischaemia is a novel process involved in ischaemic damage in patients with aneurysmal subarachnoid haemorrhage. *Brain*. 2009;132:1866-1881. doi:10.1093/brain/awp102. Available at: http://www.ncbi.nlm.nih.gov/pubmed/19420089.

23. **The answer is B.** The patient described is in nonconvulsive status epilepticus (NCSE) as seen by sustained GPDs at ~2.5 Hz. These discharges also have classic triphasic wave morphology, which have been historically associated with metabolic derangements and hepatic encephalopathy. Approximately one quarter of patients with GPDs will go on to have seizures and the triphasic morphology of discharges does not influence the risk of seizures. Although metabolic derangements and intoxication are a common cause of GPDs with triphasic morphology, patients with acute brain injuries such as tuberculous meningoencephalitis and central nervous system (CNS) Lyme disease, as well as with epilepsy, may also display such morphology of discharges. These patterns also respond to both benzodiazepine and nonsedating antiseizure medications.

Foreman B, Mahulikar A, Tadi P, et al. Generalized periodic discharges and 'triphasic waves': a blinded evaluation of inter-rater agreement and clinical significance. *Clin Neurophysiol*. 2016;127:1073-1080. doi:10.1016/j.clinph.2015.07.018. Available at: http://www.ncbi.nlm.nih.gov/pubmed/26294138 Accessed August 15, 2017.

O'Rourke D, Chen PM, Gaspard N, et al. Response rates to anticonvulsant trials in patients with triphasic-wave EEG patterns of uncertain significance. *Neurocritical Care* 2016;24:233-239. doi:10.1007/s12028-015-0151-8. Available at: http://www.ncbi.nlm.nih.gov/pubmed/26013921.

24. **The answer is A.** EDB is a novel EEG finding seen in approximately 30% patients with anti-NMDA receptor encephalitis. While its presence raises the suspicion for this autoimmune encephalitis, it is not considered diagnostic and further confirmatory workup is necessary. EDB may also have prognostic implications, as it is associated with status epilepticus (SE) and a prolonged illness course. Seizures and NCSE are not uncommon in anti-NMDA receptor encephalitis, and do warrant aggressive treatment with antiseizure medications and immunotherapy. Anti-NMDA receptor encephalitis is associated with ovarian teratoma, not small-cell lung cancer.

Schmitt SE, Pargeon K, Frechette ES, et al. Extreme delta brush: a unique EEG pattern in adults with anti-NMDA receptor encephalitis. *Neurology*. 2012;79:1094-1100. doi:10.1212/WNL.0b013e3182698cd8. Available at: http://www.ncbi.nlm.nih.gov/pubmed/22933737.

Veciana M, Becerra JL, Fossas P, et al. EEG extreme delta brush: an ictal pattern in patients with anti-NMDA receptor encephalitis. *Epilepsy & Behavior*. 2015;49:280-285. doi:10.1016/j.yebeh.2015.04.032. Available at: http://www.ncbi.nlm.nih.gov/pubmed/26071995.

25. **The answer is B.** LPDs and LRDA are independent predictors of acute seizures with approximately 60% of patients having seizures during acute illness. Moreover, patterns exhibiting higher frequencies than 1.5 Hz and those associated with a "plus" modifier seem to be associated with a higher risk. Such seizures are nonconvulsive in the majority of cases (80%–90%) and monitoring for up to 48 hours is indicated in patients with alteration of consciousness to maximize the yield of the recording.

Gaspard N, Manganas L, Rampal N, et al. Similarity of lateralized rhythmic delta activity to periodic lateralized epileptiform discharges in critically ill patients. *JAMA*. 2013;70:1288-1295. doi:10.1001/jamaneurol.2013.3475. Available at: http://www.ncbi.nlm.nih.gov/pubmed/23921464.

Rodriguez Ruiz A, Vlachy J, Lee JW, et al. Association of periodic and rhythmic electroencephalographic patterns with seizures in critically ill patients. *JAMA*. 2017;74:181-188. doi:10.1001/jamaneurol.2016.4990. Available at: http://www.ncbi.nlm.nih.gov/pubmed/27992625.

Struck AF, Osman G, Rampal N, et al. Time-dependent risk of seizures in critically ill patients on continuous electroencephalogram. *Ann Neurol*. 2017;82:177-185. doi:10.1002/ana.24985. Available at: http://www.ncbi.nlm.nih.gov/pubmed/28681492.

26. **The answer is C.** Neuroprognostication in cardiac arrest should rely on a multimodal approach, as no single predictor (not even pupillary reflex) carries a 100% positive predictive value for poor outcome across all studies. Several features of EEG have neuroprognostic implications: presence or absence of epileptiform activity, abnormal variability, abnormal reactivity, and burst suppression. Of these, reactivity has been the most traditionally studied and reliable EEG parameter for neuroprognostication. Of importance, EEG interpretation is a factor to take into consideration as it is a user-dependent tool, and can be affected by hypothermia and sedatives, all of which are significant confounding factors. More recently, the use of quantitative EEG to reduce the subjectivity of reactivity interpretation is increasing, and holds promise in improving accuracy of neuroprognostication.

Hermans MC, Westover MB, van Putten MJ, et al. Quantification of EEG reactivity in comatose patients. *Clin Neurophysiol*. 2016;127:571-580. doi:10.1016/j.clinph.2015.06.024. Available at: http://www.ncbi.nlm.nih.gov/pubmed/26183757.

Hofmeijer J, van Putten MJ. EEG in postanoxic coma: prognostic and diagnostic value. *Clin Neurophysiol*. 2016;127:2047-2055. doi:10.1016/j.clinph.2016.02.002. Available at: http://www.ncbi.nlm.nih.gov/pubmed/26971488.

Rossetti AO, Tovar Quiroga DF, Juan E, et al. Electroencephalography predicts poor and good outcomes after cardiac arrest: a two-center study. *Crit Care Med*. 2017;45:e674-e682. doi:10.1097/CCM.0000000000002337. Available at: http://www.ncbi.nlm.nih.gov/pubmed/28406812.

Tjepkema-Cloostermans MC, Hofmeijer J, Beishuizen A, et al. Cerebral recovery index: reliable help for prediction of neurologic outcome after cardiac arrest. *Crit Care Med*. 2017;45:e789-e97. doi:10.1097/CCM.0000000000002412. Available at: http://www.ncbi.nlm.nih.gov/pubmed/28430695.

Westhall E, Rossetti AO, van Rootselaar AF, et al. Standardized EEG interpretation accurately predicts prognosis after cardiac arrest. *Neurology*. 2016;45:e674-e682. doi:10.1097/CCM.0000000000002337. Available at: http://www.ncbi.nlm.nih.gov/pubmed/26865516.

27. **The answer is E.** The case describes a patient who exhibits rapid neurologic deterioration in the setting of osmotic shifts during renal replacement therapy for refractory hyperammonemia. Dialysis disequilibrium syndrome is a neurologic emergency due to acute diffuse

cerebral edema precipitated by osmolar shifts. Moreover, patients with acute liver failure or decompensated cirrhosis are at high risk for developing cerebral edema. Diffuse attenuation of cerebral rhythms is seen in the raw EEG and in the quantitative EEG (qEEG) trends, with diffuse loss of power and high suppression percentage. Although patients with hepatic failure are at high risk for seizures and SE, this EEG is not consistent with seizures and benzodiazepines are not the next step in the management of this patient. The most appropriate next step is to stop renal replacement therapy and obtain a CT of the head on an emergent basis for the prompt diagnosis of cerebral edema and downward herniation. Prompt osmotic therapy should be considered once this is diagnosed. An MRI of the brain is also diagnostic for cerebral edema; however, the patient is too unstable to lie flat for a prolonged period of time. Extensor posturing is not compatible with a brain-death diagnosis.

Fantaneanu T, Alvarez V, Lee JW. Teaching neuroImages: acute generalized suppression on continuous EEG heralds clinical and radiologic deterioration. *Neurology*. 2015;84:e119-e120. doi:10.1212/WNL.0000000000001490. Available at: http://www.ncbi.nlm.nih.gov/pubmed/25901064.

Newey CR, Sarwal A, Hantus S. Continuous electroencephalography (cEEG) changes precede clinical changes in a case of progressive cerebral edema. *Neurocritical Care*. 2013;18:261-265. doi:10.1007/s12028-011-9650-4. Available at: http://www.ncbi.nlm.nih.gov/pubmed/22108782.

28. **The answer is D.** LRDA and LPDs carry a similar risk for the development of acute seizures during acute brain illness and patients with these findings on initial recording should be monitored for at least 24 hours or longer if they are comatose. TIRDA is a characteristic interictal pattern associated with temporal lobe epilepsy and is not a benign variant. Although this patient is at risk for seizures and NCSE, prophylactic midazolam is not indicated.

Gaspard N, Manganas L, Rampal N, et al. Similarity of lateralized rhythmic delta activity to periodic lateralized epileptiform discharges in critically ill patients. *JAMA*. 2013;70:1288-1295. doi:10.1001/jamaneurol.2013.3475. Available at: http://www.ncbi.nlm.nih.gov/pubmed/23921464.

29. **The answer is B.** Initially thought to be pathognomonic of outcomes incompatible with meaningful recovery; the recent recognition of distinct electroclinical patterns in postanoxic myoclonus is changing the landscape of neuroprognostication in hypoxic–ischemic encephalopathy. The presence of midline/vertex predominant epileptiform discharges correlating with myoclonus in a reactive continuous background has been associated with a favorable postanoxic myoclonus profile and indicates patients that benefit from aggressive initial care, such as this case.

Elmer J, Rittenberger JC, Faro J, et al. Clinically distinct electroencephalographic phenotypes of early myoclonus after cardiac arrest. *Ann Neurol*. 2016;80:175-184. doi:10.1002/ana.24697. Available at: http://www.ncbi.nlm.nih.gov/pubmed/27351833.

Mikhaeil-Demo Y, Gavvala JR, Bellinski, II, et al. Clinical classification of post anoxic myoclonic status. *Resuscitation*. 2017;119:76-80. doi:10.1016/j.resuscitation.2017.07.035. Available at: http://www.ncbi.nlm.nih.gov/pubmed/28800888.

5

Critical Care EEG

HIBA A. HAIDER

■ QUESTIONS

1. A 65-year-old right-handed woman is brought to the ED with acute onset of right hemiparesis (leg>arm), and right-sided facial droop. According to eyewitness's accounts, she is a professional gymnastics coach who fell to the ground an hour ago at the gym while lifting weights. There had been no antecedent trauma, and she was noted to have vomited and moaning in pain, muttering incomprehensible sounds and markedly weaker on her right side. The patient has never had a prior stroke or head trauma, has had no prior surgeries, takes no blood thinners, and her prothrombin time (PT)/partial thromboplastin time (PTT)/International Normalized Ratio (INR) is normal. Her serum glucose is 155, platelets are 240 (normal), blood pressure (BP) is 180/71, and she progressively gets more obtunded. A head CT scan in the ED shows a Hunt and Hess grade 4 diffuse subarachnoid hemorrhage (SAH) with intraventricular extension. While being transported to the angiography suite for possible intervention, she is noted to have a 40-second episode of orofacial twitching and right gaze/head deviation. A 7 mm left middle cerebral artery (MCA) ruptured aneurysm is identified and clipped. Which of the following is true of patients with aneurysmal SAH?

   A. Poor Hunt and Hess grade, high Fisher score, surgical clipping, and aneurysmal rebleed are predictors of in-hospital seizures
   B. In-hospital seizures have no clear relationship to outcome if they are controlled early
   C. In the absence of any documented in-hospital seizures, seizure prophylaxis is not typically recommended
   D. In-hospital seizures are more common than delayed seizures

2. A 45-year-old male patient suffered an aneurysmal subarachnoid hemorrhage (SAH; Hunt and Hess grade 3 on presentation) 5 days ago. He was transferred from an outside hospital due to concerns of rebleeding after craniotomy and clipping of an anterior communicating artery aneurysm on postbleed day 1. He has a Glasgow Coma Scale (GCS) of 4, and requires urgent external ventricular drain (EVD) placement for obstructive hydrocephalus. MRI reveals patchy regions of subacute infarction in the left and right anterior cerebral artery territories with some hemorrhagic conversion. A STAT EEG is initiated which reveals frequent brief (10–20 second) nonevolving runs of the following EEG pattern in the left anterior head region. Management of this patient should include all of the following, **except**:

   A. Initiation of continuous EEG to monitor for nonconvulsive seizures (NCS) and delayed cerebral ischemia
   B. Initiate seizure prophylaxis with levetiracetam, if no contraindications
   C. Initiate seizure prophylaxis with phenytoin, if no contraindications
   D. Daily screening Transcranial Dopplers (TCDs)

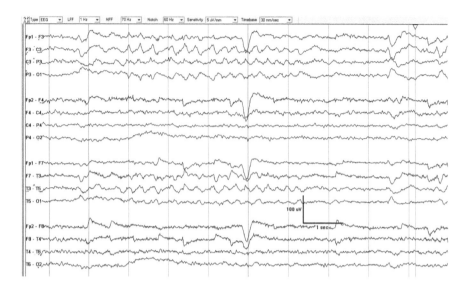

Source: Image courtesy ACNS Standardized Critical Care EEG Nomenclature Training Module, available at https://www.acns.org/research/critical-care-eeg-monitoring-research-consortium-ccemrc/education

3. Which of the following features on EEG is **not** associated with an increased risk of seizures?

   A. Generalized periodic discharges (GPD) with triphasic morphology (previously known as triphasic waves)
   B. GPDs without triphasic morphology
   C. Lateralized periodic discharges (LPD)
   D. Generalized rhythmic delta activity in the bifrontal regions (GRDA)

4. A 70-year-old man with hypertension and renal failure is admitted to the ICU after cardiac arrest. The time period from cardiac arrest to initiation of cardiopulmonary resuscitation (CPR) was approximately 5 minutes. CPR was performed for 25 minutes before the return of spontaneous circulation. Approximately 3 days after admission, the patient is normothermic and not on any sedative medication. On neurologic exam, he remains unresponsive to all noxious stimuli, and pupillary and corneal reflexes are present. The EEG shows the following pattern, and the EEG findings are nonreactive to environmental stimuli. Later in the record this pattern is intermittently seen at regular intervals of 5 to 8 seconds. Which statement correctly describes the pattern seen?

   A. Generalized periodic discharges (GPDs), good prognosis for meaningful neurologic recovery
   B. Burst-suppression (BS) pattern, indeterminate prognosis for meaningful neurologic recovery
   C. Myoclonic status epilepticus (MSE), indeterminate prognosis for meaningful neurologic recovery
   D. GPDs, poor prognosis for meaningful recovery

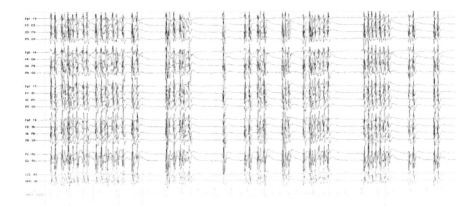

Source: Image courtesy A. Rodriguez Ruiz, MD

5. A patient with grade 4 subarachnoid hemorrhage (SAH) with the following EEG tracing had no EEG background reactivity to auditory, nailbed, nasal tickle, or trapezius stimuli but was reactive to nipple stimulation. Which of the following EEG findings are associated with patient outcomes in SAH?

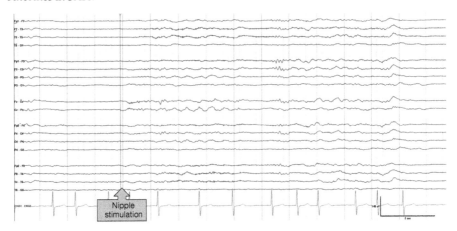

A. Nonconvulsive status epilepticus (NCSE) within the first 24 hours
B. Seizure burden
C. Presence or absence of sleep architecture
D. All of the above

6. At least 24 hours of continuous EEG (cEEG) monitoring to rule out nonconvulsive seizures (NCS) is indicated in which of the following:

A. Comatose patient with aneurysmal subarachnoid hemorrhage (SAH)
B. Obtunded (otherwise healthy) patient after an unwitnessed fall
C. Obtunded patient with sepsis and multiorgan failure slow to improve clinically
D. Confused but awake patient with stimulus-induced focal motor myoclonic jerks
E. All of the above

7. What characteristic of a periodic pattern on EEG in a critically ill patient would confirm that it is an ictal phenomenon?

   A. Triphasic morphology
   B. Lateralized (as opposed to generalized)
   C. "Plus" modifiers
   D. Clinical correlate

8. You are consulted on a 35-year-old man admitted to the medical ICU with a history of generalized epilepsy who was found unconscious at home by his partner, appearing to have vomited on himself. Upon further probing you find out that he has a history of generalized epilepsy since his teens, and was well controlled on topiramate until recently. Over the past year he has had episodes of wandering and intermittent confusion and, because of this, recently established care with a neurologist who transitioned him to valproic acid 250 mg TID about 1 month ago. He has an elevated ammonia level (120 micromol/L), valproate serum level within normal range (55 mg/L), and normal liver function tests. STAT routine EEG shows this pattern:

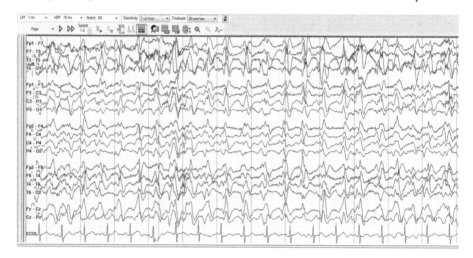

   Which of the following is the next best step?

   A. Intravenous (IV) lorazepam plus IV loading dose of levetiracetam; continue valproic acid at maintenance dose of 250 mg TID and initiate continuous EEG (cEEG)
   B. IV lorazepam plus IV loading dose of valproic acid, aiming for a serum level of 100 or more and initiate cEEG
   C. Hold valproic acid, treat hyperammonemia, and initiate cEEG
   D. Continue maintenance valproic acid, treat hyperammonemia with lactulose, and initiate cEEG

9. A patient with a left centro-parietal subdural hemorrhage status postcraniotomy for evacuation might be expected to show which of the following findings on EEG?

   A. Focal slowing, attenuation of faster frequencies, and lower amplitudes in the left centro-parietal region
   B. Higher voltage, spiky waveforms with irregular morphology over the left centro-parietal region
   C. Left centro-parietal lateralized periodic discharges (LPDs)
   D. Rhythmic slowing in the left centro-parietal region
   E. All of the above

10. You are consulted on a 32-year-old man with end-stage liver disease due to nonalcoholic steatohepatitis and septic shock, who progressively becomes more obtunded in the medical step-down unit, necessitating intubation and transfer to the ICU. MRI shows multifocal embolic strokes with hemorrhagic conversion. Continuous EEG (cEEG) is initiated and shows the following pattern. How would you best describe the patterns shown on the following EEG?

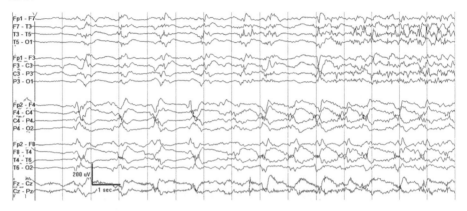

A. Bilateral independent periodic discharges (BIPDs)
B. Lateralized periodic discharges (LPDs)
C. Generalized periodic discharges (GPDs)
D. Periodic artifact

11. This question pertains to the image seen in the previous Question #10. What is the most accurate interpretation of the pattern shown in the EEG?

A. Bilateral independent foci of cortical irritability
B. Bilateral independent foci of cortical irritability and/or structural abnormality
C. Generalized structural abnormality, most severe over the right hemisphere
D. Periodic artifact

12. A 20-year-old man is admitted to the ICU because of coma of unclear etiology. There is no history of trauma and no structural lesion on neuroimaging. Which of the following findings on EEG would be associated with a uniformly unfavorable prognosis?

A. Spindle-like discharges with variability and reactivity
B. Moderately discontinuous background with polymorphic delta slowing
C. Diffuse monomorphic nonreactive alpha activity
D. Diffuse monomorphic rhythmic delta activity

13. What is the incidence of electroclinical dissociation or subclinical seizures in neonates during continuous EEG (cEEG) monitoring after the administration of anticonvulsant medications?

A. 5%–15%
B. 25%–35%
C. 55%–65%
D. 75%–85%

14. An 18-year-old boy with chronic renal disease presents in status epilepticus (SE) that is refractory to treatment with benzodiazepines, fosphenytoin, phenobarbital, and valproic acid. An intravenous (IV) pentobarbital drip is initiated and burst suppression (BS) is achieved on EEG. Thirty-six hours later, he is found to have cardiac arrhythmias, hypotension, and an increased anion gap. Which of the following is correct?

A. He has refractory SE and needs an increase in pentobarbital drip rate
B. He has worsening refractory SE and needs to be transitioned to another anesthetic agent such as propofol.
C. He has propylene glycol toxicity and needs discontinuation of pentobarbital
D. A spinal tap and broad spectrum antibiotic coverage are indicated

15. The following figure shows a quantitative EEG (qEEG) trend panel of 1-hour duration processed from the continuous EEG record of a 35-year-old previously healthy male patient who presented with fever and new onset seizures of undetermined cause. Seizures are refractory to intravenous (IV) fosphenytoin, levetiracetam, and lacosamide. He is started on a midazolam infusion. Which of the following statements about this record is **false**?

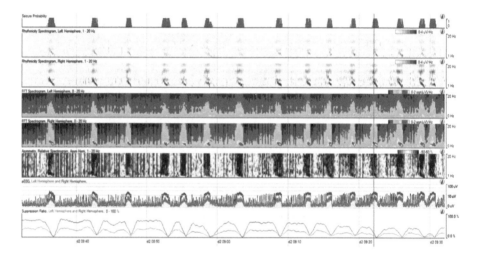

A. Fifteen events visualized on this trend panel are concerning for seizures.
B. The seizures are very likely focal in onset but conventional EEG review is needed to confirm this.
C. The background is one of asymmetric burst suppression (BS), with the right hemisphere more suppressed compared to the left.
D. Seizure onset alternates between the left and the right hemispheres.

16. The figure shows a 2-hour quantitative EEG trend panel processed from continuous EEG (cEEG) of a 70-year-old woman admitted for left hemi-body focal motor clonic seizures that are controlled with a combination of fosphenytoin and lacosamide. She remains altered and "dazed" after motor seizures are clinically controlled, and becomes progressively more obtunded requiring noninvasive ventilatory support. You are called to evaluate her for the need for intubation. While evaluating her case, you consult with the EEG fellow on call at time point X, and he informs you that there are 1-Hz lateralized periodic discharges (LPDs) maximal in the right frontocentral region, often with superimposed rhythmic and fast components. In the subsequent 2-hour epoch shown:

A. Seizures begin at time point B and continue through C
B. Seizures begin during A and continue through B and C
C. There is increasing amplitude, rhythmicity, and power of frequencies over the right hemisphere that could signify worsening metabolic distress
D. Making a diagnosis of nonconvulsive status epilepticus (NCSE) in this patient may require a trial of an intravenous (IV) loading dose of an antiepileptic drug
E. Both C and D are correct

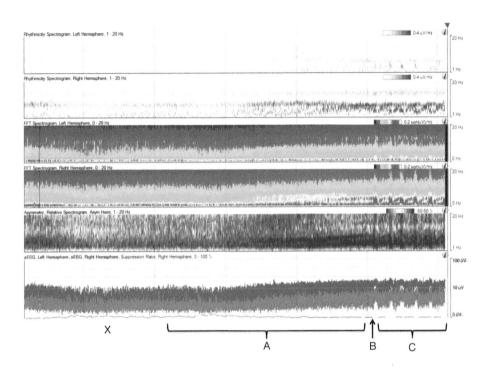

17. All of the following sets of medications are associated with nonconvulsive status epilepticus (NCSE), **except**:

    A. Baclofen and tiagabine
    B. Cephalosporins and fluoroquinolones
    C. Ifosfamide and bevacizumab
    D. Cyclobenzaprine and cisplatin

18. All of the following statements are true about the pattern shown, **except**:

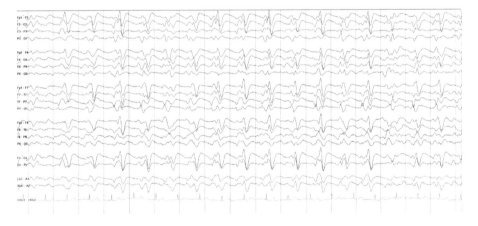

    A. The pattern morphology is specific for encephalopathies of toxic metabolic origin
    B. In some cases, treatment with nonsedating antiepileptic drugs or benzodiazepines can result in clinical improvement
    C. The pattern is a nonspecific marker of diffuse cortical–subcortical dysfunction
    D. This pattern can be associated with an increased risk of seizures

■ ANSWERS

1. **The correct answer is A.** Risk factors known to be associated with the development of seizures include younger than 40 years, loss of consciousness greater than 1 hour or low Glasgow Coma Scale (GCS) at onset, middle cerebral artery aneurysm rupture, clot burden on head CT, associated intracerebral hemorrhage, rebleeding, cerebral infarction, surgical clipping and craniotomy, and poor Hunt and Hess grade. B is incorrect: several studies have found an association between seizures and worse functional outcome without an impact on overall mortality (summarized in Maciel & Gilmore, 2016). After excluding patients with a history of epilepsy, Claassen et al. found a strong relationship between in-hospital seizures and 12-month mortality from SAH onset. C is incorrect: American Heart Association guidelines suggest using postseizure prophylaxis in the immediate posthemorrhagic period with a class IIb, level B recommendation. In the absence of in-hospital seizures, consensus guidelines by the Neurocritical Care Society recommend limiting postseizure prophylaxis to 3 to 7 days in addition to avoiding phenytoin, since there is evidence that phenytoin can impact cognitive outcomes in patients with SAH (Naidech et al., 2005). In SAH patients suffering a seizure during hospitalization, the literature supports continuation of antiepileptic drug therapy for a variable period (6 weeks to 6 months) and there is no consensus to support a particular treatment duration. D is incorrect: the incidence of delayed in-hospital seizures (onset >14 days postbleed) has been reported to be up to 25% with prolonged follow-up, compared to the reported 4% to 10% in the initial 4 weeks after SAH. A recent meta-analysis showed overall incidences of 2.3% for in-hospital seizures and 5.5% for delayed in-hospital seizures with a mean onset latency of 7.45 months (Raper et al., 2013).

Claassen J, Peery S, Kreiter KT, et al. Predictors and clinical impact of epilepsy after subarachnoid hemorrhage. *Neurology*. 2003;60(2):208-214. doi:10.1212/01.WNL.0000038906.71394.DE

Connolly ES Jr, Rabinstein AA, Carhuapoma JR, et al. Guidelines for the management of aneurysmal subarachnoid hemorrhage: a guideline for healthcare professionals from the American Heart Association/American Stroke Association. *Stroke*. June 2012;43(6):1711-1737. doi:10.1161/STR.0b013e3182587839

Diringer MN, Bleck TP, Claude Hemphill J 3rd, et al. Critical care management of patients following aneurysmal subarachnoid hemorrhage: recommendations from the Neurocritical Care Society's Multidisciplinary Consensus Conference. *Neurocrit Care*. September 2011;15(2):211-240. doi:10.1007/s12028-011-9605-9

Lanzino G, D'Urso PI, Suarez J, et al. Seizures and anticonvulsants after aneurysmal subarachnoid hemorrhage. *Neurocrit Care*. 2011;15:247. doi:10.1007/s12028-011-9584-x

Maciel CB, Gilmore EJ. Seizures and epileptiform patterns in SAH and their relation to outcomes. *J Clin Neurophysiol*. June 2016;33(3):183-195. doi:10.1097/WNP.0000000000000268

2. **The answer is C.** This question pertains to the standardized American Clinical Neurophysiology Society (ACNS) terminology for the description of rhythmic and periodic patterns seen in critically ill patients. The EEG shows lateralized rhythmic delta activity with superimposed sharp (LRDA+S), which is a rhythmic pattern highly associated with seizures. A is true: this patient with poor grade aneurysmal SAH is at postbleed day 5, and is entering the window for delayed cerebral ischemia (DCI); vasospasm is one contributing mechanism for DCI but is not the only one implicated. EEG changes consistent with DCI include a decline in alpha-delta ratio (ADR) and relative alpha variability, thus continuous EEG (cEEG) can be a useful adjunctive diagnostic modality for DCI and has been shown to precede findings consistent with vasospasm on TCD studies. Poor-grade SAH patients are also at high risk for NCS. While the majority of NCS are detected within 48 hours of monitoring in comatose patients, patients with SAH who develop DCI may have emergence of NCS and periodic patterns later in their course (during the time window when they are at highest risk of DCI). Thus, continuous EEG (cEEG) is indicated for both seizure and ischemia monitoring at this time, the former being endorsed as a clinical indication by a consensus statement from the ACNS. B is true: while there is no high-quality data to guide decision making with regard to antiepileptic drug prophylaxis, consensus guidelines by the Neurocritical Care Society recommend limiting postseizure prophylaxis to 3 to 7 days in addition to avoiding phenytoin use. A study investigating the impact of phenytoin on cognitive outcomes in patients with SAH led to abandonment of

its routine use for postseizure prophylaxis in patients with SAH (Naidech et al., 2005). Despite the lack of adequate head-to-head comparisons in patients with SAH, the preferred drug for prophylaxis seems to be levetiracetam because it seems noninferior to phenytoin in acute brain injury and postcraniotomy patients, is noninferior to valproate, does not interact with nimodipine and seems more tolerable by patients. Continued antiepileptic drug use once the aneurysm is secured should be driven by clinical status and EEG findings; this patient not only has LRDA+S on EEG (a rhythmic pattern highly associated with seizures), but also is status post clipping and postcraniotomy, with rebleeding of the aneurysm, obstructive hydrocephalus, and infarction of brain tissue in the relevant vascular distribution. These are all risk factors for increased seizure occurrence, and thus it is reasonable to continue postseizure prophylaxis during the hospitalization, preferably with levetiracetam.

Connolly ES Jr, Rabinstein AA, Carhuapoma JR, et al. Guidelines for the management of aneurysmal subarachnoid hemorrhage: a guideline for healthcare professionals from the American Heart Association/american Stroke Association. *Stroke*. June 2012;43(6):1711-1737. doi: 10.1161/STR.0b013e3182587839

Diringer MN, Bleck TP, Claude Hemphill, J 3rd et al. Critical care management of patients following aneurysmal subarachnoid hemorrhage: recommendations from the Neurocritical Care Society's Multidisciplinary Consensus Conference. *Neurocrit Care*. September 2011;15(2):211-240. doi:10.1007/s12028-011-9605-9

Hirsch LJ, LaRoche SM, Gaspard N, et al. American Clinical Neurophysiology Society's standardized critical care EEG terminology: 2012 version. *J Clin Neurophysiol*. February 2013;30(1):1-27. doi:10.1097/WNP.0b013e3182784729

Muniz CF, Shenoy AV, O'Connor KL, et al. Clinical development and implementation of an institutional guideline for prospective EEG monitoring and reporting of delayed cerebral ischemia. *J Clin Neurophysiol*. June 2016;33(3):217-226. doi:10.1097/WNP.0b013e3182784729

3. **The answer is D**. GPDs with and without triphasic morphology and LPDs are all associated with a higher risk of seizures. Lateralized rhythmic delta activity (LRDA) is associated with a higher risk of seizures, but generalized rhythmic delta activity (GRDA) is not. GRDA can be bifrontally predominant.

Foreman B, Claassen J, Abou Khaled K, et al. Generalized periodic discharges in the critically ill: a case-control study of 200 patients. *Neurology*. November 6, 2012;79(19):1951-1960. doi: 10.1212/WNL.0b013e3182735cd7

Rodriguez Ruiz A, Vlachy J, Lee JW, et al. Association of periodic and rhythmic electroencephalographic patterns with seizures in critically ill patients. *JAMA Neurol*. February 1, 2017;74(2):181-188. doi:10.1001/jamaneurol.2016.4990

4. **The answer is D**. The EEG shows GPDs at a frequency of up to 5 Hz on a suppressed and reportedly nonreactive background. Based on the description of the record, the GPDs likely transition to a BS pattern, which is characterized by high-amplitude cerebral activity alternating with an isoelectric background, with the periods of suppression comprising at least 50% of the record. In the absence of hypothermia or sedative medications (both of which can result in a BS pattern), BS is usually associated with poor neurologic outcome, so B is incorrect. A is incorrect: specific characteristics of BS associated with poor outcome include the presence of GPDs within bursts on an otherwise suppressed background (as in this case), identical bursts, and GPDs time-locked with myoclonic jerks, which would be consistent with MSE and which also portends a poor prognosis. C is incorrect: since myoclonus is not reported as a physical finding on examination, there is not enough information to make a diagnosis of MSE.

Hofmeijer J, Tjepkema-Cloostermans MC, van Putten MJ. Burst-suppression with identical bursts: a distinct EEG pattern with poor outcome in postanoxic coma. *Clin Neurophysiol*. 2014;125(5):947-954. doi:10.1016/j.clinph.2013.10.017

Young GB. The EEG in coma. *J Clin Neuro*. 2000;17(5):473-485. doi:10.1097/00004691-200009000-00006

5. **The answer is D.** A study by Claassen et al. evaluated 116 patients with SAH who underwent continuous EEG (cEEG; 88% with a Hunt and Hess grade of 3 or worse on admission). In this study, EEG findings associated with poor functional outcome at 3 months included

absence of sleep architecture during the first 24 hours of cEEG hookup (odds ratio10.4, 95% confidence interval 1.4–78.1) or at any time of the hospital stay (odds ratio 4.3., 95% confidence interval 1.1–17.2); presence of lateralized periodic discharges (LPDs) at any time (odds ratio 18.8, 95% confidence interval 1.6–214.6); presence of any type of periodic discharges, even after controlling for age; Hunt and Hess grade; and intraventricular hemorrhage (IVH; odds ratio 9.0, 95% confidence interval 1.7–49.0). Additionally, poor outcome at 3 months was seen in all patients with the following characteristics: (a) no EEG reactivity, (b) absence of state changes within the first 24 hours, (c) NCSE within the first 24 hours, (d) generalized periodic discharges (GPDs), and (e) bilateral independent periodic discharges (BIPDs).

DeMarchis et al. analyzed 402 patients with SAH undergoing cEEG monitoring and found a dose–response relationship between seizure burden and outcome: the detection of any seizure on cEEG was associated with more than a three-fold increased odds of unfavorable functional outcome at 3 months. Every hour of nonconvulsive seizures (NCS) was associated with 10% higher odds of disability or death at 3 months. Seizure burden was also associated with unfavorable functional and cognitive outcome at 3 months. For every hour of seizure on cEEG, the Telephone Interview for Cognitive Status (TICS) score decreased by 0.19 points (TICS score ranges from 0 [worst] to 51 [best]).

Claassen J, Hirsch LJ, Frontera JA, et al. Prognostic significance of continuous EEG monitoring in patients with poor-grade subarachnoid hemorrhage. *Neurocrit Care.* April 2006;4(2):103-112. doi:10.1385/ncc: 42: 103

De Marchis GM, Pugin D, Meyers E, et al. Seizure burden in subarachnoid hemorrhage associated with functional and cognitive outcome. *Neurology.* January 19, 2016;86(3):253-260. doi:10.1212/WNL.0000000000002281

6. **The answer is E.** The most common indications for ICU cEEG are diagnosis of NCS and other paroxysmal events; assessment of efficacy of treatment of NCS; identification of cerebral ischemia; monitoring of sedation and high-dose suppressive therapy; and assessment of severity of encephalopathy and prognostication. The American Clinical Neurophysiology Society (ACNS) Consensus Guidelines summarized a list of medical conditions where the likelihood of capturing seizures on cEEG is considerably high.

Recent convulsive status epilepticus (SE) or clinical seizure without return to baseline; acute brain injury (including aneurysmal SAH, intraparenchymal hemorrhage [IPH], moderate to severe traumatic brain injury [TBI], central nervous system [CNS] infections, brain tumors, acute ischemic stroke, and hypoxic–ischemic injury); epilepsy-related; sepsis associated encephalopathy; and status post extracorporeal membrane oxygenation.

Herman ST, Abend NS, Bleck TP, et al. Consensus statement on continuous EEG in critically ill adults and children, part I: indications. *J Clin Neurophysiol.* 2015;32(2):87-95. doi: 10.1097/WNP.0000000000000166

7. **The answer is D.** This question pertains to the definition of nonconvulsive status epilepticus (NCSE). The most unequivocal NCSE pattern is one with epileptiform discharges that evolve in frequency, amplitude, or location, or have persistent frequencies faster than 2.5 Hz. Additionally, based on the Salzburg criteria, epileptiform discharges less than or equal to 2.5 Hz would meet criteria for NCSE if they exhibit either (a) an associated clinical correlate (e.g., limb jerking; facial, axial, or limb myoclonus; gaze or head deviation; nystagmus) or (b) clinical and EEG improvement after administering an intravenous (IV) antiepileptic drug. A is incorrect: triphasic morphology alone is not sufficient to determine whether or not a pattern is ictal. B is incorrect: periodic discharges of all distributions (lateralized or generalized) can be ictal. C is incorrect: the presence of plus modifiers is associated with increasing epileptogenicity but is not a confirmatory finding.

Beniczky S, Hirsch LJ, Kaplan PW, et al. Unified EEG terminology and criteria for nonconvulsive status epilepticus. *Epilepsia.* September 2013;54(suppl 6):28-29. doi:10.1111/epi.12270

Rodriguez Ruiz A, Vlachy J, Lee JW, et al. Association of periodic and rhythmic electroencephalographic patterns with seizures in critically ill patients. *JAMA Neurol.* February 1, 2017;74(2):181-188. doi:10.1001/jamaneurol.2016.4990

Sutter R, Kaplan PW. Electroencephalographic criteria for nonconvulsive status epilepticus: synopsis and comprehensive survey. *Epilepsia*. August 2012;53(suppl 3):1-51. doi:10.1111/j.1528-1167.2012.03593.x

8. **The answer is C.** This patient has hyperammonemic encephalopathy secondary to valproic acid. The EEG shows generalized periodic discharges (GPDs) at a frequency of 1 Hz, with triphasic morphology. Based on the frequency and nonevolving pattern, this would not fit criteria for nonconvulsive status epilepticus (NCSE) and so options A and B are incorrect. GPDs with triphasic morphology in this patient likely are associated with toxic–metabolic derangement (high ammonia), hence correcting this and discontinuing the offending drug should take priority.

9. **The answer is E.** Focal slowing, attenuation of faster frequencies, and lower amplitudes in the left centro-parietal region would be due to structural dysfunction related to the small subdural hematoma (SDH). Higher voltage and spiky waveforms with irregular morphology over the left centro-parietal region is a description consistent with a breach rhythm, which would be an expected finding after craniotomy. LPDs and rhythmic slowing in the left centro-parietal region, a description consistent with lateralized rhythmic delta activity (LRDA), are also likely findings, as patients with SDH and recent neurosurgery are both at higher risk for seizures, and rhythmic periodic patterns such as LPDs and lateral rhythmic delta activity (LRDA) are thus frequently encountered.

10. **The answer is A.** The pattern shown is bilateral independent periodic discharges with superimposed fast and rhythmic activity (BIPDs + FR). 1-Hz periodic discharges with superimposed rhythmicity (+R) are seen maximally over the right centro-parietal region (bottom half of page); independently occurring 1-Hz PDs with superimposed fast activity (+F) are seen over the left frontotemporal region (top half of page). In the last 5 seconds of the epoch, the left-sided BIPDs attenuate and give way to a buildup of rhythmic activity over the left, which was the onset of a seizure.

11. **The answer is B.** Periodic discharges of all distributions are associated with a higher risk of seizures. In addition to signifying increased epileptogenic potential, periodic patterns can also accompany structural injury. Bilateral independent periodic discharges (BIPDs) per se do not imply the presence of generalized dysfunction, although the bilateral abnormalities do result in some form of generalized (but likely) asymmetric dysfunction.

12. **The answer is C.** Diffuse monomorphic nonreactive alpha activity (option C) is consistent with alpha coma. Nonreactive coma patterns are typically associated with an unfavorable prognosis. Option A (Spindle-like discharges with variability and reactivity) is a description consistent with spindle coma; best outcomes are seen when spindle coma is due to drugs or seizures; intermediate outcomes are seen with trauma, hypoxic brain injury, and cardiopulmonary arrest; and poor outcomes occur with brainstem and cerebral infarctions. Option B is incorrect. Polymorphic delta slowing and moderately discontinuous background signify more severe brain dysfunction but have not shown to be independently associated with unfavorable outcomes. Option D is consistent with a description of generalized rhythmic delta activity (GRDA), which has not been shown to be associated with an increased risk of seizures or predictive of outcome.

Synek VM. Prognostically important EEG coma patterns in diffuse anoxic and traumatic encephalopathies in adults. *J Clin Neurophysiol*. April 1988;5(2):161-174. doi:10.1097/00004691-198804000-00003

13. **The answer is C.** About 50% to 60% of neonates will have subclinical seizures detected on EEG monitoring after antiepileptic drug administration. In neonates with clinical signs associated with seizures (i.e., electro-clinical seizures), a clinical correlate is seen in only some of the seizures; the majority are electrographic only. The persistence of electrographic seizures is termed uncoupling or decoupling.

Scher M, Alvin J, Gaus L, et al. Uncoupling of EEG-clinical neonatal seizures after antiepileptic drug use. *Pediatr Neurol.* 2003;28(4):277-280. doi:10.1016/s0887-8994(02)00621-5

Shellhaas R, Chang T, Tsuchida T. The American clinical neurophisiology society's guideline on continuous electroencephalography monitoring in neonates. *J Clin Neurophysiology.* 2011;28(6):611-617. doi:10.1097/WNP.0b013e31823e96d7

14. **The answer is C.** Pentobarbital contains 40% v/v of propylene glycol, and is the most likely cause of the patient's high anion gap metabolic acidosis and clinical deterioration. Propylene glycol toxicity related to IV phenobarbital, lorazepam, and diazepam has also been described. Underlying renal insufficiency and hepatic dysfunction both increase the risk for developing toxicity.

15. **The answer is D.** This qEEG panel shows a compressed hour of conventional EEG data (timescale at the bottom).

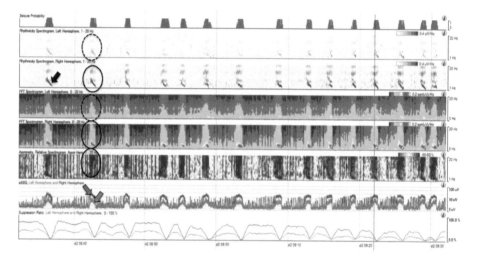

From top to bottom, the trends pictured include seizure probability (automated seizure detection algorithm), rhythmicity spectrogram (left and right hemispheres), color density spectral array (CDSA) (left and right hemispheres), relative asymmetry spectrogram, amplitude-integrated EEG (aEEG) and suppression ratio. A is true; 15 paroxysmal increases in signal are marked (see black arrow; the first one of the 15 events is marked with a black arrow); this arch-shaped appearance is typical of a seizure. B is true; it appears that the seizures involve the right hemisphere, as there is increased signal seen on the right hemispheric rhythmicity spectrogram, CDSA, and relative asymmetry spectrogram (black ovals). There is signal also over the left hemispheric trends; however, this is lower in intensity (grey dotted ovals) and likely signifies partial involvement of or volume conduction of electrographic activity over the left hemisphere. On aEEG there an increase in amplitude over the right hemisphere (red arrow) compared to the left (blue arrow), again suggesting a focal, right hemispheric seizure. All seizures appear similar, with right-side changes most apparent and preceding any left-sided changes in signal, hence all the onsets are right hemispheric, and do not alternate between left and right (D is false, hence the correct answer).

16. **The answer is E.** This quantitative EEG (qEEG) panel shows 2 hours of processed data. From top to bottom, the trends pictured include rhythmicity spectrogram (left and right hemispheres), FFT spectrogram or color density spectral array (left and right hemispheres), relative asymmetry spectrogram, amplitude-integrated EEG (aEEG), and suppression ratio. While the five brief arch-shaped deflections starting at time point B are suggestive of seizures, there is also slowly increasing amplitude, rhythmicity, and power of frequencies over the right hemisphere during A that is concerning for a slow evolving change in the electrographic pattern (described as right hemispheric lateralized periodic discharges [LPDs] in the question). An assessment of whether or not seizures start at B or at some point before this (i.e., during A), cannot be made by looking at qEEG alone (hence A and B are both incorrect). Raw EEG and video footage would need to be reviewed to determine whether the LPDs over the

right hemisphere are slowly evolving to a more ictal-appearing pattern during A (as would be suggested by increasing superimposed fast frequencies and rhythmicity or LPDs + FR), and whether they are associated with a neurologic decline (worsening exam) or clinical correlate. If a clinical correlate is confirmed, the pattern could qualify as an ictal phenomenon even in the absence of an unequivocal NCSE pattern (i.e., ≥2.5 Hz evolving epileptiform discharges). Such equivocal patterns are said to lie on the ictal–interictal continuum. Most commonly these comprise of periodic discharges between 1 and 2.5 Hz that exhibit slow evolving changes in morphology, frequency, location, or amplitude, or superimposed fast/rhythmic activity, can appear as a slowly intensifying bar of color (as in "A"). Multimodality monitoring can be helpful in determining the significance of unequivocal patterns but is not in routine clinical use at this time.

Beniczky S, Hirsch LJ, Kaplan PW, et al. Unified EEG terminology and criteria for nonconvulsive status epilepticus. *Epilepsia*. September 2013;54(suppl 6):28-29. doi:10.1111/epi.12270

Chong DJ, Hirsch LJ. Which EEG patterns warrant treatment in the critically ill? Reviewing the evidence for treatment of periodic epileptiform discharges and related patterns. *J Clin Neurophysiol*. 2005;22:79-91. doi:10.1097/01.wnp.0000158699.78529.af

Claassen J. How I treat patients with EEG patterns on the ictal-interictal continuum in the neuro ICU. *Neurocrit Care*. 2009;11:437-44. doi:10.1007/s12028-009-9295-8

Sivaraju A, Gilmore EJ. Understanding and managing the ictal-interictal continuum in neurocritical care. *Curr Treat Options Neurol*. February 2016;18(2):8. doi:10.1007/s11940-015-0391-0

17. **The answer is D.** Drug-induced NCSE is an important consideration in critically ill patients. NCSE due to beta-lactam antibiotics, particularly cefepime, has been well described, most often in association with renal dysfunction. Other drugs that have been associated with NCSE include fluoroquinolones, ifosfamide, L-asparaginase, busulfan, and cisplatin. In some cases, NCSE is a presentation of drug-induced reversible posterior leukoencephalopathy syndrome (RPLS); among the more common culprits are tacrolimus, cyclosporine, and bevacizumab. Of the given options, cyclobenzaprine is the only one not associated with NCSE.

18. **The answer is A.** The EEG shows generalized periodic discharges (GPDs) with triphasic morphology, previously known simply as triphasic waves. *Triphasic morphology* is a minor modifier that describes GPDs that present with three phases: negative–positive–negative in polarity. GPDs with triphasic morphology were traditionally considered to be associated with a toxic–metabolic encephalopathy, and therefore were thought to have low association with seizures. However, in a recent study, GPDs *without* triphasic morphology were more likely to be seen during a pure toxic–metabolic encephalopathy. In a retrospective matched case-control cohort study of 200 patients with GPDs, patients with GPDs experienced seizures more commonly than controls without GPDs (46% vs. 34%, respectively; $p = .014$) and this was replicated in other uncontrolled studies. B is true; in a retrospective series of 64 patients with GPDs with triphasic morphology, 10/53 (19%) had a clear response (clinical and EEG improvement) to benzodiazepines and 19/45 (42%) had a positive response to nonsedating antiseizure drugs. In many cases, GPDs appear in an encephalopathic patient and it may not be clear whether or not GPDs are ictal in nature, particularly when there is a known severe toxic or metabolic disturbance. In these cases, a trial of antiseizure drug therapy should be considered.

Foreman B, Claassen J, Abou Khaled K, et al. Generalized periodic discharges in the critically ill: a case-control study of 200 patients. *Neurology*. 6, 2012;79(19):1951-1960. doi: 10.1212/WNL.0b013e3182735cd7

Foreman B, Mahulikar A, Tadi P, et al. Generalized periodic discharges and "triphasic waves": a blinded evaluation of inter-rater agreement and clinical significance. *Clin Neurophysiol*. February 2016;127(2):1073-1080. doi:10.1016/j.clinph.2015.07.018

O'Rourke D, Chen PM, Gaspard N, et al. Response rates to anticonvulsant trials in patients with triphasic-wave EEG patterns of uncertain significance. *Neurocrit Care*. April 2016;24(2):233-239. doi:10.1007/s12028-015-0151-8

Rodriguez Ruiz A, Vlachy J, Lee JW, et al. Association of periodic and rhythmic electroencephalographic patterns with seizures in critically ill patients. *JAMA Neurol*. February 1, 2017;74(2):181-188. doi:10.1001/jamaneurol 2016.4990 Availablec at: http://archneur.jamanetwork.com/article.aspx?doi=10.1001/jamaneurol.2016.4990.

6 Neuromuscular Medicine

*SUUR BILICILER, JUSTIN KWAN, CECILE L. PHAN,
AND MITHILA VULLAGANTI*

QUESTIONS

1. A 48-year-old woman presented to the emergency room with increasing shortness of breath. In the past 14 months, she had a 25-pound weight loss, slurred speech, swallowing difficulty, and arm and leg muscle weakness. On examination, she had tongue weakness and fasciculations, proximal and distal limb muscle weakness, atrophy, and fasciculations, and hyperreflexia. Her sensory examination was normal. What is the best intervention for her respiratory symptoms?

   A. Noninvasive positive pressure ventilation
   B. Bronchodilator
   C. Corticosteroid
   D. High-flow oxygen

2. A 24-year-old woman with an eating disorder consisting of binge eating followed by self-induced vomiting presented with a 6-month history of generalized weakness and exercise intolerance. The examination revealed generalized weakness affecting proximal more than distal muscles, muscle atrophy, and normal sensation. The serum creatine phosphokinase (CPK) was 620 units/L. ECG showed sinus tachycardia and inverted T waves. What is the most likely cause of this patient's muscular symptoms?

   A. Polymyositis
   B. Emery–dreifuss muscular dystrophy
   C. Complication of bulimia
   D. Ipecac-induced myopathy

3. Which of the following is an important intervention in the management of rhabdomyolysis to prevent acute renal injury?

   A. Aggressive fluid repletion
   B. Antioxidant therapy
   C. Peritoneal dialysis
   D. Rapid infusion of hypertonic saline

4. Which of the following conditions are susceptible to succinylcholine-induced hyperkalemia?

   A. Muscular dystrophy
   B. Inflammatory myopathy
   C. Critical illness neuropathy
   D. All of the above

5. A 35-year-old African American woman presented to the emergency room with respiratory failure, difficulty swallowing, and slurred speech. These symptoms had been present for the past several weeks, but recently worsened after she contracted a viral upper respiratory tract infection. On examination the patient was in respiratory distress with increased work of breathing, significant facial weakness and atrophy, weak neck flexors, and severe flaccid dysarthria. Extraocular movements were intact, and her limbs were strong with normal tendon reflexes. She had seen by an outside neurologist who diagnosed her with seronegative myasthenia gravis. Which of the following study is useful to confirm her diagnosis?

   A. GM1 antibody
   B. Muscle-specific-kinase (MuSK) antibody
   C. GQ1b antibody
   D. Striational antibody

6. An 80-year-old man recently diagnosed with myasthenia gravis had worsening weakness, slurred speech, excessive drooling, as well as severe muscle cramps and diarrhea. He was taking regular pyridostigmine 180 mg every 4 hours four times a day and extended release pyridostigmine 180 mg at bed time. In addition, he was recently started on prednisone 20 mg daily. His worsening symptoms are caused by:

   A. Steroid-induced weakness in myasthenia gravis
   B. Current gastrointestinal (GI) infection with diarrhea
   C. Excessive cholinergic activity from overdosing of acetylcholine esterase inhibitors
   D. He does not have myasthenia gravis (MG) because cramps and diarrhea are not clinical features of MG

7. A 20-year-old woman with seropositive myasthenia gravis was admitted to the ICU with respiratory failure, severe dysphagia, and weakness. The best treatment option for this patient is:

   A. Plasma exchange because it works faster than intravenous immunoglobulin (IVIg) and is better tolerated than IVIg
   B. IVIg since it is easily available and does not require the placement of a central line
   C. Either plasma exchange or IVIg
   D. IV pyridostigmine 2 mg every 4 hours

8. A patient who was previously diagnosed with myasthenia gravis is in the emergency room with respiratory insufficiency and altered mentation. His bedside spirometry values are as follows: forced vital capacity (FVC) 1.6 L (he weighs 83 kg), negative inspiratory force (NIF) −18 cm H_2O, peak expiratory flow (PEF) −35 cm H_2O. His oxygen saturation is 95% on room air. What should be done next?

   A. Intubate the patient immediately for airway protection
   B. Obtain a STAT arterial blood gas (ABG) as bedside spirometry is not as accurate at predicting respiratory failure
   C. Place the patient on high-flow oxygen using a nonrebreather mask
   D. Observe the patient closely with FVC and NIF every 2 hours and intubate once FVC drops below 15 mL/kg

9. For patients with myasthenic crisis in the ICU on mechanical ventilation, which of the following statements is **true** regarding initiation of steroid therapy?

   A. High-dose steroid should be avoided because it can cause transient worsening of the myasthenia
   B. High-dose prednisone 60 to 80 mg PO daily should be initiated in conjunction with plasma exchange or intravenous immunoglobulin (IVIg)

C. Steroid should be started at the lowest dose possible and slowly titrate up to alternate day dosing of 60 to 80 mg QOD

D. Intravenous (IV) methylprednisolone is the preferred drug since prednisone tablets cannot be given via percutaneous endoscopic gastrostomy (PEG) tube

Please read the following clinical presentation paragraph and answer Questions 10 to 15.
A 66-year-old gentleman with no significant past medical history presented to the emergency room complaining of progressive numbness and weakness in his legs for 5 days after an episode of diarrhea. He denied recent foreign travel or outdoor activities. He was not taking any medications. On his general examination, he was afebrile and had a heart rate of 120 per minute, blood pressure of 100/70 mmHg, and a respiratory rate of 13 breaths per minute. His neurological examination showed normal mental status, intact cranial nerves except for mild facial weakness, proximal and distal weakness in both upper and lower extremities, decreased light touch and pinprick in lower extremities and hands, diffuse loss of muscle stretch reflexes, and no sensory level and flexor plantar responses. His chest x-ray, complete blood count (CBC), thyroid function testing, liver function studies, cardiac enzymes, serum and urine toxicity screens, and comprehensive metabolic panel including sodium, calcium, potassium, serum protein, blood urea nitrogen (BUN), and creatinine (Cr) were normal. His ECG showed sustained sinus tachycardia. During his medical evaluation, the patient became increasingly short of breath and was admitted to the neurologic ICU after intubation.

10. What is the most likely diagnosis?

   A. Guillain–Barré syndrome (GBS)
   B. Chronic inflammatory demyelinating polyradiculoneuropathy (CIDP)
   C. Spinal cord injury
   D. Multiple sclerosis (MS)

11. What is the next diagnostic study that needs to be ordered?

   A. Cranial MRI
   B. Transthoracic echocardiogram
   C. Lumbar puncture (LP)
   D. Evoked potentials

12. What is the best treatment for this patient?

   A. Intravenous immunoglobulin (IVIg)
   B. Plasmapheresis and oral steroids
   C. IVIg followed by plasma exchange
   D. Intravenous (IV) steroids

13. The day after admission to the neurologic ICU, the patient's serum sodium level was 128 mEq/L. What is/are the possible explanation(s) for the hyponatremia?

   A. Syndrome of inappropriate antidiuretic hormone (SIADH)
   B. Pseudohyponatremia secondary to the best treatment option patient received for his disease
   C. Both A and B
   D. None of the above

14. What are the common cardiovascular complications in this disorder?

   A. Sustained sinus tachycardia
   B. Hypotension
   C. Atrial and ventricular arrhythmias
   D. All of the above

15. A week after his last treatment, he noticed increasing numbness and weakness in his arms and legs that had previously improved. What is the most likely cause for his symptom?

    A. Recurrent Guillain–Barré syndrome (GBS)
    B. Side effect from treatment for GBS
    C. Treatment-related fluctuation (TRF)
    D. Critical illness neuropathy

16. A 72-year-old man was admitted with bacteremia and altered mental status. His hospital course was complicated by aspiration pneumonia, causing respiratory difficulty and oxygen desaturation for which he was intubated. After 5 days, it was noted he had difficulty weaning off the ventilator. On exam he had flaccid weakness involving both arms and both legs with normal tone and +1 reflexes throughout. He nodded his head consistently to light touch sensation which was reproducible. Which of the following pathophysiologic mechanisms have been implicated in this diagnosis?

    A. Preferential loss of myosin
    B. Muscle necrosis
    C. Sodium channel dysfunction
    D. All of the above

17. A 54-year-old woman is admitted for urosepsis. On exam she is noted to have flaccid weakness involving both arms and both legs with normal tone, absent reflexes, and sensory exam was not reliably reproducible. Which of the following pathophysiologic mechanisms have been implicated in this diagnosis?

    A. Edema of the endoneurium
    B. Direct ischemic injury to the endoneurium
    C. Direct toxic effects due to hypoglycemia
    D. All of the above

18. The following electrodiagnostic findings on nerve conduction studies are **most** likely to be seen in critical illness polyneuropathy (CIP) and critical illness myopathy (CIM), respectively:

    A. Preferential loss of sensory nerve action potential (SNAP) amplitudes over compound muscle action potential (CMAP) amplitudes; increased CMAP duration
    B. Equal loss of SNAP and CMAP amplitudes; temporal dispersion
    C. Equal loss of SNAP and CMAP amplitudes; slowed conduction velocities
    D. Preferential loss of CMAP more than SNAP amplitudes; conduction block

19. The following class of antibiotics medications is **least** likely to cause exacerbation of myasthenia gravis symptoms:

    A. Aminoglycosides
    B. Fluoroquinolones
    C. Ketolides
    D. Penicillins

20. The following are typical clinical features shared by serotonin syndrome (SS), neuroleptic malignant syndrome (NMS), and malignant hyperthermia (MH):

    A. Fever
    B. Altered mental status
    C. Rigidity
    D. All of the above

■ ANSWERS

1. **The answer is A.** This is a case of typical amyotrophic lateral sclerosis (ALS). In ALS, noninvasive positive pressure ventilation has been shown to reduce shortness of breath, improve ventilation, and prolong survival. Early treatment with noninvasive positive-pressure ventilation has also been suggested to prolong survival and slow the rate of decline in the respiratory function in ALS patients. Bronchodilator and corticosteroid therapy has not been shown to be helpful in alleviating respiratory symptoms in ALS. Oxygen therapy is not recommended to alleviate dyspnea unless there is an alternative medical indication.

Bourke SC, Tomlinson M, Williams TL, et al. Effects of non-invasive ventilation on survival and quality of life in patients with amyotrophic lateral sclerosis: a randomised controlled trial. *Lancet Neurol.* 2006;5:140-147. doi:10.1016/S1474-4422(05)70326-4

Carratu P, Spicuzza L, Cassano A, et al. Early treatment with noninvasive positive pressure ventilation prolongs survival in Amyotrophic Lateral Sclerosis patients with nocturnal respiratory insufficiency. *Orphanet J Rare Dis.* 2009;4:10. doi:10.1186/1750-1172-4-10

Hardiman O, van den Berg LH, Kiernan MC. Clinical diagnosis and management of amyotrophic lateral sclerosis. *Nat Rev Neurol.* October 11, 2011;7(11):639–649. doi:10.1038/nrneurol.2011.153

Miller RG, Jackson CE, Kasarskis EJ, et al. Practice parameter update: the care of the patient with amyotrophic lateral sclerosis: drug, nutritional, and respiratory therapies (an evidence-based review): report of the Quality Standards Subcommittee of the American Academy of Neurology. *Neurology.* October 13, 2009;73(15):1218-1226. doi:10.1212/WNL.0b013e3181bc0141

2. **The answer is D.** Ipecac syrup can be used as an emetic in large doses, especially in accidental poisoning. Ipecac-induced myopathy should be considered in an individual who has progressive myopathy and a history of eating disorder. Patients may have myopathy and cardiomyopathy due to excessive ipecac use. Discontinuation of ipecac can result in resolution of the symptoms.

Mastaglia FL. Iatrogenic myopathies. *Curr Opin Neurol.* October 2010;23(5):445-449. doi:10.1097/WCO.0b013e32833c2054

3. **The answer is A.** Early and aggressive fluid repletion can be an effective intervention to prevent acute renal injury in rhabdomyolysis. Water retention by damaged muscle can deplete intravascular fluid in the patients who have severe muscle injury. The quantity of fluids needed depends on the severity of the muscle injury, and the optimal composition of the fluid to be used remains controversial. Antioxidant therapy and hypertonic saline are not used to prevent renal failure in rhabdomyolysis. Dialysis may be necessary in patients who have electrolyte disturbance, fluid overload, or acidosis in the setting of acute renal failure.

Bosch X, Poch E, Grau JM. Rhabdomyolysis and acute kidney injury. *N Engl J Med.* July 2, 2009;361(1):62-72. doi:10.1056/NEJMra0801327

4. **The answer is D.** Muscular dystrophy, muscle inflammation, disuse atrophy, denervation, thermal trauma, and severe infection have all been identified as potential risk factors for succinylcholine-induced hyperkalemia. Spread of the acetylcholine receptors throughout the muscle membrane and upregulation of acetylcholine receptors with resultant efflux of potassium during activation of the receptors is the proposed mechanism for hyperkalemia. Fatal arrhythmia may be the consequence of this underrecognized condition.

Martyn JA, Richtsfeld M. Succinylcholine-induced hyperkalemia in acquired pathologic states: etiologic factors and molecular mechanisms. *Anesthesiology.* January 2006;104(1):158-169. doi:10.1097/00000542-200601000-00022

5. **The answer is B.** This patient has myasthenia gravis associated with anti-MuSK antibody. Forty percent of "seronegative MG" patients who test negative for acetylcholine receptor antibodies have MuSK antibody. Myasthenic patients with anti-MUSK antibodies are predominantly women and have several distinctive features, including prominent facial weakness and atrophy, significant pharyngeal and respiratory involvement with frequent crises,

and good response to plasma exchange for acute crises and rituximab for long-term immuno suppression.

Martyn JA, Richtsfeld M. Succinylcholine-induced hyperkalemia in acquired pathologic states: etiologic factors and molecular mechanisms. *Anesthesiology*. January 2006;104(1):158-169. doi:10.1097/00000542-200601000-00022

6. **The answer is C.** In patients who with myasthenia gravis who have with worsening symptoms, it is important to distinguish the disease itself from cholinergic crisis or paradoxical worsening due to high-dose steroid use. In this case the patient has other signs of cholinergic overdose (excessive cramps and diarrhea), and the steroid dosage is likely not high enough to cause worsening of symptoms.

Hetherington KA, Losek JD. Myasthenia gravis: myasthenia vs. cholinergic crisis. *Pediatr Emerg Care*. August 2005;21(8):546-548. doi:10.1097/01.pec.0000173353.76142.81

7. **The answer is C.** A recent class I randomized controlled trial showed that IVIg has comparable efficacy to plasma exchange in moderate to severe myasthenia gravis. Both are well tolerated, and the duration of effects is comparable.

Barth D, Nabavi Nouri M, Ng E, et al. Comparison of IVIg and PLEX in patients with myasthenia gravis. *Neurology*. June 7, 2011;76(23):2017-2023. doi:10.1212/WNL.0b013e31821e5505

8. **The answer is A.** Indications for mechanical ventilation in myasthenia gravis patients include an FVC ≤15 mL/kg (normal ≥60 mL/kg), a NIF ≤20 cm H_2O (normal ≥70 cm H_2O), or PEF ≤40 cm H_2O (normal ≥100 cm H_2O). One should not wait for the ABG to become abnormal before securing the airway because this occurs late in the course of myasthenia gravis crisis, after the patient has already decompensated.

Bershad EM, Feen ES, Suarez JI. Myasthenia gravis crisis. *South Med J*. January 2008;101(1):63-69. doi:10.1097/SMJ.0b013e31815d4398

9. **The answer is B.** A high-dose initiation therapy is recommended for patients in myasthenic crisis who are already in the controlled setting of an ICU and in need of rapid improvement. This should be done in parallel with IVIg or plasma exchange because high-dose corticosteroid can cause transient worsening of the myasthenia symptoms.

Jani-Acsadi A, Lisak R. Myasthenic crisis: guidelines for prevention and treatment. *J Neurol Sci*. October 15, 2007;261(1-2):127-133. doi:10.1016/j.jns.2007.04.045

10. **The answer is A.** In spinal cord injury, a sensory level is often present on the neurological examination. Patients usually have extensor plantar responses suggesting corticospinal tract dysfunction. In addition, the presentation is sudden rather than progressive. Similar findings including long tract signs are observed in MS. Loss of reflexes is more suggestive of a peripheral nervous system disorder although in acute spinal cord injury reflexes could also be absent. The findings in this patient do not localize to the spinal cord. CIDP presents with similar findings but the clinical course is more insidious. The diagnosis of CIDP requires that symptoms are present for at least 8 weeks or more in a progressive fashion. In this case, the most likely diagnosis is GBS. GBS is an acute immune-mediated disorder of the peripheral nervous system, usually presenting as an acute ascending paralysis. GBS is the most common cause of postinfectious neuromuscular paralysis worldwide with an incidence between 0.6 and four cases per 100,000. The most commonly identified precipitant is *Campylobacter jejuni*. Epstein-Barr virus, cytomegalovirus, HIV, and mycoplasma pneumoniae have all been associated with GBS. The weakness reaches nadir at 2 to 4 weeks followed by recovery, which may occur over the course of several months or be partial. Respiratory weakness and dysautonomia are potential life-threatening complications. Variants of GBS are acute inflammatory demyelinating polyradiculoneuropathy (AIDP), which is the most frequent type; acute motor axonal neuropathy (AMAN); acute motor and sensory axonal neuropathy (AMSAN); acute pandysautonomia; and Miller Fisher syndrome. Miller Fisher syndrome classically presents

with ophthalmoplegia, ataxia, and hyporeflexia in a descending fashion rather than ascending paralysis.

Uncini A, Kuwabara S. Electrodiagnostic criteria for Guillain-Barré syndrome: a critical revision and the need for an update. *Clin Neurophysiol.* August 2012;123(8):1487-1495. doi:10.1016/j.clinph.2012.01.025

Vucic S, Kiernan MC, Cornblath DR. Guillain-Barré syndrome: an update. *J Clin Neurosci.* June 2009;16(6):733-741. doi:10.1016/j.jocn.2008.08.033

11. **The answer is A.** Lumbar puncture is an important investigative tool in diagnosing GBS. Elevated cerebrospinal fluid (CSF) protein with a normal CSF cell count (albumin-cytologic dissociation) is seen. Even though cell counts up to 50 cells/mm^3 are reported, an abnormal CSF cell count warrants further CSF studies to exclude underlying infections. In such cases, the patient's HIV status must be assessed. Of note, CSF studies can be normal in the first week of the disease. Other important studies that are necessary to evaluate this patient's symptoms include electromyography (EMG) and nerve conduction velocity (NCV) studies. EMG is performed to assess axonal injury and is more meaningful in the later phases of the disease. NCV studies can show prolongation of H-reflex latencies, prolonged F-wave latencies, or absence of F-wave responses. These findings may be the only abnormalities in the initial study, particularly early in the disease course. Prolongation of latencies and slowing of conduction velocities can be seen either initially or later on as the disease progresses. If the NCV studies are normal, the study should be repeated in 1 to 2 weeks. The clinical presentation will dictate infectious disease evaluation that may include stool cultures and serology for *Campylobacter jejuni*, HIV serology, Epstein-Barr virus, mycoplasma pneumonia, or cytomegalovirus.

Vucic S, Kiernan MC, Cornblath DR. Guillain-Barré syndrome: an update. *J Clin Neurosci.* June 2009;16(6):733-741. doi:10.1016/j.jocn.2008.08.033

12. **The answer is A.** Based on class 1 studies, IVIg and plasmapheresis are both equally efficacious for treating GBS. Trials of treatment with plasma exchange followed by IVIg have failed to reveal additional clinical benefit. There is currently no evidence that a second course of IVIg is effective in patients who continue to deteriorate, although ongoing trials are investigating the benefits of a second IVIg course in selected patients with poor prognosis. The most common side effects encountered with IVIg are headache, nausea, chills, fever, and hypertension. Hypercoagulability and renal failure are more serious adverse effects related to IVIg treatment. The most common side effects encountered with plasmapheresis are hypotension, bleeding, and allergic reaction. Each patient should be evaluated individually regarding adverse effect profile before choosing IVIg or plasmapheresis. Corticosteroids do not modify the long-term outcome and are found to be ineffective in most studies. Therefore, corticosteroids are not recommended for the treatment of GBS.

Hughes RA, Swan AV, van Doorn PA. Corticosteroids for Guillain-Barré syndrome. *Cochrane Database Syst Rev.* February 17, 2010;(2):CD001446. doi:10.1002/14651858.CD001446.pub2

Patwa HS, Chaudhry V, Katzberg H, et al. Evidence-based guideline: intravenous immunoglobulin in the treatment of neuromuscular disorders: report of the Therapeutics and Technology Assessment Subcommittee of the American Academy of Neurology. *Neurology.* March 27, 2012;78(13):1009-1015. doi:10.1212/WNL.0b013e31824de293

Willison HJ, Jacobs BC, van Doorn PA. Guillain-Barré syndrome. *Lancet.* August 13, 2016;388(10045):717-727. doi:10.1016/S0140-6736(16)00339-1

13. **The answer is C.** SIADH is a well-known and usually overlooked electrolyte disorder associated with GBS. Many patients are asymptomatic. The pathophysiology of SIADH in GBS is unknown; however several hypotheses have been offered, including downward osmotic resetting and enhanced renal tubular sensitivity to antidiuretic hormone (ADH). Some studies have suggested that GBS is more severe in patients who developed SIADH. Pseudohyponatremia due to laboratory artifact can also occur in GBS patients who have been treated with IVIg.

Saifudheen K, Jose J, Gafoor VA, et al. Guillain-Barré syndrome and SIADH. *Neurology.* February 22, 2011;76(8):701-704. doi:10.1212/WNL.0b013e31820d8b40

14. **The answer is D.** Cardiovascular abnormalities seen in GBS are attributed to autonomic neuropathy. Common cardiovascular complications are rhythm abnormalities (bradyarrhythmias, sustained sinus tachycardia, atrial and ventricular arrhythmias), blood pressure variability (hypotension or hypertension), myocardial involvement (myocarditis, neurogenic stunned myocardium, heart failure), acute coronary syndromes (ST-elevation myocardial infarction [STEMI]), and electrocardiographic changes (giant T waves, prolonged QT intervals, ST–T changes, U waves, atrioventricular block, bradycardia, and tachycardia).

Mukerji S, Aloka F, Farooq MU, et al. Cardiovascular complications of the Guillain-Barré syndrome. *Am J Cardiol.* November 15, 2009;104(10):1452-1455. doi:10.1016/j.amjcard.2009.06.069

15. **The answer is C.** This patient has TRF. Up to 16% of patients with GBS can have one or more episodes of worsening motor or sensory symptoms after an initial improvement or stabilization of symptoms. The fluctuations are unrelated to the treatment modality and are suggested to be due to a prolonged immune attack on the peripheral nervous system. Acute onset chronic inflammatory demyelinating polyneuropathy (CIDP) should be considered if a patient deteriorates more than three times or if symptoms continue to worsen after 8 weeks from the onset of the initial symptoms.

Ruts L, Van Koningsveld R, Van Doorn PA. Distinguishing acute-onset CIDP from Guillain-Barré syndrome with treatment-related fluctuations. *Neurology.* 2005;65:138-140. doi:10.1212/WNL.0b013e3181e07d14

Visser LH, van der Meché FG, Meulstee J, et al. Risk factors for treatment related clinical fluctuations in Guillain-Barré syndrome. Dutch Guillain-Barré study group. *J Neurol Neurosurg Psychiatry.* 1998;64:242-244. doi:10.1136/jnnp.64.2.242

Willison HJ, Jacobs BC, van Doorn PA. Guillain-Barré syndrome. *Lancet.* August 13, 2016;388(10045):717-727. doi:10.1016/S0140-6736(16)00339-1

16. **The answer is D.** This patient has critical illness myopathy (CIM), which typically presents as flaccid weakness and failure to wean from the ventilator. Patients who have been mechanically ventilated for as little as 4 to 7 days duration can develop CIM; other risk factors include sepsis, systemic inflammatory response syndrome (SIRS), and multiorgan failure. The clinical features may be indistinguishable from critical illness polyneuropathy (CIP), although there is typically lack of sensory involvement in CIM. An electrodiagnostic study can be helpful in distinguishing between the two. Preferential loss of muscle myosin, muscle necrosis, and sodium channelopathy causing reduced muscle membrane excitability are thought to play a role in CIM.

de Letter MA, Schmitz PI, Visser LH, et al. Risk factors for the development of polyneuropathy and myopathy in critically ill patients. *Crit Care Med.* 2001;29:2281-2286. doi:10.1097/00003246-200112000-00008

Latronico N, Bolton CF. Critical illness polyneuropathy and myopathy: a major cause of muscle weakness and paralysis. *Lancet Neurol.* 2011;10:931-941. doi:10.1016/S1474-4422(11)70178-8

Sher JH, Shafiq SA, Schutta HS. Acute myopathy with selective lysis of myosin filaments. *Neurology.* 1979;29:100-106. doi:10.1212/wnl.29.1.100

17. **The answer is A.** This patient likely has critical illness polyneuropathy (CIP). While CIP can mimic critical illness myopathy (CIM), this patient had absent reflexes suggestive of a neuropathic process. Microvascular changes (caused by sepsis) lead to vascular permeability and edema of the nerve endings, facilitating the passage of neurotoxic factors into the endoneurium and formation of endoneural edema. This causes impaired energy delivery to the axon, leading to axonal death. Neurotoxic effects of hyperglycemia may impair the microcirculation to peripheral nerves, and consequent axonal degeneration (which might explain the improvement in CIP that occurs with intensive insulin therapy). There is no direct evidence that peripheral nerve microcirculation is impaired.

Bolton CF. Neuromuscular manifestations of critical illness. *Muscle Nerve.* 2005;32:140-163. doi:10.1002/mus.20304

Hermans G, Van den Berghe G. Clinical review: intensive care unit acquired weakness. *Critical Care.* 2015;19:274. doi:10.1186/s13054-015-0993-7

18. **The answer is A.** The presence of sensory abnormalities (clinically and electrically) can help distinguish CIP from CIM. In CIM, there is a reduction in the CMAP (or motor) amplitudes and an increase in duration; the increased CMAP duration is an important electrical feature of CIM. Alternatively, an increased CMAP duration may be seen in demyelinating neuropathy; however, in this setting it is typically accompanied by conduction block and slowing of conduction velocities in the demyelinating range.

Goodman BP, Harper CM, Boon AJ. Prolonged compound muscle action potential duration in critical illness myopathy. *Muscle Nerve*. 2009;40:1040-1042. doi:10.1002/mus.21445

19. **The answer is D.** Aminoglycosides are well established to impair neuromuscular transmission and produce clinically significant weakness. Microelectrode studies on nerve muscle preparations suggest that the effect is presynaptic, postsynaptic, or both, and may depend on the specific aminoglycoside used. Telithromycin (Ketek), a ketolide antibiotic, has been observed to cause severe myasthenia gravis exacerbation in some patients and is not recommended for use in myasthenia. Fluoroquinolones have also been associated with anecdotal reports of increased weakness in myasthenic patients. Acute worsening of myasthenia gravis has been reported following administration of ciprofloxacin, a fluoroquinolone. Penicillin generally has a low risk of mysasthenia gravis exacerbation.

Capute AJ, Kim YI, Sanders DB. Neuromuscular blocking effects of therapeutic concentrations of various antibiotics on normal rat skeletal muscle. A quantitative comparison. *J Pharmacol Exp Ther*. 1981;217:369-378.

Jennett AM, Bali D, Jasti P, et al. Telithromycin and myasthenic crisis. *Clin Infect Dis*. 2006;43:1621-1622. doi:10.1086/509646

Omar A, Latronico N. Neurologic aspects of systemic disease. In: Biller J, Ferro JM, eds. *Handbook of Clinical Neurology (3rd Series): Neurologic Aspects of Systemic Disease Part III*. Vol. 121. Elsevier; 2014.

Pittinger CB, Eryasa Y, Adamson R. Antibiotic induced paralysis. *Anesth Analg*. 1970;49:487-501. doi:10.1213/00000539-197005000-00033

20. **The answer is D.** NMS and SS are rare, life-threatening disorders that are typically medication-induced. Both share similar clinical features such as fever, altered mental status, and hypertonicity. The presence of neuromuscular excitation such as clonus, hyperreflexia, tremor, and hyperkinesia are strongly suggestive of SS. In contrast, NMS is characterized by muscular "lead-pipe" rigidity, extrapyramidal symptoms, and hyporeflexia. MH is a potentially life-threatening clinical syndrome of hypermetabolism involving the skeletal muscle, which can present with fever, tachycardia, and muscle rigidity leading to rhabdomyolysis. MH is an autosomal dominant myopathy, most commonly due to mutation within the ryanodine receptor (*RYR1*) resulting in large quantities of calcium to be released from the sarcoplasmic reticulum of skeletal muscle causing a hypermetabolic state after exposure to triggering agents (typically by the volatile inhalational anesthetic agents and the muscle relaxant succinylcholine, though other drugs have also been implicated).

Keary CJ, Nejad SH, Rasimas JJ, et al. Intoxications associated with agitation, tachycardia, hypertension, and fever: differential diagnosis, evaluation, and management. *Prim Care Companion CNS Disord*. 2013;15(3):PCC.12f01459. doi:10.4088/PCC.12f01459

MacLennan DH, Duff C, Zorzato F, et al. Ryanodine receptor gene is a candidate for predisposition to malignant hyperthermia. *Nature*. February 8, 1990;343(6258):559-561. doi:10.1038/343559a0

Sokoro AA, Zivot J, Ariano RE. Neuroleptic malignant syndrome versus serotonin syndrome: the search for a diagnostic tool. *Ann Pharmacother*. 2011;45:e50. doi:10.1345/aph.1P787

7 CNS Infections

DORIS KUNG AND ROHINI SAMUDRALWAR

▪ QUESTIONS

1. A 40-year-old male traveling from Colombia developed 2 days of progressive facial weakness, followed by difficulty swallowing, and started experiencing numbness in his fingers. One week prior to presentation, he had headache, myalgias, and conjunctivitis without fevers. Physical examination on arrival showed facial diplegia, tachypnea, and drooling. He was alert and able to follow commands but had weakness of head flexion, minimal weakness of the extremities, and diminished reflexes in all extremities. Cerebrospinal fluid (CSF) showed elevated protein and normal white blood cells. Diagnostic imaging studies of the brain and spine returned negative. What infectious agent would **not** likely cause his clinical picture?

   A. Dengue virus
   B. West Nile virus (WNV)
   C. Chikungunya virus
   D. Zika virus (ZIKV)
   E. Powassan virus (POW)

2. A 45-year-old man presents with 2 to 3 days of altered behavior, fever, seizures, and headaches. His EEG reveals left temporal periodic lateralized epileptiform discharges (PLEDs) and slowing in that region. Cerebrospinal fluid (CSF) studies are obtained. What is **not** a poor prognostic factor?

   A. Initial poor level of consciousness
   B. Generalized seizures on presentation
   C. Age
   D. Delayed initiation of treatment
   E. Diffusion restriction on MRI

3. A 65-year-old male presents with headache and altered mental status (AMS). He is found to have an intracranial hemorrhage with associated intraventricular involvement and subsequent hydrocephalus requiring an external ventricular drain (EVD). Although there is initial improvement in his mentation, he develops fever 1 week later and becomes more somnolent. Repeat imaging does not reveal any significant changes. Cerebrospinal fluid (CSF) analysis reveals low glucose and positive CSF culture for *Staphylococcus aureus*. Which empiric therapy has the highest level of evidence for this condition?

   A. Meropenem and fluoroquinolone
   B. Vancomycin and antipseudomonal beta lactam
   C. Second- or third-generation cephalosporin
   D. Vancomycin and metronidazole
   E. Ertapenem and vancomycin

4. Which central nervous system (CNS) complications can occur with infective endocarditis (IE), in order from the most to least common?

   A. Meningitis, embolic stroke, hemorrhagic stroke
   B. Embolic stroke, hemorrhagic stroke, meningitis
   C. Embolic stroke, intracranial mycotic aneurysm, hemorrhagic stroke
   D. Intracranial mycotic aneurysm, hemorrhagic stroke, embolic stroke
   E. Hemorrhagic stroke, embolic stroke, intracranial mycotic aneurysm

5. A 3-week-old infant is brought in with decreased alertness, lethargy, and fever. Which is the **least** likely cause of infection in this patient?

   A. *Neisseria meningitidis*
   B. *Streptococcus agalactiae*
   C. *Listeria monocytogenes*
   D. *Haemophilus influenzae*
   E. *Escherichia coli*

6. A 40-year-old man returned from Ghana and admitted to forgetting to take his mefloquine. He complained of headache, fever, and abdominal pain, and these quickly progressed to a comatose state. What stain is used to confirm the infection?

   A. Hematoxylin and eosin (H&E)
   B. India ink
   C. Gram stain
   D. Congo red
   E. Giemsa

7. A 40-year-old man presents with acute onset of left leg more than arm and facial weakness. His family member reports he had a vesicular rash of the face 2 weeks ago. What is the hazard ratio (HR) for patients with herpes zoster ophthalmicus developing an ischemic stroke in 1 year?

   A. 1.31
   B. 2.61
   C. 3.13
   D. 4.28
   E. 5.14

8. A 47-year-old HIV patient presents with headache, stiff neck, and altered mental status (AMS). A lumbar puncture (LP) is done showing opening pressure of 38 cmH_2O. Cerebrospinal fluid (CSF) studies reveal a positive India ink stain; white cell count, protein, and glucose are normal. MRI brain shows enhancing lesions with little mass effect. What is the best treatment for this patient?

   A. Amphotericin B × 2 weeks
   B. Amphotericin B + flucytosine × 1 week
   C. Amphotericin B + flucytosine × 2 weeks
   D. Amphotericin B + flucytosine × 2 weeks + fluconazole for 10 weeks
   E. Amphotericin B + flucytosine × 10 weeks + fluconazole for 10 weeks

9. The patient in the preceding question develops worsening altered mentation 2 weeks following his presentation to the hospital. Which factor(s) would **not** increase the risk of morbidity or mortality?

   A. High baseline cerebrospinal fluid (CSF) opening pressures greater than or equal to 250 mmH_2O
   B. Altered mental status (AMS) on presentation

C. Treatment with antiretroviral therapy (ART) along with antifungal treatment upon presentation

D. CSF study with white blood cell (WBC) count of 30 cells/mL and protein of 67 mg/dL

E. All of the above would increase the risk of morbidity and mortality

10. A 32-year-old man from Mexico presents with generalized tonic–clonic seizures. CT scan shows characteristic diffuse lesions in the parenchyma. On examination, he also has focal weakness, parkinsonian symptoms, and papilledema, and complains of decreased vision. Which symptom(s) is/are **not** typical of neurocysticercosis?

A. Focal weakness

B. Decreased vision

C. Seizures

D. Parkinsonian symptoms

E. None of the above

11. A 15-year-old girl with myasthenia gravis presents with difficulty breathing. Her family reports that she had a urinary tract infection (UTI) and was on trimethoprim–sulfamethoxazole. She is admitted in crisis and intubated. While in the ICU, she receives 5 days of intravenous immunoglobulin (IVIg). Her weakness and shortness of breath improve, but she develops a mild headache, which is treated with ibuprofen. Before discharge, she is administered a pneumococcal vaccine. Two days later, she presents with altered mental status (AMS), fever, and neck stiffness. Cerebrospinal fluid (CSF) shows a mildly elevated protein of 53 (normal range = 12–45 mg/dL), normal glucose of 60 (normal range = 40–80 mg/dL), normal red blood cell (RBC) count, elevated white blood cell (WBC) count of 50 (normal <10 per µL) with lymphocytic predominance, and a negative Gram stain. What is the likely cause of her symptoms?

A. IVIg

B. Trimethoprim–sulfamethoxazole

C. Vaccine

D. Ibuprofen

E. Any of the above

12. A 67-year-old man presents with neck stiffness, headache, right leg weakness, and fever. His symptoms progress rapidly to flaccid paralysis and areflexia. Cerebrospinal fluid (CSF) studies show elevated white blood cell (WBC) count with lymphocytic predominance, normal red blood cell (RBC) count, elevated protein (85 mg/dL), and normal glucose. CSF Gram stain and bacterial cultures are negative. What is a possible viral agent responsible for this man's meningitis?

A. Flavivirus family

B. Adenovirus family

C. Enterovirus family

D. Herpes virus family

E. Hanta virus family

13. A 45-year-old man with HIV, on antiretroviral therapy (ART) inconsistently, presents with 1 month of worsening mental status, left visual field deficit, and right-sided weakness. His MRI shows two nonenhancing subcortical white matter lesions in the left parietal and right occipital areas without surrounding edema. On T2-weighted imaging, the lesions are hyperintense, and on T1-weighted imaging, the lesions are hypointense. Which factors may increase the risk of worsening the disease?

A. CD4 greater than 100 cells/uL

B. Hepatitis C

C. Intravenous (IV) drug use

D. Highly active antiretroviral therapy (HAART)

E. Steroid treatment

14. A 30-year-old woman presents with back pain and fever. On examination, she has some mild lower extremity weakness, but the examination is limited by pain. She admits to intravenous (IV) drug use in the past month. What is the most likely causative organism?

A. *Mycobacterium tuberculosis*

B. *Pseudomonas aeruginosa*

C. *Staphylococcus aureus*

D. *Cryptococcus*

E. *Haemophilus influenza*

15. A 47-year-old woman is brought into the hospital for chest pain. Having been admitted, she is noted to have altered behavior the next morning. Her neurological examination is nonfocal except that when she is shown a pen, she says it is a button; when asked what color shirt the doctor is wearing, she states an incorrect color; when she walks to the bathroom, she runs into the walls; when asked how many fingers are held up in front of her face, she is always incorrect in all quadrants. Her CT scan shows bilateral occipital strokes, and transthoracic echocardiogram shows a mobile mass on the mitral valve. Blood cultures confirm bacteremia. Which factor is the least likely to increase her risk for embolism?

A. Vegetation of 15 mm

B. Mitral valve vegetation

C. *Streptococcus agalactiae* infection

D. *Staphylococcus aureus* infection

E. Tricuspid valve vegetation

16. In the preceding case, which factor may delay surgery for valve replacement?

A. Uncontrolled infection

B. Ischemic stroke

C. Intracranial hemorrhage

D. Heart failure

E. Prosthetic valve endocarditis

17. A 65-year-old woman with Alzheimer's dementia presents with fever, flank pain, pyuria, seizures, and altered mental status (AMS). She is found to have a single ring-enhancing lesion with mass effect in the right frontal region on brain imaging. She is also noted to have a facial fracture possibly resulting from a fall after a seizure. What would be your initial choice in treatment?

A. First- or second-generation cephalosporin, carbapenem, and stereotactic aspiration

B. Third- or fourth-generation cephalosporin, metronidazole, Diflucan, craniotomy, and anticonvulsant

C. Third- or fourth-generation cephalosporin, metronidazole, carbapenem, craniotomy, and anticonvulsant

D. Third- or fourth-generation cephalosporin, metronidazole, vancomycin, stereotactic aspiration, and anticonvulsant

E. None of the above

18. A patient with AIDS presents with headaches and altered mental status (AMS) for the past 2 days. The MRI of the brain shows a single ring-enhancing lesion in the parenchyma with some mass effect. What percentage of patients with toxoplasmosis in the central nervous system (CNS) have multiple ring-enhancing lesions on presentation?

A. 40%
B. 50%
C. 60%
D. 70%
E. 80%

19. A 12-year-old child who recently emigrated from India presents with headache, neck stiffness, fever, and multiple cranial neuropathies. Two weeks before, the patient had been complaining of malaise, anorexia, cough, and weight loss. A chest x-ray shows hilar adenopathy. The patient's MRI with contrast reveals hydrocephalus, basal cistern enhancement, and several ring-enhancing lesions. What is the best treatment of choice for this patient?

A. Rifampin and isoniazid
B. No treatment; wait for biopsy
C. Rifampin, isoniazid, pyrazinamide, ethambutol, and dexamethasone
D. Rifampin, isoniazid, pyrazinamide, and ethambutol
E. Dexamethasone alone

20. A 56-year-old male who had a recent aortic valve replacement with a bioprosthetic valve was admitted for sudden onset left-sided headache, right hemiplegia, and altered mentation. On admission, he had a fever of 102°F and blood pressure was 192/85. CT of the head showed a left cortical intracerebral hemorrhage (ICH). Given his history and presentation, the most concerning etiology of the ICH is:

A. Hypertension-related
B. Mycotic aneurysm
C. Anticoagulation
D. Hemorrhagic conversion of ischemic infarction
E. Abscess

21. A 55-year-old male presented with drainage from his right ear, swelling of his right face, and severe headaches. He was found to have a large phlegmon in his right maxillary sinus and leptomeningeal enhancement. On further evaluation, he was found to have a large unruptured mycotic aneurysm of the right middle cerebral artery (MCA) on arterial angiography. What is the optimal therapeutic strategy for unruptured mycotic aneurysms?

A. Bactericidal antibiotic therapy for 4 to 6 weeks and surgical intervention in cases with focal symptoms, serial angiography every 2 weeks
B. Endovascular intervention immediately followed by antibiotic therapy for 4 weeks
C. Surgical intervention so no antibiotic treatment is necessary
D. Antibiotic therapy for 4 to 6 weeks and clinical monitoring

22. A 33-year-old female diagnosed with glioblastoma (GBM) multiforme, on high-dose steroids, presented with status epilepticus (SE) requiring intravenous (IV) phenytoin and intubation for airway protection. Prior to seizure onset, her family reported that she was complaining of severe headaches for the past several days. On examination, she remains sedated, unresponsive, and withdraws to noxious stimuli more prominently on the left. Contrast CT imaging shows a ring-enhancing lesion in the left paracentral gyrus with vasogenic edema. Further workup reveals pulmonary infiltrates described to be in a halo shape. Laboratory findings show neutropenia. Given these clinical manifestations, what is the likely etiology of the focal lesion seen on imaging?

A. Aspergillosis
B. Cryptococcus
C. Candida

D. Blastomyces

E. Coccidioides

23. Assuming a nontraumatic lumbar puncture, what characteristics in the cerebrospinal fluid (CSF) can be present to suggest the earlier etiology?

A. Elevated glucose, normal protein, normal opening pressure, elevated white count, no red blood cell (RBC) count

B. Decreased glucose concentration, elevated protein, elevated opening pressure, few RBCs

C. Normal glucose, elevated protein, normal opening pressure, normal white blood cells (WBCs), and no RBCs

D. Normal glucose, elevated protein, elevated opening pressure, normal WBCs, and few RBCs

■ ANSWERS

1. **The answer is E.** POW is a tick-borne virus and is found in the northeastern part of the United States, Canada, and Russia. Previously rare, POW infections have become more common in recent years. If a patient is infected, POW can cause devastating encephalitis or meningioencephalitis. Although it can cause muscle weakness and respiratory failure with death in up to 10% of patients affected, it has not been linked directly to acute inflammatory demyelinating polyradiculoneuropathy (AIDP) as this patient's case suggests. All other viruses listed in the answer choices are mosquito-borne viruses and can cause AIDP.

   The ZIKV, which is the most likely cause of this patient's symptoms, was linked to cases of AIDP in Colombia based on epidemiological data collected by Parra and colleagues in 2016. In the 6 years prior to their study only 20 per month cases of AIDP infection occurred compared to 90 cases per month in the first 12 weeks of 2016 corresponding to the time of an outbreak in ZIKV infections. A total of 68 patients were included in this study and the majority of these patients (97%) had symptoms compatible with ZIKV infection before the onset of the Guillain–Barré syndrome (GBS).

   Dengue virus is known to cause several neurological manifestations, most commonly encephalitis, often in the setting of hemorrhagic fever. AIDP has also been reported. Chikungunya has been prevalent in India and La Reunion Island off the coast of Africa and presents with encephalitis, seizures, and myelopathy. Most recently in 2013 to 2014, AIDP has also been reported in French Polynesia and La Reunion Island. WNV most commonly presents as a polio-like syndrome with acute flaccid paralysis and can also present as AIDP.

   Brizzi, K. Neurologic manifestation of chikungunya virus. *Curr Infect Dis Rep.* 2017;19(2):6. doi:10.1007/s11908-017-0561-1

   Carod-Artal, FJ, Wichmann O, Farrar J, et al. Neurological complications of dengue virus infection. *Lancet Neurol.* 2013;12(9):906-919. doi:10.1016/S1474-4422(13)70150-9

   Ebel GD. Update on Powassan virus: emergence of a North American tick-borne flavivirus. *Annu Rev Entomol.* 2010;55:95-110. doi:10.1146/annurev-ento-112408-085446

   Parra B, Lizarazo J, Jiménez-Arango JA, et al. Guillain–Barré syndrome associated with Zika virus infection in Colombia. *N Engl J Med.* 2016;375(16):1513-1523. doi:10.1056/NEJMoal605564

   Petersen, LR, Brault AC, Nasci RS. West Nile virus: review of the literature. *JAMA.* 2013;310(3):308-315. doi:10.1001/jama.2013.8042

2. **The answer is B.** Herpes simplex encephalitis (HSE) is rare; however, it carries a high rate of death in up to 70% of patients. Almost all cases of HSE are caused by herpes simplex virus-1 (HSV-1). The virus, for unknown reasons, has a predilection for the temporal lobes. It can affect the temporal lobes and adjacent limbic areas usually asymmetrically in adults. In neonates, there can be more diffuse involvement. Diagnosis can be confirmed on the basis of a combination of neuroimaging, CSF polymerase chain reaction (PCR) studies, and EEG. Poor prognostic factors have been determined to be older age, diffusion restriction on MRI, poor level of consciousness at presentation, and delaying initiation of treatment more than 1 day after presentation. Factors that were not definitively associated with poor prognosis included focal neurological deficits, seizures, and extent of central nervous system (CNS) lesions on imaging.

   Singh TD, Fugate JE, Hocker S, et al. Predictors of outcome in HSV encephalitis. *J Neurol.* February 2016;263(2):277-289. doi:10.1007/s00415-015-7960-8

3. **The answer is B.** This patient is likely suffering from ventriculitis after EVD placement. Although there is not a standard for defining infection to diagnose meningitis or ventriculitis after neurosurgery, the Centers for Disease Control's National Healthcare Safety Network suggests at least one of the following criteria: positive CSF culture, CSF pleocytosis, low CSF glucose concentration, positive Gram stain of CSF, positive blood culture, or two of the following symptoms: fever greater than 38°, headache, meningeal signs, or cranial nerve signs in patients older than 1 year. First choice for empiric treatment of healthcare-associated ventriculitis and meningitis is vancomycin plus an antipseudomonal beta-lactam. Vancomycin

trough concentrations should be maintained at 15 to 20 μg/mL in seriously ill adults who are receiving intermittent boluses.

Tunkel AR, Hasbun R, Bhimraj A, et al. 2017 Infectious Diseases Society of America's clinical practice guidelines for healthcare-associated ventriculitis and meningitis. *Clin Infect Dis.* 2017;64(6):34-65. doi:10.1093/cid/ciw861

4. **The answer is B.** IE can cause multiple organ complications. Neurologic complications from IE portend a poor prognosis and occur in about 20% to 55% of IE cases. Left-sided valve IE with *Staphylococcus aureus* infection is a major risk factor for neurologic complications. Embolic strokes occur in 20% to 50% of cases, hemorrhagic strokes occur in 12% to 30% of cases, meningitis occurs in 2% to 20% of cases, and intracranial mycotic aneurysms occur in less than 10% of cases. Embolic strokes can be clinically silent or the presenting symptom of IE. The risk of embolic events is 20% to 50% but decreases significantly to 6% to 21% after antibiotic treatment is started. However, there is an increase in embolic events in the first few days after initiation of antibiotics, and thus surgery is often recommended within the first few days of presentation. Intracranial hemorrhage may result from hemorrhagic transformation of an embolic stroke, ruptured mycotic aneurysm, or even erosion of the vessel walls from septic emboli. Microbleeds have also been observed. Cerebral hemorrhage management is discussed in a later question. In meningitis cases associated with IE, the cerebrospinal fluid (CSF) is only transiently positive for the infective agent. Patients often present with fever, heart murmur, petechiae, and meningeal signs. Mycotic aneurysms are thought to result from arterial emboli that travel into the intraluminal space, or possibly from the spread of the infection hematogenously through the intimal vessels. Vessel imaging with CT or magnetic resonance angiography (MRA) is necessary. Four-vessel angiography should be performed if noninvasive imaging is negative and suspicion is high. Some unruptured mycotic aneurysms will resolve with antibiotic treatment and can be clinically silent. Ruptured, large, or enlarging aneurysms need to have neurosurgical or endovascular intervention.

Sonneville R, Mourvillier B, Bouadma L, et al. Management of neurological complications of infective endocarditis in ICU patients. *Ann Intensive Care.* 2011;1(1):10. doi:10.1186/2110-5820-1-10

5. **The answer is A.** When a patient comes in with symptoms of meningitis, it is important that it is recognized and treated appropriately. A lumbar puncture (LP) and blood cultures should be obtained immediately. The LP should not be delayed unless there is suspicion of possible herniation. If there is a possible risk of mass lesions or increased intracranial pressure, then empiric antibiotic treatment is recommended. Empiric treatment should be chosen on the basis of the age of the patient. *Listeria monocytogenes* is more common in patients younger than 1 month or older than 50 years. Ampicillin is recommended plus cefotaxime or aminoglycoside for coverage of *S. agalactiae, E. coli,* and *Klebsiella* species in patients younger than 1 month. *N. meningitidis* is not considered a common organism of infection in patients younger than 1 month. In patients age 1 to 23 months, the recommendation is to use vancomycin plus a third-generation cephalosporin to cover *Streptococcus pneumoniae, N. meningitidis, S. agalactiae, H. influenzae,* and *E. coli.* In patients age 2 to 50 years, the recommendation is again vancomycin and a third-generation cephalosporin to cover *N. meningitidis* and *S. pneumoniae.* Finally, vancomycin, ampicillin, and a third-generation cephalosporin are recommended in patients older than 50 years to cover *S. pneumoniae, N. meningitidis, L. monocytogenes,* and aerobic Gram-negative bacilli. In children, the use of dexamethasone is still debated, but may be recommended as adjunctive treatment in infants and children with *H. influenzae B* infection.

Tunkel AR, Hartman BJ, Kaplan SL, et al. Practice guidelines for the management of bacterial meningitis. *Clin Infect Dis.* 2004;39(9):1267-1284. doi:10.1086/425368

6. **The answer is E.** Malaria is transmitted to humans via a female *Anopheles* mosquito that carries the *Plasmodium* organism. Four different species of the genus *Plasmodium* are known to cause malaria: *Plasmodium falciparum, Plasmodium ovale, Plasmodium vivax,* and *Plasmodium*

malariae. Clinically, the symptoms of malaria can be characterized by cyclic fevers. The most severe infection is caused by *P. falciparum.* Complications of malaria can involve the nervous system, causing seizures, altered mentation, and coma. Diagnosis of malaria can be suspected in patients with anemia and elevated levels of bilirubin, lactate dehydrogenase, and reticulocyte counts. Malaria is confirmed by Giemsa stains on thick and thin blood smears and can also be detected with Wright's and Field's stains. Rapid diagnostic tests (RDTs) are also available, which detect plasmodial antigens or enzymes. Currently, most RDTs target *P. falciparum*–specific proteins.

Tangpukdee N, Duangdee C, Wilairatana P, et al. Malaria diagnosis: a brief review. *Korean J Parasitol.* 2009;47(2):93-102. doi:10.3347/kjp.2009.47.2.93
Wilson W, Sande M. *Current Diagnosis and Treatment in Infectious Diseases.* New York, NY: Lange Medical Books/McGraw-Hill; 2001:888-889.

7. **The answer is D.** Varicella-Zoster virus (VZV) infection of the central nervous system (CNS) can manifest in many ways. As noted in this case, the patient suffered an ischemic stroke likely due to large vessel vasculopathy from viral invasion of the endothelial cells. VZV can also cause meningitis, encephalitis, cerebellitis, myelitis, ischemic and hemorrhagic strokes, and even demyelinating polyradiculoneuropathies. This patient suffered an episode of herpes zoster ophthalmicus. The exact percent of patients developing ischemic strokes due to zoster infection is not known. A Taiwanese group did a population study of patients known to have had zoster infection and looked at the rate of strokes in 1 year. Patients with the history of zoster infection had an adjusted HR of 1.31 as compared to those without zoster infection. Furthermore, the adjusted HR for patients with herpes zoster ophthalmicus and development of stroke in 1 year was 4.28. Treatment of patients with CNS vasculitis due to VZV infection is intravenous (IV) acyclovir for a minimum of 14 days, with or without addition of corticosteroid.

Grahn A, Studahl M. Varicella-Zoster virus infections of the central nervous system—prognosis, diagnostics, and treatment. *J Infect.* 2015;71(3):281-293. doi:10.1016/j.jinf.2015.06.004
Kang JH, Ho JD, Chen YH, et al. Increased risk of stroke after a herpes zoster attack: a population-based follow-up study. *Stroke.* 2009;40(11):3443-3448. doi:10.1161/STROKEAHA.109.562017

8. **The answer is D.** Diagnosis of cryptococcal central nervous system (CNS) infection in HIV patients is dependent on a high index of suspicion. CNS infection can involve the brain parenchyma and cause single or multiple focal mass lesions called cryptococcomas. CSF evaluation is essential for the diagnosis. The CSF pressure, cryptococcal antigen titer, CSF India ink positivity for *Cryptococcus*, and fungal culture can be helpful. Induction and consolidation treatment of patients with CNS cryptococcal disease is amphotericin B, 0.7 to 1 mg/kg/d plus flucytosine 100 mg/kg/d for 2 weeks, followed by fluconazole 400 to 800 mg/d for at least 10 weeks. Maintenance treatment with fluconazole 200 mg orally daily is recommended lifelong in patients with a history of cryptococcal CNS infection, and CD4 count less than 100 cells/uL. Discontinuing suppressive therapy can be considered in patients on highly active antiretroviral therapy (HAART) who have a CD4 count greater than 100 cells/uL and undetectable or very low HIV ribonucleic acid (RNA) level for greater than or equal to 3 months (minimum of 12 months of treatment).

Perfect JR, Dismukes WE, Dromer F, et al. Clinical practice guidelines for the management of cryptococcal disease: 2010 update by the Infectious Diseases Society of America. *Clin Infect Dis.* 2010;50(3):291-322. doi:10.1086/649858

9. **The answer is D.** This patient likely suffered from immune reconstitution inflammatory syndrome (IRIS). Fortunately, central nervous system (CNS) involvement from IRIS occurs in only about 1% of patients after starting ART. In some studies, the percentage of cryptococcal-related IRIS is 10% to 45% in ART-naïve HIV patients and most occur within the first month of treatment in those also treated for cryptococcal meningitis. Presenting with altered mentation predicts poor prognosis. Initial CSF studies in cryptococcal meningitis patients showed that patients with CSF white blood cell counts of ≤25 cells/mL and protein count ≤50 mg/dL had

higher risk of developing IRIS. Based on the Cryptococcal Optimal ART Timing (COAT) trial, delaying treatment with ART by more than 5 weeks is recommended. Additionally, treatment of increased intracranial pressures (ICPs) in cryptococcal meningitis may be very difficult and not as responsive to standard treatment. A retrospective observational study of 381 AIDS patients with cryptococcal meningitis showed that patients with high baseline CSF opening pressures greater than or equal to 250 mmH$_2$O were at higher risk for death in the first 2 weeks of diagnosis.

Boulware DR, Bonham SC, Meya DB, et al. Paucity of initial cerebrospinal fluid inflammation in cryptococcal meningitis is associated with subsequent immune reconstitution inflammatory syndrome. *J Infect Dis.* 2010;202(6):962-970. doi:10.1086/655785

Bowen LN, Smith B, Reich D, et al. HIV-associated opportunistic CNS infections: pathophysiology, diagnosis and treatment. *Nat Rev Neurol.* 2016;12:662-674. doi:10.1038/nrneurol.2016.149

Graybill JR, Sobel J, Saag M, et al. Diagnosis and management of increased intracranial pressure in patients with AIDS and cryptococcal meningitis. The NIAID Mycoses Study Group and AIDS Cooperative Treatment Groups. *Clin Infect Dis.* 2000;30(1):47-54. doi:10.1086/313603

10. **The answer is E.** Neurocysticercosis remains a very serious health problem in the world, especially in developing countries. In a majority of patients (70%) with neurocysticercosis, the primary manifestation is seizures, making it the leading cause of acquired epilepsy in the developing world. However, manifestations of neurocysticercosis are varied and numerous, depending on the number and location of central nervous system (CNS) lesions. Cysts can be located in the parenchyma, subarachnoid space, eyes, ventricles, and so on. Massive infection can even affect the muscles of the body. In the acute phase, cysts can cause surrounding edema and inflammation, resulting in increased intracranial pressure (IP) usually due to hydrocephalus. If there are numerous cysticerci, there can be a severe immune response from the host resulting in an encephalitis picture and intracranial hypertension. All of these symptoms (seizures, focal weakness, decreased vision, parkinsonian symptoms, etc.) can be manifestations of neurocysticercosis.

Del Brutto OH. Neurocysticercosis: a review. *Sci World J.* 2011;2012:1-8. doi:10.1100/2012/159821

11. **The answer is E.** Ruling out bacterial meningitis is the obvious first step in the approach to this patient. The Bacterial Meningitis Score developed in 2002 for pediatric patients can be used to risk stratify a patient. The variables that are considered are (a) positive CSF Gram stain, (b) CSF absolute neutrophil count 1,000 cells/μL, (c) CSF protein 80 mg/dL, (d) peripheral blood absolute neutrophil count 10,000 cells/μL, and (e) history of seizure before or at the time of presentation. If the patient does not present with any of these variables, the risk of bacterial meningitis is very low, with a negative predictive value of 100% and a 95% confidence interval (97%–100%). Any of these medications, including IVIg and the pneumococcal vaccine, that the patient received could have caused her to have aseptic meningitis. Once bacterial meningitis is ruled out, drug-induced aseptic meningitis is very likely, given the number of possible causative medications she took.

Jolles S, Sewell WA, Leighton C. Drug-induced aseptic meningitis: diagnosis and management. *Drug Saf.* 2000;22(3):215-226. doi:10.2165/00002018-200022030-00005

Nigrovic LE, Kuppermann N, Macias CG, et al. Clinical prediction rule for identifying children with cerebrospinal fluid pleocytosis at very low risk of bacterial meningitis. *JAMA.* 2007;297(1):52-60. doi:10.1001/jama.297.1.52

12. **The answer is A.** The man most likely has West Nile virus (WNV) infection causing poliomyelitis and meningitis. WNV belongs to the flavivirus family and is transmitted to humans by infected mosquitoes. Neurologic manifestations of WNV infection include meningitis, encephalitis, and myelitis, including acute flaccid (polio-like) monoplegia without other signs of neuroinvasive disease. Patients with West Nile poliomyelitis may present with fever myalgias, encephalopathy, and asymmetric weakness, which can progress quickly to quadriplegia. CSF studies may show lymphocytic pleocytosis and elevated protein. Electrodiagnostic studies show acute denervation in affected muscles with low-amplitude compound muscle action potentials and normal sensory nerve action potentials, representing axonal loss

in motor neurons. Limbs with no motor response or no voluntary muscle activity on needle examination have a poor prognosis for recovery.

Leis AA, Stokic DS. Neuromuscular manifestations of West Nile virus infection. *Front Neurol.* 2012;37(3):1-10. doi:10.3389/fneur.2012.00037

Preston D, Shapiro B. *Electromyography and Neuromuscular Disorders.* Philadelphia, PA: Elsevier; 2005.

13. **The answer is D.** This patient has progressive multifocal leukoencephalopathy (PML), which is caused by a reactivation of the John Cunningham (JC) virus in the central nervous system (CNS). PML is a serious disease that unfortunately has no effective treatment. HAART treatment can lead to immune reconstitution inflammatory syndrome (IRIS) and in some cases can lead to reactivation or enhanced immune response to an inactive or active infection, respectively. IRIS is defined as a paradoxical decline in the clinical status of a patient following immune restoration with ART and has been commonly associated with *Mycobacterium tuberculosis*, cryptococcal, and cytomegalovirus infections. Several factors have been shown to increase the risk of developing IRIS, including first introduction of antiretroviral drugs, active or subclinical opportunistic infection at the time of initiation of combined ART, low CD4 count (<50 cells/mm^3), and rapid immune recovery based on a rapid decrease in HIV plasma viral load. Steroid treatment has been tried but shown to be definitely effective in only one study for the treatment of tuberculosis (TB) associated with IRIS. Although it may improve outcomes in other reactivated infections, adequate treatment trials have not been done to determine this.

Meintjes G, Wilkinson RJ, Morroni C, et al. Randomized placebo-controlled trial of prednisone for paradoxical tuberculosis-associated immune reconstitution inflammatory syndrome. *AIDS.* 2010;24(15):2381-2390. doi:10.1097/QAD.0b013e32833dfc68

Müller M, Wandel S, Colebunders R, et al. Immune reconstitution inflammatory syndrome in patients starting antiretroviral therapy for HIV infection: a systematic review and meta-analysis. *Lancet Infect Dis.* 2010;10(4):251-261. doi:10.1016/S1473-3099(10)70026-8

Tan K, Roda R, Ostrow L, et al. PML-IRIS in patients with HIV infection: clinical manifestations and treatment with steroids. *Neurology.* 2009;72(17):1458-1464. doi: 10.1212/01.wnl.0000343510.08643.74

14. **The answer is C.** The most common cause of spinal epidural abscess is still *Staphylococcus aureus* (two-thirds of patients). However, *Pseudomonas* and *M. tuberculosis* have been increasingly associated with IV drug use. Presentation of a spinal epidural abscess may start with back pain at the level of infection (Stage 1), and cause radicular-type pain in the same dermatomal level (Stage 2), progressing to weakness, sensory symptoms, or bladder and bowel dysfunction (Stage 3), and finally paralysis (Stage 4). The classic clinical triad is back pain, fever, and neurological signs, but these symptoms may not present in every patient. On laboratory testing, many patients will have leukocytosis and positive blood cultures for the offending bacteria. Cerebrospinal fluid (CSF) studies are not routinely recommended because of the risk of meningitis or subdural infection. MRI with IV contrast of the spine is the diagnostic evaluation of choice and can help differentiate the mass from other types of tumors of the spine. Treatment includes emergency decompressive laminectomy if there are focal neurologic deficits and no contraindications and concurrent antibiotic (IV route usually) treatment for 6 weeks. Antimicrobial treatment is started with empiric antibiotics for staphylococcal infection (vancomycin for possible methicillin-resistant *S. aureus*) and Gram-negative bacilli, usually third- or fourth-generation cephalosporins.

Chuo CY, Fu YC, Lu YM, et al. Spinal infection in intravenous drug abusers. *J Spinal Disord Tech.* 2007;20(4):324-328. doi:10.1097/BSD.0b013e31802c144a

Darouiche RO. Spinal epidural abscess. *N Engl J Med.* 2006;355(19):2012-2020. doi:10.1056/NEJMra055111

15. **The answer is E.** This patient suffers from Anton's syndrome or cortical blindness, which is a stroke that affects both occipital cortices from occlusion of bilateral posterior cerebral arteries. Patients with this syndrome will often deny blindness and are not aware of their deficit. Stroke

or transient ischemic attacks (TIAs) comprise 40% to 50% of cases of neurologic complications due to infective endocarditis (IE). Several factors that predispose patients to cerebral emboli include vegetations measuring greater than 10 to 15 mm in size, mobile vegetations, *S. aureus* infection, *S. agalactiae* or fungal infection (due to the size of the vegetation with these latter two infections), and/or mitral valve involvement. Right-sided IE is less likely to cause embolic strokes unless there is a right-to-left shunt. Appropriate treatment with antibiotics early after the recognition of IE can decrease the incidence of stroke.

Brazis PW, Masdeu JC, Biller J. *Localization in Clinical Neurology*. 5th ed. Philadelphia, PA: Lippincott Williams & Wilkins; 2007.

Sonneville R, Mourvillier B, Bouadma L, et al. Management of neurological complications of infective endocarditis in ICU patients. *Ann Intensive Care*. 2011;1(1):10. doi:10.1186/2110-5820-1-10

16. **The answer is C.** The timing of surgery after an embolic event has been debated. Recommendations for management of infective endocarditis (IE) complications have been set forth by the Task Force on the Prevention, Diagnosis, and Treatment of Infective Endocarditis of the European Society of Cardiology (2015) and by the American Association for Thoracic Surgery (AATS) consensus guidelines:

   i. Surgery is recommended without delay (within a few days) after a silent cerebral embolism or transient ischemic attacks (TIAs).

   ii. Neurosurgery or endovascular therapy is recommended for any large, enlarging, or ruptured intracranial infectious aneurysms.

   iii. After a stroke, surgery is indicated for heart failure, uncontrolled infection, abscess, or persisting high embolic risk and should not be delayed (within a few days), unless there is coma or if there is confirmed cerebral hemorrhage on imaging.

   iv. After intracranial hemorrhage, surgery should be postponed for at least 1 month or more.

   Current recommendations do not suggest the use of anticoagulation treatment in patients with IE with and without a stroke or intracranial bleeding. However, if there are compelling reasons for anticoagulation such as atrial fibrillation or mechanical prosthetic valve, then careful consideration of risks and benefits must be discussed and perhaps a lowered International Normalized Ratio (INR) or partial thromboplastin time (PTT) level may be necessary. Antiplatelets may be continued if there is no evidence of major hemorrhage.

Habib G, Lancellotii P, Antunes MJ, et al. 2015 ESC Guidelines on the management of infective endocarditis: the Task Force for the Management of Infective Endocarditis of the European Society of Cardiology (ESC). Endorsed by the European Association for Cardio-Thoracic Surgery (EACTS), the European Association of Nuclear Medicine (EANM). *Eur Heart J*. November 21, 2015;36(44):3075-3128. doi:10.1093/eurheartj/ehv319

Pettersson GB, Coselli JS, Hussain ST, et al. 2016 The American Association for Thoracic Surgery (AATS) consensus guidelines: surgical treatment of infective endocarditis: executive summary. *J Thorac Cardiovasc Surg*. January 24, 2017;153(6):1241-1258.e.29. doi:10.1016/j.jtcvs.2016.09.093

17. **The answer is D.** Cerebral abscesses are fortunately rare. Patients can present with headaches, altered mentation, focal neurological symptoms, and fever. Abscesses can be complications of penetrating trauma of the cranium or neurosurgical operations. Hematogenous or contiguous spread from infections of the oropharynx, paranasal sinuses, and the middle ear are also possible sources of abscesses. Infections can be bacterial, opportunistic, fungal, protozoal, or helminthic. Bacterial infection usually depends on the origin of the infection and the patient's comorbidities. For example, streptococcal infection is usually due to infection from the nasopharynx or oropharynx. Staphylococci can be seen in cases associated with infective endocarditis (IE), trauma, or iatrogenic procedures. Opportunistic and fungal infections are more commonly encountered in immunocompromised patients. Initial antimicrobials are chosen empirically to treat polymicrobial etiologies, since these can be a common cause of abscesses. Choices are usually a third- or fourth-generation cephalosporin, metronidazole, and vancomycin to cover Gram-positive, Gram-negative, and anaerobic organisms.

Open craniotomy versus closed stereotactic drainage has been controversial in the past, but recent reviews have found that stereotactic aspiration in the age of CT imaging has dramatically improved mortality rates compared with excision (6.6% vs. 12.7% mean mortality rates, respectively). Anticonvulsants are recommended early in the treatment, with or without a history of seizures, since they can occur in up to a quarter of patients with cerebral abscesses.

Honda H, Warren DK. Central nervous system infections: meningitis and brain abscess. *Infect Dis Clin North Am.* 2009;23(3):609-623. doi:10.1016/j.idc.2009.04.009

Ratnaike TE, Das S, Gregson BA, et al. A review of brain abscess surgical treatment—78 years: aspiration versus excision. *World Neurosurg.* 2011;76(5):431-436. doi:10.1016/j.wneu.2011.03.048

18. **The answer is D.** CNS toxoplasmosis infection is a common neurologic complication of AIDS. Reactivation of latent toxoplasmosis parasite causes cerebral toxoplasmosis and occurs usually in AIDS patients with CD4 cell counts below 200/μL. Patients often present with fever, headaches, seizures, and focal neurological deficits. Cerebral toxoplasmosis presents with multiple ring-enhancing lesions in about 70% of patients, typically involving the parenchymal white matter or the subcortical gray matter, especially the thalamus and basal ganglia. Unfortunately, distinguishing cerebral toxoplasmosis from lymphoma can often be difficult, and although lesions of primary CNS lymphoma are often multifocal and periventricular, more often standard neuroimaging is insufficient to distinguish the two diseases. Ultimately, antitoxoplasmosis treatment with pyrimethamine and sulfadiazine remains the most revealing method of distinguishing the two. Response to treatment for toxoplasmosis can be seen in 5 days with significant improvement in more than 90% of patients in 14 days.

Berger JR. Mass lesions of the brain in AIDS: the dilemmas of distinguishing toxoplasmosis from primary CNS lymphoma. *AJNR Am J Neuroradiol.* 2003;24(4):554-555.

Chang L, Cornford ME, Chiang FL, et al. Radiologic-pathologic correlation. Cerebral toxoplasmosis and lymphoma in AIDS. *Am J Neuroradiol.* 1995;16(8):1653-1663.

Kiderlen TR, Liesenfeld O, Schürmann D, et al. Toxoplasmic encephalitis in AIDS-patients before and after the introduction of highly active antiretroviral therapy (HAART). *Eur J Clin Microbiol Infect Dis.* 2011;30(12):1521-1525. doi:10.1007/s10096-011-1254-6

19. **The answer is C.** Tuberculous meningitis is a serious, devastating manifestation of extrapulmonary tuberculosis (TB) infection. The exact incidence of extrapulmonary TB is not well known, but is expected to be high because of high rates of pulmonary TB in developing countries. One study in Germany found that out of 26,302 patients, 21.6% had extrapulmonary TB. In this study, risk of extrapulmonary TB was highest in females, children younger than 15 years, and patients immigrating from Asia or Africa. In patients with HIV, the rate of progression to extrapulmonary TB is five times higher than in non-HIV patients. TB meningitis is thought to result from hematogenous spread from pulmonary TB resulting in small granulomas in the brain parenchyma and the meninges. Patients with TB meningitis often present with advanced disease, with fever, headache, altered mental status (AMS), and meningismus. Cranial neuropathies, focal neurological symptoms, and raised intracranial pressure (IP) are seen in more severe cases. The gold standard of diagnosis for tuberculous meningitis is a culture positive for *Mycobacterium tuberculosis* from the spinal fluid; however, time and low sensitivity make this difficult. Polymerase chain reaction (PCR) for the organism has moderate sensitivity and excellent specificity, 58% and 98%, respectively. Neuroimaging of TB meningitis often shows hydrocephalus, parenchymal and/or basilar cistern enhancement, infarctions, edema, and tuberculomas in decreasing frequency. Treatment of tuberculous meningitis relies on early recognition and antituberculous drugs, including isoniazid, rifampicin, ethambutol, and pyrazinamide, for 2 months. Isoniazid and rifampin are then continued for 7 or 10 months; some recommend longer, up to 12 months. A recent Cochrane Database review even suggested that 6 months of treatment may be sufficient; however, there are no randomized controlled trials comparing the safety and efficacy of durations of treatment in TB meningitis. A 2008 Cochrane review of the treatment of tuberculous meningitis shows that the use of steroids in the setting of tuberculous meningitis is recommended to decrease death and disability, but this was found to be significant in only non-HIV patients. Studies in HIV patients

were small and not powered to detect a significant result, so a recommendation could not be made for this patient population.

Garg RK. Tuberculous meningitis. *Acta Neurol Scand*. 2010;122(2):75-90. doi:10.1111/j.1600-0404.2009.01316.x

Jullien S, Ryan H, Modi M, et al. Six months therapy for tuberculous meningitis. *Cochrane Database Syst Rev*. 2016;9:CD012091. doi:10.1002/14651858.CD012091.pub2

Prasad K, Singh B. Corticosteroids for managing tuberculous meningitis. *Cochrane Database Syst Rev*. 2008;1:CD002244. doi:10.1002/14651858

20. **The answer is B.** Mycotic aneurysms are rare complications of infective endocarditis (IE) and have been reported to occur in 2% of IE patients. In a large literature review of patients with IC and mycotic intracranial aneurysms from 2001, several clinical presentations were described. The most common appeared to be the presence of hemorrhage (52%), followed by infarction (20%), or infarction with hemorrhage (6%). Mycotic aneurysms typically are located in the anterior circulation, often within distal branches of the middle cerebral artery (MCA). Cerebral mycotic aneurysms are formed when septic emboli migrate and lodge within the vasa vasorum or intraluminal space of the of the cerebral vasculature. The septic emboli then produce inflammatory destruction of the arterial wall, through the adventitial layer resulting in arterial dilatation. Of note, mycotic aneurysms tend to involve distal vasculature which helps distinguish them from the proximally occurring congenital/berry aneurysms. The most common pathogen is streptococci and less commonly staphylococci. Fungal aneurysms may be seen in immunocompromised patients and can occur in proximal vessels.

Mylonakis, E, Calderwood SB. Infective endocarditis in adults. *N Eng J Med*. 2001;345(18):1318-1330. doi:10.1056/NEJMra010082

Roos, KL. *Principles of Neurologic Infectious Diseases: Principles and Practice*. New York, NY: McGraw-Hill Professional; 2004.

21. **The answer is A.** Management of mycotic aneurysms remains controversial. No randomized controlled trials exist. Several reviews, including one by Chun and colleagues, presented a patient treatment algorithm based on the review of 27 cases of mycotic aneurysms and suggested nonmedical intervention as the first option for unruptured aneurysms. Endovascular intervention can be undertaken for ruptured aneurysms in cases with low risk of intervention. Surgical treatment of a ruptured aneurysm is suggested in unstable patients. An aneurysm has a high surgical risk if there is circumferential vessel involvement, if the location is proximal, or if parent artery sacrifice cannot be done due to considerable neurological deficits. Expert recommendation is to start with antibiotic therapy for 4 to 6 weeks with serial angiography every 2 weeks. If there is failure of shrinkage of aneurysm, neurosurgical intervention may be needed. One third of repeat angiographies show disappearance of aneurysm. Most common pathogens include *Streptococci viridans* and *Staphylococcus aureus*.

Chun JY, Smith W, Halbach VV, et al. Current multimodality management of infectious intracranial aneurysms. *Neurosurgery*. June 2001;48(6):1203-1213; discussion 1213-1214. doi:10.1097/0006123-200106000-00001

Roos, KL. *Principles of Neurologic Infectious Diseases: Principles and Practice*. New York, NY: McGraw-Hill Professional; 2004:461-462.

22. **The answer is A.** (The rationale is in Answer 23.)

23. **The answer is B.** Typically fungal meningitis presents as a progressive, chronic, or subacute meningitis, more commonly in immunosuppressed individuals, and involving other organ systems. Invasive pulmonary aspergillosis has a typical "halo" like appearance on radiography. Sustained neutropenia is also a risk factor for invasive aspergillosis. A major complication of invasive aspergillosis includes central nervous system (CNS) involvement and is associated with a mortality rate of 90%. Dissemination can occur through hematogenous spread from a pulmonary focus or from direct extension of paranasal sinus infection. CNS aspergillosis is the most lethal manifestation of infection due to *Aspergillus* species and can be difficult to treat. Cryptococcus, can present with intracranial lesions, typically involving

cranial nerves; however, it does not have the pulmonary features seen in this patient. *Candida* typically colonizes through alterations in mucosa or skin rather than through the pulmonary system, but is more prevalent in patients with neutropenia. Coccidioides rarely presents as CNS mass lesions whereas blastomyces does in the setting of pneumonitis or genitourinary infections rather than discrete pulmonary lesions. Fungal meningitis can appear nonspecific clinically and radiographically. CSF typically shows lymphocytic pleocytosis, elevated protein, and low glucose. A rapid diagnosis is necessary to avoid further complications, which include seizures, cerebral infarction, hydrocephalus, and elevated CSF pressure.

Roos, KL. *Principles of Neurologic Infectious Diseases: Principles and Practice.* New York, NY: McGraw-Hill Professional; 2004:175-177.

8

Toxic–Metabolic Disorders

ELISSA K. FORY

■ QUESTIONS

1. A 68-year-old woman with bipolar disorder, depression, and hypertension was admitted to the hospital after a fall. Her home medications included lithium and fluoxetine. She had never consumed alcohol. On initial examination, she had expressive aphasia but no weakness. A CT scan of the head revealed an acute left fronto-temporo-parietal subdural hematoma with mass effect and midline shift. The subdural was evacuated by craniotomy, and her aphasia improved. Three days after evacuation, she became confused and agitated. A CT scan of the head showed expected postoperative changes. A 24-hour EEG had diffuse slowing, with occasional sharp waves seen from the left temporal lobe. She was given small intermittent doses of haloperidol and lorazepam for agitation. On postoperative day 4, vital signs were temperature 100.8°F, pulse 120 beats/min, respiratory rate (RR) 18 breaths/min, and blood pressure (BP) fluctuated from 90/50 mmHg to 150/80 mmHg. She was agitated, more confused, and diaphoretic. Her pupils were 6 mm and reactive in ambient light. She held both arms up antigravity without drift but was tremulous. Muscle tone was increased in bilateral lower extremities, and she had clonus on both patellar and ankle reflex testing. Liver function tests and creatine phosphokinase (CPK) were normal. A lithium level was 0.7 mmol/L. What is the most likely diagnosis?

   A. Ethanol withdrawal
   B. Lithium toxicity
   C. Serotonin syndrome (SS)
   D. Neuroleptic malignant syndrome (NMS)
   E. Malignant hyperthermia (MH)

2. What is the most common cause of acute liver failure in the United States?

   A. Acute hepatitis B infection
   B. Acute hepatitis C infection
   C. Idiosyncratic drug reactions to drugs such as phenytoin, valproic acid, ribavirin, and nucleoside reverse transcriptase inhibitors
   D. Autoimmune hepatitis
   E. Acetaminophen overdose

3. A 30-year-old man was admitted to an inpatient psychiatric hospital for depression with psychotic features. He was on escitalopram and quetiapine as an outpatient, and these medications were continued. Due to acute psychosis, he received multiple doses of intravenous (IV) haloperidol and the quetiapine was up titrated. One week after his hospitalization, he had gradual onset of slowed movements and decreased motor activity. On neurologic examination 10 days after admission, he was awake but nonconversant. His pupils were 4 mm and briskly

reactive. There was rigidity in all four extremities without cogwheeling, decreased deep tendon reflexes, and no clonus. His vitals were temperature 103°F, pulse 105 beats/min, and blood pressure (BP) 165/100 mmHg. Laboratory studies included a white blood cell (WBC) count of $12 \times 10^3/\mu$L and a creatine phosphokinase (CPK) of 10,000 units/L. All the following are reasonable options in the treatment of this patient's condition **except:**

A. Start cyproheptadine 4 mg PO q8h
B. Start dantrolene 1 mg/kg IV push
C. Start bromocriptine 2.5 mg PO q8h
D. Stop haloperidol and quetiapine
E. Start lorazepam 1 mg IV or intramuscular (IM) q6h

4. Which of the following choices best describes the inheritance pattern and the associated molecular abnormality in malignant hyperthermia (MH)?

A. Autosomal dominant, myosin kinase
B. Autosomal dominant, peripheral myelin protein 22 (PMP 22)
C. X-linked, dystrophin protein
D. Autosomal recessive, alpha-sarcoglycan protein
E. Autosomal dominant, ryanodine receptor

5. A 45-year-old man is brought to the ED after being found unresponsive on a city sidewalk. The ECG shown is obtained. What is the most likely diagnosis?

A. Benzodiazepine overdose
B. Hypothermia
C. Tricyclic antidepressant (TCA) overdose
D. Subarachnoid hemorrhage (SAH)
E. Hypercalcemia

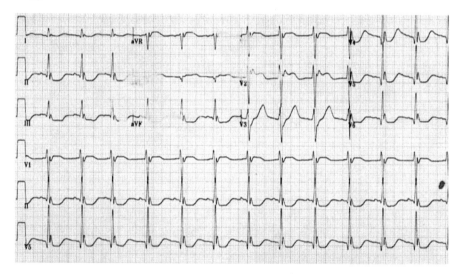

Source: From Stahmer SA. Arrhythmia. In: Rehm CGR, Fuhrman TMF, eds. Adult Problem-Based Learning Discussions. Mt. Prospect, IL: Society of Critical Care Medicine; 2008:8. Reproduced with permission of the publisher. Copyright 2008 Society of Critical Care Medicine.

6. A 35-year-old woman with a medical history only of depression is admitted with lethargy and acute respiratory failure after taking 60 100 mg tablets of amitriptyline. She had last been seen 4 hours prior to being discovered with altered mental status (AMS). Her initial vital signs were temperature 38°C, pulse 120 beats/min, respiratory rate (RR) 20 breaths/min, and blood

pressure (BP) 120/60 mmHg. In the ED, a large-bore nasogastric tube was placed after intubation, but no pill fragments were recovered after water lavage. Normal saline was started at 75 mL/hr. An ECG showed sinus tachycardia with PR interval 0.18 seconds, QRS interval 0.12 seconds, and QTc 0.60 seconds. Which of the following treatments is classically initiated in this scenario?

A. Beta-blockers such as esmolol or metoprolol
B. Amiodarone
C. Calcium gluconate
D. Sodium bicarbonate
E. Magnesium sulfate

7. Which of the following is **not** found in the clinical presentation of serotonin syndrome (SS)?

A. Miosis
B. Clonus
C. Diarrhea
D. Fever
E. Hypertension

8. Because of the short half-life of naloxone, patients with opiate overdose may be placed on continuous intravenous (IV) infusions of naloxone. What is the most accurate statement about the half-life of IV naloxone and its duration of action when given as a one-time dose?

A. 5 to 7 minutes; 5 to 7 minutes
B. 5 to 7 minutes; 20 to 30 minutes
C. 60 to 90 minutes; 10 to 90 minutes
D. 60 to 90 minutes; 60 to 90 minutes
E. 60 to 90 minutes; 240 to 360 minutes

9. The risk for clinically significant arrhythmias such as atrial fibrillation or ventricular fibrillation increases when the body temperature falls below:

A. 36°C
B. 34°C
C. 32°C
D. 30°C
E. 28°C

10. A 30-year-old woman with no medical or surgical history undergoes an emergent appendectomy. Thirty minutes after extubation, she is noted to be hot to touch and to have muscle rigidity in her jaw and extremities. Her vital signs are temperature 41°C, pulse 140 beats/min, respiratory rate (RR) 30 breaths/min, and blood pressure (BP) 100/50 mmHg. A portable chest x-ray was clear. Brown urine is noted in the catheter bag. What is the best treatment for her underlying condition?

A. Succinylcholine
B. Dantrolene
C. Broad-spectrum antibiotics
D. Rocuronium
E. Lorazepam

11. A 45-year-old physician from Seattle travels to Houston in July for a medical conference. His regular exercise schedule is running approximately 3 miles, two to three times per week. He wants to take advantage of his extra time away from work and goes on a 5-mile run at noon. He carries a 1-L bottle of water with him. After the run, he has generalized weakness and

feels nauseated. He is walking back to his hotel room when he vomits and then has syncope. Emergency medical service (EMS) is called, and he is taken to the ED. There, he is awake and fully oriented, but feels generally weak. His vital signs are temperature 38.5°C, pulse 120 beats/min, respiratory rate (RR) 12 breaths/min, blood pressure (BP) 90/55 mmHg. His neurologic examination is normal. Laboratory data include sodium of 130 mmol/L, creatinine of 1.0 mg/dL, creatine phosphokinase (CPK) of 400 units/L, white blood cell (WBC) $8 \times 10^3/\mu$L, and a normal urinalysis. Which of the following best describes this patient's condition?

A. Heat syncope
B. Heat cramp
C. Heat exhaustion
D. Exertional heat stroke
E. Nonexertional heat stroke

12. A young adult is brought to the ED for altered mental status (AMS) and combative behavior. The police were called after he was wandering drunkenly on the street, shouting paranoid phrases about the government and his parents. When the officers tried to take him into custody, he flew into a rage and it took five men to restrain him and place him in handcuffs. The police officers called emergency medical service (EMS) because they were concerned about his altered mentation. Initial vital signs in the ED were temperature 37°C, pulse 130 beats/min, respiratory rate (RR) 14 breaths/min, and blood pressure (BP) 180/100 mmHg. The patient would alternate between being quiet and staring with eyes open to being extremely agitated and requiring leather four-point restraints. His skin was flushed, he had copious saliva manifested by drooling, and there were mild expiratory wheezes. His pupils were 2 mm and reactive, and there was spontaneous rotatory nystagmus noted and vertical nystagmus on upward gaze. Face was symmetrical, and strength was full and symmetrical. Which of the following is most likely to be positive on urine toxicology screening?

A. Cocaine
B. Opiates
C. Methylenedioxymethamphetamine (MDMA; "Ecstasy")
D. Phencyclidine (PCP)
E. Amphetamines

13. Several unrelated persons in a large metropolitan city are brought into a local ED because of illness after they exited the subway at the same stop. All patients had marked miosis. Other symptoms and signs varied among the patients and included headache, rhinorrhea, salivation, nausea, vomiting, diarrhea, cough, shortness of breath, blurry vision, and muscle twitching. One patient developed seizures and respiratory failure requiring mechanical ventilation. What is the mechanism of action of the toxin responsible for this clinical scenario?

A. Anticholinergic activity
B. Excessive cholinergic activity
C. Antidopaminergic activity
D. Excessive dopaminergic activity
E. Excessive histaminergic activity

14. In the clinical scenario described in Question 13, what is the treatment of choice?

A. Pralidoxime
B. Flumazenil
C. Naltrexone
D. Physostigmine
E. Methylene blue

15. Which of the following is **not** a side effect of barbiturate overdose, either accidental or therapeutic (such as thiopental or pentobarbital coma for status epilepticus)?

    A. Hypotension
    B. Immunosuppression
    C. Gastroparesis
    D. Hypokalemia
    E. Ventricular tachycardia

16. Due to the current opiate epidemic in the United States, basic life support (BLS) guidelines now include administration of naloxone in the field for suspected opiate overdose leading to unresponsiveness and/or respiratory depression in patients with a pulse. Which of the following is a recommended dose and route of naloxone in this setting?

    A. Naloxone 0.4 mg intranasal
    B. Naloxone 0.4 mg intravenous
    C. Naloxone 2 mg intramuscular
    D. Naloxone 2 mg intranasal
    E. Naloxone 4 mg intramuscular

17. An unknown young man presents to the ED after being found by police on a sidewalk with agitation and bizarre behavior. No family is available for history, but the patient was reportedly found in an area known to have common "spice" usage. Temperature is 38°C, P 110 beats/min, blood pressure (BP) 170/90. He moves all extremities equally and antigravity. Which of the following is **true** regarding "spice"?

    A. "Spice" is legal and safe
    B. The main active ingredient in "spice" is delta 9-tetrahydrocannibinol
    C. Neurologic complications of "spice" include ischemic stroke, seizures, and psychosis
    D. "Spice" is also known as "bath salts"
    E. Since "spice" is a synthetic cannabinoid, a routine urine drug screen can detect "spice"

18. An 18-year-old woman is brought to the ED by her friends after a rave. She had used "Ecstasy" about 6 hours prior to presentation. She complains of diffuse headache which was insidious in onset, nausea, and vomiting. She becomes progressively somnolent while in the ED but is able to be awakened. Vital signs are temperature 38.5°C, pulse 100 beats/min, respiratory rate (RR) 26 breaths/min, blood pressure (BP) 140/80 mmHg, oxygen saturation 96% on 4-L nasal cannula. Serum sodium is 123 mEq/L. Chest x-ray shows mild diffuse pulmonary edema. Noncontrast head CT on admission to the ED showed a young, full brain without overt pathology. In addition to close monitoring of respiratory status and level of alertness, what is the next best step?

    A. Free water restriction
    B. 3% sodium chloride bolus of 100 mL
    C. Normal saline (NS) infusion at 75 mL/h
    D. Intubation
    E. High-flow oxygen therapy

19. Which of the following are well-known physiologic effects of "bath salts" or synthetic cathinones?

    A. Euphoria, psychosis, seizures, tachycardia, hypertension, and rhabdomyolysis
    B. Somnolence, respiratory depression, miosis, and constipation
    C. Miosis, bradycardia, hypotension, rhinorrhea, and bronchospasm
    D. Somnolence, apnea, hypotension, and decreased intracranial pressure
    E. Anesthesia, analgesia, bronchodilation, nausea, and vomiting

■ ANSWERS

1. **The answer is C.** Serotonin Syndrome (SS) is a clinical diagnosis and requires that the patient had been recently exposed to a serotonergic agent. Common symptoms of SS include agitation or confusion, fever, hypertension, tachycardia, diaphoresis, mydriasis, tremor, akathisia, clonus, and muscle rigidity. Many drugs have been implicated in the development of SS, including selective serotonin reuptake inhibitors (SSRIs), monoamine oxidase inhibitors, other antidepressants, opiates such as meperidine and tramadol, lithium, and triptans. Although some of the clinical features of SS overlap with NMS, NMS is associated with normal pupil size, rigidity in all limbs, hyporeflexia, and a state of quiet delirium or mutism. Therefore, NMS would not be the best answer for this patient. Alcohol withdrawal can indeed have symptoms of delirium and autonomic instability. However, hyperreflexia does not develop over time, and muscle tone and pupils should be normal. Lithium toxicity is not the correct answer, as the lithium level was within therapeutic range. Clinical signs and symptoms of acute lithium toxicity include dysarthria, ataxia, nystagmus, nausea, vomiting, diarrhea, and nephrogenic diabetes insipidus (DI). MH is not the correct answer, as it develops soon after general anesthesia and is associated with very high fever, pipe-like rigidity, and hyporeflexia.

Boyer EW, Shannon M. The serotonin syndrome. *N Engl J Med.* 2005;352(11):1112-1120. doi:10.1056/NEJMra041867

Grandjean EM, Aubry JM. Lithium: updated human knowledge using an evidence-based approach: part III: clinical safety. *CNS Drugs.* 2009;23(5):397-418. doi:10.2165/00023210-200923050-00004

2. **The answer is E.** Viral hepatitides are the most common cause of acute liver failure worldwide, but in the United States acetaminophen overdose is the culprit in 39% to 51% of cases. Idiosyncratic drug reactions are the second most common reason for acute liver failure, accounting for 13% of the cases.

Khashab M, Tector AJ, Kwo PY. Epidemiology of acute liver failure. *Curr Gastroenterol Rep.* 2007;9(1):66-73. doi:10.1007/s11894-008-0023-x

Larson AM, Polson J, Fontana RJ, et al. Acetaminophen-induced acute liver failure: results of a United States multicenter, prospective study. *Hepatology.* 2005;42(6):1364-1372. doi:10.1002/hep.20948

Ostapowicz G, Fontana RJ, Schiødt FV, et al. Results of a prospective study of acute liver failure at 17 tertiary care centers in the United States. *Ann Intern Med.* 2002;137(12):947-954. doi:10.7326/0003-4819-137-12-200212170-00007

3. **The answer is A.** This patient has neuroleptic malignant syndrome (NMS). Cyproheptadine is a histamine and serotonin antagonist, and can be used in the treatment of serotonin syndrome (SS), but does not have action on dopamine receptors. Choices B through E are reasonable options in the treatment of NMS. Dantrolene is a skeletal muscle relaxant that works by decreasing the release of intracellular calcium from the sarcoplasmic reticulum. It is used in the treatment of malignant hyperthermia (MH) and moderate to severe NMS. In cases of significant rigidity, dantrolene at doses of 1 to 2.5 mg/kg IV push can be given. Bromocriptine is a dopamine receptor agonist and also has indications for treatment in Parkinsonism and in prolactinomas. Certainly, all dopamine antagonists should be discontinued in the setting of NMS. Lorazepam is considered a first-line agent for sedation and to promote muscle relaxation. Finally, isotonic IV fluids should be given to all patients due to insensible losses from fever and to prevent acute renal failure from rhabdomyolysis.

Strawn JR, Keck PE Jr, Caroff SN. Neuroleptic malignant syndrome. *Am J Psychiatry.* 2007;164(6):870-876. doi:10.1176/ajp.2007.164.6.870

4. **The answer is E.** Autosomal dominant is the inheritance pattern, and ryanodine receptor is the associated molecular abnormality. Choice A describes the inheritance of myotonic dystrophy. Choice B describes the inheritance of Charcot–Marie–Tooth disease (CMT-1a) or hereditary neuropathy with liability to pressure palsies when there is a gene duplication or deletion,

respectively. Choice C describes inheritance of Duchenne muscular dystrophy. Choice D is the defect in one of the limb girdle muscular dystrophies.

Bird TD, Tapscott SJ. Clinical neurogenetics. In: Bradley WG, Daroff RB, Fenichel GM, Jankovic J, eds. *Neurology in Clinical Practice*. Philadelphia, PA: Butterworth-Heinemann; 2004:803-807.

5. **The answer is B.** The ECG shows Osborn waves, a characteristic J-point elevation of at least 1-mm elevation at the end of the QRS complex found in patients with hypothermia. In one study, Osborn waves were found in every patient whose temperature was less than or equal to 30.5°C. The height of the Osborn wave is inversely related to body temperature. Benzodiazepine overdose is infrequently associated with reversible atrioventricular block. TCA overdose does not cause Osborn waves, but rather leads commonly to QT prolongation and prolongation of the QRS interval. Common ECG changes seen after SAH include ST-segment elevation or depression, inverted or peaked T waves, Q waves, or prolonged QTc interval. Severe hypercalcemia can cause lethargy and even coma; the ECG shows a shortened QTc interval.

Arroyo Plasencia AM, Ballentine LM, Mowry JB, et al. Benzodiazepine-associated atrioventricular block. *Am J Ther*. 2012;19(1):e48-e52. doi:10.1097/mjt.0b013e3181dcf572

Diercks DB, Shumaik GM, Harrigan RA, et al. Electrocardiographic manifestations: electrolyte abnormalities. *J Emerg Med*. 2004;27(2):153-160. doi:10.1016/j.jemermed.2004.04.006

Harrigan RA, Brady WJ. ECG abnormalities in tricyclic antidepressant ingestion. *Am J Emerg Med*. 1999;17(4):387-393. doi:10.1016/s0735-6757(99)90094-3

Sommargren CE. Electrocardiographic abnormalities in patients with subarachnoid hemorrhage. *Am J Crit Care*. 2002;11(1):48-56. doi:10.1136/bcr.08.2010.3253

Vassallo SU, Delaney KA, Hoffman RS, et al. A prospective evaluation of the electrocardiographic manifestations of hypothermia. *Acad Emerg Med*. 1999;6(11):1121-1126. doi:10.1111/j.1553-2712.1999.tb00114.x

6. **The answer is D.** The evidence to use sodium bicarbonate in tricyclic antidepressant (TCA) poisoning is from case series and animal studies; there have been no randomized clinical trials testing this treatment. One series showed that a majority of patients treated had normalization or near-normalization of the QRS complex after being treated with sodium bicarbonate. Bicarbonate should be given for wide complex tachyarrhythmias after TCA overdose and may be considered to a pH goal of 7.45 to 7.55 in patients with a wide QRS or prolonged QTc interval.

Body R, Bartram T, Azam F, et al. Guidelines in Emergency Medicine Network (GEMNet): guideline for the management of tricyclic antidepressant overdose. *Emerg Med J*. 2011;28(4):347-368. doi:10.1136/emj.2010.091553

Kerr GW, McGuffie AC, Wilkie S. Tricyclic antidepressant overdose: a review. *Emerg Med J*. 2001;18(4):236-241. doi:10.1136/emj.18.4.236

7. **The answer is A.** Miosis is *not* a part of SS; rather, pupils tend to be dilated and reactive (mydriasis). Clonus may be present, especially in the lower extremities. Bowel function tends to be increased in SS, with diarrhea and hyperactive bowel sounds.

Boyer EW, Shannon M. The serotonin syndrome. *N Engl J Med*. 2005;352(11):1112-1120. doi:10.1056/NEJMra041867

8. **The answer is C.** Naloxone has a half-life of about 60 to 90 minutes. In some studies, the duration of action of naloxone has been shown to be as long as its half-life. However, in other studies and in clinical practice, the duration of effect seems to be much shorter than the pharmacokinetic elimination, as the drug may be redistributed out of the brain more rapidly than opiates.

Clarke SF, Dargan PI, Jones AL. Naloxone in opioid poisoning: walking the tightrope. *Emerg Med J*. 2005;22(9):612-616. doi:10.1136/emj.2003.009613

Glass PS, Jhaveri RM, Smith LR. Comparison of potency and duration of action of nalmefene and naloxone. *Anesth Analg*. 1994;78(3):536-541. doi:10.1213/00000539-199403000-00021

Kaufman RD, Gabathuler ML, Bellville JW. Potency, duration of action and pA2 in man of intravenous naloxone measured by reversal of morphine-depressed respiration. *J Pharmacol Exp Ther.* 1981;219(1):156-162.

9. **The answer is D.** Clinically significant arrhythmias are rare with body temperatures greater than 30°C. Atrial fibrillation is more commonly seen than ventricular fibrillation or ventricular tachycardia.

Polderman KH, Herold I. Therapeutic hypothermia and controlled normothermia in the intensive care unit: practical considerations, side effects, and cooling methods. *Crit Care Med.* 2009;37(3):1101-1120. doi:10.1097/ccm.0b013e3181962ad5

Vassallo SU, Delaney KA, Hoffman RS, et al. A prospective evaluation of the electrocardiographic manifestations of hypothermia. *Acad Emerg Med.* 1999;6(11):1121-1126. doi:10.1111/j.1553-2712.1999.tb00114.x

10. **The answer is B.** This patient has malignant hyperthermia (MH). MH is a syndrome of muscle hypermetabolism that follows the administration of succinylcholine or inhaled anesthetic agents. Various muscle protein abnormalities predispose persons to MH, with the most common being a ryanodine receptor mutation. The clinical syndrome can begin during induction of anesthesia, intraoperatively, or in the several hours after surgery. Clinical signs and symptoms include marked hyperpyrexia, tachycardia, cyanosis, masseter muscle spasm, muscle rigidity, a rise in end-tidal CO_2, and rhabdomyolysis. Dantrolene is the mainstay of therapy, which decreases the excitation–contraction coupling in skeletal muscle by reducing the amount of calcium released from the sarcoplasmic reticulum, with no effect on the neuromuscular junction. With aggressive recognition and treatment, mortality from MH has fallen from 70% to less than 10%. Succinylcholine would be the wrong answer, as it is associated with MH and could worsen the syndrome. Broad-spectrum antibiotics would be used in the setting of sepsis. Although sepsis could cause fever, tachycardia, tachypnea, and hypotension, it does not cause muscle rigidity and rhabdomyolysis. Therefore, antibiotics would not treat the underlying condition, making them an incorrect response. In a real-life scenario, it is likely that antibiotics would be given (in addition to dantrolene) while cultures were pending. Nondepolarizing muscle blockers such as rocuronium are generally considered safe in MH, but would not treat the MH itself. Finally, benzodiazepines can be used to promote muscle relaxation and are the first-line treatment in the rigidity associated with neuroleptic malignant syndrome (NMS). However, benzodiazepines alone would not sufficiently treat the severe muscle rigidity of MH.

Hopkins PM. Malignant hyperthermia: advances in clinical management and diagnosis. *Br J Anaesth.* 2000;85(1):118-128. doi:10.1093/bja/85.1.118

Krause T, Gerbershagen MU, Fiege M, et al. Dantrolene—a review of its pharmacology, therapeutic use and new developments. *Anaesthesia.* 2004;59(4):364-373. doi:10.1111/j.1365-2044.2004.03658.x

Strawn JR, Keck PE Jr, Caroff SN. Neuroleptic malignant syndrome. *Am J Psychiatry.* 2007;164(6):870-876. doi:10.1055/s-0035-1553246

11. **The answer is C.** Heat exhaustion describes a syndrome of generalized weakness, nausea, vomiting, and syncope without neurologic dysfunction or tissue damage. The core temperature may be somewhat elevated, but is not extremely elevated. In heat exhaustion, salt and/or water losses from sweating lead to hypovolemia and syncope. Heat syncope describes syncope due to peripheral vasodilation from elevated environmental temperature. Heat cramp refers to exertional cramping in the heat due to dehydration. It would not be the right answer here, as the patient had no cramps. Heat stroke is a loss of thermoregulation, which leads to an extremely elevated core body temperature (generally defined as greater than 40.6°C); neurologic dysfunction (such as delirium, lassitude, seizures, and coma); and anhidrosis. There may be signs or symptoms of other end-organ or tissue damage such as acute renal failure, elevated liver function tests, cardiac conduction defects, disseminated intravascular coagulopathy, or rhabdomyolysis. Heat stroke is important to recognize, as early treatment—decreasing the core temperature to below 38.9°C within 30 minutes—may decrease mortality.

Heat stroke may be exertional or nonexertional. Exertional heat stroke is usually seen in previously healthy persons exercising or working in a hot and humid environment. Nonexertional heat stroke is generally seen in debilitated or elderly persons with a prolonged exposure to high temperatures and humidity. The two most reasonable answers for this patient's condition are heat exhaustion or exertional heat stroke. Since his core temperature was well below 40.6°C and he had no overt neurologic dysfunction other than syncope, heat exhaustion is the better answer.

Dematte JE, O'Mara K, Buescher J, et al. Near-fatal heat stroke during the 1995 heat wave in Chicago. *Ann Intern Med*. 1998;129(3):173-181. doi:10.7326/0003-4819-129-3-199808010-00001

Grogan H, Hopkins PM. Heat stroke: implications for critical care and anaesthesia. *Br J Anaesth*. 2002;88(5):700-707. doi:10.1093/bja/88.5.700

12. **The answer is D.** PCP is a hallucinogen, which has an affinity for multiple types of neurotransmitter receptors. It antagonizes *N*-methyl-D-aspartate receptors, inhibits monoamine reuptake, and has cholinergic effects via both nicotinic and muscarinic receptors. Persons intoxicated with PCP classically have periods of super-human strength and seem anesthetized to painful stimuli. They often have ataxia and vertical or rotatory nystagmus. Owing to monoamine reuptake inhibition, PCP has a sympathomimetic effect with hypertension and tachycardia. Cholinergic activity can lead to miosis, salivation, bronchospasm, and diaphoresis. Although cocaine or amphetamines can cause sympathomimetic effects and paranoia, they do not cause ataxia or bizarre nystagmus. Opiate intoxication would cause sedation, depressed RR, miosis, constipation, and analgesia. MDMA is both a stimulant and a hallucinogen; it increases the release of serotonin, dopamine, and norepinephrine and then decreases their metabolism via monoamine oxidase inhibition. Classically, MDMA intoxication is associated with severe hyperthermia. Like cocaine and PCP, MDMA can cause sympathomimetic effects, paranoia, and hallucinations. The lack of ataxia, nystagmus, and cholinergic signs helps to distinguish MDMA intoxication from PCP intoxication.

Bey T, Patel A. Phencyclidine intoxication and adverse effects: a clinical and pharmacological review of an illicit drug. *Cal J Emerg Med*. 2007;8(1):9-14.

Smith KM, Larive LL, Romanelli F. Club drugs: methylenedioxymethamphetamine, flunitrazepam, ketamine hydrochloride, and gamma-hydroxybutyrate. *Am J Health Syst Pharm*. 2002;59(11):1067-1076.

13. **The answer is B.** This scenario describes a hypothetical sarin nerve gas attack, as occurred in Japan in the mid-1990s. Sarin is an organophosphate and acts via acetyl-cholinesterase inhibition, leading to excessive acetylcholine action and cholinergic crisis. Sarin acts on both the peripheral and the central nervous system (CNS) and on both the nicotinic and the muscarinic acetylcholine receptors. Symptoms include neuromuscular weakness, loss of deep tendon reflexes, muscle fasciculations, seizures, altered mental status (AMS), miosis, blurred vision, ocular pain, tachycardia or bradycardia, and the SLUDGE symptoms of salivation, lacrimation, urination, diarrhea, gastrointestinal upset (nausea), and emesis. Serum cholinesterase or erythrocyte acetyl-cholinesterase activity may be measured, but treatment should not be delayed for the results. Anticholinergic syndrome would be manifested peripherally with decreased bowel sounds, dry and warm skin, dry mouth, mydriasis, urinary retention, and tachycardia. Central signs of anticholinergic syndrome include either a depressed level of consciousness (sedation or coma) or agitation, anxiety, and disorientation. Excessive anti-dopaminergic activity could result in parkinsonism, tardive dyskinesia, and/or hyperprolactinemia. Excessive dopaminergic activity, such as in overdoses of dopamine agonists such as pramipexole or bromocriptine, can lead to psychosis, orthostasis, nausea, hyperkinetic movement disorders (dyskinesias), and pathological addictive behaviors. Finally, excessive histamine release can lead to bronchoconstriction, vasodilation, nasal congestion and rhinorrhea, hives, erythema, and gastric acid secretion.

Torline RL. Extreme hyperpyrexia associated with central anticholinergic syndrome. *Anesthesiology.* 1992;76(3):470-471. doi:10.1097/00000542-199203000-00023

Yanagisawa N, Morita H, Nakajima T. Sarin experiences in Japan: acute toxicity and long-term effects. *J Neurol Sci.* 2006;249(1):76-85. doi:10.1016/j.jns.2006.06.007

14. **The answer is A.** Pralidoxime is the antidote to organophosphates and was effective in reversing the signs of cholinergic poisoning (miosis and respiratory depression) in the patients in Japan when given up to 6 hours after exposure to sarin. One should note that the most current Cochrane Review does not support giving oximes for organophosphate poisoning because of lack of sufficient evidence. Flumazenil is the antidote to benzodiazepines. Naltrexone is an oral opiate antagonist. Physostigmine is an anticholinesterase inhibitor and can be used to treat overdoses of anticholinergic agents, but would worsen these patients' current symptoms. Finally, methylene blue is given for the treatment of methemoglobinemia.

Buckley NA, Eddleston M, Li Y, et al. Oximes for acute organophosphate pesticide poisoning. *Cochrane Database Syst Rev.* 2011;2:CD005085. doi:10.1002/14651858.CD005085.pub2

Dart RC, Goldfrank LR, Chyka PA, et al. Combined evidence-based literature analysis and consensus guidelines for stocking of emergency antidotes in the United States. *Ann Emerg Med.* 2000;36(2):126-132. doi:10.1067/mem.2000.108182

Yanagisawa N, Morita H, Nakajima T. Sarin experiences in Japan: acute toxicity and long-term effects. *J Neurol Sci.* 2006;249(1):76-85. doi:10.1016/j.jns.2006.06.007

15. **The answer is E.** High-dose barbiturate therapy is known to be associated with gastroparesis, immunosuppression, respiratory failure, hypotension, and poikilothermia. Infusions of thiopental have also been associated with life-threatening hypokalemia and rebound hyperkalemia on infusion discontinuation. Ventricular tachycardia is not associated with barbiturate therapy, and in fact, barbiturates have been associated with decreased incidence of torsades de points in animal models with prolonged QT intervals.

Neil MJ, Dale MC. Hypokalaemia with severe rebound hyperkalaemia after therapeutic barbiturate coma. *Anesth Analg.* 2009;108(6):1867-1868. doi:10.1213/ane.0b013e3181a16418

Weissenburger J, Nesterenko VV, Antzelevitch C. Transmural heterogeneity of ventricular repolarization under baseline and long QT conditions in the canine heart in vivo: torsades de pointes develops with halothane but not pentobarbital anesthesia. *J Cardiovasc Electrophysiol.* 2000;11(3):290-304. doi:10.1111/j.1540-8167.2000.tb01798.x

16. **The answer is D.** The recommended doses of naloxone during a suspected opiate overdose leading to unresponsiveness or cardiac arrest in the field are 2 mg intranasal or 0.4 mg intramuscular. There is no recommendation for intravenous administration in the prehospital setting. If the patient responds, the dose may be repeated every 4 minutes as needed.

Lavonas EJ, Drennan IR, Gabrielli A, et al. Part 10: special circumstances of resuscitation. 2015 American Heart Association guidelines update for cardiopulmonary resuscitation and emergency cardiovascular care. *Circulation.* 2015;132(suppl 2):S504-S506. doi:10.1161/CIR.0000000000000264

17. **The answer is C.** "Spice" refers to any number of illegal synthetic cannabinoids, which are not chemically the same as the active ingredient in marijuana (delta 9-tetrahydrocannabinol) or legal synthetic cannabinoids. There are many other street names for "spice," including "K2," "fake weed," "Scooby snax," and "Mr. nice guy." "Spice" does not show up as marijuana on a urine toxicology screen. Well-documented neurologic effects include ischemic stroke, seizures, and psychosis. Many chemical compounds marketed as "spice" are illegal by various states. "Bath salts" refers to synthetic cathinones, a new group of psychoactive stimulants.

Kemp AM, Clark MS, Dobbs T, et al. Top 10 facts you need to know about synthetic cannabinoids: not so nice spice. *Am J Med.* 2016;129(3):240-244. doi:10.1016/j.amjmed.2015.10.008

NIDA. Synthetic cathinones ("Bath Salts"). National Institute on Drug Abuse Web site. Available at: https://www.drugabuse.gov/publications/drugfacts/synthetic-cathinones-bath-salts. January 6, 2016. Accessed August 9, 2017.

18. **The answer is B.** "Ecstasy," or 3,4-methylenedioxymethamphetamine (MDMA), is known to cause acute, symptomatic hyponatremia by promoting the inappropriate secretion of arginine vasopressin. Additionally, patients often drink large amounts of water during a rave—possibly due to "Ecstasy"-induced hyperthermia or fluid losses from sweating while dancing. These two factors ("Ecstasy"-induced syndrome of inappropriate antidiuretic hormone [SIADH] and large amounts of free water intake) can lead to symptomatic acute hyponatremia with cerebral edema. It is more common in females. Signs and symptoms include headache, nausea, vomiting, somnolence, seizure, coma, herniation, and death. Neurogenic pulmonary edema may accompany and exacerbate the cerebral edema. Acute symptomatic hyponatremia with cerebral edema is life-threatening and should be treated aggressively with hypertonic saline boluses and/or drips, as appropriate. Per oral fluid restriction is likely also a reasonable step but will not correct the sodium and cerebral edema quickly enough in this situation. Therefore, B is the correct answer.

    Moritz ML, Kalantar-Zadeh K, Ayus JC. Ecstacy-associated hyponatremia: why are women at risk? *Nephrol Dial Transplant*. 2013;28:2206-2209. doi:10.1093/ndt/gft192

19. **The answer is A.** Synthetic cathinones have amphetamine-like effects and modulate serotonin. Sympathomimetic effects such as those seen with amphetamine or cocaine use are common in hospitalized patients. Rhabdomyosis has been well described with cathinones. Mydriasis, not miosis, is seen with use of bath salts. B describes effects of opiates. C describes the muscarinic side effects of organophosphate poisoning. D describes effects of propofol. E describes effects of ketamine.

    Prosser JM, Nelson LS. The toxicology of bath salts: a review of synthetic cathinones. *J Med Toxicol*. 2012;8:33-42. doi:10.1007/s13181-011-0193-z

9

Inflammatory and Demyelinating Diseases

CARLOS PEREZ, SHIVIKA CHANDRA, AND FLAVIA NELSON

■ QUESTIONS

1. What is the mechanism of action related to a reduction in the total lymphocyte number for Gilenya, an oral disease–modifying therapy for multiple sclerosis (MS)?

   A. Attaches to VLA-1 and blocks interaction with its ligand on central nervous system (CNS) endothelium vascular cell adhesion molecule-1 (VCAM-1)
   B. Induces Th2 lymphocytes
   C. Blocks capacity of lymphocytes to egress from lymph nodes by binding to sphingosine-1-phosphate receptors on cell membrane
   D. Suppresses T-cell activation by inhibiting binding of T-cell receptor complexes
   E. Unknown

2. A 20-year-old woman presented with a 2-week history of headache, low-grade fever, and anxiety, rapidly followed by homicidal ideation, aggressive agitation, seizures, oral dyskinesias, hypoventilation, hyperthermia, and prominent autonomic instability requiring intubation and sedation. In the ICU, she developed episodes of hypotension and bradycardia with periods of asystole lasting up to 15 seconds. Upon weaning off sedation, she would open her eyes but was otherwise unresponsive to external stimuli. Subsequently, she was noted to have frequent facial grimacing, lip smacking, rhythmic abdominal contractions, kicking motions of the legs, and intermittent dystonic postures of the right arm. Cerebrospinal fluid (CSF) showed a white blood cell (WBC) count of 28 with lymphocytic pleocytosis, a mildly elevated protein of 30, normal glucose and normal immunoglobulin G (IgG) index, no oligoclonal bands (OCBs), negative herpes simplex virus (HSV) polymerase chain reaction (PCR), and negative cytology. Blood cultures were also negative. EEG showed diffuse slowing without focal temporal lobe abnormalities. Cranial MRI showed no abnormalities. Conventional angiography was normal. Brain biopsy was inconclusive. An ovarian teratoma was found on further workup. What is the most likely diagnosis?

   A. Limbic encephalitis
   B. Rabies
   C. Acute disseminated encephalomyelitis (ADEM)
   D. *N*-methyl-ᴅ-aspartate (NMDA) receptor encephalitis
   E. Central nervous system (CNS) vasculitis

3. A 35-year-old Hispanic woman is admitted to the medical ICU for plasma exchange (PLEX) for the treatment of vision loss refractory to intravenous (IV) steroids. She originally presented to the ED with a 6-day history of painful vision loss in her right eye. A 5-day course of IV methylprednisolone was given without clinical improvement after a 2-week period. Two years ago, she was evaluated because of severe refractory nausea, hiccups, and difficulty walking

from weakness in her left leg. These symptoms lasted several weeks. Her weakness never fully improved. Her brain MRI was normal at that time. Which would be the next step in managing this patient?

A. Spinal tap
B. Initiate treatment with PLEX and order brain MRI w/wo contrast
C. Initiate treatment with PLEX and order brain and spine MRI w/wo contrast
D. Initiate treatment with a disease-modifying therapy for multiple sclerosis (MS)
E. Treat the patient with PLEX and observe

4. The patient from Question 3 was treated with PLEX with significant improvement. Brain MRI was normal. Spinal MRI showed a hyperintense T2 lesion extending from C2 to C6. The gold standard for diagnosis of this entity is:

A. Presence of oligoclonal bands (OCBs)
B. Positive immunoglobulin G (IgG) for aquaporin 4 antibody
C. Low glucose levels with increased white blood cell (WBC) count
D. Protein 14–3-3
E. Increased IgG index and synthesis rate

5. Which of the following medications has shown to be beneficial in the treatment of neuromyelitis optica (NMO)?

A. Chronic use of oral prednisone
B. Glatiramer acetate
C. Natalizumab
D. Rituximab
E. Interferon-beta1a

6. A 30-year-old woman with a history of recurrent aphthous mouth ulcerations, uveitis, and skin ulcers presents with headache and ataxia. In the ED, she has a generalized tonic–clonic seizure and is intubated. MRI of the brain shows lesions predominantly in the brainstem. Cerebrospinal fluid (CSF) analysis shows pleocytosis, elevated protein, and normal glucose. This disease has been associated to which of the following?

A. Human leukocyte antigen (HLA)-DR15
B. HLA-B5 and HLA-B1
C. HLA-DQB1–0602
D. Cytoplasmic antineutrophil cytoplasmic antibodies (C-ANCA)
E. HLA B27

7. A 40-year-old woman with a 1-year medical history of worsening symptoms manifested by skin abnormalities, difficulty breathing, and hearing loss presents to the ED with cognitive decline and seizures. She has been diagnosed with a condition associated to antibodies Scl-70. Biopsy shows thickening of the skin as well as fibrosis. The patient is most likely suffering from:

A. Progressive systemic sclerosis
B. Sjögren's syndrome
C. Systemic lupus erythematosus (SLE)
D. Rheumatoid arthritis
E. Thromboangiitis obliterans

8. Which of the following medications has been associated with aseptic meningitis?

A. Amphotericin B
B. Nalidixic acid

    C. Ethambutol
    D. Vancomycin
    E. Penicillins

9. A 50-year-old man on treatment with tacrolimus for an autoimmune condition develops mental changes, seizures, and blindness. This medication has been associated to which of the following diseases?

    A. Acute demyelinating encephalomyelitis (ADEM)
    B. Posterior reversible encephalopathy syndrome (PRES)
    C. Multiple sclerosis (MS)
    D. Benign intracranial hypertension
    E. Vestibular damage

10. A 70-year-old woman presents with a 2-week history of jaw claudication, neck pain, and vertigo. Brain imaging studies (CT and MRI) were reported as normal. Patient was treated symptomatically with poor response. Which is the most likely diagnosis?

    A. Cerebrovascular disease
    B. Polymyalgia rheumatica
    C. Takayasu's arteritis
    D. Temporal arteritis
    E. Wegener's granulomatosis

11. A 45-year-old right-handed man with a history of relapsing remitting multiple sclerosis (RRMS) being treated with natalizumab (Tysabri) presents to the ED with a 4-week history of cognitive decline, ataxia, and recent right hemiparesis and vision disturbances. He deteriorates over the next couple of days and is transferred to the ICU after intubation for airway protection. Initial head CT scan showed multiple foci of hypodensities. Brain MRI showed new large T2 hyperintense white matter lesions beginning at gray–white matter junctions and coalescing to form confluent lesions. No enhancements were noted in the postcontrast imaging. Cerebrospinal fluid (CSF) examination would most likely show which of the following?

    A. Protein kinase inhibitor (protein 14–3-3)
    B. Depressed glucose levels
    C. Positive capsular polysaccharide antigen titer
    D. John Cunningham (JC) virus by polymerase chain reaction (PCR)
    E. Presence of oligoclonal bands (OCBs) and increased immunoglobulin G (IgG) index

12. Despite appropriate management, the patient in Question 11 dies a few months later. Which finding would you expect to find by brain pathology?

    A. Leptomeningeal inflammatory infiltrates with enlarged cystic spaces
    B. Reactive astrocytosis with bizarre appearance of giant astrocytes
    C. Caseating granulomas with multinucleated giant cells and activated macrophages
    D. Intracellular vacuolation of neuropil primarily affecting gray matter

13. From the following options, please choose the one that best fits the following description: An aggressive form of demyelinating disease that presents with extensive white matter lesions in the brain and spine. On MRI, the demyelinating lesions tend to show homogeneous enhancement with gadolinium. This entity has an acute onset, rapid progression, and may cause death.

    A. Devic's disease neuromyelitis optica (NMO)
    B. Acute disseminated encephalomyelitis (ADEM)
    C. Marburg's variant

D. Tumefactive multiple sclerosis (MS)

E. Posterior reversible encephalopathy syndrome (PRES)

14. A 23-year-old woman with a history of migraines presents to the ED with concerns for a stroke. She reports right arm numbness that began 3 days ago and right arm weakness since this morning, both becoming progressively worse. She is only on oral contraceptives. She also describes a tingling sensation traveling down her right arm when bending her neck forward. Hypercoagulable and cardiovascular workup are normal. Brain MRI shows six nonenhancing white matter lesions in both cerebral hemispheres—five perpendicular to the ventricles and one juxtacortical—all of which are seen on T2w fluid attenuated inversion recovery (FLAIR), with no enhancements on T1w postcontrast series. Cervical MRI shows a small lesion on T2w sagittal and axial imaging on the left side of the spinal cord at the level of C6 with gadolinium enhancement on T1w postcontrast imaging. What would be the best next step?

A. She meets the 2010 McDonald diagnostic criteria for multiple sclerosis (MS) and needs treatment with intravenous (IV) methylprednisolone

B. She needs to have cerebrospinal fluid (CSF) analysis to confirm diagnosis of MS and evoked potentials prior to the administration of IV methylprednisolone

C. She needs repeated hypercoagulable workup for possible stroke as she is on oral contraceptives

D. Start aspirin

E. She has acute disseminated encephalomyelitis (ADEM) and needs treatment with IV methylprednisolone

15. A 35-year-old woman with aggressive multiple sclerosis (MS) is admitted to the ICU to receive her first rituximab infusion. Shortly after beginning the infusion, she becomes tachycardic and febrile. She is immediately taken off the drug and is given a histamine blocker. She improves within 30 minutes and becomes stable again. The best next step is:

A. To not give her rituximab ever again, as she had an anaphylactic reaction to it

B. To wait 30 to 60 minutes, give intravenous (IV) corticosteroids, and start the rituximab infusion at half of the rate it was given and titrated to tolerance

C. To give her dopamine to prevent further blood pressure (BP) drop

D. To try rituximab infusion at half the dose and over a longer infusion time

E. To premedicate with IV corticosteroids and an H2 blocker and try rituximab infusion at half the dose and over a longer infusion time

16. A 27-year-old woman presents with a 2-week history of progressive right hemiparesis. MRI of the brain demonstrates a 4.5-cm enhancing mass in the left posterior frontal white matter, with several smaller lesions in the periventricular white matter of the contralateral hemisphere. A stereotactic biopsy shows no evidence of neoplasia, but reveals demyelinated neurons with axonal sparing and an infiltrate of foamy macrophages and perivascular lymphocytes. What would be the most appropriate diagnosis?

A. Marburg's variant

B. Primary progressive multiple sclerosis (MS)

C. Tumefactive MS

D. False negative for malignancy

E. Balo's concentric sclerosis

17. A 30-year-old man with an unremarkable medical history wakes up with right upper extremity weakness. He is also experiencing tingling sensation along his spine when he moves his neck forward. He has never experienced these symptoms before. He recalls that for the past month, he has been feeling more tired than usual and that a year ago, he had tingling sensation on his left leg that lasted for a week and resolved. A cervical MRI shows a 4.5-mm lesion on

T2w images, in the right anterior horn at the level of C6–C8 with mild enhancement on post-gadolinium T1w images. Thoracic MRI shows multiple patch-like lesions on T2w images at the levels of T2–T3, T5–T6, and T9–T11, none of them enhancing. Brain MRI shows two small white matter lesions perpendicular to the left ventricle. What is the most likely diagnosis?

A. Relapsing remitting multiple sclerosis (RRMS)
B. Acute partial transverse myelitis (APTM)
C. Devic's disease
D. Vitamin B$_{12}$ deficiency
E. Idiopathic transverse myelitis

18. A 7-year-old boy with no significant medical history is taken to the ED by his parents for altered mental status (AMS) and right hemiparesis. One week ago, he had new onset of persistent headaches followed by personality changes and lethargy for 2 days. Last night, his mother noted mild weakness on the right side. Three weeks ago, he missed 2 days of school because of a cold that he caught from his little sister. Brain MRI shows large, confluent white matter lesions in both cerebral hemispheres that enhance with gadolinium. What is the most likely diagnosis?

A. Guillain–Barré syndrome (GBS)
B. Multiple sclerosis (MS)
C. Clinically isolated syndrome
D. Acute disseminated encephalomyelitis (ADEM)
E. Viral encephalitis

19. Infection with which pathogen carries the highest risk for acute disseminated encephalomyelitis (ADEM)?

A. Measles
B. Epstein–Barr syndrome (EBS)
C. Varicella–Zoster virus (VZV)
D. *Haemophilus influenzae*
E. Cytomegalovirus (CMV)

20. The following symptoms are typical of acute disseminated encephalomyelitis (ADEM) **except**:

A. Sensory deficit
B. Encephalopathy
C. Seizures
D. Ataxia
E. Ascending paralysis

21. The most typical presentation of acute disseminated encephalomyelitis (ADEM) is

A. Sudden loss of consciousness, fever, headache, and malaise after the development of neurological symptoms
B. Ascending paralysis, fever, diarrhea, and personality changes that develop over hours
C. Headache, low-grade fever, myalgias, and malaise prior to the onset of neurological symptoms
D. Rapidly progressing paraparesis with initial flaccidity followed by spasticity

22. The following are in the differential diagnosis of acute disseminated encephalomyelitis (ADEM) **except**:

A. Multiple sclerosis (MS)
B. Neuromyelitis optica (NMO)

C. Guillain–Barré syndrome (GBS)

D. Balo's concentric sclerosis

E. Posterior reversible encephalopathy syndrome (PRES)

23. A 40-year-old African American man with a medical history of hypertension was seen by his ophthalmologist for subacute loss of vision in his left eye. During the eye examination, he was found to have papilledema and visual field defects. He was sent to a neurologist for evaluation and started on intravenous (IV) steroids for 5 days. His vision improved promptly. A brain MRI showed abnormal hyperintense T2 signal in the left optic nerve. A month later, he again presented with subacute vision loss in his left eye and mild changes in his right eye vision. A second round of steroids was given, with improvement in both eyes. A new MRI of the brain shows faint enhancement of both optic nerves and meningeal enhancement. Cerebrospinal fluid (CSF) analysis is done and is positive for oligoclonal bands (OCBs), elevated protein, elevated white blood cell (WBC) count, and elevated angiotensin-converting enzyme (ACE) levels in CSF and blood. What is the most likely diagnosis?

A. Neuromyelitis optica (NMO)

B. Multiple sclerosis (MS)

C. Neurosarcoidosis

D. Recurrent viral optic neuritis (ON)

E. Ischemic ON

24. Which of the following is the **most common** central nervous system (CNS) manifestation(s) of systemic lupus erythematosus (SLE)?

A. Stroke (arterial)

B. Acute confusional state, psychosis

C. Ataxia

D. Venous thrombosis

E. Chorea, parkinsonism

25. A 64-year-old woman admitted to the ICU for severe hyponatremia secondary to diuretic use develops worsening confusion, dysarthria, and dysconjugate gaze over 24 hours. She has a history of an upper respiratory tract infection 3 weeks earlier, at which time the serum sodium was normal. MRI of the brain is most likely to show

A. Brainstem ischemic infarction

B. Abnormal hyperintense signal in the pons on T2w imaging

C. Cerebral edema

D. Multiple T2 hyperintense lesions in the white matter

E. Cerebellar tonsillar herniation

26. A 23-year-old woman presents with a 1-week history of fever and worsening headache associated with photophobia, nausea, and vomiting. Physical examination revealed nuchal rigidity but no focal neurologic signs. Brain MRI was unremarkable. Cerebrospinal fluid (CSF) studies showed pleocytosis with predominant neutrophils, normal glucose, and increased protein. All other studies, including a Gram stain, as well as bacterial, fungal, and viral CSF cultures were negative. On further investigation, the patient reported a 2-week history of mild low back pain treated with ibuprofen. What is the most likely diagnosis?

A. Bacterial meningitis

B. HIV encephalitis

C. Drug-induced aseptic meningitis (DIAM)

D. Central nervous system (CNS) tuberculosis (TB)

E. Cryptococcal meningitis

■ ANSWERS

1. **The answer is C.** Currently, three oral therapies are approved for relapsing remitting multiple sclerosis (RRMS; fingolimod—United States/Russia, teriflunomide—United States/European Union, and dimethyl fumarate—United States). Fingolimod itself is not bioactive, but when phosphorylated by sphingokinase 2, it becomes active through modulation of four of the five known G protein–coupled sphingosine-1-phosphate (S1P) receptors and alters lymphocyte trafficking by trapping them in the peripheral lymph nodes. Circulating lymphocyte counts reduce rapidly when therapy is started, remain stable during chronic treatment, and on average return to the normal range within 6 weeks after therapy is stopped.

   Brinkmann V, Billich A, Baumruker T, et al. Fingolimod (FTY720): discovery and development of an oral drug to treat multiple sclerosis. *Nat Rev Drug Discov.* 2010;9(11):883-897. doi:10.1038/nrd3248

   Freedman MS, Montalban X, Miller AE, et al. Comparing outcomes from clinical studies of oral disease-modifying therapies (dimethyl fumarate, fingolimod, and teriflunomide) in relapsing MS: assessing absolute differences using a number needed to treat analysis. *Mult Scler Relat Disord.* 2016;10:204-212. doi:10.1016/j.msard.2016.10.010

2. **The answer is D.** NMDA receptor encephalitis typically begins as a fulminant encephalopathy, with prominent neuropsychiatric manifestations, seizures, language dysfunction (verbal reduction, mutism, pressured speech), movement disorders (including dyskinesias or rigidity), decreased level of consciousness, and autonomic instability or central hypoventilation in young people. After this often-dramatic presentation, one to three relapses may occur. Most patients either die or recover from the disease. It is associated with antibodies against NR1–NR2 heteromers of the NMDA receptor (IgG GluN1 antibodies). It can be associated with tumors, especially ovarian teratoma. Tumor removal and immunotherapy can reverse the symptoms.

   Dalmau J, Gleichman AJ, Hughes EG, et al. Anti-NMDA-receptor encephalitis: case series and analysis of the effects of antibodies. *Lancet Neurol.* 2008;7(12):1091-1098. doi:10.1016/S1474-4422(08)70224-2

   Graus F, Titulaer MJ, Balu R, et al. A clinical approach to diagnosis of autoimmune encephalitis. *Lancet Neurol.* 2016;15(4):391-404. doi:10.1016/S1474-4422(15)00401-9

3. **The answer is C.** See explanation with Answer 5.

4. **The answer is B.** See explanation with Answer 5.

5. **The answer is D.** The classical presenting clinical features of NMO are optic neuritis (ON) and acute transverse myelitis. These events can occur simultaneously or in close succession. ON associated with NMO can be severe and steroid resistant. Myelitis is often, but not always clinically severe, and accompanied by a contiguous lesion that spans three or more vertebral segments on MRI. Bilateral limb paresis, spinal cord sensory syndromes, and bowel and bladder dysfunction are hallmarks of individual events. Events that involve the brainstem can be manifested by refractory nausea, vomiting, or hiccups owing to lesions in the periventricular region of the medulla, likely affecting the area postrema and medial lateral portions of the nucleus tractus solitarius. Diagnostic criteria for NMO have recently been revised to incorporate the high specificity of NMO immunoglobulin G (IgG; aquaporin 4) antibody testing. Two of the elements of the NMO diagnostic criteria are based on neuroimaging assessments. Most patients with NMO have normal brain MRI or only nonspecific white matter lesions that fail to meet multiple sclerosis (MS) imaging criteria, especially early in the disease. Second and more specific is the finding of a longitudinally extensive spinal cord lesion in association with acute transverse myelitis. Such lesions are defined by a contiguous T2 hyperintensity extending over three or more vertebral segments of the spinal cord and often have a core of T1 hypointensity. Treatment of the acute clinical relapses include intravenous (IV) corticosteroids, such as methylprednisolone. Oral azathioprine and chimeric anti-CD20 monoclonal protein rituximab are now commonly used for long-term management.

Trebst C, Jarius S, Berthele A, et al. Update on the diagnosis and treatment of neuromyelitis optica: recommendations of the Neuromyelitis Optica Study Group (NEMOS).*J Neurol.* 2014;261: 1-16. doi:10.1007/s00415-013-7169-7

Wingerchuk DM. Neuromyelitis optica spectrum disorders. *Continuum (Minneap Minn).* 2010;16(5 Multiple Sclerosis):105-121. doi:10.1093/med/9780199341016.003.0023

6. **The answer is B.** Behcet's disease is a relapsing inflammatory disorder without a defined cause. It may affect the central nervous system (CNS), and has a preference for the brainstem and diencephalon. Vasculitis is a characteristic feature (a third of the cases) with narrowing, occlusion, and aneurysm formation (88% venous). The brainstem is vulnerable because of poor venous collaterals. Behcet's may have a postviral or autoimmune pathophysiology, although familial cases and an association with HLA-B5 and HLA-B1 support a genetic role. HLA-DR15 has been associated to multiple sclerosis (MS). HLA-DQB1–0602 has been associated to narcolepsy, and C-ANCA to Wegener's granulomatosis. HLA-B27 is associated with ankylosing spondylitis.

Bartt R, Shannon K. Autoimmune and inflammatory disorders. In: Goetz CG, ed. *Textbook of Clinical Neurology.* 2nd ed. Philadelphia, PA: Elsevier Science; 2003:1124-1125.

Grossman RI, Yousem DM. *Neuroradiology: The Requisites.* 2nd ed. Philadelphia, PA: Mosby; 2003:201.

7. **The answer is A.** Progressive systemic sclerosis is a condition associated with thickening of the skin and subcutaneous tissues as well as smooth muscle atrophy and fibrosis of internal organs such as the gastrointestinal tract, lungs, heart, and kidneys. Antinuclear antibodies are typically found, usually in a nucleolar pattern; antibodies to Scl-70 are specific. Central nervous system (CNS) disease has been reported and may present as global cognitive decline or as a focal lesion. Encephalopathy, migraine, psychiatric changes, seizures, and focal neurological deficits have also been reported.

Bartt R, Shannon K. Autoimmune and inflammatory disorders. In: Goetz CG, ed. *Textbook of Clinical Neurology.* 2nd ed. Philadelphia, PA: Elsevier Science; 2003:1116-1117.

8. **The answer is E.** Penicillins and cephalosporins have been associated with aseptic meningitis. Amphotericin B and nalidixic acid have been associated with benign intracranial hypertension. Ethambutol has been associated with cerebellar ataxia and optic neuritis (ON). Vancomycin may cause cochlear and vestibular damage.

Kompoliti K, Horn S. Drug-induced and iatrogenic neurological disorders. In: Goetz CG, ed. *Textbook of Clinical Neurology.* 2nd ed. Philadelphia, PA: Elsevier Science; 2003:1233.

9. **The answer is B.** Neurotoxicity is a significant complication of the use of immunosuppressive medications, especially tacrolimus and cyclosporine, both of which have been associated with PRES. This syndrome is characterized clinically by mental status changes, seizures, and cortical blindness that are usually reversible with discontinuation of the offending medication.

Hodnett P, Coyle J, O'Regan K, et al. PRES (posterior reversible encephalopathy syndrome), a rare complication of tacrolimus therapy. *Emerg Radiol.* 2009;16(6):493-496. doi:10.1007/s10140-008-0782-6

Lessig S, Corey-Bloom J. Systemic diseases. In: Corey J, David R, eds. *Clinical Adult Neurology.* 3rd ed. New York, NY: Demos Medical Publishing; 2009:429.

10. **The answer is D.** Giant cell arteritis (temporal arteritis, GCA) is a large vessel, T-cell-mediated vasculitis. CD4 cells aggregate with a response centered on the internal elastic lamina. Pain is commonly experienced by patients with GCA. Headache, painful visual loss, sometimes with scalp tenderness (most common symptom), jaw claudication, and neck pain have been associated to the disease. Erythrocyte sedimentation rate (ESR) is usually more than 30 mm/hr. Symptoms usually last for at least 2 weeks. Diagnosis can be confirmed by biopsy.

Slevin J, Ryan M. Headaches. In: Corey J, David R, eds. *Clinical Adult Neurology.* 3rd ed. New York, NY: Demos Medical Publishing; 2009:143.

11. **The answer is D.** Progressive multifocal leukoencephalopathy (PML) is an opportunistic infection caused by the JC virus. It usually occurs in the late stages of HIV infection and has recently been associated with the use of natalizumab in patients with multiple sclerosis (MS). Clinical manifestations are variable, depending on the location and extent of lesions. Common features include cognitive deficits, focal paralysis or generalized weakness, visual disturbances, and gait abnormalities. The most common manifestation in AIDS patients is hemiparesis. Brain MRI shows hyperintense T2 subcortical white matter multifocal lesions beginning at the gray–white matter junction and coalescing to form confluent lesions. Lesions appear hypointense in T1 images. Typically, there is little or no enhancement unlike active MS lesions. The prognosis of natalizumab-associated PML is better than in AIDS patients. Diagnosis can be made by CSF analysis, which shows the presence of JC virus by PCR. This test has a sensitivity of more than 80% and specificity of more than 90%. Once the test is positive, plasma exchange (PLEX) can be done to remove natalizumab from the system. A negative test does not exclude diagnosis.

Tracy J, Mowzoon N. Neurology of infectious diseases. In: Mowzoon N, Flemming K, eds. *Neurology Board Review: An Illustrated Study Guide*. Rochester, MN: Mayo Foundation for Medical Education and Research. Mayo Clinic Scientific Press; 2007:613-614.

12. **The answer is B.** In progressive multifocal leukoencephalopathy (PML) pathology, macroscopic appearance shows confluent demyelination predominantly at juxtacortical white matter or near the deep gray matter (in contrast to multiple sclerosis [MS] lesions, which have predilection for periventricular white matter). Microscopically, there are enlarged oligodendrocytes filled with virions and reactive astrocytosis with bizarre-appearing giant astrocytes.

Tracy J, Mowzoon N. Neurology of infectious diseases. In: Mowzoon N, Flemming K, eds. *Neurology Board Review: An Illustrated Study Guide*. Rochester, MN: Mayo Foundation for Medical Education and Research. Mayo Clinic Scientific Press; 2007:613-614.

13. **The answer is C.** Marburg's variant is a rapidly progressive demyelinating process, with extensive lesions that can be multifocal, located in the cerebral hemispheres. It can also involve brainstem and optic nerves. It can present as a pseudotumor variant with headache, vomiting, altered mental status, and/or focal neurological deficits depending on the sites of the lesions. It differentiates from the tumefactive form by the contrast uptake, which is homogeneous in the Marburg's variant. Pathological studies will show extensive necrosis, massive macrophage infiltration in the acute lesions, and severe and extensive demyelination. Cerebrospinal fluid (CSF) analysis may show mononuclear pleocytosis. Oligoclonal bands (OCBs) are usually absent.

Barahona-Strauch J. Encefalomielitis diseminada aguda y sclerosis multiple. In: Arriagada CR, Nogales-Gaete J, eds. *Esclerosis Multiple Una Mirada Ibero-Panamericana*. New York, NY: Demos Medical; 2008:555-563.

14. **The answer is A.** The patient meets the criteria of dissemination in place and time (previous possible left optic neuritis [ON]) and new episode of partial transverse myelitis at the level of C6. In addition, she has at least six other white matter lesions in the typical location for diagnosis of MS. CSF is not necessary to confirm diagnosis in her case. IV methylprednisolone treatment is suggested. The possibility of a stroke is reduced given the imaging findings, which are diagnostic for MS.

Polman CH, Reingold SC, Banwell B, et al. Diagnostic criteria for multiple sclerosis: 2010 revisions to the McDonald criteria. *Ann Neurol*. 2011;69(2):292-302. doi:10.1002/ana.22366

15. **The answer is B.** This patient most likely experienced an infusion reaction due to cytokine release, which is common in patients who take rituximab for the very first time. The appropriate treatment is to wait 30 to 60 minutes and give corticosteroids before starting the rituximab infusion at half of the previous rate and titrate to tolerance. Repeating the medication challenge depends on the severity of the reaction. It is absolutely contraindicated if the patient experienced a severe or true anaphylactic reaction.

Vogel WH. Infusion reactions: diagnosis, assessment, and management. *Clin J Oncol Nurs.* 2010;14(2):E10-E21. doi:10.1188/10.CJON.E10-E21

16. **The answer is C.** Tumefactive MS may mimic the clinical and MRI characteristics of glioma or a cerebral abscess. Typically, tumefactive MS lesions are 2 cm or more in diameter, with perilesional edema on MRI. In addition, more than 50% of the lesions are gadolinium enhancing (closed-ring, open-ring, arc-like, punctate, or nodular appearance) and tend to respond to intravenous (IV) steroids. The gold standard for diagnosis and proper treatment is a biopsy, which will show typical histopathology of demyelinating disease.

Dagher AP, Smirniotopoulos J. Tumefactive demyelinating lesions. *Neuroradiology.* 1996;38(6):560-565. doi:10.1007/s002340050308

Totaro R, Di Carmine C, Splendiani A, et al. Ocurrence and long-term outcome of tumefactive demyelinating lesions in multiple sclerosis. *Neurol Sci.* 2016;37:1113-1117. doi:10.1007/s10072-016-2558-1

17. **The answer is B.** The patient is experiencing an episode of APTM. These patients may have patchy sensory impairment, mild to moderate weakness of asymmetric distribution, and occasional bladder dysfunction. Patients with APTM have greater chances of converting to MS. Earlier studies have clearly shown that patients with asymmetric and patchy spinal cord abnormal signal had converted to clinically definite multiple sclerosis (CDMS) within 3 years. Thirteen out of 15 patients (87%) who converted had abnormal brain MRI at the onset of disease. The length of the lesions is typically shorter than two vertebral segments.

Pandit L. Transverse myelitis spectrum disorders. *Neurol India.* 2009;57(2):126-133. doi:10.4103/0028-3886.51278

18. **The answer is D.** ADEM is often a monophasic demyelinating disorder that usually begins within 6 weeks after a viral infection or immunization. It causes rapid development of multifocal or focal neurological symptoms, as well as encephalopathy. Brain MRI shows enlarged and confluent white matter edematous lesions which are characteristically multiple, bilateral but asymmetric, and tend to enhance simultaneously or nearly simultaneously with gadolinium.

Krupp LB, Tardieu M, Amato MP, et al. International Pediatric Multiple Sclerosis Study Group criteria for pediatric multiple sclerosis and immune-mediated central nervous system demyelinating disorders: revisions to the 2007 definitions. *Mult Scler.* 2013;19:1261. doi:10.1177/1352458513484547

Pirko I, Noseworthy JH. Demyelinating disorders of the central nervous system. In: Goetz CG, ed. *Textbook of Clinical Neurology.* Philadelphia, PA: Elsevier Science; 2003:1059-1082.

19. **The answer is A.** ADEM has been reported to follow a number of immunizations, usually within 6 weeks, including those for pertussis, diphtheria, measles, mumps, rubella, influenza, tetanus, and yellow fever. Parainfectious ADEM usually follows onset of the infectious illness, often during the recovery phase, but because of the latency between pathogen exposure and illness, it may precede clinical symptoms of infection or the two may occur simultaneously. Measles carries the highest risk for ADEM of any infection, occurring in 1 per 400 to 1,000 cases, and measles-associated ADEM has a high rate of morbidity and mortality. ADEM MRI lesions are expected to resolve in 3 to 6 months, unlike typical multiple sclerosis (MS) lesions.

Pirko I, Noseworthy JH. Demyelinating disorders of the central nervous system. In: Goetz CG, ed. *Textbook of Clinical Neurology.* Philadelphia, PA: Elsevier Science; 2003:1059-1082.

20. **The answer is E.** From all of the symptoms listed, ascending paralysis is not typical of ADEM. Ascending paralysis is seen more commonly in Guillain–Barré syndrome (GBS), porphyria, and tick-borne paralysis.

Pirko I, Noseworthy JH. Demyelinating disorders of the central nervous system. In: Goetz CG, ed. *Textbook of Clinical Neurology.* Philadelphia, PA: Elsevier Science; 2003:1059-1082.

21. **The answer is C.** Typical clinical features of ADEM are prodrome of headache, low-grade fever, myalgia, and malaise, often preceding the onset of ADEM by a few days. The most frequent clinical signs are motor deficits followed by sensory deficits, brainstem signs, and cerebellar signs. Neurological symptoms develop rapidly in the acute phase and are commonly associated with encephalopathy, stupor, coma, meningismus, and seizures. Peak severity occurs within several days, and recovery may begin soon afterward.

Pirko I, Noseworthy JH. Demyelinating disorders of the central nervous system. In: Goetz CG, ed. *Textbook of Clinical Neurology*. Philadelphia, PA: Elsevier Science; 2003:1059-1082.

22. **The answer is C.** GBS is a peripheral nervous system demyelinating disease. ADEM, MS, and NMO are central nervous system (CNS) demyelinating diseases. ADEM is usually distinguished from MS by a history of antecedent vaccination or infection. ADEM usually has a rapid onset, commonly presenting with seizures and altered consciousness, with involvement of the gray and white matter structures as well as the cerebellum on MRI.

Cree BA. Diagnosis and differential diagnosis of multiple sclerosis. *Continuum (Minneap Minn)*. 2010;16(5 Multiple Sclerosis):19-36 doi:10.1212/01.CON.0000389932.38919.c7

23. **The answer is C.** Recurrent steroid-dependent ON is a presenting form of neurosarcoidosis. The presence of elevated ACE levels in the CSF and serum is suggestive of the disease. Further tests, such as gallium 67 scan and biopsy, must be done to confirm the diagnosis and establish a definite treatment. Visual recovery often follows corticosteroid treatment, but some patients may have permanent vision loss. Relapsing vision loss following a short course of corticosteroids for presumed optic neuritis is a clue to this disorder.

Zajicek JP, Scolding NJ, Foster O, et al. Central nervous system sarcoidosis—diagnosis and management. *QJM*. 1999;92(2):103-117. doi:10.1093/qjmed/92.2.103

24. **The answer is B.** SLE is an autoimmune disease manifested by malar rash, photosensitivity, arthritis, sclerosis, mucosal ulcers, and many other systemic symptoms. CNS involvement is common. Fifty percent of the patients can have a neuropsychiatric presentation. The most common symptom is acute confusional state, psychosis, and dementia. Other CNS symptoms are stroke, venous thrombosis, ataxia, and movement disorders.

Kanttarci OH. Inflammatory and demyelinating disorders of the central nervous system. In: Mowzoon N, Flemming K, eds. *Neurology Board Review: An Illustrated Study Guide*. Rochester, MN: Mayo Foundation for Medical Education and Research. Mayo Clinic Scientific Press; 2007:576-578.

25. **The answer is B.** Central pontine myelinolysis is, in most cases, associated with rapid correction of hyponatremia or hyperosmolar states. It typically presents in a devastating fashion as quadriplegia and pseudobulbar palsy, partial forms present as confusion, dysarthria, and/or disturbances of conjugate gaze without quadriplegia. MRI is useful in establishing the diagnosis, showing a symmetric area of abnormal high signal intensity in the pons on T2-weighted images; occasional cases present with lesions outside the brainstem. Therapeutic guidelines for restoration of severe hyponatremia should aim for gradual correction, that is, by 10 mmol/L (10 mEq/L) within 24 hours and 20 mmol/L (20 mEq/L) within 48 hours.

Hauser SL, Josephson SA. *Harrison's Neurology in Clinical Medicine*. 2nd ed. New York, NY: McGraw-Hill; 2010:290.

26. **The answer is C.** DIAM can be caused by medications such as nonsteroidal anti-inflammatory drugs (NSAIDs), antimicrobials (amoxicillin, cephalosporins, isoniazid), intravenous immunoglobulins (IVIg), monoclonal antibodies, and vaccines. The mechanism is not currently understood but the clinical presentation is often indistinguishable from infectious meningitis, including signs of meningism, and in severe cases, papilledema. Brain neuroimaging is normal and CSF studies typically show a pleocytosis with neutrophil predominance and increased protein. DIAM is a diagnosis of exclusion. Symptoms will persist until the causative drug is withdrawn and will then resolve within a few days.

Kepa L, Oczko-Grzesik B, Stolarz W, et al. Drug-induced aseptic meningitis in suspected central nervous system infections. *J Clin Neurosci*. 2005;12(5):562-564. doi:10.1016/j.jocn.2004.08.024

10 Neuroendocrine Disorders

MATTHEW FLAHERTY, HOWARD J. FAN, AND ANH NGUYEN

▦ QUESTIONS

1. An 18-year-old African American woman, with no medical history, presented with a temperature of 101.2°F, photophobia, and nuchal rigidity. Cerebrospinal fluid (CSF) was collected with an elevated opening pressure and the following chemistries: white blood cells (WBCs) 234 mm^3, glucose 23 mg/dL, and protein 300 mg/dL. She was diagnosed with bacterial meningitis and started on vancomycin and ceftriaxone. On hospital day 2, she developed polyuria. Serum sodium was 158 mEq/L (135–145 mEq/L), urine osmolality (UOsm) 240 mOsmol/kgH$_2$O (50–1,200 mOsmol/kgH$_2$O), and urine sodium (Una) 20 mEq/L (40–200 mEq/L/d). What is the most likely cause of her polyuria?

   A. Syndrome of inappropriate antidiuretic hormone (SIADH)
   B. Cerebral salt wasting (CSW)
   C. Diabetes insipidus (DI)
   D. Psychogenic polydipsia
   E. None of the above

2. A 35-year-old man with recent diagnosis of von Hippel–Lindau disease presents to the ICU with respiratory failure secondary to pulmonary edema and blood pressure (BP) of 193/110. Prior to admission, he had been complaining of a 3-day history of episodic headaches and palpitations. What is the most likely diagnosis?

   A. Hyperaldosteronism
   B. Pheochromocytoma
   C. Renal artery stenosis
   D. Fibromuscular dysplasia
   E. Medication noncompliance

3. What is the most appropriate test to establish a diagnosis for the patient in Question 2?

   A. Renal ultrasound with doppler
   B. Ratio of plasma aldosterone to plasma renin activity
   C. Plasma metanephrines
   D. Restart home antihypertensives
   E. None of the above

4. A 40-year-old man has been complaining of increasing fatigue and loss of libido. He denies symptoms of headache, diplopia, and changes in urination or thirst. The patient underwent an elective transsphenoidal surgery 6 months before to remove a nonfunctioning pituitary adenoma; results of postoperative pituitary functioning were normal. Three months after the

surgery, he had stereotactic radiation to treat the residual tumor. What is the most likely diagnosis?

A. Regrowth of the adenoma
B. Diabetes insipidus (DI)
C. Hydrocephalus
D. Hypopituitarism

5. A 24-year-old woman with a history of bipolar disorder, on lithium, presented to the ICU intubated and in a coma. Two days before admission, she had been suffering from "the flu." Her vitals are blood pressure (BP) 101/68 mmHg, heart rate (HR) 65 beats/min, and temperature 96°F. Physical examination revealed no scars, dry skin, no eye opening to noxious stimuli, localizing throughout, and absent deep tendon reflexes. Pertinent laboratory findings are negative for influenza A/B and West Nile antigen, lithium level 1 mEq/L (0.8–1.2 mEq/L), thyroid-stimulating hormone (TSH) 10 µU/mL (0.4–4.0 µU/mL), and free T4 0.09 ng/dL (0.7–2.0 ng/dL). What is the most likely cause of her presentation?

A. Hyperthyroidism
B. Hypothyroidism
C. Lithium toxicity
D. West Nile infection
E. None of the above

6. A 74-year-old African American man with a history of atrial fibrillation is transferred to the ICU from an outside hospital after experiencing acute symptoms of right middle cerebral artery (MCA) syndrome and receiving intravenous (IV) tissue plasminogen activator (tPA). For a month before admission, he had been complaining of heat intolerance, diarrhea, and weight loss. He also stated that he felt like his neck was enlarging. Upon arriving to the ICU, he is found to have a rapid ventricular rate (RVR) and is subsequently started on an amiodarone drip with good rate control. The next morning, he has a generalized motor seizure lasting 20 minutes before being controlled, is back in RVR, and has a temperature of 104°F. What is the likely diagnosis for his acute decompensation?

A. Cerebral infection
B. Reinfarction
C. Hypothyroidism
D. Thyroid storm

7. A 72-year-old Asian man with a history of hypertension, hyperlipidemia, noninsulin-dependent diabetes, and gout presents to the ED with signs of left middle cerebral artery (MCA) syndrome. On brain CT, there appears to be a hyperdense left MCA sign. Serum glucose is found to be 980 mg/dL with a mild ketoacidosis. On arterial blood gas (ABG), there is a base deficit of −11. What is the most likely diagnosis?

A. Hyperosmolar hyperglycemic syndrome (HHS)
B. Diabetic ketoacidosis (DKA)
C. Cushing syndrome
D. Addison's disease

8. A 42-year-old female who has been out of medical care presents to the ED with complaints of double vision and lethargy. She also endorses palpitations, generalize weakness, and unintentional weight loss for the past month. She denies substance abuse and does not take any medications or supplements. Her vitals are significant for: temperature 39°C, blood pressure (BP) 175/88 mmHg, heart rate (HR) 120 beats/min, respiratory rate (RR) 18, and saturating 100% on room air. Exam is notable for mild agitation, supple neck, warm extremities, and brisk

reflexes but without clonus. A noncontrast CT of the head reveals no overt abnormalities and ECG shows atrial fibrillation with rapid response rate. She is given metoprolol 5 mg intraveneously (IV) × 2 with some improvement in her HR and is transferred to the ICU for further management. What is the most appropriate treatment of the patient's underlying condition?

A. Propylthiouracil, propranolol
B. Levothyroxine
C. Lugol's solution
D. Bromocriptine mesylate, Dantrolene sodium
E. A and C
F. B and D

9. An elderly male patient presents with urine osmolality (UOsm) greater than 100 mOsm/L (reference 50–1,200) and urine sodium (Una) greater than 30 mmol/L (reference 15–250), consistent with which of the following etiologies of hyponatremia?

A. Syndrome of inappropriate secretion of antidiuretic hormone (SIADH), hypothyroidism, adrenal insufficiency
B. Polydipsia, inappropriate water administration to children
C. Vomiting, diarrhea, and third spacing
D. Congestive heart failure (CHF), cirrhosis, renal failure
E. Diuretic use, renal tubular dysfunction

10. A 52-year-old male is admitted to the ICU with a high grade aSAH secondary to a ruptured anterior communicating artery aneurysm. An external ventricular drain (EVD) is emergently placed and he is taken for successful clipping of the aneurysm the following morning. On postbleed day 5, a basic metabolic panel revealed sodium 130mEq/L, potassium 3.5 mEq/L, chloride 105 mEq/L, bicarbonate 22 mEq/L, blood urea nitrogen (BUN) 10 mg/dL, and creatinine (Cr)1 mg/dL. The patient is receiving nimodipine 60 mg q4hr and maintenance fluids with 0.9 normal saline (NS) at 75 cc/hr. Which of the following features is most useful in establishing the etiology of the patient's hyponatremia?

A. Hypovolemia and negative sodium balance
B. Hypernatremia and positive fluid balance
C. Hypotonic plasma
D. High urine output
E. Intracellular volume depletion

11. The treatment of cerebral salt wasting (CSW) typically includes:

A. Hypotonic volume replacement
B. Restoration of positive sodium balance with hypertonic saline
C. Fludrocortisone
D. Treatment of underlying etiology

12. A 40-year-old man with renal insufficiency in the ICU is found to have symptomatic hyponatremia of 119 mmol/L on his second day of admission. He is given hyperosmolar saline, and his sodium rises to 128 mmol/L the next day. After tube feeding is started, his sodium falls to 122 mmol/L. What is the next best step in normalizing his sodium over the long term?

A. High-protein diet
B. Demeclocycline
C. Conivaptan
D. Tolvaptan
E. Hypertonic saline

13. Which of the following comorbidities can predispose to the development of osmotic demyelination syndrome (ODS)?

   A. Chronic alcoholism
   B. Malnutrition
   C. Renal insufficiency
   D. Liver cirrhosis
   E. All of the above

14. The most important risk factors for the development of osmotic demyelination syndrome (ODS) include:

   A. Duration of hyponatremia
   B. Serum sodium at presentation
   C. Rate of serum sodium correction
   D. All of the above

15. A 55-year-old male with past medical history significant for hypertension, chronic obstructive pulmonary disease (COPD), and type 2 diabetes is admitted to the ICU due to concerns for aspiration pneumonia with sepsis physiology. His initial vitals include temperature 39°C, blood pressure (BP) 105/70, heart rate (HR) 110, respiratory rate (RR) 22, and saturating 92% on 2 L nasal cannula. He was pan cultured and started on broad spectrum antibiotics including vancomycin, cefepime, and azithromycin. In the ICU, he has increased work of breathing and is intubated for airway protection using etomidate 0.3 mg/kg and rocuronium 15 mcg/kg. He is sedated with propofol 30 mcg/kg/min and placed on fentanyl drip at 75 mcg/hr. Over the next 24 hours, he develops persistent hypotension with systolic BP in the low 80s requiring initiation of pressors. Which of the following is contributory to the patient's hypotension?

   A. Etomidate use during induction
   B. Septic shock
   C. Sedative/analgesia
   D. Positive pressure mechanical ventilation (PPV)
   E. All of the above

16. An elderly unconscious immigrant female presents with low serum, unbound thyroxine (fT4), and triiodothyronine (fT3), with associated sinus bradycardia and hypothermia. Which of the following therapies should be considered?

   A. Rewarming
   B. Corticosteroids
   C. Intravenous (IV) fluids and vasopressors
   D. Mechanical ventilation
   E. All of the above

17. A 35-year-old female is admitted to the ICU for observation overnight after a motor vehicle accident in which she developed trace traumatic subarachnoid hemorrhage (tSAH). On review of systems, she endorses galactorrhea, decreased libido, and irregular menses for the past 4 months. Beta human chorionic gonadotropin (beta-HCG) testing is negative and she is not taking any medications or herbal supplements. Workup is significant for a prolactin level of 200 ng/L and a MRI brain with and without contrast reveals a 2.5-cm pituitary macroadenoma. Which of the following is the most appropriate initial treatment?

   A. Cabergoline
   B. Transphenoidal surgery
   C. Temozolomide
   D. Bromocriptine

18. The patient in the previous question declines treatment and is discharged the following morning. She is lost to follow-up and returns to the ED 2 years later with complaints of diplopia with worsening galactorrhea and continued amenorrhea. Beta human chorionic gonadotropin (beta-HCG) is negative and MRI brain with and without contrast shows an interval increase of the pituitary macroadenoma to 3 cm. Thyroid-stimulating hormone (TSH), free T4, and basal cortisol levels are normal but the prolactin level is now 30 ng/L. Which of the following is the most likely explanation for the decreased prolactin level?

A. Decreased mass effect on the pituitary stalk
B. Hook effect
C. Panhypopituitarism
D. Transition from secreting to nonsecreting macroadenoma

■ ANSWERS

1. **The answer is C.** Although not a common etiology, meningitis can cause central DI. Other etiologies of DI include cranial trauma, brain surgery (transsphenoidal), sellar and suprasellar tumors, pituitary apoplexy, Sheehan's syndrome, and sarcoidosis. Typically, laboratory values seen in DI are hypernatremia, low UOsm, normal Una, and low urine specific gravity. With SIADH and CSW, there is hyponatremia, high Uosm, and high Una. Psychogenic polydipsia will show hyponatremia, low to normal UOsm, and low to normal Una.

   James K. An endocrinology consult. In: Torbey M, ed. *Neurocritical Care.* New York, NY: Cambridge University Press; 2010:397-409.

2. **The answer is B.** Von Hippel–Lindau syndrome is an autosomal dominant disease consisting of cerebellar and spinal cord hemangioblastomas, retinal angiomas, renal cell carcinoma, and pheochromocytoma. Given the patient's presentation and history, the most likely diagnosis is pheochromocytoma. Fibromuscular dysplasia is most commonly seen in females.

   Pacak K, Linehan WM, Eisenhofer G, et al. Recent advances in genetics, diagnosis, localization, and treatment of pheochromocytoma. *Ann Intern Med.* 2001;134(4):315-329. doi:10.7326/0003-4819-134-4-200102200-00016

3. **The answer is C.** Plasma metanephrines are the most useful test if the pretest probability is high, as in this case. When normal, it effectively excludes the diagnosis of pheochromocytoma, and mild elevations can be false positives. Renal ultrasound with doppler helps in the diagnosis of both renal artery stenosis and fibromuscular dysplasia. Serum aldosterone to renin ratio will diagnose hyperaldosteronism.

   Pacak K, Linehan WM, Eisenhofer G, et al. Recent advances in genetics, diagnosis, localization, and treatment of pheochromocytoma. *Ann Intern Med.* 2001;134(4):315-329. doi:10.7326/0003-4819-134-4-200102200-00016

4. **The answer is D.** Radiation therapy to the pituitary gland can cause deficiencies of anterior pituitary hormones. Cortisol deficiency, hypothyroidism, and hypogonadism could be possible causes of his symptoms. Regrowth of the adenoma is unlikely, as radiation therapy is effective in "curing" nonfunctioning adenomas. DI usually manifests 24 to 48 hours after surgery to the pituitary. Radiation to the pituitary generally does not damage the posterior pituitary. Neither transsphenoidal surgery nor radiation causes hydrocephalus.

   Corenblum B. Hypopituitarism (panhypopituitarism). In: Griffing GT, ed. *Medscape.* 2011. Available at: http://emedicine.medscape.com/article/122287-overview.

5. **The answer is B.** One of lithium's many side effects is hypothyroidism. Myxedema coma is a life-threatening manifestation of hypothyroidism. This patient presenting in a coma after 2 days of being ill likely is in myxedema coma manifested by the side effect of lithium and the added stress of illness. Her high TSH and low free T4 help to validate her etiology. Hyperthyroidism is unlikely, as TSH is low and free T4 is high in this disease. Given the normal lithium level, her coma is unlikely to be a manifestation of lithium toxicity. A negative West Nile antigen can help rule out West Nile infection as an etiology.

   James K. An endocrinology consult. In: Torbey M, ed. *Neurocritical Care.* New York, NY: Cambridge University Press; 2010:397-409.

6. **The answer is D.** The most likely diagnosis is thyroid storm characterized by seizure, RVR, and hyperthermia. For a month, the patient had been experiencing symptoms of thyrotoxicosis, which could be secondary to Graves' disease given his neck mass. Amiodarone has been associated with thyrotoxicosis with two major forms: type 1 seen in patients with preexisting or latent thyroid disease, while type 2 occurs due to unrestrained release of thyroid hormone from an inflamed, previously normal thyroid gland. Given the patient's likelihood of Graves' disease, the amiodarone drip that was started to control his rate precipitated a thyroid storm. Cerebral infection such as meningitis can cause seizure and hyperthermia; given the history

and presentation, thyroid storm is more likely. Reinfarction may cause a seizure and cardiac arrhythmias, but is unlikely to cause extreme hyperthermia. Symptoms of hypothyroidism are cold intolerance, constipation, and bradyarrhythmia, and these are not present in this patient.

Kannan CR, Seshadri KG. Thyrotoxicosis. *Dis Mon.* 1997;43(9):601-677.

7. **The answer is A.** This patient has presented with a stroke that has precipitated HHS. This syndrome is typically seen in elderly patients with precipitating factors such as stroke and myocardial infarction. With HHS, the patient may or may not have a history of non–insulin-dependent diabetes, extreme hyperglycemia greater than 1,000 mg/dL, and decreased sensorium/coma secondary to osmotically mediated cellular dehydration. DKA is typically manifested in younger insulin-dependent diabetics with hyperglycemia in the range of 400 to 800 mg/dL, marked ketoacidosis, and hyperkalemia. The treatment for HHS and DKA are similar with the goal to maintain normoglycemia while correcting hypovolemia and any electrolyte derangements. Cushing syndrome is manifested after prolonged exposure to high doses of corticosteroids, which is not the case in this patient. Addison's disease is a disorder of the adrenal gland not producing sufficient glucocorticoids or mineralocorticoids. Hypoglycemia is a symptom of Addison's disease.

Lorber D. Nonketotic hypertonicity in diabetes mellitus. *Med Clin North Am.* 1995;79(1):39-52. doi:10.1016/s0025-7125(16)30083-9

8. **The answer is E.** Thyroid storm is a difficult diagnosis to make but can be life threatening if missed. It requires a high clinical index of suspicion with prompt treatment often occurring prior to confirmatory laboratory values becoming available. Propylthiouracil inhibits the production of thyroid hormones by inhibiting the conversion of T4 to T3. Lugol's solution (sodium ipodate or potassium iodide) inhibits the release of thyroid hormones and is typically started after an hour following the first dose of antithyroidal drug to avoid stimulating thyroid hormone synthesis. Propranolol, a beta-adrenergic blocker, is used to treat the hypertension and tachycardia associated with thyroid storm. In larger doses, greater than 240 mg, it too can inhibit the conversion of T4 to T3. Levothyroxine is a synthetic T4 used to treat hypothyroidism. Dopamine agonists such as bromocriptine and muscle relaxants have been used in the treatment of neuroleptic malignant syndrome (NMS) but this diagnosis is unlikely in this case scenario given lack of medication history for antipsychotic or dopamine receptor antagonist medications.

Kannan CR, Seshadri KG. Thyrotoxicosis. *Dis Mon.* 1997;43(9):601-677.

9. **The answer is A.** Euvolemic hyponatremia, typically associated with SIADH, hypothyroidism, and adrenal insufficiency, is characterized by a USom greater than 100 mOsm/L (usually >300) and a Una greater than 30 mmol/L. Other causes of euvolemic hyponatremia include polydipsia and inappropriate water administration, which have UOsm less than 100 Osm/L and a Una greater than 30 mmol/L. Vomiting, diarrhea, and third spacing can cause hypovolemic hyponatremia (UOsm >300 mOsm/L, Una <20 mmol/L, and FeNa <1%). CHF and cirrhosis present with hypervolemic hyponatremia (UOsm > 300 mOsm/L, Una <20 mmol/L, and FeNa <1%). Excessive diuretic use typically presents with an elevated UOsm greater than 300 mOsm/L, Una greater than 20 mmol/L, and elevated FeNa greater than 1%.

Adrogué HJ, Madias NE. Hyponatremia. *N Engl J Med.* 2000;342(21):1581-1589. doi:10.1056/nejm200005253422107

10. **The answer is A.** Hyponatremia is the most common electrolyte abnormality occurring after subarachnoid hemorrhage (SAH) with etiologies including diuretic use, excessive intravenous (IV) fluid therapy, cerebral salt wasting (CSW), and syndrome of inappropriate secretion of antidiuretic hormone (SIADH). The patient is not taking diuretics and is only receiving 0.9 NS maintenance fluids at 75 cc/hr making CSW and SIADH the more likely culprits

behind the hyponatremia. CSW syndrome is defined by the development of extracellular volume depletion due to a renal sodium transport abnormality in patients with intracranial disease and normal adrenal and thyroid function. SIADH is a result of excessive secretion of antidiuretic hormone leading to increased water reabsorption in the distal convoluted renal tubules resulting in free water retention and corresponding dilutional hyponatremia. It may be difficult to distinguish from SIADH, which develops under similar circumstances and also presents with hyponatremia. The main clinical difference between these two conditions is the total fluid status of the patient: CSW patients present with hypovolemia and a negative sodium balance, whereas SIADH is associated with euvolemia or hypervolemia. Another useful tool in differentiating CSW from SIADH is a laboratory finding. Random urine sodium concentrations tend to be greater than 100 mEq/L in CSW. SIADH rarely leads to a random urine sodium of greater than 100 mEq/L. Finally, once the hyponatremia is corrected, uric acid levels normalize in SIADH with the fractional excretion of uric acid (FEUA) generally less than 10% while hypouricemia remains in CSW with FEUA greater than 10%.

Nakajima H, Okada H, Hirose K, et al. Cerebral salt-wasting syndrome and inappropriate antidiuretic hormone syndrome after subarachnoid hemorrhage. *Intern Med.* March 15, 2017;56(6):677-680. doi:10.2169/internalmedicine.56.6843

11. **The answer is B.** The treatment of CSW typically includes assessment of fluid balance and restoration of serum sodium levels with hypertonic saline. CSW refractory to hypertonic saline may require the use of fludrocortisone, a synthetic mineralocorticoid, indicated for replacement in primary adrenal insufficiency and in refractory CSW.

Woo MH, Kale-Pradhan PB. Fludrocortisone in the treatment of subarachnoid hemorrhage-induced hyponatremia. *Ann Pharmacother.* 1997;31(5):637-639. doi:10.1016/j.wneu.2017.09.182

12. **The answer is D.** High-protein diet or oral urea administration induces an osmotic diuresis, increases free water excretion, and thus ameliorates hyponatremia in syndrome of inappropriate secretion of antidiuretic hormone (SIADH). Demeclocycline, which blocks antidiuretic hormone (ADH) action through inhibition of cyclic adenosine monophosphate (cAMP) generation and thus increases free water excretion, can be an alternative for refractory hyponatremia. Demeclocycline is contraindicated in patients with renal disease, hepatic cirrhosis, or congestive heart failure (CHF). Conivaptan is for short-term use only and therefore not useful for long-term management. Tolvaptan, a selective V2 receptor blocker, is available for long-term oral use.

Oster JR, Epstein M. Demeclocycline-induced renal failure. *Lancet.* 1977;1(8001):52. doi:10.1016/s0140-6736(77)91697-x
Zietse R, van der Lubbe N, Hoorn EJ. Current and future treatment options in SIADH. *NDT Plus.* 2009;2(suppl 3):iii12-iii19. doi:10.1093/ndtplus/sfp154

13. **The answer is E.** ODS results from too rapid correction of serum sodium, causing demyelination of susceptible neurons, classically in the pons. Symptoms include spastic paralysis, pseudobulbar palsy, dysarthria, horizontal gaze paralysis, and decreased consciousness, which progresses over hours to days. Increased risk of ODS has been associated with chronic alcoholism, malnutrition, renal insufficiency, and liver cirrhosis.

Laureno R, Karp BI. Myelinolysis after correction of hyponatremia. *Ann Intern Med.* 1997;126(1): 57-62. doi:10.7326/0003-4819-126-1-199701010-00008

14. **The answer is D.** The majority of ODS cases occur in patients whose sodium concentrations at presentation are less than or equal to 105 mEq/L, and nearly all reported cases arise in patients who present with a serum sodium of 120 mEq/L or less. Studies in experimental animals showed that brain damage does not occur when hyponatremia of less than a day's duration is rapidly corrected. However, if hyponatremia persists for 2 to 3 days or more, the same treatment can result in severe demyelination. The recommended maximum rate of correction, based on numerous animal studies, is 0.5 mmol/L/hour, 10 to 12 mmol/L in the first 24 hours, and no more than 18 mmol/L in the first 48 hours.

Laureno R, Karp BI. Myelinolysis after correction of hyponatremia. *Ann Intern Med*. 1997;126(1):57-62. doi:10.7326/0003-4819-126-1-199701010-00008

15. **The answer is E.** Etomidate is a commonly used anesthetic inducing agent but its use has been controversial in septic and critically ill patients. Etomidate inhibits the 11 beta-hydroxylase enzyme responsible for converting 11 beta-deoxycortisol into cortisol in the adrenal gland leading to a cortisol-deficient state and resulting hypotension. Data from the Annane and the Corticosteroid Therapy of Septic Shock (CORTICUS) study suggest administrating stress doses of hydrocortisone within 6 hours in critically ill patients receiving etomidate as an inducing agent. Septic shock causes hypotension via cytokine- and inflammatory-mediated cascades leading to peripheral vasodilation. Fentanyl causes hypotension due to suppression of endogenous catecholamines, while propofol decreases peripheral vascular resistance. Positive pressure mechanical ventilation decreases venous return to the heart resulting in hypotension.

Arita N, Ward JL, and Marik PE. Pituitary, adrenal, and thyroid disease in the critical ill patient. In: *Comprehensive Critical Care: Adult*. 2nd ed. Mount Prospect, IL: Society of Critical Care Medicine;2012:403-410.

Ostemann ME, Keenan SP, Seiferlinget RA, et al. Sedation in the intensive care unit. *JAMA*. March 15, 2000;283(11):1451-1459. doi:10.1001/jama.283.11.1451. Available at: jamanetwork.com/journals/jama/fullarticle/192488.

16. **The answer is E.** Myxedema coma is the most extreme form of hypothyroidism, typically presenting as coma or lethargy with bradycardia, hypothermia, hyponatremia, and respiratory failure precipitated by infection, heart failure, or amiodarone exposure. It is a medical emergency associated with a high mortality rate, although rare in presentation because of widespread availability of thyroid-stimulating hormone (TSH) assays. Treatment involves ventilator support, cautious rewarming, glucocorticoid therapy 50 to 100 mg hydrocortisone q6h, and hemodynamic support. Sodium levels less than 120 mEq/L should be treated. The optimal mode of thyroid hormone therapy in patients with myxedema coma is controversial, largely because the condition is so rare that there are no clinical trials comparing the efficacy of different treatment regimens. Whether patients with myxedema coma should be treated with T4, T3, or both is controversial, but IV therapy remains a common option.

Arita N, et al. Pituitary, adrenal, and thyroid disease in the critical ill patient. In: *Comprehensive Critical Care: Adult*. 2nd ed. Mount Prospect, IL: Society of Critical Care Medicine; 2012: 403-410.

17. **The answer is A.** Hyperprolactinemia can be caused by secretory tumors (prolactinomas) but can also be seen with nonsecretory suprasellar tumors. The current theory for hyperprolactinemia involving nonsecretory suprasellar tumors is termed the "stalk effect" and revolves around prolactin inhibition by dopamine from the hypothamalmus via a negative feedback system. As such, tumors that compress the infundibular stalk dopaminergic neurons or disrupt the hypophyseal portal system by which dopamine is delivered to the lactotrophs will result in an elevation in prolactin. Prolactinomas are most commonly seen in women between the ages of 20 to 50 years and make up approximately 50% of all pituitary adenomas. Prolactinomas are initially treated with dopamine agonists which activate dopamine receptors on the tumor, leading to a reduction in tumor size and lower prolactin levels. Cabergoline is preferred over bromocriptine as it has fewer adverse effects and is more effective in normalizing prolactin levels while reducing the overall tumor size. While transsphenoidal adenoma surgery is generally the initial treatment of most pituitary adenomas, this is not the case with prolactinomas given the high efficacy and tolerability of dopamine agonists. Temozolomide is a DNA alkylating agent reserved for glioblastoma multiforme and aggressive pituitary macroadenomas.

Molitch M. Diagnosis and treatment of pituitary adenomas. *JAMA*. February 7, 2017;317(5):516-524. doi:10.1001/jama.2016.19699. Available at: jamanetwork.com/journals/jama/fullarticle/2600472.

18. **The answer is C.** In general, if the prolactin level is more than 200 ng/L, the cause of the elevated prolactin is likely a prolactinoma rather than compression of the pituitary stalk. In large prolactinomas (>3 cm), the high prolactin levels may saturate the antibodies in some assays causing a falsely diminished prolactin level. This phenomenon is known as the "hook effect" and can be corrected by running the sample in a 1:100 dilution. Although secreting macroadenomas can become nonsecreting, this is a less likely scenario given the patient's interval worsening of symptoms attributable to elevated prolactin levels. Similarly, given normal thyroid profile and basal cortisol levels, panhypopituitarism is unlikely

Molitch M. Diagnosis and treatment of pituitary adenomas. *JAMA*. February 7, 2017;317(5):516-524. doi:10.1001/jama.2016.19699. Available at: jamanetwork.com/journals/jama/fullarticle/2600472.

Neuro-Oncology

*KEITH KERR, YOSHUA ESQUENAZI, AND
NITIN TANDON*

■ QUESTIONS

1. A 54-year-old right-handed man with a medical history of hypertension and diabetes presented to the ED after an episode of confusion that lasted for about 15 minutes. On further
   questioning, the patient admitted to episodes of speech difficulty going on for about 3 weeks
   and a 2-week history of headaches. On physical examination, he was found to have a receptive
   aphasia. A noncontrast CT scan done in the ED showed evidence of a hypodense lesion in the
   left temporal lobe. The CT and MRI of the brain are shown here. What is the appropriate next
   step for the definitive management of this patient?

   A. Lumbar puncture (LP) and initiation of high-dose acyclovir
   B. Fosphenytoin load and 24-hour video EEG (vEEG)
   C. Intravenous (IV) dexamethasone and levetiracetam and plans for surgical resection
   D. Functional MRI
   E. Aspirin and CT angiogram of the brain

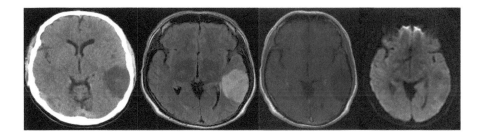

2. What is the median survival time for patients with a World Health Organization (WHO)
   grade IV glioblastoma (GBM) with the current standard of care, including adjuvant
   chemotherapy?

   A. Greater than 5 years
   B. 10 to 20 months
   C. Less than 6 months
   D. About 2 to 2.5 years
   E. Less than 9 months

3. A patient with the accompanying MRI presents as a direct transfer to the ICU from an outside hospital with a rapidly declining mental status and worsening L hemiparesis. What is the next best step in management?

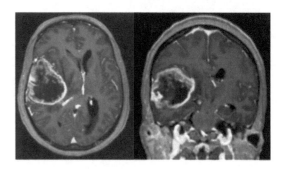

A. Emergent resection of the mass
B. High-dose steroids
C. External ventricular drain (EVD) placement
D. Intubation
E. Initiation of fluid resuscitation

4. Which of the following is the most common intracranial neoplasm in adults?

A. Glioblastoma (GBM)
B. Meningioma
C. Pituitary tumors
D. Medulloblastoma
E. Metastases

5. A 42-year-old woman with no significant medical history presents to the ED 7 hours after the sudden onset of headache associated with nausea and vomiting. On physical examination, she is confused and complaining that she is having difficulty seeing. Her blood pressure (BP) is 75/40. The accompanying MRI of the brain was obtained. What is the best next step in the management of this patient?

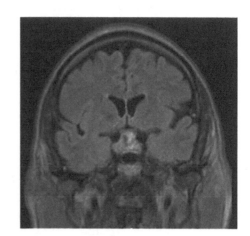

A. External ventricular drain (EVD) placement and emergent diagnostic cerebral angiogram
B. Broad-spectrum antibiotics and lumbar puncture (LP)
C. High-dose corticosteroids
D. Emergent surgical resection
E. Diagnostic cerebral angiogram and intra-arterial tissue plasminogen activator (tPA)

6. What is the most likely diagnosis in Question 5?

A. Subarachnoid hemorrhage (SAH) from a ruptured posterior communicating aneurysm
B. Cavernous sinus thrombosis
C. Bacterial meningitis
D. Benedikt syndrome
E. Pituitary apoplexy

7. After surgery the patient's blood pressure normalizes and her mental status is improved. Her vision is also back to baseline. On postoperative day (POD) 1 her laboratory values are as follows: sodium: 157, potassium: 4.0, blood urea nitrogen (BUN) 28, creatine (Cr) 0.9, glucose 110. Her urine output has been greater than 300 cc per hour for the past 4 hours. What is the source of her hypernatremia?

   A. Syndrome of inappropriate antidiuretic hormone secretion (SIADH)
   B. Diabetes insipidus (DI)
   C. Improper fluid administration
   D. Diuresis of perioperative fluids
   E. Cerebral salt wasting syndrome (CSWS)

8. Which lab values support a diagnosis of diabetes insipidus (DI)?

   A. Urine specific gravity of less than 1.005
   B. Urine osmolality (UOsm) of less than 300 mOsm/kg
   C. Plasma osmolality greater than 300 mOsm/kg
   D. Sodium level greater than 145
   E. All of the above

9. Which of the following is best characterized as an intradural extramedullary spinal cord tumor?

   A. Meningioma
   B. Ependymoma
   C. Astrocytoma
   D. Spinal metastasis
   E. Hemangioblastoma

10. Which of the following is/are the most common symptom of metastatic epidural spinal cord compression (MESCC)?

   A. Weakness
   B. Sensory deficits
   C. Back pain
   D. Autonomic symptoms
   E. Ataxia and gait disturbances

11. A 58-year-old woman with a medical history of hypertension and lung cancer undergoing chemotherapy presents to the ED with a 3-week history of worsening back pain and 4-day history of weakness in her lower extremities. On physical examination, strength in her lower extremities is 4/5 throughout, her reflexes are normal, and there is no evidence of clonus or abnormal plantar response. The accompanying CT scan and MRI of the thoracic spine, reveal a lesion at T9 level. Which of the following is the best management option for this patient?

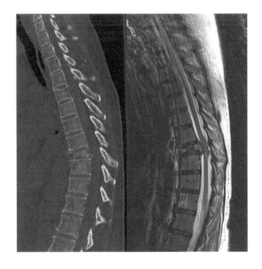

    A. Corticosteroids and radiation therapy
    B. Kyphoplasty
    C. Corticosteroids, separation surgery, and adjuvant stereotactic radiosurgery (SRS)
    D. Thoracic laminectomy and instrumentation
    E. Spinal SRS and kyphoplasty

12. Which of the following is the most common presenting symptom in carcinomatous meningitis (CM)?

    A. Photophobia
    B. Mental status changes
    C. Trigeminal neuralgia
    D. Nuchal rigidity
    E. Diplopia

13. Which of the following is the most useful laboratory test in the diagnosis of carcinomatous meningitis (CM)?

    A. Leptomeningeal biopsy
    B. Cerebrospinal fluid (CSF) examination
    C. Serology for tumor markers
    D. Flow cytometry and DNA single-cell cytometry
    E. Fluorescence in situ hybridization

14. Which of the following paraneoplastic syndromes (PNS) is associated with involuntary, arrhythmic, chaotic multidirectional saccades with horizontal, vertical, and torsional components, accompanied by myoclonic jerks in the limbs and trunk?

    A. Anti-Hu limbic encephalitis
    B. Opsoclonus-myoclonus
    C. Paraneoplastic cerebellar degeneration
    D. Lambert–Eaton syndrome
    E. Polymyositis

15. A 48-year-old male presents for elective resection of a right temporal glioma as pictured in the following MRI. Postoperatively the patient was doing well upon transfer to the neuro ICU. He received 1 g of levetiracetam during surgery. Approximately 6 hours postoperatively the patient has a complex partial seizure. The seizure lasts 30 seconds and the patient returns to his baseline. Which intervention should be performed next?

    A. CT scan of the brain
    B. Intravenous (IV) lorazepam
    C. IV levetiracetam
    D. MRI of the brain
    E. Intubation

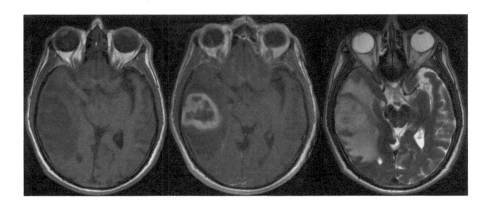

16. A similar patient as in question 15 has a grand mal seizure about 4 hours post-op that is ongoing for 3 minutes when you are called by the nurse. The seizure lasts 5 minutes and the patient has a subsequent left hemiparesis but is awake and interactive. Which intervention should be performed next?

   A. CT scan of the brain
   B. Intravenous (IV) lorazepam
   C. IV levetiracetam
   D. MRI of the brain
   E. Intubation

■ ANSWERS

1. **The answer is C.** CT of the brain shows a left posterior temporal hypodensity. MRI of the brain shows increased signal intensity on T2, without evidence of restricted diffusion or contrast enhancement, consistent with a low-grade glioma. Low-grade gliomas typically arise in and around eloquent cortex. Patients present with either seizures; symptoms of raised intracranial pressure (ICP) (headache, nausea, vomiting, lethargy); or focal neurological deficits (weakness, sensory abnormalities, neglect, visual or speech difficulty), depending on tumor size and location. The role of surgical resection is well established in patients with symptoms of local mass effect, increased ICP, or intractable seizures. Greater extent of resection correlates with improved survival time and reduces the risk of malignant transformation. An awake craniotomy with intraoperative brain mapping has shown promising results in the resection of lesions in or around eloquent structures. Functional MRI can help localize language function in patients with brain tumors, but lacks both specificity and sensitivity and cannot be used alone for language localization. There is no evidence of acute ischemia on diffusion-weighted MRI; therefore, neither a CT angiogram nor aspirin administration is indicated. The patient presented with a simple partial seizure, and even though fosphenytoin should be administered for seizure prophylaxis, a 24-hour EEG is not indicated. Herpes encephalitis is a consideration in a patient presenting with seizures and a temporal lobe mass, but patients typically have fever. Herpes encephalitis typically involves the mesial structures of the temporal lobe and can occasionally have evidence of hemorrhage within these structures.

   Bulakbasi N, Kocaoglu M. Central nervous system infections of herpesvirus family. *Neuroimaging Clin N Am.* 2008;18(1):53-84; viii. doi:10.1016/j.nic.2007.12.001

   Lubrano V, Draper L, Roux FE. What makes surgical tumor resection feasible in broca's area? Insights into intraoperative brain mapping. *Neurosurgery.* 2010;66(5):868-875; discussion 875. doi:10.1227/01.NEU.0000368442.92290.04

   Sanai N, Berger MS. Operative techniques for gliomas and the value of extent of resection. *Neurotherapeutics.* 2009;6(3):478-486. doi:10.1016/j.nurt.2009.04.005

2. **The answer is B.** Even with maximal safe resection and adjuvant therapies the median survival time is 14.6 months in patients participating in clinical trials and 10 to 11 months in the general GBM population. The current standard of care has evolved from resection followed by adjuvant radiotherapy to resection, concurrent chemotherapy (temozolomide) and radiation, and additional adjuvant chemotherapy. The expression of specific molecular biomarkers, especially *O*-6-methylguanine methyltransferase (MGMT) and isocitrate dehydrogenase mutation, may determine the response of the tumor to treatment and helps in identifying the magnitude of benefit from this regimen. Bevacizumab therapy has also had a definitive impact in slowing the progression of recurrent GBMs. Two recent phase III clinical trials have demonstrated a survival benefit with fewer systemic adverse events in both newly diagnosed and recurrent GBM using Tumor Treating Fields (TTF). The results of these trials have led to the FDA approval of TTF for recurrent and newly diagnosed GBM in 2011 and 2015, respectively.

   Quick A, Patel D, Hadziahmetovic M, et al. Current therapeutic paradigms in glioblastoma. *Rev Recent Clin Trials.* 2010;5(1):14-27. doi:10.2174/157488710790820544

   Stupp R, Mason WP, van den Bent MJ, et al. Radiotherapy plus concomitant and adjuvant temozolomide for glioblastoma. *N Engl J Med.* 2005;352(10):987-996. doi:10.1056/NEJMoa043330

   Stupp R, Taillibert S, Kanner AA, et al. Maintenance therapy with tumor-treating fields plus temozolomide vs temozolomide alone for glioblastoma: a randomized clinical trial. *JAMA.* 2015;314(23):2535-2543. doi:10.1001/jama.2015.16669

   Stupp R, Wong ET, Kanner AA, et al. NovoTTF-100A versus physician's choice chemotherapy in recurrent glioblastoma: a randomised phase III trial of a novel treatment modality. *Eur J Cancer.* 2012;48(14):2192-2202. doi:10.1016/j.ejca.2012.04.011

   Walbert T, Mikkelsen T. Recurrent high-grade glioma: a diagnostic and therapeutic challenge. *Expert Rev Neurother.* 2011;11(4):509-518. doi:10.1586/ern.11.37

3. **The answer is D.** The patient is presenting with signs of uncal herniation and increased intracranial pressure (ICP). At this time, the most important intervention is airway protection given the patient's rapidly declining mental status. Steroids and fluid resuscitation will be important parts of managing the cerebral edema, but are not the first step in management. Given the large size of the mass, surgical resection will be indicated in an urgent fashion, but not emergently. Emergent surgical resection may be indicated for tumors that present with a large hemorrhagic component, but intubation would still be the first step in management. EVD placement is useful in managing ICP, and may play a role in the management of a tumor with concurrent hydrocephalus, but since this patient does not have severe hydrocephalus it is not indicated at this time.

> Quick A, Patel D, Hadziahmetovic M, et al. Current therapeutic paradigms in glioblastoma. *Rev Recent Clin Trials*. 2010;5(1):14-27. doi:10.2174/157488710790820544

4. **The answer is E.** Metastatic brain tumors are the most common intracranial neoplasm in adults (about 30% of all tumors), arising in 10% to 15% of all patients with systemic malignancies. They are most often located at the gray–white matter junction of the cerebral and cerebellar hemispheres, but they may affect any part of the central nervous system (CNS), including the leptomeninges. The most common primary sites of origin are the lung, breast, melanoma, kidney, and gastrointestinal (GI) tract. GBM is the most common and lethal adult primary brain tumor. Meningiomas account for an estimated 13% to 26% of primary intracranial neoplasms, occurring most frequently in women in the middle decades of life. Pituitary tumors account for 10% to 15% of all primary brain tumors. Medulloblastomas account for 17% of all brain tumors in the pediatric population, but less than 1% of all adult CNS tumors.

> Al-Shamy G, Sawaya R. Management of brain metastases: the indispensable role of surgery. *J Neurooncol*. 2009;92(3):275-282. doi:10.1007/s11060-009-9839-y

5 and 6. The answers are C and E, respectively. The patient has signs and symptoms of visual compromise and pituitary endocrine dysfunction from pituitary apoplexy. The noncontrast coronal MRI of the brain shows evidence of a pituitary mass with suprasellar extension and acute intratumoral hemorrhage. Pituitary tumor apoplexy is an uncommon event characterized by the abrupt onset of severe headache, restriction of visual fields, deterioration of visual acuity, weakness of ocular motility, and clinical signs of pituitary endocrine dysfunction. Hemorrhage into or necrosis of a preexisting sellar mass, most commonly a pituitary macroadenoma, produces expansion and compression of the sellar components and surrounding structures resulting in displacement of the optic nerves and chiasm, and impingement of the cranial nerves along the cavernous sinus (III, IV, and VI). Damage and destruction of the anterior pituitary leads to multiple acute and/or chronic hormone deficiencies in many patients. In this patient, the pituitary endocrine dysfunction is manifesting as hypotension related to the lack of adrenocorticotropic hormone (ACTH) production. Medical management may be indicated in rare cases where the signs and symptoms are mild, restricted to meningismus or ophthalmoplegia, and deemed to be stable. In patients with visual compromise, hypotension, or altered level of consciousness, emergent surgical decompression, most commonly through a transsphenoidal approach, should be performed. In cases of hypotension, high-dose corticosteroids must be initiated to medically stabilize the patient prior to the operating room. There is no evidence of SAH, and hemorrhage only into the sella would be extremely unlikely from an aneurysm. The extension of blood into the suprasellar cistern may provoke the development of a chemical meningitis, but there is no evidence of other symptoms suggestive of bacterial meningitis. The constellation of signs and symptoms and the radiographic evidence of an expansive sellar mass with intratumoral hemorrhage rule out the possibility of cavernous sinus thrombosis or a midbrain infarction.

> Verrees M, Arafah BM, Selman WR. Pituitary tumor apoplexy: characteristics, treatment, and outcomes. *Neurosurg Focus*. 2004;16(4):1-7. doi:10.3171/foc.2004.16.4.7

7 and 8. The answers are B and E, respectively. The patient's symptoms and labs are characteristic of DI. Clinically, this manifests as polydipsia and polyuria. Laboratory criteria for diagnosis include a sodium level greater than 140 to 145, urine output greater than 250 to

500 cc/hr for 2 to 3 consecutive hours, a urine specific gravity less than 1.005, UOsm less than 300 mOsm/kg, and serum osmolality greater than 300 mOsm/kg. SIADH is characterized by low urine output with improper water retention and hyponatremia. Improper fluid administration can be distinguished from DI by the urine and serum osmolalities. In DI, the patient will have hypoosmolar urine and hyperosmolar serum due to inappropriate water loss. In inappropriate hypertonic saline administration one would expect both of these values to be elevated. Diuresis of perioperative fluids is a common cause of polyuria after surgery, but would not be accompanied by polydipsia or a rising sodium level. CSWS is characterized by hyponatremia instead of hypernatremia.

Schreckinger M, Szerlip N, Mittal S. Diabetes insipidus following resection of pituitary tumors. *Clin Neurol Neurosurg*. 2013;115(2):121-126. doi:10.1016/j.clineuro.2012.08.009

9. **The answer is A.** Primary tumors of the spinal cord are 10 to 15 times less common than primary intracranial tumors and represent 2% to 4% of all primary tumors of the central nervous system (CNS). Primary spinal cord tumors are divided into three categories on the basis of anatomic location:

   i. Intramedullary

   ii. Intradural extramedullary

   iii. Extradural

   Extradural tumors primarily consist of systemic cancer metastases that result in epidural spinal cord compression. Intramedullary spinal cord tumors (IMSCTs) constitute 8% to 10% of all primary spinal cord tumors, with the majority comprising gliomas (80%–90%), of which 60% to 70% are ependymomas and 30% to 40% are astrocytomas. Fifteen percent of all primary intradural spinal cord tumors are ependymal in origin and include one of three histopathologic subtypes: ependymoma, subependymoma, and myxopapillary ependymoma. The third most common IMSCT is hemangioblastoma, representing 3% to 8% of all IMSCTs. Intradural extramedullary spinal cord tumors are either meningiomas (50%) or peripheral nerve sheath tumors (50%). The clinical presentation of primary spinal cord tumors is determined in part by the location of the tumor, and in nearly all clinical instances, pain is the predominant presenting symptom.

   Chamberlain MC, Tredway TL. Adult primary intradural spinal cord tumors: a review. *Curr Neurol Neurosci Rep*. 2011;11(3):320-328. doi:10.1007/s11910-011-0190-2

10. **The answer is C.** MESCC is a devastating complication of systemic cancer that affects about 5% of all patients. Prostate, breast, and lung cancer each account for 15% to 20% of all cases; non-Hodgkin's lymphoma, renal cell cancer, and multiple myeloma account for 5% to 10%, and the remainder of cases are due to colorectal cancers, sarcomas, and tumors from unknown primaries. MESCC usually occurs in patients who have a preexisting diagnosis of cancer, although MESCC is the first manifestation of cancer in about 20% of patients. Metastatic tumors reach the epidural space and compress the spinal cord via the growth of a paravertebral tumor in about 15% of cases, a process more commonly associated with lymphomas and neuroblastomas. In the majority (85% of patients), the tumor reaches the spine via hematogenous metastasis to the vertebral body, grows into the bone, and then spreads into the epidural space, causing secondary compression of the spinal cord. The compression can be gradual, although acute compression secondary to bone destruction with vertebral body collapse and displacement of bone fragments into the epidural space can also occur. Back pain is the earliest and most common symptom of MESCC and is present in more than 95% of patients at diagnosis. Radicular pain due to compression or invasion of the nerve roots is commonly present in patients who develop MESCC. The pain is frequently unilateral, with cervical or lumbosacral spine involvement, or bilateral, with thoracic spine involvement. Weakness is the second most common symptom and is present in 35% to 75% of patients. Sensory deficits rarely occur before motor deficits or pain and are present in about 50% to 70% of patients.

Occasionally, patients may present with ataxia of gait owing to involvement of the spinocerebellar tracts without pain, motor, or sensory findings. Autonomic symptoms occur late in the progression, and isolated bowel or bladder dysfunction are rarely the presenting symptoms. MRI is the diagnostic imaging modality of choice for the diagnosis of MESCC. First-line therapy is corticosteroids, and once the diagnosis is suspected, patients with neurologic deficits should be started on high-dose corticosteroids. Definitive treatment almost always includes radiotherapy. Combination of radical surgery and radiation is superior to radiation alone in selected patients, and is preferred in patients with life expectancies of more than 6 months. Early diagnosis and appropriate treatment will prevent paraplegia in most patients.

Cole JS, Patchell RA. Metastatic epidural spinal cord compression. *Lancet Neurol.* 2008;7(5):459-466. doi:10.1016/S1474-4422(08)70089-9

Ribas ES, Schiff D. Spinal cord compression. *Curr Treat Options Neurol.* 2012;14(4):391-401. doi:10.1007/s11940-012-0176-7

11. **The answer is C.** Therapeutic options for patients with metastatic epidural spinal cord compression (MESCC) include corticosteroids, surgery, and radiation therapy. Corticosteroids decrease spinal cord edema and might have an oncolytic effect on certain tumors, including lymphoma and breast cancer. They are effective in preventing neurological deterioration in the short term. Earlier studies looking at the role of laminectomy in MESCC have suggested that posterior decompression alone may be associated with a poor outcome. Decompressive surgery addressing the anterior compressive disease from either a transpedicular or a thoracotomy approach followed by an instrumented fusion may result in better neurological outcomes compared with patients who were treated with radiation alone. New methods of delivering more focused radiation with the potential delivery of higher radiation doses to the tumor with less exposure to the spinal cord and healthy tissue have emerged. For patients with metastatic epidural spinal cord compression and high-grade spinal cord compression (such as in the current case), separation surgery is a safe and effective treatment option. During separation surgery, the spinal column is stabilized and the epidural tumor is resected without requiring significant vertebral body resection. Tumor separation from the spinal cord allows patients to undergo postoperative SRS with very high rates of local tumor control and is an effective palliative paradigm for this patient population.

Laufer I, Rubin DG, Lis E, et al. The NOMS framework: approach to the treatment of spinal metastatic tumors. *Oncologist.* 2013;18(6):744-751. doi:10.1634/theoncologist.2012-0293

Patchell RA, Tibbs PA, Regine WF, et al. Direct decompressive surgical resection in the treatment of spinal cord compression caused by metastatic cancer: a randomised trial. *Lancet.* 2005;366(9486):643-648. doi:10.1016/S0140-6736(05)66954-1

12. **The answer is E.** Clinical features of CM are caused by the obstruction of normal cerebrospinal fluid (CSF) flow or by direct tumor infiltration. The clinical signs and symptoms are associated with increased intracranial pressure (ICP) and by infiltration of the nerves producing focal neurological deficit. The most common presenting clinical features are cranial nerve palsies, followed by headaches, cerebral disturbances, spinal nerve involvement, mental status changes, and limb weakness. Diplopia is the most common symptom of cranial nerve dysfunction, with cranial nerve VI being the most frequently affected, followed by cranial nerves III and IV. Trigeminal involvement, cochlear dysfunction, and optic neuropathy are also common findings. Spinal signs and symptoms include weakness, dermatomal or segmental sensory loss, and pain in the neck, back, or a radicular pattern. Nuchal rigidity is present in only 15% of cases.

Chamberlain MC. Neoplastic meningitis. *Oncologist.* 2008;13(9):967-977. doi:10.1634/theoncologist. 2008-0138

13. **The answer is B.** The most useful laboratory test in the diagnosis of CM is the CSF examination. Abnormalities include increased opening pressure (>200 mmH$_2$O), increased leukocytes (>4/mm^3), elevated protein (>50 mg/dL), and decreased glucose (<60 mg/dL), which, though suggestive of CM, are not diagnostic. The demonstration of malignant cells in the CSF

is the cornerstone of the final diagnosis. A positive CSF cytology is found on the initial lumbar puncture (LP) in 50% to 70% and in nearly all cases after three attempts. False-positive cytologies demonstrating reactive lymphocytes are associated with infectious or inflammatory diseases. Increased CSF opening pressure is found in 50% to 70% of patients and depends on the extent of the leptomeningeal involvement. Elevated protein in the CSF and low glucose are seen in approximately 75% and 40% of the cases, respectively. Biochemical markers have also been evaluated, but their use has been limited by poor sensitivity and specificity. Among these substances are carcinoembryonic antigen (CEA), lactate dehydrogenase (LDH), alkaline phosphatase, beta-human chorionic gonadotropin (beta-HCG), and others. Cytogenetic studies, including flow cytometry, DNA single-cell cytometry, and fluorescence in situ hybridization can give additional diagnostic information, are especially useful in liquid tumors (leukemia and lymphoma), and appear more sensitive than CSF cytology. In cases where there is no manifestation of systemic cancer and CSF examinations remain inconclusive, a meningeal biopsy may be diagnostic, and the yield of this test may be higher if the biopsy is taken from an enhancing region seen on the MRI. Nevertheless, the gold standard of CM diagnosis remains the combination of the full clinical picture and positive cytology.

Pavlidis N. The diagnostic and therapeutic management of leptomeningeal carcinomatosis. *Ann Oncol.* 2004;15(suppl 4):iv285-291. doi:10.1093/annonc/mdh941

14. **The answer is B.** PNSs affecting the nervous system are rare neurologic syndromes caused by cancer but not ascribable to metastases. Any portion of the nervous system may be involved. The pathogenesis of these disorders appears to be an immune reaction against antigens shared by the cancer and the nervous system. Two clinical features shared by most PNSs affecting the central nervous system (CNS) are the rapid development of symptoms, and signs of inflammation in the cerebrospinal fluid (CSF) including moderated lymphocytic pleocytosis, increased protein concentration, high immunoglobulin G (IgG) index, and CSF-specific oligoclonal bands. In about 70% of patients with paraneoplastic neurologic disorders (PND), neurological symptoms are the first manifestation of a tumor. Of these patients, 70% to 80% will have a positive screening for cancer on initial assessment. Most tumors are identified with imaging of the chest, abdomen, and pelvis using CT, fluorodeoxyglucose-PET, or both. Opsoclonus comprises involuntary, arrhythmic, and chaotic multidirectional saccades with horizontal, vertical, and torsional components, and is commonly accompanied by myoclonic jerks in the limbs and trunk, cerebellar ataxia, tremor, and encephalopathy. Recent findings suggest that disinhibition of the fastigial nucleus of the cerebellum may be involved in the pathophysiological mechanism of opsoclonus. Opsoclonus–myoclonus can occur with infections, toxic–metabolic disorders, and paraneoplastic mechanisms. In children, the disorder is related to the presence of a neuroblastoma in about 50% of cases. In adults, the tumors most commonly involved include small-cell lung cancer and cancers of the breast and ovary. Cerebellar dysfunction is one of the most common paraneoplastic presentations of cancer. The hallmark of paraneoplastic cerebellar degeneration is an extensive loss of Purkinje cells that might be associated with inflammatory infiltrates in the cerebellar cortex, deep cerebellar nuclei, and inferior olivary nuclei. Neurological deficits are sometimes preceded by prodromal symptoms, such as viral-like illness, dizziness, nausea, or vomiting. These symptoms are followed by gait unsteadiness that rapidly develops into ataxia, diplopia, dysarthria, and dysphagia. Some patients may have blurry vision, oscillopsia, and transient opsoclonus. Limbic encephalitis is an inflammatory process confined to the limbic system. Patients may develop mood and sleep disturbances, seizures, hallucinations, and short-term memory loss that may progress to dementia. EEG usually reveals foci of epileptic activity in one or both temporal lobes or focal or generalized slow activity. In 70% to 80% of the cases, MRI fluid-attenuated inversion recovery (FLAIR) or T2 sequences show hyperintense signals in the medial portion of one or both temporal lobes. The clinical picture combined with findings of EEG, MRI, and CSF inflammatory changes suggest the diagnosis. The tumors more frequently involved are small-cell lung cancer, testicular germ-cell neoplasms, thymoma, Hodgkin's lymphoma,

or teratoma. Lambert–Eaton myasthenic syndrome is a rare presynaptic disorder of neuro-muscular transmission; unlike myasthenia gravis, the muscles of the trunk, shoulder girdle, pelvic girdle, and lower extremities are the ones that are most frequently involved.

Dalmau J, Rosenfeld MR. Paraneoplastic syndromes of the CNS. *Lancet Neurol*. 2008;7(4):327-340. doi:10.1016/S1474-4422(08)70060-7

Posner JB, Dalmau JO. Paraneoplastic syndromes affecting the central nervous system. *Annu Rev Med*. 1997;48:157-166. doi:10.1146/annurev.med.48.1.157

15 and 16. The answers are C and B, respectively. The patient in question 15 had a brief seizure 6 hours after surgery. Given the length of time since the surgery the patient is likely to have a low serum level of the drug used during surgery. Reloading the patient with levetiracetam is the best choice. A CT of the brain should be ordered to rule out a postoperative hemorrhage as a cause of this seizure, but treatment of the seizure should not be delayed. An MRI of the brain could be completed to look for residual tumor as a cause of the seizure, but similar to the CT it should not be completed prior to treatment. The patient is back to his neurologic baseline and is awake and alert, so intubation is not indicated as the patient is protecting his airway. The short duration of the seizure, and the patient's return to baseline, means the patient is unlikely to still be having seizures, therefore IV lorazepam should not be used. The patient in question 16 had a seizure long enough in duration to be classified as being in status epilepticus (SE) that has not yet been treated. IV lorazepam is therefore the proper next step to provide treatment instead of levetiracetam. This is especially true given the patient's persistent neurologic deficit. In one series, nonconvulsive status occurred in 10% to 20% of patients after convulsive SE that clinically appeared to be treated adequately as judged by lack of convulsions. Similar to the patient in 15, imaging by CT or MRI is indicated to look for cause of the seizure, but not prior to proper treatment. This patient is also protecting his airway, and therefore does not require intubation at this time.

Costello DJ, Cole AJ. Treatment of acute seizures and status epilepticus. *J Intensive Care Med*. 2007;22(6):319-347. doi:10.1177/0885066607307506

DeLorenzo RJ, Waterhouse EJ, Towne AR, et al. Persistent nonconvulsive status epilepticus after the control of convulsive status epilepticus. *Epilepsia*. 1998;39(8):833-840. doi:10.1111/j.1528-1157.1998.tb01177.x

COREY E. GOLDSMITH

QUESTIONS

1. Which of the following statements is true about eclampsia?

   A. Eclampsia can develop up to 48 hours postpartum
   B. Sudden severe throbbing headache is the most common herald of a seizure
   C. The blood pressure (BP) is elevated for several hours prior to convulsions
   D. EEG and cerebrospinal fluid (CSF) are normal
   E. All of the answers are true

2. Ammonia levels above ___ µmol/L are more often associated with cerebral herniation:

   A. 50
   B. 100
   C. 150
   D. 200
   E. 250

3. A 70-year-old man with a history of chronic kidney disease is admitted to the ICU after a motor vehicle accident with multiple fractures. He receives morphine but no other form of sedatives. Later he develops a hyperactive delirium associated with diffuse myoclonus, asterixis, and tremors. Cranial nerves are intact with antigravity movement and withdrawal to pain in all four extremities. Noncontrast CT scan of head is negative for acute intracranial pathology. Which management option is likely to be most effective?

   A. Naloxone
   B. Mild hypothermia
   C. Anticoagulation
   D. Acute hemodialysis
   E. Fosphenytoin load

4. A 29-year-old male presents with a 4-week history of progressively worsening cognitive and behavioral disturbances and new onset of multiple generalized seizures on the day of admission. He is agitated and confused with diffuse hyperreflexia but an otherwise nonfocal neurologic exam. Basic laboratories are normal with no signs of infection. Brain MRI shows T2/fluid-attenuated inversion recovery (FLAIR) hyperintensities in bilateral medial temporal lobes. Cerebrospinal fluid (CSF) analysis shows lymphocytic pleocytosis, normal protein and glucose levels, and negative viral infectious serologies including herpes simplex virus (HSV) polymerase chain reaction (PCR). EEG shows baseline diffuse slowing. He continues to have

multiple generalized tonic–clonic seizures over the next few days. What should your next step in management be?

A. Brain biopsy
B. Treat with antiepileptic agents and await CSF autoimmune encephalitis results
C. Treat with intravenous (IV) acyclovir
D. Treat with antifungals
E. Treat with IV methylprednisolone, intravenous immunoglobulins (IVIg), or plasma exchange (PLEX)

5. The most common neurologic finding in preeclampsia is:

A. Vision problems
B. Headache
C. Clonus
D. Epigastric pain
E. Seizures

6. Which of the following patients is/are at risk for developing posterior reversible encephalopathy syndrome (PRES)?

A. A 26-year-old woman with lupus being treated with high-dose steroids
B. A 62-year-old man with chronic renal failure but well-controlled blood pressure (BP) being given erythropoietin
C. A 33-year-old man with HIV on combined antiretroviral therapy (ART) presenting with hypercalcemia and found to have hyperparathyroidism
D. An 18-year-old girl receiving cyclosporine
E. All of the above

7. Targeted temperature management (TTM) has been shown to confound neuroprognostication after cardiac arrest. Which of the following statements is **false**?

A. TTM may cause the somatosensory-evoked potential (SSEP) responses to be falsely absent
B. TTM may elevate serum neuron-specific enolase, making the cutoff value inaccurate
C. TTM can delay the return of pupillary and motor function, making the previous timing of these examinations inaccurate
D. Metabolism and pharmacokinetics of the sedatives/paralytics are altered during hypothermia.
E. All of the above

8. Which of the following statements is correct in regard to management of blood pressure (BP) in hypertensive encephalopathy?

A. BP should be aggressively reduced until neurologic symptoms resolve
B. Initial treatment should lower the diastolic BP to about 100 mmHg or no more than a 25% drop
C. Antihypertensive medicines should be reduced or stopped if there is an increase in serum creatinine after initial lowering of BP
D. Nitroprusside can be given at its maximal dose of 10 mcg/kg/min for up to 30 minutes
E. Nitroglycerin is a reasonable first-line choice for BP management in hypertensive encephalopathy

9. **Brain** MRI in eclampsia typically shows:

A. Normal brain
B. Periventricular white matter T2 fluid-attenuated inversion recovery (FLAIR) lesions

    C. Multifocal parieto-occipital subcortical T2 FLAIR lesions

    D. Cortical infarctions

    E. Pontine lesions

10. Imaging findings suggestive of mitochondrial encephalopathy with lactic acidosis and stroke-like episodes (MELAS) include:

    A. Equal involvement of the deep white matter and cortex

    B. Relative sparing of the deep white matter compared with the cortex

    C. Specific involvement of the anterior temporal lobes

    D. Mainly frontal lobe involvement

    E. Magnetic resonance spectroscopy (MRS) findings that show high N-acetyl aspartate (NAA) peaks

11. Which combination of limbic encephalitis antibodies (Ab) is **incorrectly** matched with the most commonly associated tumor?

    A. Anti-N-methyl-D-aspartate (NMDA) Ab—Ovarian teratoma

    B. Anti-Hu Ab–Small-cell lung cancer

    C. Anti-gamma-aminobutyric acid (GABA)-B Ab—Thymoma

    D. Anti-contactin associated protein 2 (CASPR2) Ab—Thymoma

    E. Anti-AMPA Ab—Small-cell lung cancer and thymoma

12. Uremic encephalopathy:

    A. Usually occurs when glomerular filtration rate (GFR) is less than 10%

    B. Always occurs in association with other electrolyte disturbances

    C. Occurs in chronic renal failure more than acute renal failure

    D. Can be easily distinguished from status epilepticus (SE) by examination alone

    E. All of the above

13. Which of the following medicines should be avoided when treating hypertension in pregnancy?

    A. Enalapril

    B. Methyldopa

    C. Labetalol

    D. Nicardipine

    E. Hydralazine

Please read the following clinical presentation paragraph and answer questions from 14 to 18.

A 26-year-old woman with no significant medical history is admitted to the ICU with altered mental status (AMS). Her family reports that she has been complaining of fatigue, muscle aches, low-grade fevers, poor appetite, and nausea and vomiting for the past week. In the past 2 days, she has become progressively confused. Her family reports no alcohol use, although she may have been taking some acetaminophen in the past couple of weeks. On examination, she is arousable with vigorous stimuli, confused, and disoriented, but follows some simple commands. Her pupils are reactive, she has full extra-ocular muscle movements with nystagmus on end-gaze. Her speech is dysarthric. She is unable to ambulate because of ataxia and is noted to have asterixis. Her sclera is icteric, and she has some right upper quadrant (RUQ) tenderness to palpation but no other signs of chronic liver disease. She appears euvolemic. Noncontrast CT scan of head is normal. She has elevated bilirubin (T_{Bili} 20 mg/dL) and transaminases. Her prothrombin time (PT)/International Normalized Ratio (INR) is 112 sec/6.5, fibrinogen is 415, platelet count is 100 K/μL, blood urea nitrogen (BUN) is 70 mg/dL, and creatinine (Cr) is 3.6 mg/dL. Acetaminophen level is undetectable, and hepatitis A Immunoglobulin M (IgM) is positive.

14. This patient's condition:

    A. Usually develops in patients with chronic cirrhosis

    B. Is associated with ascites and cachexia

    C. Is most commonly caused by viral hepatitis in the United States

    D. Has a high rate of cerebral edema

    E. Has a mortality rate of 5% to 10% without liver transplantation

15. This patient's presentation is consistent with Grade ___ hepatic encephalopathy (HE):

    A. 0

    B. 1

    C. 2

    D. 3

    E. 4

16. The feature in the patient's presentation most convincing of the need for liver transplantation is:

    A. Etiology

    B. Creatinine value

    C. Bilirubin value

    D. Prothrombin time (PT) value

    E. Severity of encephalopathy

17. All of the following treatments could be recommended for this patient who was deemed to be a transplant candidate **except**:

    A. Intracranial pressure (ICP) monitoring

    B. Hyperosmotic agents such as mannitol or hypertonic saline if ICP is elevated

    C. Neomycin

    D. Prophylactic antibiotics

    E. *N*-acetylcysteine

18. In regard to the patient's renal failure:

    A. Renal failure is an unusual accompaniment to fulminant liver failure

    B. Fluid resuscitation will improve her renal failure, and no other intervention is warranted

    C. Intermittent hemodialysis is the best option for this patient

    D. Continuous renal replacement therapy (CRRT) is the best option for this patient

    E. The renal failure will self-correct with improvement in her hepatic failure

19. Which of the following physical examination findings accurately predicts poor neurological outcome after cardiac arrest in patients **not** treated with targeted temperature management (TTM)?

    A. Continued comatose state at 72 hours

    B. Hyperthermia

    C. Absent pupillary response at 8 hours

    D. Absent pupillary response at 24 hours

    E. Absent motor response at 24 hours

20. Which of the following physical examination findings accurately predicts universally poor outcomes post–cardiac arrest in patients treated with targeted temperature management (TTM)?

    A. Absent pupillary response at 72 hours

    B. Absent pupillary response at 24 hours

C. Continued comatose status at 72 hours
D. Any noted myoclonus
E. Absent motor response at 72 hours

21. A 55-year-old man with previously well-compensated hepatitis C cirrhosis presents with acute confusion and disorientation after being given a new medication. Which of the following would **not** be a possible culprit?

    A. Lorazepam
    B. Haloperidol
    C. Furosemide
    D. Hydrocodone/acetaminophen
    E. Topiramate

22. A 30-year-old woman is receiving magnesium sulfate for severe preeclampsia at 36 weeks gestation. Each of the following is a maternal effect of this treatment **except**:

    A. Sedation
    B. Hypocalcemia
    C. Sensitization to nondepolarizing muscle relaxants
    D. Cardiac dysfunction prior to respiratory depression
    E. Loss of deep tendon reflexes (DTRs) prior to significant cardiac dysfunction

23. Drugs that abolish all brainstem function and may mimic brain death include

    A. Valproic acid overdose
    B. Tricyclic antidepressant (TCA) overdose
    C. Barbituate coma
    D. Both B and C
    E. All of the above

24. A 65-year-old male presents after a generalized tonic–clonic seizure. His family reports that he has been having worsening memory for the past 2 months, forgetting conversations and tasks as well as getting lost in his neighborhood. He also has become disinhibited with excessive eating. While in the emergency room (ER), he intermittently has brief twitches of his right face and arm and momentarily stops responding during these episodes. His family says these episodes have been happening multiple times daily for the past 2 to 3 months. Which of the following diagnoses is most likely?

    A. Anti-LGI1 encephalitis
    B. Alzheimer's disease
    C. Frontotemporal dementia
    D. Creutzfeldt–Jakob disease (CJD)
    E. Hashimoto's encephalitis

25. Which of these ancillary study findings is associated with the worst neurologic outcomes after cardiac arrest with or without targeted temperature management (TTM)?

    A. Burst-suppression pattern on EEG at 24 hours
    B. Bilateral periodic lateralized discharges (BILPDs) or generalized periodic discharges (GPDs) on EEG at 72 hours
    C. Theta coma on EEG at 72 hours
    D. Absent N20 responses on somatosensory evoked potentials (SSEPs) at 72 hours
    E. Absent brainstem auditory evoked potentials at 72 hours

26. A 25-year-old man with known mitochondrial encephalopathy with lactic acidosis and stroke-like episodes (MELAS) presents 2.5 hours after sudden onset of left hemiparesis and left homonymous hemianopsia. He had initially had a headache and worsening vision to the left. He then became lethargic and developed left hemiparesis with some possible intermittent left-sided shaking. CT head is negative for acute abnormalities. What is the best step in management?

   A. Send to interventional radiology for possible thrombectomy
   B. Start daily aspirin therapy
   C. Check a computed tomography angiography (CTA) head and neck
   D. Give intravenous (IV) tissue plasminogen activator (tPA)
   E. Start an L-arginine infusion

27. A 45-year-old man without known medical history is found down in his home. He is somnolent though arousable to vigorous stimulation. On examination, he is noted to have nuchal rigidity, normal cranial nerve function, and diffuse arrhythmic twitching of his muscles. Labs show normal complete blood count, blood urea nitrogen (BUN) 90 mg/dL, and creatinine (Cr) 4.4 mg/dL. He is intubated for airway protection, and a lumbar puncture (LP) is done after a normal CT head scan without contrast. Which of the following findings would lead you **away** from the diagnosis of uremic encephalopathy as the primary etiology?

   A. Nuchal rigidity
   B. Myoclonus
   C. Hemiparesis
   D. Cerebrospinal fluid (CSF) protein greater than 60 mg/dL
   E. All could be seen in uremic encephalopathy

28. A 36-year-old gravida 2 para 1 woman at 35 weeks 3 days presents with nausea, vomiting, and muscle aches for the past 2 days. She had sudden onset of severe right upper quadrant (RUQ) pain 2 hours ago and presented to the doctor. Urine dipstick shows no proteinuria. She did have a headache. The most common maternal complication of this syndrome is:

   A. Seizures
   B. Disseminated intravascular coagulation (DIC)
   C. Liver rupture
   D. Cerebral hemorrhage
   E. Pulmonary edema

29. Which of the following statements is correct in hypertensive encephalopathy?

   A. The cerebrospinal fluid (CSF) is normal, including immunoglobulin G (IgG) studies
   B. Patients with hypertensive encephalopathy always show features of posterior reversible encephalopathy syndrome (PRES) on MRI
   C. Seizures are a more common presenting symptom than headache or visual loss in PRES
   D. Cord lesions on MRI eliminate the possibility of PRES
   E. EEG generally shows lateralized periodic discharges LPDs in the parietal and occipital areas

30. A 27-year-old woman presents with acute onset of bizarre behavior in the workplace and is initially admitted to the psychiatry floor. Over the next week she exhibited worsening bizarre behavior, intermittent confusion, and worsening memory function, and eventually became mute. She was noted to have facial twitching and then developed a generalized tonic–clonic seizure. Basic laboratories were normal without signs of infection except for an elevation in creatinine kinase (CK) to 823 prior to the seizure. Urine toxicology is negative. Cerebrospinal

fluid (CSF) showed a lymphocytic pleocytosis and an MRI brain was unremarkable. EEG showed diffuse slowing without epileptiform discharges. What is the most likely diagnosis?

A. Herpes simplex virus (HSV) encephalitis
B. Anti-*N*-methyl-D-aspartate (NMDA) receptor encephalitis
C. Drug intoxication
D. Anti-gamma-aminobutyric acid (GABA)-A receptor encephalitis
E. Contactin associated protein 2 (CASPR2) antibody–associated disease

31. The brain structures most sensitive to hypoxia include

A. Cortical layer 4 and 5 more than other cortical layers
B. Caudate/putamen more than thalami
C. Frontotemporal areas more than occipitoparietal areas
D. White matter more than gray matter
E. Hippocampus regions 3 and 4 more than other hippocampal areas

32. The nurse calls you with the laboratory results for your patient currently on a targeted temperature management (TTM) protocol status-post-cardiac arrest. Which of the following would **not** be an expected laboratory abnormality from the hypothermia alone?

A. Hypokalemia
B. Hypomagnesemia
C. Hyperglycemia
D. Thrombocytopenia
E. Leukocytosis

33. A 65-year-old man on chronic hemodialysis is found down in his home. Vitals show normothermia, blood pressure (BP) 110/70 mmHg, and pulse rate 100 beats/min. He is lethargic and confused, although he does follow simple commands and is moving all four extremities. He is noted to have bilateral abducens nerve palsies but an otherwise nonfocal neurologic examination. CT head scan is normal. Labs show creatinine (Cr) 3.1 mg/dL (baseline), blood urea nitrogen (BUN) 40 mg/dL, normal liver function tests, and ammonia 60 μmol/L. Which intervention should be done first?

A. Lactulose
B. Hemodialysis
C. Thiamine intravenously (IV)
D. EEG
E. Empiric antibiotics

34. Which of the following scenarios is **not** consistent with hypertensive encephalopathy?

A. A 48-year-old man with lupus who presents with 1 day of acute dizziness, nausea, confusion, vision problems and blood pressure (BP) 240/130 mmHg. CT scan of the head shows diffuse brainstem hypodensity
B. A 60-year-old woman who presents with sudden onset vision loss in the setting of rapidly ascending paralysis of all four extremities over the past 3 days and bilateral facial palsies
C. A 65-year-old man with uncontrolled hypertension who presents with BP 190/100 mmHg and a headache for the past month. He has a normal neurologic examination
D. A 55-year-old man with untreated hypertension who presents with drowsiness, left gaze deviation, and BP 240/140 mmHg. CT head scan shows diffuse symmetric cerebellar and brainstem hypodensities
E. All of the above

35. A 26-year-old gravida 2 para 1⟶2 woman, who delivered a healthy baby girl 8 hours ago without complications, starts to complain of a severe headache. While the nurse is getting pain medication, she suddenly becomes unresponsive and has a generalized tonic–clonic seizure that lasts 3 minutes. She does not fully return to baseline, has another seizure, and has now returned to baseline. She had not previously been hypertensive, although blood pressure (BP) now is 200/110 mmHg. CT head scan without contrast is negative. In regard to her treatment, you should:

   A. Load with fosphenytoin
   B. Start labetalol to lower BP
   C. Start high-dose magnesium sulfate
   D. Do nothing, since the patient has already delivered and will likely not seize again
   E. Both B and C

36. A 28-year-old woman with diabetes mellitus (DM) presents 6 hours after acute onset of hemisensory loss and unilateral vision loss. Her mother also has diabetes and her brother is deaf, but there is no history of early cerebrovascular disease in the family. Which of the following is true about her most likely diagnosis?

   A. Headache, memory problems, hearing loss, short stature, and diabetes are uncommon comorbidities
   B. Lactic acid level is unhelpful in making the diagnosis
   C. The most common identified mutation is a point mutation at mitochondrial nucleotide pair 3,243 (a transfer ribonucleic acid-Leu gene)
   D. Medications to be avoided include metformin and L-arginine
   E. She should be started on a daily aspirin to help prevent further neurologic episodes

■ ANSWERS

1. **The answer is B.** Sudden severe throbbing headache is the most common herald of a seizure secondary to eclampsia. While more common antepartum, eclampsia can occur up to 4 weeks postpartum. The BP is often elevated for only a short time before the convulsion, and in 20% of women, systolic BP never elevates above 140 mmHg. Interictal EEG in eclamptic patients shows diffuse or focal slowing that gradually returns to normal over several weeks. CSF analysis usually shows elevated protein and in some cases mild pleocytosis.

   Frontera JA, Ahmed W. Neurocritical care complications of pregnancy and puerperum. *J Crit Care*. 2014;29(6):1069-1081. doi:10.1016/j.jcrc.2014.07.010
   Shah AK, Rajamani K, Whitty JE. Eclampsia: a neurological perspective. *J Neurol Sci*. 2008; 271(1-2):158-167. doi:10.1016/j.jns.2008.04.010

2. **The answer is D.** Although there is no direct relationship, ammonia levels above 200 μmol/L are more often associated with cerebral herniation. High intracranial pressure (ICP) as well as uncal herniation can be seen at much lower ammonia levels, hence dependence on monitoring ammonia levels alone is not recommended.

   Clemmesen JO, Larsen FS, Kondrup J, et al. Cerebral herniation in patients with acute liver failure is correlated with arterial ammonia concentration. *Hepatology*. 1999;29(3):648-653. doi:10.1002/hep.510290309.

3. **The answer is D.** Uremic encephalopathy is the most likely etiology in a patient with known chronic kidney disease and acute development of a hyperactive delirium associated with myoclonus and asterixis but preserved cranial nerve function. Anoxic injury or status epilepticus (SE) are also possibilities and need to be ruled out, but are less likely in this scenario. Morphine overdose would not cause the myoclonus seen and would show pupillary changes.

   Brouns R, De Deyn PP. Neurological complications in renal failure: a review. *Clin Neurol Neurosurg*. 2004;107(1):1-16. doi:10.1016/j.clineuro.2004.07.012

4. **The answer is E.** Clinical presentation and MRI and CSF findings are highly suggestive of limbic encephalitis. Clinical diagnosis of autoimmune encephalitis can be made in a patient with subacute (<3 months) onset of working memory impairment, altered mental status (AMS), or psychiatric symptoms PLUS at least one of the following findings: new focal central nervous system (CNS) findings, new seizures not otherwise explained, CSF pleocytosis, or MRI features suggestive of encephalitis with reasonable exclusion of alternative causes. This patient meets the criteria for possible autoimmune encephalitis and should receive immunotherapy with IV steroids, IVIg, or PLEX. While the diagnosis is not confirmed yet, early treatment is associated with better outcomes. In addition, alternatives etiologies have been reasonably excluded. Treating with antiepileptics only is not reasonable as the results of CSF autoimmune encephalitis can take weeks. Treating with antifungals or antiviral agents is not indicated in the absence of infections. Brain biopsy is of low yield and unlikely to illuminate the diagnosis at this point.

   Graus F, Titulaer MJ, Balu R, et al. A clinical approach to diagnosis of autoimmune encephalitis. *Lancet Neurol*. 2016;15(4):391-404. doi: 10.1016/S1474-4422(15)00401-9

5. **The answer is B.** Almost all of these features are seen in high prevalence in preeclampsia, but headache is the most common, seen in 83% of patients. Clonus is seen in 46%, vision problems in 45%, and epigastric pain in 20%. Seizures are the defining feature of eclampsia, but are not seen in preeclampsia.

   Kaplan PW. Eclampsia. In: Kaplan PW, ed. *Neurologic Disease in Women*. New York, NY: Demos Medical Publishing; 2006:235-246.

6. **The answer is E.** PRES is a clinico-radiological syndrome associated with multiple clinical conditions including hypertensive encephalopathy, several autoimmune disorders such as lupus, acute or chronic renal diseases, thrombotic thrombocytopenic purpura/hemolytic

uremic syndrome (TTP/HUS), high-dose steroid therapy, liver failure and/or transplantation, endocrine dysfunctions (including primary aldosteronism, pheochromocytoma, hypercalcemia/hyperparathyroidism), bone marrow transplantation, massive blood transfusion/erythropoietin therapy, porphyria, and multiple medications/drugs (such as cyclosporine, cis-platinum, some monoclonal antibodies, ART, intravenous immunoglobulins [IVIg], contrast media, scorpion poison, stimulants, etc.).

Fischer M, Schmutzhard E. Posterior reversible encephalopathy syndrome. *J Neurol.* 2017;264(8):1608-1616. doi:10.1007/s00415-016-8377-8

Fugate JE, Rabinstein AA. Posterior reversible encephalopathy syndrome: clinical and radiological manifestations, pathophysiology, and outstanding questions. *Lancet Neurol.* 2015;14(9):914-925. doi:10.1016/s1474-4422(15)00111-8answ

7. **The answer is A.** The ability to accurately predict poor prognosis in hypoxic–ischemic brain injury after cardiac arrest has changed in the era of TTM. Hypothermia does not result in the absence of N20 responses on SSEP, and this prognostic marker seems to remain valid for universally dismal outcome more than 24 hours after arrest. However, all of the other statements are true. Several series have shown good recovery after cardiac arrest in patients treated with TTM who had high serum neuron-specific enolase values, absent pupillary function at 24 hours, or absent motor function at 72 hours. Therefore, these findings cannot be used alone for prognostication. Absent motor function, as described in the 2015 American Heart Association guidelines, has been associated with a high false positive predictive value and is not recommended to be used in neuroprognostication regardless of TTM. Hypothermia slows hepatic metabolism of sedatives; also high doses of sedatives frequently required to treat the associated shivering can further complicate the picture.

Callaway CW, Donnino MW, Fink EL, et al. Part 8: post–cardiac arrest care: 2015 American Heart Association guidelines update for cardiopulmonary resuscitation and emergency cardiovascular care. *Circulation.* 2015;132(suppl 2):S465-S482. doi:10.1161/CIR.0000000000000262

8. **The answer is B.** When treating hypertensive encephalopathy, initial treatment usually with intravenous (IV) medications should aim to drop the diastolic BP to about 100 mmHg or a 25% drop (whichever is less) within the first 2 to 6 hours. Faster or further drops may reduce the BP below the autoregulatory range and worsen neurologic symptoms. The goal is not necessarily to eliminate all neurologic symptoms. Sometimes there is an elevation in the creatinine associated with this initial BP lowering; however, antihypertensive medicines should be continued. Nitroprusside is an efficacious and quick BP-lowering agent; however, its use is limited at its maximal dose of 10 mcg/kg/min for at most 10 minutes, especially in renal insufficiency. Nitroglycerin is an effective antihypertensive agent in hypertensive emergency, but its use has been reported in multiple cases to worsen posterior reversible encephalopathy syndrome (PRES). Therefore, the use of nitroglycerin should be avoided in any case of hypertensive encephalopathy.

Marik PE, Rivera R. Hypertensive emergencies: an update. *Curr Opin Crit Care.* 2011;17(6):569-580. doi:10.1097/MCC.0b013e32834cd31d

Sheta MA, Paladugu M, Mendelson J, et al. When should nitroglycerine be avoided in hypertensive encephalopathy? *Hypertension.* 2011;58(5):e187-e188. doi:10.1161/HYPERTENSIONAHA. 111.175703

9. **The answer is C.** Multifocal parieto-occipital subcortical FLAIR lesions are seen in almost all patients with eclampsia if MRI is obtained soon after convulsions and can be seen in preeclampsia as well. The pattern is almost identical to that seen in posterior reversible encephalopathy syndrome (PRES), and similarly is usually transient and reversible.

Brewer J, Owens MY, Wallace K, et al. Posterior reversible encephalopathy syndrome in 46 of 47 patients with eclampsia. *Am J Obstet Gynecol.* 2013;208(6):468.e1-e6. doi:10.1016/j.ajog.2013.02.015

Mayama M, Uno K, Tano S, et al. Incidence of posterior reversible encephalopathy syndrome in eclamptic and patients with preeclampsia with neurologic symptoms. *Am J Obstet Gynecol.* 2016;215(2):239.e1-e5. doi:10.1016/j.ajog.2016.02.039

10. **The answer is B.** Brain MRI in MELAS usually shows asymmetric cortical lesions that do not confine to vascular territories with sparing of the deeper white matter. The parietal/temporal/occipital lobes are typically more involved than frontal lobes on imaging, although neuropsychiatric testing of MELAS patients primarily shows a frontal pattern, suggesting involvement at this level. MRS can be very useful, usually showing a low NAA peak and high lactate peak in affected areas—a very sensitive marker of metabolic disorders. There is a strong correlation between high ventricular lactate as measured by MRS and the degree of neuropsychological and neurologic impairment. Specific involvement of the anterior temporal lobes is seen in cerebral autosomal dominant arteriopathy with subcortical infarctions and leukoencephalopathy (CADASIL) but not MELAS.

El-Hattab AW, Adesina AM, Jones J, et al. MELAS syndrome: clinical manifestations, pathogenesis, and treatment options. *Mol Genet Metab*. 2015;116(1-2):4-12. doi:10.1016/j.ymgme.2015. 06.004

Kaufmann P, Engelstad K, Wei Y, et al. Natural history of MELAS associated with mitochondrial DNA m.3243A>G genotype. *Neurology*. 2011;77(22):1965-1971. doi:10.1212/WNL. 0b013e31823a0c7f

11. **The answer is C.** Limbic encephalitis are associated with autoimmune or paraneoplastic diseases. In paraneoplastic encephalitis, specific antibodies are highly associated with specific tumor types. Anti-NMDA receptor antibodies are associated with ovarian teratoma. Antibodies against CASPR2 and AMPA, but not GABA-B, receptors are associated with thymoma. Small-cell lung cancer produces a number of paraneoplastic syndromes secondary to antibodies against Hu, and GABA-B and AMPA receptors. Anti-GABA-A receptor antibodies are much less commonly associated with neoplasms.

Graus F, Titulaer MJ, Balu R, et al. A clinical approach to diagnosis of autoimmune encephalitis. *Lancet Neurol*. 2016;15(4):391-404. doi:10.1016/S1474-4422(15)00401-9

12. **The answer is A.** GFR is usually less than 10% when uremic encephalopathy occurs. Although uremic encephalopathy is often associated with electrolyte disturbances (such as hyponatremia, hyperkalemia, metabolic acidosis, and hyperthyroidism), it can also occur in isolation. The acuity of renal failure is a risk factor for the development of uremic encephalopathy more than the degree of azotemia. Uremic encephalopathy can present with multifocal myoclonus in the setting of altered mental status (AMS), which can be indistinguishable from SE without EEG.

Raskin NH. Neurologic complications of renal failure. In: Aminoff MJ, ed. *Neurology and General Medicine*. Philadelphia, PA: Churchill Livingstone; 2001:293-296.

13. **The answer is A.** Angiotensin converting enzyme (ACE) inhibitors and angiotensin-receptor blockers should be avoided in all stages of pregnancy as they increase fetal cardiac abnormalities associated with first-trimester exposure and fetal renal abnormalities in the latter half of pregnancy. Methyldopa is usually considered the drug of choice for long-term management of hypertension during pregnancy, whereas labetalol, nicardipine, and/or hydralazine are often used for acute treatment.

Kaplan PW. Eclampsia. In: Kaplan PW, ed. *Neurologic Disease in Women*. New York, NY: Demos Medical Publishing; 2006:235-246.

14. **The answer is D.** Acute hepatic failure is defined as patients with previously normal liver function developing encephalopathy within 8 weeks of onset of their liver disease. The most common cause in the United States is drug exposure, most commonly acetaminophen. Viral hepatitis is the cause in only about 10% of the cases in the United States. In the developing world, viral hepatitis remains the most common cause of acute hepatic failure. Clinical presentation is usually the acute onset of encephalopathy associated with nausea, vomiting, and abdominal pain with evidence of elevated transaminases and coagulopathy on labs. Cerebral edema occurs in 80% of comatose patients with acute hepatic failure but due to increasing awareness and improved neurocritical care only accounts for 10% to 20% of the mortality

among fulminant patients. Mortality is 30% to 80% in patients who do not receive a liver transplant, although the outcome depends on etiology and aggressiveness of management strategies. Acute liver failure from acetaminophen overdose, pregnancy, or hepatitis A has better transplant-free survival rates than other drug toxicities.

Frontera JA, Kalb T. Neurological management of fulminant hepatic failure. *Neurocrit Care*. 2011;14(2):318-327. doi: 10.1007/s12028-010-9470-y

Kandiah PA, Olson JC, Subramanian RM. Emerging strategies for the treatment of patients with acute hepatic failure. *Curr Opin Crit Care*. 2016;22(2):142-151. doi:10.1097/MCC.0000000000000291

15. **The answer is D.** Grade 1 HE involves only a trivial lack of awareness, short attention span, and possibly euphoria or anxiety. Grade 2 HE entails disorientation, inappropriate behavior, personality changes, and impaired cognition with some incoordination and dysarthria. Grade 3 HE demonstrates semistupor with gross confusion, bizarre or inappropriate behavior with fits of paranoia or rage, ataxia, nystagmus, and dysarthria, with progression to coma and posturing or signs of brain herniation in Grade 4. Asterixis can occur at any grade.

Bismuth M, Funakoshi N, Cadranel JF, et al. Hepatic encephalopathy: from pathophysiology to therapeutic management. *Eur J Gastroenterol Hepatol*. 2011;23(1):8-22. doi:10.1097/MEG.0b013e3283417567

16. **The answer is D.** The King's College criteria are most commonly used to assess prognosis and assessment for transplant in acute liver failure (ALF), though new criteria have been proposed. For acetaminophen-induced ALF, arterial pH less than 7.3 irrespective of coma grade or PT greater than 100 seconds (INR 6.5) and serum Cr greater than 300 mol/L (3.4 mg/dL) in patients with grade III/IV hepatic encephalopathy (HE) are associated with a very poor outcome without transplant. In non–acetaminophen-induced ALF, the criteria used to predict poor prognosis without transplant consist of PT greater than 100 seconds or any three of the following irrespective of HE grade: drug toxicity, indeterminate cause of ALF, age younger than 10 or older than 40, jaundice to coma interval greater than 7 days, PT greater than 50 seconds (INR >3.5), and serum bilirubin greater than 300 µmol/L (17.5 mg/dL).

Frontera JA, Kalb T. Neurological management of fulminant hepatic failure. *Neurocrit Care*. 2011;14(2):318-327. doi: 10.1007/s12028-010-9470-y

Polson J, Lee WM. AASLD position paper: the management of acute liver failure. *Hepatology*. 2005;41(5):1179-1197. doi:10.1002/hep.20703

17. **The answer is C.** Retrospective trials have shown no benefit of lactulose or neomycin on morbidity or mortality in acute hepatic failure and can cause dehydration and worsening renal failure as well as gaseous abdominal distention, which could interfere with liver transplant. Neomycin is specifically contraindicated because of its propensity for nephrotoxicity. Invasive or noninvasive ICP monitoring can be considered in all acute Grade III/IV hepatic encephalopathy (HE) patients since cerebral edema occurs in 86% to 95% of this population, though no clear mortality benefit has been shown. CT scan of head is an insensitive indicator of elevated ICP. Intracranial hypertension should be treated as in other etiologies with conservative measures and then with hyperosmolar therapy. Prophylactic antibiotics are recommended in patients with advanced stage HE, refractory hypotension, presence of systemic inflammatory response syndrome (SIRS), and candidates for organ transplant. N-acetylcysteine is known to be beneficial in acute hepatic failure regardless of etiology.

Kandiah PA, Olson JC, Subramanian RM. Emerging strategies for the treatment of patients with acute hepatic failure. *Curr Opin Crit Care*. 2016;22(2):142-151. doi:10.1097/MCC.0000000000000291

Karvellas CJ, Fix OK, Battenhouse H, et al. Outcomes and complications of intracranial pressure monitoring in acute liver failure: a retrospective cohort study. *Crit Care Med*. 2014;42(5):1157-1167. doi: 10.1097/CCM.0000000000000144

McPhail MJ, Kriese S, Heneghan MA. Current management of acute liver failure. *Curr Opin Gastroenterol*. 2015;31:209-214. doi:10.1097/MOG.0000000000000174

18. **The answer is D.** Acute renal failure complicates up to 50% of patients with acute liver failure (ALF). Renal failure results in increased urea, which is acted upon by colonic bacteria similarly to protein, resulting in increased ammonia and leading to hepatorenal syndrome. It is unlikely that fluid resuscitation will correct the renal failure. Continuous renal replacement therapy (CRRT) is the preferred modality for dialysis in patients with fulminant liver failure because of its ability to continuously address electrolyte disturbances, allow adjustments in osmotic therapy, and prevent rapid fluid shifts. CRRT can also lower the ammonia levels, hence may be considered in all ALF patients. Intermittent hemodialysis is often poorly tolerated because of hemodynamic instability, fluid shifts, and risk of increasing intracranial pressure (ICP).

Kandiah PA, Olson JC, Subramanian RM. Emerging strategies for the treatment of patients with acute hepatic failure. *Curr Opin Crit Care*. 2016;22(2):142-151. doi:10.1097/MCC.0000000000000291

McPhail MJ, Kriese S, Heneghan MA. Current management of acute liver failure. *Curr Opin Gastroenterol*. 2015;31:209-214. doi:10.1097/MOG.0000000000000174

19. **The answer is D.** According to the American Academy of Neurology (AAN) Practice Parameters, the following clinical findings accurately predict universally poor outcome: myoclonic status epilepticus (MSE) within the first 24 hours in patients with primary circulatory arrest, absence of pupillary responses within 1 to 3 days after resuscitation, absent corneal reflexes within 1 to 3 days after resuscitation, and absent or extensor motor responses after 3 days. However, the more recent American Heart Association guidelines recommend against using absent or extensor motor response alone due to a high false positive predictive value. Up to 90% of survivors of anoxic injury have awoken by 72 hours, so a continued comatose state would be a discouraging sign, but it is not an accurate predictor of universally poor outcome. Earlier pupillary or motor examination findings have not been found to be as accurate in prediction. Hyperthermia is associated with worse outcome, but is not predictive of universally poor outcome.

Callaway CW, Donnino MW, Fink EL, et al. Part 8: post–cardiac arrest care: 2015 American Heart Association guidelines update for cardiopulmonary resuscitation and emergency cardiovascular care. *Circulation*. 2015;132(suppl 2):S465-S482. doi:10.1161/CIR.0000000000000262

Wijdicks EF, Hijdra A, Young GB, et al. Practice parameter: prediction of outcome in comatose survivors after cardiopulmonary resuscitation (an evidence-based review): report of the Quality Standards Subcommittee of the American Academy of Neurology. *Neurology*. 2006;67(2):203-210. doi:10.1212/01.wnl.0000227183.21314.cd

20. **The answer is A.** Recent guidelines on neuro-prognostication in patients with hypoxic–ischemic injury after cardiac arrest treated with or without TTM suggest not offering any prognostic recommendations until at least 72 hours after return of spontaneous circulation (ROSC) or return of normothermia. The application of a multimodal approach incorporating physical exam findings as well as neurophysiological testing (EEG and somatosensory evoked potential [SSEP]) improves prognostication. Absent pupillary response, when examined very carefully and at 72 hours, is a marker of universally poor prognosis but not at 24 hours in patients treated with TTM. Myoclonus is not a poor prognostic indicator by itself though the diagnosis of MSE should be investigated. Absent or extensor motor responses have a high false-positive predictive value and should not be used as prognostic markers.

Callaway CW, Donnino MW, Fink EL, et al. Part 8: post–cardiac arrest care: 2015 American Heart Association guidelines update for cardiopulmonary resuscitation and emergency cardiovascular care. *Circulation*. 2015;132(suppl 2):S465-S482. doi:10.1161/CIR.0000000000000262

Oddo M, Friberg H. Neuroprognostication after cardiac arrest in the light of targeted temperature management. *Curr Opin Crit Care*. June 2017;23(3):244-250. doi:10.1097/MCC.0000000000000406

21. **The answer is B.** Benzodiazepines, diuretics, and narcotics are all associated with worsening or decompensation of hepatic encephalopathy (HE). Topiramate can also cause hyperammonemia. Haloperidol is generally considered safer in patients at risk for or with HE.

Bismuth M, Funakoshi N, Cadranel JF, et al. Hepatic encephalopathy: from pathophysiology to therapeutic management. *Eur J Gastroenterol Hepatol*. 2011;23(1):8-22. doi:10.1097/MEG.0b013e3283417567

22. **The answer is D.** Magnesium sulfate administration is associated with predictable maternal effects including loss of DTRs (>4–6 mEq/L), followed by somnolence and respiratory depression (>8 mEq/L), and then cardiotoxicity (>15 mEq/L). Magnesium sulfate infusion also causes flushing (likely secondary to its vasodilatory effect) and hypocalcemia. Magnesium sulfate can sensitize patients to nondepolarizing muscle relaxants (and to a lesser extent depolarizing muscle relaxants), so smaller doses are recommended.

Kaplan PW. Eclampsia. In: Kaplan PW, ed. *Neurologic Disease in Women*. New York, NY: Demos Medical Publishing; 2006:235-246.

23. **The answer is E.** Many drug overdoses may present with coma, with preserved pupillary function often the distinguishing feature from an examination consistent with brain death. However, some drug overdoses, including TCAs, barbiturates, and valproic acid, have been associated with complete abolition of brainstem function including pupillary responses.

Auinger K, Müller V, Rudiger A, et al. Valproic acid intoxication imitating brain death. *Am J Emerg Med*. 2009;27(9):1177. e5-1177.e6. doi:10.1016/j.ajem.2009.02.019
Wijdicks EF, Hijdra A, Young GB, et al. Practice parameter: prediction of outcome in comatose survivors after cardiopulmonary resuscitation (an evidence-based review): report of the Quality Standards Subcommittee of the American Academy of Neurology. *Neurology*. 2006;67(2): 203-210. doi:10.1212/01.wnl.0000227183.21314.cd

24. **The answer is A.** The patient described has many classic features of anti-LGI1 encephalitis. LGI1 autoimmune encephalitis presents classically in males in their 60s with initial faciobrachial dystonic or subtle focal seizures that can be very frequent throughout the day but are often not recognized as seizures. Memory problems and cognitive deficits develop over the next few months. Problems with spatial disorientation, insomnia, apathy, and disinhibition are common. Most patients develop generalized tonic–clonic seizures later in the disease course. This syndrome is important to recognize because patients can recover almost completely with appropriate immunosuppressant therapy. The rapidly progressive course and the prominent seizures are not consistent with Alzheimer's disease and fronto-temporal dementia. CJD should be a consideration and can progress over this time course; however, the semiology is more consistent with seizures than myoclonus and other common features of CJD are not present. Hashimoto's encephalitis should also be a consideration as it can also present as subacute dementia with seizures or myoclonus. However, these seizures are usually less frequent and more generalized.

Graus F, Titulaer MJ, Balu R, et al. A clinical approach to diagnosis of autoimmune encephalitis. *Lancet Neurol*. 2016;15(4):391-404. doi:10.1016/S1474-4422(15)00401-9
Van Sonderen A, Thijs RD, Coenders EC, et al. Anti-LGI1 encephalitis: clinical syndrome and long-term follow-up. *Neurology*. 2016;87:1449-1456. doi:10.1212/WNL.0000000000003173

25. **The answer is D.** Although most of these findings are associated with poor outcome, only absent N20 responses within days 1 to 3 are associated with an invariably poor prognosis regardless of TTM. Spontaneous Burst suppression on EEG after 72 hours (rather than 24) or after rewarming is also almost invariably associated with a poor prognosis. BIPLDs, GPDs, and alpha or theta coma on EEG are associated with worse outcomes but not universally poor. Brainstem auditory evoked potentials have not been shown to have prognostic value post–cardiac arrest.

Callaway CW, Donnino MW, Fink EL, et al. Part 8: post–cardiac arrest care: 2015 American Heart Association guidelines update for cardiopulmonary resuscitation and emergency cardiovascular care. *Circulation.* 2015;132(suppl 2):S465-S482. doi:10.1161/CIR.0000000000000262

Wijdicks EF, Hijdra A, Young GB, et al. Practice parameter: prediction of outcome in comatose survivors after cardiopulmonary resuscitation (an evidence-based review): report of the Quality Standards Subcommittee of the American Academy of Neurology. *Neurology.* 2006;67(2):203-210. doi:10.1212/01.wnl.0000227183.21314.cd

26. **The answer is E.** Patients with MELAS present with stroke-like episodes often associated with a headache, vision changes, as well as seizure activity as in the patient described. Patients with a diagnosis of MELAS who present with seizure, headache, altered mental status (AMS), focal weakness, visual loss, sensory loss, dysarthria, or ataxia should receive a loading dose of IV L-arginine 0.5g/kg immediately as well as D5 or D10 normal saline (NS) to reverse the catabolism. This therapy is recommended to begin within 3 hours of onset and should not be delayed by imaging studies; therefore, vessel imaging should not be the next step. The bolus dose of L-arginine should be followed by an additional 0.5g/kg infusion over the next 3 days with continued IV fluids. Stroke-like episodes in MELAS result from low levels of nitric oxide leading to vasoconstriction and hypoxemia. L-arginine is converted to nitric oxide and has been shown to be beneficial in patients with MELAS to decrease the severity of stroke-like episodes. A STAT EEG should also be obtained to assess for nonconvulsive status epilepticus (NCSE). While large vessel ischemic stroke is possible at this age, the constellation of symptoms is not consistent with a vascular distribution. IV thrombolysis or thrombectomy would not be expected to work and could cause harm. Daily aspirin is not recommended in MELAS.

Koenig MK, Emrick L, Karaa A, et al. Recommendations for the management of stroke like episodes in patients with mitochondrial encephalomyopathy, lactic acidosis, and strokelike episodes. *JAMA Neurol.* May 1, 2016;73(5):591-594. doi:10.1001/jamaneurol.2015.5072

27. **The answer is E.** Neurologic manifestations of uremic encephalopathy include delirium, agitation, visual hallucination, and stupor evolving to coma. Seizures (partial or generalized) are seen in one-third of uremic encephalopathy patients, as are signs of meningeal irritation. Multifocal myoclonus and asterixis are very common in later stages of uremic encephalopathy that could progress to total body multifocal myoclonus—the described "uremic twitch syndrome." Hemiparesis occurs in almost half of the patients, which may alternate sides during the illness. Papilledema and dysarthria can also be seen. CSF findings include elevated protein and pleocytosis, mimicking aseptic meningitis.

Burn DJ, Bates D. Neurology and the kidney. *J Neurol Neurosurg Psychiatry.* 1998;65(6):810-821.

Raskin NH. Neurologic complications of renal failure. In: Aminoff MJ, ed. *Neurology and General Medicine.* Philadelphia, PA: Churchill Livingstone; 2001:293-296.

28. **The answer is B.** This vignette describes the presentation of a patient with hemolysis, elevated liver enzymes, low platelet (HELLP) syndrome, which is defined as hemolysis with a microangiopathic blood smear, elevated liver enzymes, and a low platelet count. It usually occurs in the third trimester, although it can occur earlier or postpartum. It is often associated with severe preeclampsia and eclampsia. Maternal complications include DIC most frequently, but also liver rupture, cerebral hemorrhage, and pulmonary edema. Fatal pontine hemorrhage and cerebellar infarctions have been described. Neonatal complications include placental abruption, intrauterine growth retardation (IUGR), preterm labor, and perinatal death. If the syndrome develops after 34 weeks, delivery is usually recommended.

Altamura C, Vasapollo B, Tibuzzi F, et al. Postpartum cerebellar infarction and haemolysis, elevated liver enzymes, low platelet (HELLP) syndrome. *Neurol Sci.* 2005;26(1):40-42. doi: 10.1007/s10072-005-0380-2

Haram K, Svendsen E, Abildgaard U. The HELLP syndrome: clinical issues and management. A review. *BMC Pregnancy Childbirth.* 2009;9:8. doi:10.1186/1471-2393-9-8

Zeidman LA, Videnovic A, Bernstein LP, et al. Lethal pontine hemorrhage in postpartum syndrome of hemolysis, elevated liver enzyme levels, and low platelet count. *Arch Neurol.* 2005;62(7):1150-1153. doi:10.1001/archneur.62.7.1150

29. **The answer is C.** Hypertensive encephalopathy often shows MRI fluid-attenuated inversion recovery (FLAIR) lesions consistent with PRES; however, the MRI can be normal. When PRES is present radiographically, however, encephalopathy is noted in up to 90% of patients, seizures in greater than 75%, headache in 53%, and visual symptoms in 20% to 67%. There is usually much more extensive radiologic involvement than clinical symptoms—the "clinical-radiological dissociation." The MRI can show brain or cord abnormalities. EEG most commonly shows generalized slowing, not LPDs. Although lumbar puncture (LP) is not usually recommended or required in hypertensive encephalopathy due to cerebral edema, the CSF usually reveals normal or mildly elevated protein and albumin, and normal cell count.

Fischer M, Schmutzhard E. Posterior reversible encephalopathy syndrome. *J Neurol.* 2017;264(8):1608-1616. doi:10.1007/s00415-016-8377-8

Fugate JE, Rabinstein AA. Posterior reversible encephalopathy syndrome: clinical and radiological manifestations, pathophysiology, and outstanding questions. *Lancet Neurol.* 2015;14(9): 914-925. doi:10.1016/s1474-4422(15)00111-8

30. **The answer is B.** While all of these choices should be considered in the differential diagnosis, this patient has a classic presentation for anti-NMDA receptor encephalitis. Anti-NMDA receptor encephalitis usually presents in children or young adults with acute onset of psychiatric symptoms. It often progresses from psychosis, memory problems, and seizures to catatonia or agitation with autonomic instability and oro–facial–lingual dyskinesias. MRI brain may show fluid-attenuated inversion recovery (FLAIR) hyperintensity in the mesial temporal lobes but can be normal. EEG usually shows generalized or frontotemporal slowing and CSF usually demonstrates a lymphocytic pleocytosis. HSV encephalitis should always be considered on the differential with acute mental status change and seizures; however, the presentation is atypical and no changes are seen on the MRI brain. Drug intoxication should be improving after more than a week. Anti-GABA-A receptor encephalitis presents in young patients with acute altered behavior and mentation in the setting of frequent seizures similar to this patient but usually has multifocal cortical–subcortical FLAIR changes on MRI as well as abnormalities on EEG and CSF. CASPR2 antibody–associated disease usually presents in elderly men with a limbic encephalitis associated with cerebellar dysfunction, peripheral nervous system hyperexcitability, dysautonomia, insomnia, neuropathic pain, or weight loss.

Graus F, Titulaer MJ, Balu R, et al. A clinical approach to diagnosis of autoimmune encephalitis. *Lancet Neurol.* 2016;15(4):391-404. doi:10.1016/S1474-4422(15)00401-9

Spatola M, Petit-Pedrol M, Simabukuro MM, et al. Investigations in GABA$_A$ receptor antibody-associated encephalitis. *Neurology.* 2017;88(11):1012-1020. doi:10.1212/WNL.0000000000003713

31. **The answer is B.** Different brain structures show variable sensitivity to hypoxic injury. The gray matter is more sensitive than the white matter, and the occipitoparietal regions are more sensitive than the frontotemporal regions. Of the six cortical layers, layer 3 (the external pyramidal layer) is the most sensitive to hypoxia, explaining the laminar necrosis sometimes seen as sequelae of hypoxic injury. Hippocampal region 2 is the most vulnerable of the hippocampal regions. The caudate and putamen are more sensitive to hypoxia than the thalami.

Longstreth WT. Neurologic complications of cardiac arrest. In: Aminoff MJ, ed. *Neurology and General Medicine.* Philadelphia, PA: Churchill Livingstone; 2001:151-170.

32. **The answer is E.** Hypothermia is associated with a "cold diuresis" leading to hypovolemia and resultant hypokalemia and hypomagnesemia directly and from intracellular shifts. Hypothermia also decreases insulin secretion and increases insulin resistance, resulting in hyperglycemia that may be resistant to treatment. A mild bleeding diathesis is well described in hypothermia secondary to usually mild thrombocytopenia as well as impairment of qualitative platelet function and the clotting cascade. Leukopenia and increased susceptibility to

infections are well known in hypothermia, but leukocytosis is not an expected side effect of the hypothermia itself.

Polderman KH, Herold I. Therapeutic hypothermia and controlled normothermia in the intensive care unit: practical considerations, side effects, and cooling methods. *Crit Care Med.* 2009;37(3):1101-1120. doi:10.1097/CCM.0b013e3181962ad5

33. **The answer is C.** Differential diagnosis includes intracranial hemorrhage (ICH) resulting in elevated intracranial pressure (ICP), basilar meningitis (especially *Listeria* given known immunosuppressed status), Wernicke's encephalopathy, nonconvulsive status epilepticus (NCSE), alcohol withdrawal, and uremic and/or hepatic encephalopathy (HE), among others. A brain CT scan should be done in all chronic dialysis patients presenting with focal deficits due to the high risk of subdural hemorrhage secondary to platelet dysfunction and brain atrophy, and is normal in this case. Stroke is also a possibility, but more focal findings would be expected. Basilar meningitis, especially *Listeria* given the patient's risk factors, should be considered, but the lack of other suggestive features makes this less likely. NCSE is always a possibility, and seizures occur in up to one-third of uremic patients; however, this would not explain the cranial nerve six palsies. Uremic and HE may be contributing, but do not explain the entire picture. This patient has two of the triad for Wernicke's encephalopathy, and this should be considered early and be treated as in this case. Wernicke's encephalopathy is rare, but patients on dialysis are at higher risk because of low thiamine intake and accelerated loss of thiamine by hemodialysis. Because it can mimic uremic encephalopathy and often remains unrecognized, Wernicke's encephalopathy needs to be treated early.

Ihara M, Ito T, Yanagihara C, et al. Wernicke's encephalopathy associated with hemodialysis: report of two cases and review of the literature. *Clin Neurol Neurosurg.* 1999;101(2):118-121. doi:10.1016/s0303-8467(99)00014-1

34. **The answer is C.** Hypertensive encephalopathy is defined as the presence of signs of cerebral edema caused by breakthrough hyperperfusion from severe and sudden rises in BP and classically presents with relatively rapid onset of headache, nausea, vomiting, and vision changes followed by nonlocalizing neurologic symptoms such as restlessness and confusion. If the hypertension is not treated, seizures and coma may pursue. However, atypical presentations may include focal neurologic signs and brainstem (rather than parieto-occipital) radiologic involvement. Development of frank noncommunicating hydrocephalus necessitating external ventricular drainage has been reported and improved with hypertensive management. The autonomic instability associated with Guillain–Barre syndrome (GBS) and other autonomic neuropathies can also precipitate hypertensive encephalopathy. The absolute level of BP may not be as important as the rate of increase, and patients with long-standing hypertension can tolerate higher mean arterial pressures (MAPs) without the development of hypertensive encephalopathy. The patient described in C does not have progressive symptoms and does not have hypertensive encephalopathy.

Fischer M, Schmutzhard E. Posterior reversible encephalopathy syndrome. *J Neurol.* 2017;264(8):1608-1616. doi: 10.1007/s00415-016-8377-8

Fugate JE, Rabinstein AA. Posterior reversible encephalopathy syndrome: clinical and radiological manifestations, pathophysiology, and outstanding questions. *Lancet Neurol.* 2015;14(9):914-925. doi: 10.1016/s1474-4422(15)00111-8

Marik PE, Rivera R. Hypertensive emergencies: an update. *Curr Opin Crit Care.* 2011;17(6):569-580. doi:10.1097/MCC.0b013e32834cd31d

35. **The answer is E.** Eclampsia can occur up to 4 weeks postpartum. Magnesium sulfate should be started and continued for 24 hours to prevent further seizures. Multiple trials comparing magnesium sulfate to benzodiazepines and phenytoin have shown superiority of magnesium sulfate in preventing further seizures in eclampsia as well as preventing the development of seizures in severe preeclampsia. Labetalol or other antihypertensive should also be started to control this patient's BP.

Sibai BM. Magnesium sulfate prophylaxis in preeclampsia: lessons learned from recent trials. *Am J Obstet Gynecol*. 2004;190(6):1520-1526. doi:10.1016/j.ajog.2003.12.057

36. **The answer is C.** This patient most likely has mitochondrial encephalopathy with lactic acidosis and stroke-like episodes (MELAS) given her family history and presentation. Headache, exercise intolerance, memory problems, hearing loss, short stature, and diabetes are common comorbidities in addition to recurrent vomiting, epilepsy, and neuropathies. The point mutation at mitochondrial nucleotide pair 3,243 (a transfer ribonucleic acid-Leu gene) has been identified as likely responsible for 80% of patients with MELAS. This mutation has also been identified as a cause of diabetes and cardiomyopathy in patients who never manifest the entire MELAS syndrome. It is estimated that this mutation accounts for 2% of all type 2 DM cases. Lactic acid elevation is very common, especially during the stroke-like episodes. Given its propensity to cause lactic acidosis, it is recommended that metformin be avoided in patients with DM and MELAS. Patients with known MELAS who present with stroke-like episodes should be treated acutely with L-arginine infusion and then arginine 0.15 to 0.3g/kg divided three times a day (TID) should be given orally for prophylaxis against further episodes. Aspirin has no role in prophylaxis for patients with MELAS.

El-Hattab AW, Adesina AM, Jones J, et al. MELAS syndrome: clinical manifestations, pathogenesis, and treatment options. *Mol Genet Metab*. 2015;116(1-2):4-12. doi:10.1016/j.ymgme.2015.06.004

Kaufmann P, Engelstad K, Wei Y, et al. Natural history of MELAS associated with mitochondrial DNA m.3243A>G genotype. *Neurology*. 2011;77(22):1965-1971. doi:10.1212/WNL.0b013e31823a0c7f

Koenig MK, Emrick L, Karaa A, et al. Recommendations for the management of strokelike episodes in patients with mitochondrial encephalomyopathy, lactic acidosis, and strokelike episodes. *JAMA Neurol*. 2016;73(5):591-594. doi:10.1001/jamaneurol.2015.5072

13 Clinical Syndromes in Neurocritical Care

HOWARD J. FAN AND ASMA ZAKARIA

■ QUESTIONS

1. A 50-year-old man with no vascular risk factors presents to the ED with a low Glasgow Coma Scale (GCS) score and noted systolic blood pressure (BP) 220 mmHg, pulse 50 beats/min, and abnormal respirations. Before neuroimaging, the nurse reports episodic extensor posturing, poor mentation, and cardiac dysrhythmias but no lateralizing motor signs or pupillary changes. She is concerned that the patient is herniating. What can be expected on CT scan?

    A. Transtentorial (uncal) herniation
    B. Central herniation
    C. Upward herniation
    D. Cerebellar herniation
    E. External herniation

2. An overnight resident concerned with intracranial pressure (ICP) waveforms on an ICU patient wakes you with a picture of the waveform. It shows elevation of P2 wave greater than P1. What would you tell the resident?

    A. P1 pressure wave is produced from venous pulsations
    B. P1 pressure wave is typically lower than P2
    C. P2 pressure wave results from restriction of ventricular expansion
    D. Small increases in intracranial volume may cause large increases in ICP
    E. Both C and D

3. A male patient in the ICU presents with a right hemispheric mass with minimal edema and a poor Glasgow Coma Scale (GCS) score on initial evaluation. The cause(s) of his poor mental status can be attributed to:

    A. Small brainstem lesion
    B. Metabolic encephalopathy
    C. Drug overdose
    D. Dominant hemispheric infarct
    E. All of the above

4. All of the following clinical or radiographic features are more common in oral anticoagulant–associated intracranial hemorrhage (ICH) than in spontaneous hypertensive intracerebral hemorrhage **except:**

    A. Presence of a fluid level
    B. Focal neurologic deficit
    C. Multiple discrete areas of hemorrhage

    D. Papilledema and headache

    E. Rapid expansion of the hematoma

5. An external ventricular drain (EVD) is indicated in which of the following scenarios?

    A. Obstructive hydrocephalus

    B. Communicating hydrocephalus with signs of elevated intracranial pressure (ICP)

    C. Subarachnoid hemorrhage (SAH) with altered mental status (AMS)

    D. Traumatic brain injury (TBI) with Glasgow Coma Scale (GCS) score less than 8

    E. Intracerebral hemorrhage (ICH) with intraventricular involvement of the third and fourth ventricles

    F. All of the above

6. A 40-year-old patient presents with a focal parietal lesion with increased signal intensity on T2, diffusion-weighted imaging, apparent diffusion coefficient, and primarily white matter edema with maintenance of gray–white matter interface on CT and MRI imaging. Which of the following is/are true?

    A. 4 mg dexamethasone intravenously (IV) every 6 hours

    B. 0.5 to 1 g/kg mannitol IV every 6 hours to maintain serum sodium (Na) 145 to 155 mEq/L

    C. Fever, if present, should be treated with acetaminophen 650 mg PO q4h or external cooling devices if required

    D. Both B and C

    E. Both A and C

7. A 20-year-old man with traumatic brain injury (TBI) and uncontrolled intracranial hypertension undergoes prolonged hyperventilation for 8 hours overnight. At what $PaCO_2$ would you begin to worry about provoking or worsening cerebral ischemia?

    A. $PaCO_2$ 35

    B. $PaCO_2$ 30

    C. $PaCO_2$ 28

    D. $PaCO_2$ 25

8. The respiratory rate for the patient in Question 7 is lowered, and the intracranial pressure (ICP) starts spiking soon thereafter. You are now concerned for

    A. Refractory intracranial hypertension

    B. Inadequate sedation

    C. Rebound intracranial hypertension

    D. Reflex cerebral vasoconstriction

9. The intracranial pressure (ICP) monitor placed in a young traumatic brain injury (TBI) patient is reviewed the next morning by the attending on service. Sustained, high-amplitude elevation of ICP at 55 mmHg is seen for 30 minutes. Which of the following should there be concern about?

    A. Lundberg A wave

    B. Lundberg B wave

    C. Lundberg C wave

    D. Plateau wave

    E. Both A and D

10. A 62-year-old man with unknown medical history presents to the ED with headache and emesis. A CT scan of the head shows dilated lateral ventricles and bowing of the third ventricle

with absence of fourth ventricular dilation. MRI of the brain shows increased T2 signal in the periventricular area. Compression of the quadrigeminal plate will cause which of the following focal neurological deficits?

A. Parinaud's syndrome
B. Abducens nerve palsy
C. Oculomotor palsy
D. Visual field deficit

11. A 37-year-old man with a history of recent intravenous (IV) drug abuse presents with progressive obtundation leading to coma. He is febrile with a grade 3 systolic ejection murmur and Janeway lesions. His head CT scan demonstrates multifocal abnormalities consistent with embolic infarctions in multiple vascular territories of the brain. Injury to which of the following areas would be sufficient to cause coma?

A. Basis pontis
B. Bilateral occipital lobes
C. Bilateral parietal lobes
D. Right frontal lobe and left occipital lobe
E. Bilateral thalami

12. In which of the following conditions has therapeutic hypothermia (TH) been documented to improve clinical outcomes?

A. Acute cerebral infarction
B. Acute spinal cord trauma
C. Cardiac arrest
D. Subarachnoid hemorrhage (SAH)
E. Traumatic brain injury (TBI)

13. Specific consideration during the induction phase of therapeutic hypothermia (TH) includes:

A. Shivering
B. Core temperature maintenance
C. Electrolyte disturbance
D. Induction time

14. A 50-year-old woman suffers a massive embolic stroke during cardiac valve surgery. She is treated with hypothermia to a temperature of 32°C. After 6 hours, she is rewarmed. Which of the following is a risk specific to the rewarming phase of hypothermia treatment?

A. Asystole
B. Coagulopathy
C. Hypotension
D. Thrombocytopenia
E. Increased intracranial pressure (ICP)

15. A 73-year-old woman presents with sudden onset of left hemiparesis and right gaze preference. Her family wishes to know more when informed of the prognosis for early death from her condition. Which of the following is a known risk factor for fatal brain edema as a complication of acute ischemic stroke?

A. Blood glucose of 120 mg/dL
B. High National Institutes of Health (NIH) Stroke Scale score
C. Diastolic blood pressure (BP) greater than 110 mmHg
D. Diffusion lesion volume greater than 40 mL in 24 hours
E. Elevated creatinine (Cr)

16. A 61-year-old man with vascular risk factors for hypertension, coronary artery disease (CAD), and hyperlipidemia was witnessed collapsing at a gas station. He was found to be in ventricular fibrillation by emergency medical service (EMS). After achievement of return of spontaneous circulation (ROSC), he was treated with hypothermia for 24 hours. Which of the following tests might provide predictive discrimination of outcome?
    A. Brain imaging
    B. Duration of CPR at scene
    C. EEG
    D. Neuron-specific enolase level
    E. Absent pupillary reflexes and motor response at 3 days

17. Undergoing therapeutic hypothermia (TH) portends which of the following complications?
    A. Autoimmune renal injury
    B. Coagulopathy
    C. Hepatic failure
    D. Hypertension
    E. Seizures

18. A 56-year-old man presents with sudden onset of severe headache and sleepiness. His medical history is remarkable for alcohol and tobacco abuse. On triage, his blood pressure (BP) is 130/80 mmHg, Glasgow Coma Scale (GCS) score is 13, and the pupils are both 3 mm and reactive. A CT scan of the head reveals a 12 cm³ left basal ganglia hemorrhage with extension into the left lateral and third ventricles. Two hours later, he is poorly responsive, and his GCS score falls to 9. Repeat CT scan shows no change in hematoma size, but marked enlargement of the third and lateral ventricles. Which of the following interventions is most likely to improve his clinical status?
    A. Intravenous (IV) mannitol
    B. IV thiamine
    C. External ventricular drain (EVD)
    D. Therapeutic hypothermia (TH)
    E. Lowering mean arterial pressure (MAP)

19. A 61-year-old man with a history of coronary artery disease (CAD), dyslipidemia, and well-controlled hypertension presents with acute onset of left hemiparesis, hemisensory deficit, and left-sided neglect. His initial blood pressure (BP) is 260/120 mmHg, but it is reduced to 205/110 mmHg with a single dose of labetalol. Head CT scan is unremarkable, and he is treated with tissue plasminogen activator (tPA). He is then transferred to a stroke unit for careful monitoring. National Institute of Neurological Disorders and Stroke (NINDS) guidelines recommend treatment of elevated BP equal to or greater than which of the following values (in mmHg)?
    A. Systolic 160, diastolic 90
    B. Systolic 180, diastolic 105
    C. Systolic 200, diastolic 110
    D. Systolic 220, diastolic 120
    E. Systolic 240, diastolic 130

20. Which of the following EEG patterns best correlates with better prognosis after cardiac arrest?
    A. Dominant theta–delta activity without detectable normal alpha
    B. Dominant nonreactive alpha activity
    C. Burst suppression (BP)
    D. Suppressed background with continuous periodic discharges
    E. Abundant periodic lateralizing discharges

21. A 70-year-old woman presents to the hospital with acute onset of left hemiparesis and hemisensory loss. Her blood pressure (BP) is 205/100 mmHg. On examination, she is drowsy, but can follow commands with effort. Her Glasgow Coma Scale (GCS) score is 13. A non-contrast brain CT scan shows a 15 cm^3 right basal ganglia hemorrhage with no ventricular involvement. She is started on a nitroprusside infusion, reducing her BP to 165/90 mmHg. Her mental status deteriorates, with the GCS score falling to 8. Repeat CT scan shows no change in the hemorrhage size, no hydrocephalus, and no subarachnoid or intraventricular blood. Which of the following is the most likely etiology of her altered mental status (AMS)?

   A. Hypertensive encephalopathy
   B. Seizure
   C. Vasospasm
   D. Pressure-dependent reinfarction
   E. Nitroprusside-induced intracranial pressure (ICP) elevation

22. A 54-year-old woman develops a rapidly progressive paraparesis with a sensory level at T6. Which of the following features would be most suggestive of an etiology other than idiopathic transverse myelitis (TM)?

   A. Asymmetrical weakness
   B. Cerebrospinal fluid (CSF) pleocytosis
   C. Elevated immunoglobulin G (IgG) index
   D. Enhancing spinal cord lesion on spinal imaging
   E. Progression to nadir within 2 hours

23. A 32-year-old man with a history of chronic thrombocytopenia presents to the ED with an abrupt onset of headache, vomiting, and left hemiparesis. A CT scan of the brain demonstrates a 45 cm^3 hematoma within the right lenticular nucleus and internal capsule. He has been tak-ing warfarin for the past year. A "spot sign" is seen on neuroimaging. Which of the following has the **least** supporting evidence in terms of the next best clinical step?

   A. Fresh-frozen plasma (FFP)
   B. Vitamin K
   C. Factor VII
   D. Platelet transfusion or 1-deamino-8-D-arginine vasopressin
   E. Blood pressure (BP) control

24. A 49-year-old man is involved in a motor vehicle accident and sustains a significant closed traumatic brain injury (TBI). He presents to the ED with a Glasgow Coma Scale (GCS) score of 3 and remains unchanged for weeks until he is transferred to a long-term care facility. He has responsive pupils, makes conjugate roving eye movements, grimaces inconsistently to noxious stimuli, and withdraws to pain but does not make a localized response. Which of the following terms best describes this man's state of consciousness?

   A. Catatonia
   B. Locked-in state
   C. Minimally conscious state
   D. Persistent vegetative state (PVS)
   E. Coma

25. A 50-year-old man with hypertension, coronary artery disease (CAD), and prior myocardial infarction 1 year ago is brought to the ED within 30 minutes of onset of acute right hemi-paresis and dysarthria. His family reports no other medical history. Blood pressure (BP) is 175/90 mmHg. A brain CT scan shows effacement of the gray–white interface in the left insula. ECG, blood glucose, and platelet count are normal. Coagulation studies are pending. His home

regimen includes metoprolol, aspirin, and simvastatin. What is the recommended approach regarding treatment with intravenous (IV) tissue plasminogen activator (tPA)?

A. Administer tPA as soon as possible
B. Await the results of coagulation studies before administering
C. Do not administer tPA in this patient since he has been taking aspirin
D. Obtain written informed consent
E. Reduce arterial BP to reduce the risk of intracerebral hemorrhage (ICH)

26. An 80-year-old man is found collapsed in a parking lot. Emergency medical service (EMS) arrives at the scene and finds no respirations or palpable pulse. CPR is started with an initial rhythm of ventricular fibrillation. A pulse is restored after 15 minutes, with a subsequent Glasgow Coma Scale (GCS) score of 3. On examination, pupils are 2 mm sluggishly reactive, but oculocephalic reflex and corneal reflexes are absent. During his hospital stay, he develops myoclonic jerks of his face, tongue, and upper extremities but no improvement in GCS score or brainstem reflexes. An EEG is most likely to demonstrate which of the following patterns?

A. Delta–theta coma
B. Atypical spike-and-wave activity
C. Alpha coma
D. Burst suppression (BP)
E. Electrocerebral silence

27. A 60-year-old woman experiences a cardiac arrest after a run of ventricular tachycardia. Emergency resuscitation requires 30 minutes of effort before stabilization. Emergency services report the absence of pupillary response in either eye after the code. On morning rounds, the intern cites a study in which a nonreactive pupillary response is almost uniformly predictive of severe deficit and poor neurological outcome. Which of the following is/are marker(s) of poor outcome after cardiac resuscitation?

A. Initial absence of pupillary light response
B. Extensor or no motor response after 3 days
C. Myotonic status epilepticus (SE)
D. Burst suppression (BP) on EEG
E. Bilaterally absent cortical somatosensory evoked potential (SSEP) responses
F. Elevated serum neuron-specific enolase
G. All of the above

28. A 75-year-old woman involved in a motor vehicle accident while wearing a lap belt is brought into the ED and found to have a low-resting blood pressure (BP), bradycardia, and systemic signs of shock. Which of the following underlying etiologies is the likely cause?

A. Vasodilation
B. Heart failure
C. Sudden epinephrine release
D. Volume depletion

29. A 64-year-old man is brought to the ED by family after he was found confused at home. The onset of the event was not witnessed. Examination reveals left hemiparesis and dysarthria. A CT head scan without contrast is ordered. Which of the following would be a contraindication for thrombolytic therapy?

A. Hyperdense right middle cerebral artery (MCA) sign
B. Loss of gray–white differentiation in right insula
C. Loss of gray–white differentiation in right temporal cortex
D. Sulcal effacement in right hemisphere
E. Delineated hypodensity in right MCA territory

30. An 80-year-old man underwent a prolonged abdominal aortic aneurysm repair. After anesthesia wears off, he notices difficulty moving his legs. Neurology service is consulted and documents a flaccid paraplegia with a sensory level at T10. Upon follow-up with the same neurologist 3 months later, his examination reveals lower extremity weakness, bilateral ankle clonus, absent knee jerks, and plantar toe extension. Which of the following examination findings is also to be expected?

    A. Fasciculations
    B. Abnormal tibial sensory-evoked potentials
    C. Decreased amplitudes in gastrocnemius
    D. Fibrillations in sural nerve
    E. Bladder detrusor–sphincter dysfunction

31. A 62-year-old male with hypertension and atrial fibrillation, on warfarin, presents to ED with left-sided hemiparesis and cortical neglect. Triage CT imaging demonstrates a 65-ml volume right-sided lobar hemorrhage and Glasgow Coma Scale (GCS) 11. Which of the following is the most appropriate next step in management?

    A. Fresh frozen plasma (FFP)
    B. Desmopressin
    C. Vitamin K
    D. Prothrombin complex concentrate (PCC)
    E. Idarucizumab

32. A 32-year-old female with past medical history of methamphetamine abuse and hypertension is brought to emergency room (ER) by her boyfriend. She was found on the ground after a tonic–clonic seizure, was initially arousable to voice and complaining of a headache, but progressively became more obtunded en route to the ER. Triage blood pressure (BP) is 206/100 with a Glasgow Coma Scale (GCS) score of 7. Once intubated, mannitol and CO_2 hyperventilation are administered. CT of the head demonstrates ventriculomegaly with prominent dilated temporal horns and effacement of basilar cisterns, and casting of blood within the third and fourth ventricle. A nicardipine infusion is initiated by the ER staff. What is the next best step?

    A. Fosphenytoin bolus loading
    B. Dexamethasone initiation
    C. External ventricular drain (EVD) insertion
    D. Factor VII infusion
    E. Head elevation to 30 degrees

33. A 22-year-old male with past medical history of traumatic brain injury (TBI) from a motor vehicle accident presents to the ED unresponsive after a witnessed generalized convulsion lasting 3 minutes at a late-night study session. Four milligrams of lorazepam were initially administered by emergency medical service (EMS) personnel. En route to the hospital, another 4 mg of lorazepam were given for a second generalized convulsion and he was loaded with fosphenytoin 20 mg/kg intravenously (IV) upon arrival to the ED. CT of the head demonstrates right temporal encephalomalacia. Vitals are normal. Examination reveals a poor sensorium with eyes closed, no response to verbal stimuli, hippus in both pupils, and withdrawal response to appendicular pain bilaterally. Given the poor Glasgow Coma Score (GCS) and concern for airway protection, he is intubated by ED staff. What is the next best step?

    A. IV levetiracetam loading
    B. Lorazepam 2 mg IV administration
    C. Midazolam infusion
    D. Routine EEG
    E. MRI of the brain

34. After an automobile accident on the freeway, a 24-year-old male is found by emergency medical service (EMS) unable to move his arms or legs bilaterally. He is placed in spinal precautions and brought to the ED, where examination reveals lack of pain and temperature sensation but intact vibration and proprioception below the neck. No imaging is available yet. Which of the following best describes his physical exam findings?

    A. Central cord syndrome
    B. Anterior spinal cord syndrome
    C. Posterior spinal cord syndrome
    D. Brown–Sequard cord syndrome
    E. Cauda equina syndrome

35. A 21-year-old male involved in a boating accident is emergently flown to a tertiary care hospital where clinical examination reveals a Glasgow Coma Score (GCS) of 7 and CT imaging demonstrates bifrontal cortical hemorrhagic contusions. The patient is intubated and hyperventilated for CO_2 control, and hyperosmolar therapy is initiated. An intracranial pressure (ICP) monitor is placed but the neurosurgeon on call does not believe a bifrontal craniectomy would be beneficial. The patient's cerebral perfusion pressure (CPP) is 55 and he is currently being sedated with a midozalam infusion titrated to a burst-suppression (BS) pattern on continuous EEG. The ICU resident reports a sodium level of 165 and a serum osmolality of 340 mOsm. ICP remains high and CPP low. What would be the next best step for ICP control?

    A. Increase sedation with pentobarbital-induced coma
    B. Higher doses of mannitol
    C. Hypothermia induction to 32°C to 34°C
    D. Jugular bulb monitor insertion
    E. High-dose corticosteroids

■ ANSWERS

1. **The answer is D.** Cerebral herniation refers to displacement of brain tissue into nearby compartments from local intracranial pressure (ICP) gradients (see accompanying illustration). Clinical findings of cerebellar/tonsillar herniation include episodic extensor posturing and cardiac dysrhythmias from downward displacement of cerebellar tonsils through the foramen magnum with compression of the medulla. Uncal herniation classically presents with ipsilateral pupillary dilation secondary to compression of cranial nerve (CN) III from herniation of the medial temporal lobe under the tentorium cerebelli, thereby displacing the midbrain. Central herniation can present with bilateral pupillary dilation and extensor posturing with obliteration of the suprasellar cistern on imaging as both medial temporal lobes herniate through the tentorial notch. Similarly, upward herniation of posterior fossa contents through the tentorial notch presents with bilateral pupillary dilation and extensor posturing, typically as a result of excessive cerebrospinal fluid (CSF) ventricular drainage.

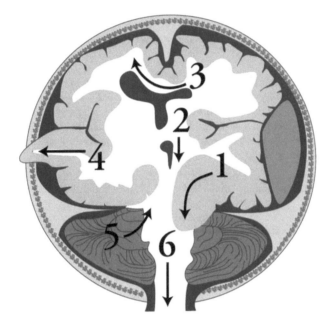

Herniation Syndromes. (1) Uncal herniation can result in third cranial nerve, posterior cerebral artery and midbrain compression; (2) central herniation can cause downward displacement of the entire brainstem with lateral gaze palsy; (3) subfalcine herniation can result in strangulation of the anterior cerebral artery under the falx; (4) extracranial herniation can occur through a traumatic skull defect or therapeutic craniectomy; (5) upward tentorial herniation can occur due to posterior fossa masses; (6) tonsillar herniation can result in brainstem compression, pupillary dilation, and cardio respiratory arrest. Used with permission from Zakaria A, Aisiku I. Management of acute intracranial hypertension. In: Farey D, Flaxman A, Chiu W, eds. *Critical Care Emergency Medicine.* New York, NY: McGraw-Hill; 2017.

2. **The answer is E.** ICP waveforms originate from transient increases in pressure from transmission of arterial pulses to the brain. P1 (percussion wave) is produced by local increases in ICP from arterial pulse pressure waves in the choroid plexus. P2 (elastance or tidal wave) results from a restriction of ventricular expansion by a closed rigid skull. P3 (dicrotic wave) is produced by closure of the aortic valve associated with the arterial dicrotic notch. Under normal circumstances, P1 >P2 >P3. Elevation of P2 greater than P1 is concerning for disturbed intracranial elastance and loss of nonlinear dynamics such that small increases in intracranial volume may dramatically increase ICP.

Lee KR, Hoff JT. Intracranial pressure. In: Youmans JR, ed. *Neurological Surgery.* Vol 1. Philadelphia, PA: Saunders; 1996:491-518.

3. **The answer is E.** A unilateral hemispheric lesion rarely causes a disturbance in consciousness. Exceptions include a large dominant hemispheric stroke or a small lesion in the brainstem or thalamus, either of which can cause significant alteration of consciousness. Otherwise, classically a disturbance in consciousness must involve a process that affects the reticular activating system (RAS) or a diffuse process that affects the cortex bilaterally, for example, metabolic encephalopathy, paraneoplastic disorders, head trauma, and posterior reversible encephalopathy syndrome.

4. **The answer is B.** Intracerebral hemorrhage of any etiology is likely to be associated with headache and a focal neurologic deficit. Oral anticoagulant–associated ICH is more likely to expand over a longer period (up to 7 days), have a fluid level and multiple discrete areas of hemorrhage compared to spontaneous ICH. Continued elevation of blood pressure (BP) is considered a risk factor for hematoma expansion. The majority of ICH expansion occurs in the first 6 hours after initial hemorrhage.

Kazui S, Minematsu K, Yamamoto H, et al. Predisposing factors to enlargement of spontaneous intracerebral hematoma. *Stroke.* 1997;28(12):2370-2375. doi:10.1161/01.str.28.12.2370

5. **The answer is F.** An EVD is the gold standard for ICP monitoring. It consists of a fluid-coupled transducer placed in the lateral ventricle, with the tip ideally located in the foramen of Monro. Placement allows for continuous ICP monitoring and intermittent drainage of cerebrospinal fluid (CSF) for ICP control. Potential complications include catheter tract hemorrhage, infection, or injury to eloquent brain tissue. The catheter should be calibrated or zeroed at the level of the foramen of Monro (external tragus of the ear). Contraindications include collapsed ventricles acute injury along trajectory tract, or ongoing coagulopathy. Determination of lateralization of placement (right vs. left) should consider the side of least intraventricular burden to minimize EVD failure due to clotting, cortical dominance, and prior structural encephalomalacia.

Lang EW, Chesnut RM. Intracranial pressure: monitoring and management. *Neurosurg Clin North Am.* 1994;5:573-605. doi:10.1016/S1042-3680(18)30488-1

6. **The answer is E.** Vasogenic edema is defined as excess fluid within the interstitial space and can be readily identified by the preservation of gray–white junction on neuroimaging. Common causes include malignant brain tumors, abscesses, meningitis, and contusions, with the mechanism believed to be disruption of blood–brain barrier perivascular tight junctions leading to the movement of water from the vascular space to the interstitium. Dexamethasone will rapidly decrease vasogenic edema, but will have minimal or no effect on cytotoxic edema. Osmolar therapy with mannitol or hypertonic saline has never been shown to alter outcomes for vasogenic edema. Hyperthermia is considered an independent risk factor for worse neurological outcomes and should be managed by antipyretics, or if necessary surface or intravascular cooling.

Lang EW, Chesnut RM. Intracranial pressure: monitoring and management. *Neurosurg Clin N Am.* 1994;5(4):573-605. doi:10.1016/S1042-3680(18)30488-1

7. **The answer is C.** Decreased carbon dioxide tension is a potent vasoconstricting trigger to the cerebral arteries. A decrease in CO_2 tension by 10 mmHg can produce sufficient reduction in cerebral blood volume (CBV) to significantly reduce intracranial pressure (ICP). Hyperventilation reduces ICP by reflex cerebral vasoconstriction secondary to cerebrospinal fluid (CSF) alkalosis. Unfortunately, it may produce sufficient decrease in CBV to induce ischemia. A $PaCO_2$ less than 28 mmHg may provoke or worsen cerebral ischemia. In patients with ICP crisis, a target $PaCO_2$ of 28 to 32 mmHg can be utilized with the effect of hyperventilation starting within 10 minutes and lasting as long as 4 to 8 hours. Hyperventilation should generally not be used prophylactically, and most patients should be maintained at a target $PaCO_2$ of 35 mmHg.

Lang EW, Chesnut RM. Intracranial pressure: monitoring and management. *Neurosurg Clin N Am.* 1994;5(4):573-605. doi:10.1016/S1042-3680(18)30488-1

Stringer WA, Hasso AN, Thompson JR, et al. Hyperventilation-induced cerebral ischemia in patients with acute brain lesions: demonstration by xenon-enhanced CT. *Am J Neuroradiol.* 1993;14(2):475-484.

8. **The answer is C.** Prolonged hyperventilation (>4 hours) can lead to rebound intracranial hypertension due to cerebrospinal fluid (CSF) buffering. Hypocarbia, once induced, should be slowly weaned over 6 to 24 hours to minimize the rebound hyperemia of reequilibration. Maintenance of deliberate respiratory alkalosis for a sustained time can worsen the outcomes in head-injury patients.

Frank JL. Management of intracranial hypertension. *Med Clin North Am.* 1993;77:61-76. doi: 10.1016/S0025-7125(16)30272-3

Muizelaar JP, Marmarou A, Ward JD, et al. Adverse effects of prolonged hyperventilation in patients with severe head injury: a randomized clinical trial. *J Neurosurg.* 1991;75(5):731-739. doi: 10.3171/jns.1991.75.5.0731

9. **The answer is E.** First described by Lundberg, plateau waves, also known as Lundberg A waves, are considered essentially pathognomonic of intracranial hypertension. A waves are 5- to 20-minutes long, high-amplitude (50–100 mmHg) increases in ICP, and are indicative of decreased intracranial compliance. The danger of plateau waves is the abolishment of cerebral perfusion pressure; waves of sufficient severity and duration to produce global cerebral ischemia must be reversed. B and C waves are of less clinical significance. B waves last 1 to 2 minutes, are of 20 to 50 mmHg in amplitude, and do not necessarily represent any pathological disturbance. C waves last 4 to 5 minutes, are less than 20 mmHg in amplitude, and have no pathological consequence.

Lundberg N. Continuous recording and control of ventricular fluid pressure in neurosurgical practice. *Acta Psychiatr Scand Suppl.* 1960;36(149):1-19.

10. **The answer is A.** Acute hydrocephalus can be seen on neuroimaging, in particular on CT imaging, with dilated lateral ventricles, bowing or enlargement of the third ventricle, and a dilated fourth ventricle (communicating hydrocephalus) or nondilated fourth ventricle suggesting noncommunicating hydrocephalus. MRI findings can show increased T2 intensity in the periventricular area, revealing transependymal cerebrospinal fluid (CSF) flow. Compression of the quadrigeminal plate can result in Parinaud's syndrome (vertical gaze palsy). Hydrocephalus is also associated with abducens nerve deficits, which can be a false localizing sign. Any process (brain tumor, hydrocephalus, pseudotumor cerebri, edema) that exerts downward pressure on the brainstem can stretch the nerve along the clivus, causing indirect damage to the sixth nerve. Early clinical signs of acute worsening hydrocephalus include deterioration of sensorium and upgaze palsy.

11. **The answer is E.** Substantive dysfunction of one of three areas of the brain can be sufficient to cause coma: the reticular activating system (RAS), bilateral frontal lobes, and bilateral temporal lobes (see CT scans on the following page). Injury to the basal or ventral pons might cause a locked-in syndrome, but would spare the RAS. Bilateral injury to the parietal and

occipital lobes is much less likely to cause severe impairment of consciousness compared to the temporal and frontal lobes where smaller incremental increases in stroke or intracerebral hemorrhage (ICH) volume can lead to more clinical deterioration than lobar injury.

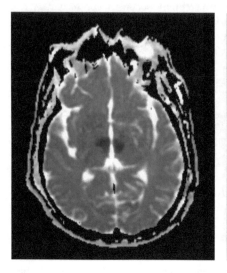 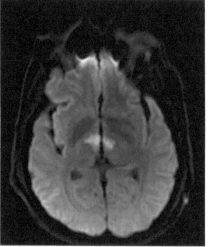

Bilateral thalamic infarctions seen after embolism to the artery of Percheron can affect the reticular activating system (RAS) and result in a comatose state.

12. **The answer is C.** Although it has been documented that fever is associated with poorer outcomes in patients with cerebral infarction, spinal cord injury, subarachnoid hemorrhage (SAH), and TBI, no studies have determined the utility of therapeutic hypothermia in these conditions. Several studies have shown a clear benefit from TH (32°C–34°C) in the first 24 hours after cardiac arrest. The neuroprotective effects of TH were most pronounced when treatment was started early, and conversely the benefits waned as treatment was delayed. The role of hypothermia in head injury is less clear. Large multicenter trials, the National Acute Brain Injury Study: Hypothermia (NABISH) I and II, appear to confirm smaller studies that induced hypothermia after severe head injury does not improve long-term outcome.

Hypothermia After Cardiac Arrest Study Group. Mild therapeutic hypothermia to improve the neurological outcome after cardiac arrest. *N Eng J Med.* 2002;346:557-563. doi:10.1056/NEJMoa012689

13. **The answer is A.** A major challenge during the induction phase is the occurrence of shivering, which produces heat, increases oxygen consumption, and prevents/slows cooling to target temperature. Combination of meperidine/buspirone, dexmedetomidine, and paralytics may control shivering. One of the most effective pharmacologic therapies to combat shivering is meperidine, which in combination with buspirone has been shown to lower the shivering threshold to 33.4°C—two degrees below normal and significantly lower than either drug alone. It has specific antishivering properties resulting from kappa-receptor activity. Meperidine should be used with caution, however, as it may depress the sensorium and complicate patient monitoring. Meperidine may also lower the seizure threshold, particularly in patients with renal dysfunction. Although the optimal rewarming rate is unknown, current consensus suggests a rewarming rate of 0.25°C to 0.5°C/hr; rapid rewarming should be avoided because of a higher incidence of electrolyte abnormalities and cardiac arrhythmias.

Mokhtarani M, Mahgoub AN, Morioka N, et al. Buspirone and meperidine synergistically reduce the shivering threshold. *Anesth Analg.* 2001;93(5):1233-1239. doi:10.1097/00000539-200111000-00038

14. **The answer is E.** Several potential complications of hypothermia must be guarded against if any therapeutic utility is to be realized. A rebound increase in ICP may occur with rewarming after hypothermia and can worsen herniation syndromes. Risk of this complication may be reduced by a slower-controlled warming phase. The other options are risks of hypothermia itself and are more commonly seen at deeper levels of hypothermia.

15. **The answer is B.** Clinical and radiologic predictors of fatal brain edema as a complication of ischemic stroke include high NIH Stroke Scale score, early nausea and vomiting, 12-hour systolic BP greater than or equal to 180 mmHg, early hypodensity of greater than 50% of the middle cerebral artery (MCA) territory on CT scan, diffusion lesion volume greater than 82 mL within 6 hours of stroke onset, involvement of additional vascular territories, elevated white blood cell (WBC) count, and a history of hypertension or heart failure. Caudate involvement in large territory MCA strokes can help predict progression to malignant MCA syndrome.

Thomalla G, Hartmann F, Juettler E, et al. Prediction of malignant middle cerebral artery infarction by magnetic resonance imaging within 6 hours of symptom onset: a prospective multicenter onservational study. *Ann Neurol.* 2010;68:435-445. doi:10.1002/ana.22125

16. **The answer is E.** A study group of the Quality Standards Subcommittee of the American Academy of Neurology reviewed the literature and reported in 2006 that tests such as CT and MRI scans, EEG, and duration of CPR had insufficient evidence for predictive discrimination of outcome after cardiac arrest. Two tests were found to be predictive of outcome: a blood test for neuron-specific enolase and the median nerve somatosensory evoked potentials (SSEP) study. However, in the posthypothermia era the prediction of outcome is more complicated. While absence of pupillary reflexes, corneal reflexes, and extensor or absent motor response at 3 days remained an accurate predictor of poor outcome in patients treated with hypothermia, a higher false positive rate was seen with neuron-specific enolase (NSE) greater than 33 ng/mL.

Fugate FE, Wijdicks EF, Mandrekar J, et al. Predictors of neurologic outcome in hypothermia after cardiac arrest. *Ann Neurol.* 2010;68(6):907-914. doi:10.1002/ana.22133

Wijdicks EF, Hijdra A, Young GB, et al. Practice parameter: prediction of outcome in comatose survivors after cardiopulmonary resuscitation (an evidence-based review): report of the Quality Standards Subcommittee of the American Academy of Neurology. *Neurology.* 2006;67(2):203-210. doi:10.1212/01.wnl.0000227183.21314.cd

17. **The answer is B.** There is evidence from several randomized clinical trials that induced hypothermia with a target temperature of 32°C to 34°C for 24 hours improves neurologic outcome in patients who are unconscious after successful resuscitation from ventricular fibrillation–associated cardiac arrest. Profound hypothermia has been shown to cause coagulopathy, suppression of cortical function, hypotension, cardiac dysrhythmia, and immunosuppression. The risk of these adverse effects is lower in therapeutic temperature ranges. Autoimmunity and renal and hepatic dysfunction are not associated with hypothermia.

Poldermna KH. Hypothermia and coagulation. *Crit Care.* 2012;16(suppl 2):A20. doi:10.1186/cc11278

Rohrer MJ, Natale AM. Effect of hypothermia on the coagulation cascade. *Crit Care Med.* 1992;20(10):1402-1405. doi:10.1097/00003246-199210000-00007

18. **The answer is C.** This patient's clinical deterioration is likely caused by progressive hydrocephalus from obstruction of the ventricular system. The next step in management would be the placement of an EVD. Osmotic therapy would not produce a meaningful or lasting reduction in intracranial pressure (ICP). Unless the patient is febrile, lowering his body temperature is unlikely to improve clinical outcome. The patient's systolic BP is within target range and further reduction is unlikely to be beneficial.

Frank JI. Management of intracranial hypertension. *Med Clin North Am.* 1993;77(1):61-76. doi:10.1016/S0025-7125(16)30272-3

Zakaria A, Aisiku I. Management of acute intracranial hypertension. In: Farey D, Flaxman A, Chiu W, eds. *Critical Care Emergency Medicine.* 2nd ed. New York, NY: McGraw Hill; 2017:chap 32.

19. **The answer is B.** NINDS guidelines for management of BP after treatment of acute ischemic stroke with (tPA) recommend monitoring BP every 15 minutes during and for 2 hours after treatment, then every 30 minutes for 6 hours, and then every hour for 18 hours. Strict parameters are recommended for BP prior to administration of rt-PA. Systolic BP should be controlled less than 180 and diastolic less than 105 during and prior to administration with intravenous (IV) labetalol PRN or nicardipine infusion. Monitor BP every 15 minutes during the antihypertensive therapy.

Powers WJ, Rabinstein AA, Ackerson T, et al. Guidelines for the early management of patients with acute ischemic stroke: a guideline for healthcare professionals from the American Heart Association/American Stroke Association. *Stroke.* 2018;49:e46-e110. doi:10.1161/STR.0000000000000158

20. **The answer is A.** Dominant theta–delta activity without detectable normal alpha activity (absence of malignant features) offers the possibility of good recovery. In one review (Scollo-Lavizzari & Bassetti, 1987), 27% of patients with this EEG pattern experienced a full neurological recovery after resuscitation from cardiac arrest. All the other choices can be categorized as malignant EEG patterns which are associated with worse outcomes after anoxic injury.

Scollo-Lavizzari G, Bassetti C. Prognostic value of EEG in post-anoxic coma after cardiac arrest. *Eur Neurol.* 1987;26(3):161-170. doi: 10.1159/000116329
Westhall E, Rossetti AO, van Rootselaar AF, et al. Standardized EEG interpretation accurately predicts prognosis after cardiac arrest. *Neurology.* 2016;86(16):1482-1490. doi:10.1212/WNL.0000000000002462

21. **The answer is E.** A variety of antihypertensives can be safely used to lower the BP in patients with intracranial hemorrhage (ICH). Nitroprusside is a nitric oxide donor, a potent vasodilator, and an inhibitor of circulating platelets, thereby reducing both preload and afterload. It is not often the antihypertensive of choice because of its potent venodilatory effects and risk of ICP elevation. Alternative agents include beta-blockers, nicardipine, and fast-acting angiotensin-converting enzyme inhibitors.

Marrietta M, Pedrazzi P, Girardis M, et al. Intracerebral hemorrhage: an often neglected medical emergency. *Intern Emerg Med.* 2007;2(1):38-45. doi:10.1007/s11739-007-0009-y

22. **The answer is E.** TM is a heterogeneous focal inflammatory disorder of the spinal cord characterized by acute or subacute development of motor weakness, sensory impairment, and autonomic dysfunction. Inflammation of the spinal cord (e.g., cerebrospinal fluid [CSF] pleocytosis, elevated IgG index, or an enhancing spinal cord lesion on MRI) is highly suggestive of TM. Most patients with idiopathic TM have some degree of weakness, either symmetric or asymmetric. Asymmetric cases are likely to be diagnosed with multiple sclerosis (MS). Neurological function usually worsens progressively over the course of 4 to 21 days, with the vast majority of cases reaching their clinical nadir within 2 weeks. Progression to nadir within 4 hours of symptom onset is one of the exclusion criteria for idiopathic or postinfectious TM.

Brinar VV, Habek M, Brinar M, et al. The differential diagnosis of acute transverse myelitis. *Clin Neurol Neurosurg.* 2006;108(3):278-283. doi:10.1016/j.clineuro.2005.11.008

23. **The answer is C.** Contrast extravasations seen on initial CT imaging are associated with the presence of hematoma progression. In the setting of anticoagulation use, the risk of intracranial hemorrhage (ICH) increases by five- to 10-fold and carries a poor prognosis. High-dose intravenous (IV) vitamin K can reverse warfarin-induced anticoagulation, but may take up to 12 to 24 hours to take effect. FFP is well accepted in the effort to reverse the coagulopathy but newer prothrombin concentrates including 3- or 4-factor prothrombin complex concentrate (PCC) and activated PCC (factor eight inhibitor bypassing activity [FEIBA]) have been shown to rapidly and reliably reverse vitamin K coagulopathy more rapidly than FFP, with

less intravascular volume loading. Such agents should be used in conjunction with vitamin K especially in liver-competent patients, to maintain correction of drug-induced coagulopathy after the acute phase. In contrast to these products, Factor VII replaces only one of the vitamin K–dependent coagulants and has not been shown to improve the outcomes (focused assessment with sonography for trauma [FAST] trial) in ICH patients.

Fredriksson K, Norrving B, Strömblad LG. Emergency reversal of anticoagulation after intracerebral hemorrhage. *Stroke*. 1992;23(7):972-977. doi:10.1161/01.str.23.7.972

Hanger HC, Geddes JA, Wilkinson, et al. Warfarin-related intracerebral haemorrhage: better outcomes when reversal includes prothrombin complex concentrates. *Intern Med J*. March 2013;43(3):308-316. doi:10.1111/imj.12034

Joseph B, Pandit V, Khalil M, et al. Use of prothrombin complex concentrate as an adjunct to fresh frozen plasma shortens time to craniotomy in traumatic brain injury patients. *Neurosurgery*. May 2015;76(5):601-607. doi:10.1227/NEU.0000000000000685

Mayer SA, Brun NC, Begtrup K, et al. Efficacy and safety of recombinant activated factor VII for acute intracerebral hemorrhage. *N Engl J Med*. 2008;358:2127-2137. doi:10.1056/NEJMoa0707534

Wintzen AR, de Jonge H, Loeliger EA, et al. The risk of intracerebral hemorrhage during oral anticoagulant treatment: a population study. *Ann Neurol*. 1984;16(5):553-558. doi: 10.1002/ana.410160505

24. **The answer is D.** Coma implies a profound disturbance in consciousness that affects both the reticular activating system (RAS) and the cerebral hemispheres. Patients in a coma have a disturbance in their sleep–wake cycle and exhibit no meaningful interaction with the environment. Minimally conscious state refers to impairment of consciousness but with discernible evidence of some level of awareness to self or environment. The hallmark of the vegetative state is a lack of evidence of interaction with the physical environment, but the patient has retained sleep–wake cycles mediated through the RAS. Behaviors commonly seen in the vegetative states include roving eye movements, purposeless smiles, and occasional verbalizations. The vegetative state is deemed *persistent* when it exceeds 1 month in duration. There is potential for recovery from the PVS, especially in cases of trauma. After 12 months post-traumatic injury and 3-month post-nontraumatic injury, the chance of recovery is exceedingly low (PVS).

Multi-Society Task Force on PVS. Medical aspects of the persistent vegetative state. *N Engl J Med*. 1994;330:1572-1578. doi:10.1056/NEJM199405263302107

25. **The answer is A.** The National Institute of Neurological Disorders and Stroke (NINDS) recommends administration of IV tPA within 60 minutes from arrival to hospital to patients who are eligible according to current American Heart Association criteria. The patient has not been taking anticoagulants or received heparin in the previous 48 hours, has no clinical or CT evidence of bleeding, and has no previous conditions that may predispose to bleeding. Therefore, tPA can be administered even before results of the prothrombin time (PT) and activated partial thromboplastin times (aPTTs) are available. Although the patient or family members should understand the potential risks and benefits of IV tPA treatment, informed consent is not required since tPA is considered the standard of care.

Powers WJ, Rabinstein AA, Ackerson T, et al. Guidelines for the early management of patients with acute ischemic stroke: a guideline for healthcare professionals from the American Heart Association/American Stroke Association. *Stroke*. 2018;49:e46-e110. doi: 10.1161/STR.0000000000000158

26. **The answer is D.** Myoclonus is the most common type of convulsive activity after cardiac arrest and usually suggests a poor prognosis. It is not clear whether this represents true seizure activity or random firing of uninhibited cortical neurons. BP is the most common EEG pattern associated with generalized myoclonus after cardiac arrest.

Wijdicks EF, Parisi JE, Sharbrough FW. Prognostic value of myoclonus status in comatose survivors of cardiac arrest. *Ann Neurol*. 1994;35:239-243. doi:10.1002/ana.410350219

27. **The answer is G.** The Multi-Society Task Force on persistent vegetative state (PVS) concluded that a patient diagnosed with a vegetative state 1 year after a traumatic brain injury (TBI) or 3 months after anoxic brain injury is very unlikely to improve. All of the options are indicators of poor outcome after cardiopulmonary resuscitation.

Levy DE, Caronna JJ, Singer BH, et al. Predicting outcome from hypoxic-ischemic coma. *JAMA*. 1985;253(10):1420-1426. doi:10.1001/jama.1985.03350340072020
Multi-Society Task Force on PVS. Medical aspects of the persistent vegetative state. *N Engl J Med*. 1994;330:1572 1578. doi:10.1056/NEJM199405263302107

28. **The answer is A.** Lap belt injuries are associated with thoracolumbar flexion distraction injuries. Multiple-level injuries occur in as high as 20% of cases. The sympathetic nervous system exits the spinal cord from the thoracolumbar segment. Injury to the thoracolumbar segment may cause loss of supraspinal regulatory control and reduced sympathetic activity. The sympathetic nervous system is compromised, and the parasympathetic nervous system dominates, causing massive vasodilation or neurogenic shock. This risk of hypotension and bradycardia is greatest soon after injury.

Teasell RW, Arnold JM, Krassioukov A, et al. Cardiovascular consequences of loss of supraspinal control of the sympathetic nervous system after spinal cord injury. *Arch Phys Med Rehabil*. 2000;81(4):506-516. doi:10.1053/mr.2000.3848

29. **The answer is E.** The presence of a region of clearly delineated hypodensity with associated mass effect is indicative of established infarction and inconsistent with an acute ischemic insult within 3 hours as established by National Institute of Neurological Disorders and Stroke (NINDS) criteria.

Demaerschalk BM, Kleindorfer DO, Adeoye OM, et al. Scientific rationale for the inclusion and exclusion criteria for intravenous alteplase in acute ischemic stroke. stroke. 2016;47:581-641. doi:10.1161/STR.0000000000000086

30. **The answer is E.** The spinal cord is perfused by two posterior spinal arteries, which supply the posterior one-third of the cord, and the single anterior spinal artery, which supplies the anterior two-thirds of the cord. The artery of Adamkiewicz typically arises between T8 and L4 and is a significant anterior spinal artery feeder. The middle and lower thoracic cord and central gray matter of the cord are particularly vulnerable to watershed injuries. A sensory level at T10 and his abnormal reflexes suggest a lesion extending to L4 but sparing the lower segments. This can produce a spastic bladder with detrusor–sphincter dyssynergia.

Blumenfeld H. *Neuroanatomy Through Clinical Cases*. Sunderland, MA: Sinauer Associates; 2010.

31. **The answer is D.** Anticoagulant reversal in intracerebral hemorrhage (ICH) is emergent and should be initiated once CT imaging demonstrates acute intracranial hemorrhage. Warfarin inhibits vitamin K–dependent Y-carboxylation of coagulation factors II, VII, IX, and X, has a half-life of 20 to 60 hours, and is not dialyzable. FFP has historically been the mainstay of warfarin reversal but has been more recently replaced by prothrombin complex concentrates (PCC, factor eight inhibitor bypassing activity [FEIBA], Kcentra). Vitamin K administration alone is insufficient for reversal in the first hours. Praxbind (idarucizumab) is a specific neutralizing monoclonal antibody fragment for the reversal of dabigatran. A one-time dose of desmopressin 0.4 mcg/kg has been shown to increase platelet membrane glycoprotein expression, promoting platelet adhesion in cases of dysfunction or antiplatelet exposure.

32. **The answer is C.** The patient has clear imaging signs of obstructive hydrocephalus. Effacement of basilar and prepontine cisterns is concerning for eventual progression to downward (central) brain herniation, necessitating CSF diversion through emergent placement of an EVD. Steroids have no role in the management of intracerebral hemorrhage (ICH) or intraventricular hemorrhage (IVH). There is limited data for the use of factor VII in reduction of ICH expansion. Seizure medications are indicated in this case but the hydrocephalus is life threatening and needs to be addressed emergently.

Hemphill JC, Greenberg SM, Anderson CS, et al. Guidelines for the management of spontaneous intracerebral hemorrhage: a guideline for healthcare professionals from American Heart Association. *Stroke.* July 2015;46(7):2032-2060. doi:10.1161/STR.0000000000000069

33. **The answer is C.** The patient is likely in status epilepticus (SE), defined as 5 minutes of continuous clinical or electrographic seizures or recurrent seizures without recovery in between. The algorithm for SE management includes initial benzodiazepine administration followed by antiepileptic medications (phenytoin, valproate, or levetiracetam). Additional lorazepam is incorrect as the patient already received the recommended lorazepam dose. If the patient remains in SE, he should be started on propofol or midazolam infusions and continuous EEG (cEEG) monitoring initiated. MRI imaging is unlikely to provide additional clinical benefit at this time given the known encephalomalacia on CT imaging, which is likely the ictal focus in this sleep-deprived patient.

Brophy GM, Bell R, Claassen J, et al. Guidelines for the evaluation and management of status epilepticus. *Neurocrit Care.* August 2012;17(1):3-23. doi:10.1007/s12028-012-9695-z

34. **The answer is B.** Anterior spinal cord syndrome occurs due to loss of blood supply to the anterior spinal artery, which supplies the anterior two-thirds of the spinal cord, typically due to a thrombotic or embolic event. Ischemia of the corticospinal, spinothalamic, and corticobulbar tracts results in motor paralysis and loss of pain and temperature sensation below the lesion or injury level.

Foo D, Rossier AB. Anterior spinal artery syndrome and its natural history. *Paraplegia.* February 1983;21(1):1-10. doi:10.1038/sc.1983.1

35. **The answer is C.** The patient has refractory ICP with poor CPP. With the option of cranial decompression removed, the next best step would be to reduce cerebral metabolic demand in an attempt to reduce metabolic stress. Mannitol loses its effectiveness and carries additional risk of acute tubular necrosis at high serum osmolality. Addition of pentobarbital for sedation is not indicated as the patient is already burst suppressed on cEEG. Hypothermia has been shown to be effective in reducing cerebral metabolic demand and ICPs, although no clear improvement in functional outcomes has been identified. Steroids have no role in traumatic brain injury and steroid-induced hyperglycemia is likely harmful.

Clifton GL, Valadka A, Zygun D, et al. Very early hypothermia induction in patients with severe brain injury (the National Acute Brain Injury Study: Hypothermia II): a randomised trial. *Lancet Neurol.* 2011;10(2):131. doi:10.1016/S1474-4422(10)70300-8

Perioperative Neurosurgical Care

BRETT SIMPSON, YOSHUA ESQUENAZI, AND
NITIN TANDON

QUESTIONS

1. A 56-year-old woman with a medical history of diabetes presented to the ED after the acute onset of headache, nausea, and vomiting. On physical examination, she was somnolent, opened her eyes to commands, and was oriented only to herself. The accompanying CT scan of the head was obtained, and an emergent external ventriculostomy was placed. The patient was then taken immediately to the endovascular suite, and a cerebral angiogram showed a small right posterior communicating aneurysm. The patient underwent a successful balloon-assisted coil embolization and was transferred to the ICU. Which of the following measures are recommendations for the prevention of delayed cerebral ischemia (DCI) secondary to vasospasm?

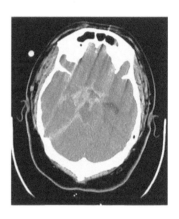

   A. Hypervolemic hemodynamic augmentation
   B. Euvolemia
   C. Hypothermia
   D. Prophylactic balloon angioplasty on postbleed day 7
   E. Prophylactic intra-arterial vasodilator therapy on postbleed day 7

2. A 72-year-old woman with a medical history of atrial fibrillation and congestive heart failure was admitted to the hospital for an elective three-level anterior cervical discectomy and fusion (ACDF) due to progressive spondylotic cervical myelopathy. She had stopped her warfarin 5 days before surgical intervention and had normal coagulation studies before the procedure. The intraoperative course was uncomplicated, and the patient was transferred from the operating room to the recovery area, and subsequently to the ICU for observation. Seven hours after the procedure, you receive a call from the nurse telling you that for the past 1 hour, the patient has been complaining of neck discomfort and has recently developed stridor. On physical examination, the patient has significant swelling in the anterior aspect of the neck, has stridor, and is marginally hypoxic. What is the next step in the management of this patient?

   A. Intravenous (IV) dexamethasone and diphenhydramine
   B. Chest x-ray, intravenous furosemide, and nonrebreather oxygen face mask
   C. ECG, CT scan of the chest, and IV heparin
   D. Emergent bedside surgical intervention
   E. Reassurance and high-dose nonsteroidal anti-inflammatory agents

3. Which of the following is the most common complication from an anterior cervical discectomy and fusion (ACDF)?

   A. Postoperative hematoma
   B. Wound infection
   C. Recurrent laryngeal nerve palsy
   D. Esophageal perforation
   E. Dysphagia

4. A 55-year-old right-handed man with a medical history of atrial fibrillation is brought to the ED after the acute onset of headache, vomiting, and left hemiparesis. CT scan of the head shows a 30-cc^3 intracerebral hemorrhage (ICH) in the right basal ganglia, with extension into the ventricular system and mild hydrocephalus. On physical examination, he is somnolent but arousable to pain. Further history reveals that 2 months ago, the patient was switched from warfarin to dabigatran etexilate (Pradaxa) for stroke prevention because of his atrial fibrillation. The following laboratory values were obtained: International Normalized Ratio (INR) = 1.32; prothrombin time (PT) = 1.13; partial thromboplastin time (PTT) = 90.2. Which of the following is the best next step to address this patient's coagulopathy?

   A. Emergent hemodialysis
   B. Vitamin K 10 mg administered intravenously (IV) along with fresh frozen plasma (FFP)—15 mL/kg administered stat
   C. Platelet transfusion—10 mL/kg
   D. Recombinant factor VIIa (rFVIIa) 80 mcg/kg
   E. Emergent administration of the monoclonal antibody idarucizumab

5. All of the following are risk factors for the development of an infection related to external ventricular drainage (EVD) **except**:

   A. Presence of intraventricular hemorrhage (IVH)
   B. Duration of the EVD placement beyond 4 days
   C. Routine daily cerebrospinal fluid (CSF) sampling
   D. Manipulation of the catheter to relieve clogging or improve flow
   E. Steroid use

6. A 31-year-old right-handed man with a previous gunshot wound to the head 2 years ago and medically refractory seizures since then was admitted electively to the hospital as part of a phase II epilepsy surgery evaluation for left-sided platinum–iridium subdural grid placement and video EEG monitoring. The intraoperative course was uncomplicated, and the patient was transferred from the operating room to the recovery area, and subsequently to the ICU, where he was doing well. Seven hours after the procedure, the patient complains of worsening headaches, vomiting, and weakness in his right arm. On physical examination, the patient has a drift in his right upper extremity but is able to hold his arm up against gravity. Which of the following is the most appropriate next step in the management of this patient?

   A. Check antiepileptic levels
   B. Mannitol administration
   C. MRI of the brain without contrast
   D. CT scan of the head without contrast
   E. Thromboelastogram

7. A 68-year-old woman underwent an elective clipping of a left 9-mm unruptured posterior communicating artery aneurysm. An intraoperative angiogram showed evidence of complete aneurysm obliteration. The intraoperative course was uncomplicated, and the patient was extubated in the operating room successfully. She was then transferred to the neurosurgical ICU for observation. Ten hours after the procedure, the patient started complaining of nausea, vomiting, and headaches. On physical examination, the patient was confused as to place and time, but no focal findings were found. Baseline laboratory and coagulation studies were normal, and her blood pressure (BP) at the time of the examination was 160/90 mmHg. The accompanying CT scan of the head was obtained. What is the most likely explanation for her condition?

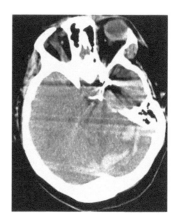

A. Aneurysm rupture due to clip misplacement
B. Hypertensive cerebellar hemorrhage
C. Remote cerebellar hemorrhage (RCH)
D. Normal postoperative CT scan
E. Contrast extravasation from diagnostic angiography

8. A 72-year-old man with a greater than 90% symptomatic right carotid artery stenosis was admitted to the hospital for an elective carotid endarterectomy (CEA). Which of the following is the correct management of this patient in the immediate postoperative period?

A. Head of bed 30 to 45 degrees, nothing by mouth (NPO), continue antiplatelet therapy, systolic blood pressure (SBP) 100 to 150 mmHg
B. Head of bed 30 to 45 degrees, regular diet, stop antiplatelet therapy, SBP 160 to 180 mmHg
C. Head of bed 30 to 45 degrees, activity as tolerated, intravenous (IV) heparin drip, SBP less than 100
D. Head of bed 15 to 30 degrees, NPO, stop antiplatelet therapy, SBP less than 100
E. Head of bed 30 to 45 degrees, regular diet, warfarin administration, SBP 100 to 150

9. A 69-year-old woman with a medical history of hypertension and diabetes was found to have a 9-mm basilar aneurysm as part of the workup for new onset of vertigo. The patient was admitted to the hospital electively and underwent a balloon-assisted coil embolization of her cerebral aneurysm. Which of the following would decrease the patient's risk of developing the most common complication of this procedure?

A. Keep systolic blood pressure (SBP) less than 140 mmHg in the immediate postoperative period
B. Intravenous (IV) heparin during the immediate postoperative course
C. Oral antiplatelet agents in the perioperative course
D. Coumadin administration in the perioperative course
E. Keep SBP greater than 140 mmHg in the immediate postoperative period

10. A 35-year-old male is admitted to the ICU following a craniotomy and interhemispheric approach to the removal of colloid cyst. The patient is neurologically intact following arrival to the unit. Overnight you are called and the patient is now having a severe headache, nausea, vomiting, and elevated systolic blood pressures (SBPs). On examination the patient is unchanged except for bilateral lateral gaze palsy. What is the most likely diagnosis?

A. Left parietal intracerebral hemorrhage (ICH)
B. Acute hydrocephalus

C. Adverse reaction to anesthetic medications
D. Damage to the mesencephalon
E. Diffuse cerebral edema

11. A 67-year-old female is admitted to ICU following right-sided craniotomy for insular glioma resection. Upon arrival to the ICU the patient's vitals are heart rate (HR) 65, blood pressure (BP) 118/80, respirations 12, oxygen saturation 99%, and temperature of 98.7°F. Overnight the patient spiked a fever to 101.5°F and white count increased from 7,000 postoperatively to 12,000. What is the next best step to management?

    A. CT of the brain
    B. Apply cooling blanket to patient
    C. Get a chest x-ray and start incentive spirometry therapy
    D. Start broad spectrum antibiotics
    E. Give a 1-L bolus of 0.9% normal saline

12. A 55-year-old female is brought to the ICU following resection of a right frontal glioma. She is neurologically intact upon arrival; however, over the next 12 hours she develops a left upper extremity drift and hemiparesis but otherwise her neurologic exam is unchanged. Stat CT of the brain is ordered which displays increase in hypodensity surrounding the tumor bed and not respecting one vascular territory. What is the best treatment for her condition at this time?

    A. MRI with T2 flair sequence to further assess the surgical cavity
    B. Initiate hyperosmolar therapy with mannitol with a goal of serum osmolarity of 500
    C. 23.4% sodium chloride bolus delivered over 30 minutes
    D. Start dexamethasone at 4 mg every 6 hours
    E. Change fluids from normal saline (NS) to D5 with ½ NS

13. A 45-year-old male comes to the ICU following left-sided superficial temporal artery to middle cerebral artery (MCA) bypass. Upon arrival, the patient is neurologically intact. Two hours after arrival, the patient develops a severe expressive aphasia and right-sided drift. What is the most likely cause of the patient's neurologic deterioration?

    A. The patient developed a right MCA occlusion
    B. The patient developed cerebral edema from brain manipulation
    C. Thrombosis of left superficial temporal artery
    D. The patient has a new right hemispheric intracerebral hemorrhage (ICH)
    E. None of the above

■ ANSWERS

1. **The answer is B.** Vasospasm of major cerebral arteries after aneurysmal subarachnoid hemorrhage (SAH) is common; it occurs most frequently 7 to 10 days after aneurysm rupture and resolves spontaneously after 21 days. DCI, associated with arterial vasospasm, remains a major cause of death and disability in patients with this condition. There is class I level evidence that oral nimodipine should be administered to all patients with aneurysmal SAH, and this agent has been shown to improve neurological outcomes, but does not prevent cerebral vasospasm. Maintenance of euvolemia and normal circulating blood volume is recommended to prevent DCI, but when this condition is diagnosed, the initial treatment is the induction of hemodynamic augmentation to improve cerebral perfusion. No randomized trials have been performed, but the quick improvement of patients with this therapy and their worsening when it is stopped prematurely are convincing proof of efficacy. Prophylactic hypervolemia or balloon angioplasty before the development of angiographic spasm is not recommended. Induction of hypertension is recommended for patients with DCI unless blood pressure is elevated at baseline or cardiac status precludes it. Cerebral angioplasty and/or selective intra-arterial vasodilator therapy is reasonable in patients with symptomatic cerebral vasospasm, particularly those who are not rapidly responding to hypertensive therapy.

   Connolly ES, Jr, Rabinstein AA, Carhuapoma JR, et al. Guidelines for the management of aneurysmal subarachnoid hemorrhage: a guideline for healthcare professionals from the American Heart Association/American Stroke Association. *Stroke.* 2012;43(6):1711-1737. doi: 10.1161/STR.0b013e3182587839

2 **and 3. The answers are D and E, respectively.** ACDF represents one of the most commonly performed spinal procedures for the management of patients with cervical radiculopathy and/or myelopathy secondary to degenerative disk disease and/or spondylosis. The clinical outcome of this procedure is good or excellent in the majority of cases. However, on rare occasions, a complication may occur, which can be catastrophic. Early identification and prompt management of these potential complications are imperative. The most commonly reported complications include postoperative dysphagia (9.5%), postoperative hematoma (5.6%), and symptomatic recurrent laryngeal nerve palsy (3.1%); other less common complications (<1%) include cerebrospinal fluid (CSF) leak, esophageal perforation, Horner syndrome, and superficial wound infections. The patient described in this vignette has the signs and symptoms of an enlarging postoperative hematoma. Postoperative hematomas from ACDF have been reported to occur in up to 5% of patients; the management of this condition can be conservative, but when there is evidence of respiratory compromise or hematoma expansion, immediate emergent surgical re-intervention should be done, including reopening the wound at bedside to decompress the upper airway, prior to efforts at endotracheal intubation.

   Fountas KN, Kapsalaki EZ, Nikolakakos LG, et al. Anterior cervical discectomy and fusion associated complications. *Spine.* 2007;32(21):2310-2317. doi:10.21037/jss.2017.08.03

4. **The answer is E.** Direct coagulation factor inhibitors, such as dabigatran, have demonstrated superior stroke and systemic embolism prevention without the burdensome monitoring and drug–drug interactions seen with agents such as warfarin. Although dabigatran has been shown to have a lower incidence of major bleeding than warfarin, in the event of catastrophic hemorrhage these events may prove to be fatal. Dabigatran etexilate (Pradaxa) is an oral anticoagulant that acts as a direct, competitive thrombin inhibitor. In 2010, the U.S. Food and Drug Administration (FDA) approved the use of dabigatran for the prevention of stroke and systemic embolism in patients with atrial fibrillation. Patients who are taking dabigatran do not require routine monitoring with PTs or INRs. As a direct thrombin (factor II) inhibitor, dabigatran exerts its mechanism of action at the very end of the coagulation cascade, and therefore neither rFVIIa nor FFP is effective as a treatment option. Because dabigatran is primarily excreted through the renal system, dialysis is an alternative for drug clearance and can remove approximately 35% to 60% of the drug in 2 to 3 hours. Until 2015, dialysis was the only and thus best reversal option for patients on this drug. In 2015, the FDA approved

the use of idarucizumab (Praxabind), a monocolonal antibody used for dabigatran reversal. Dabigatran is different from warfarin, whose inhibitory effect on clotting factors II, VII, IX, and X can be reversed by FFP, vitamin K, and factor VII.

Arbit B, Nishimura M, Hsu JC. Reversal agents for direct oral anticoagulants: a focused review. *Int J Cardiol.* 2016;223(15):244-250. doi:10.1016/j.ijcard.2016.07.304

Garber ST, Sivakumar W, Schmidt RH. Neurosurgical complications of direct thrombin inhibitors— catastrophic hemorrhage after mild traumatic brain injury in a patient receiving dabigatran. *J Neurosurg.* 2012;116(5):1093-1096. doi:10.3171/2012.2.JNS112132

5. **The answer is E.** Hydrocephalus is a common problem encountered in neurosurgical patients. EVD is frequently used in the acute treatment of these patients. The major complication of this procedure is an EVD-related infection (meningitis or ventriculitis). Manipulation, or daily sampling from the EVD, are associated with increased infection risks. Infection may lead to removal and reinsertion of a new EVD, prolonged hospital stay, treatment with antibiotics, and associated cost and morbidity. There is a well-established relationship between the duration of EVD and the occurrence of EVD-related infections that start at about 4 days after EVD insertion.

Hoefnagel D, Dammers R, Ter Laak-Poort MP, et al. Risk factors for infections related to external ventricular drainage. *Acta Neurochir (Wien).* 2008;150(3):209-214; discussion 214. doi: 10.1007/s00701-007-1458-9

6. **The answer is C.** The occurrence of a delayed and progressive neurological deficit suggests the presence of a postoperative hematoma, which can occur especially in patients with multiple prior cranial procedures. CT scan is significantly degraded by beam-hardening artifacts and is of little value in predicting the development of symptoms and possible postoperative complications after subdural grid implantation. If the electrodes are MRI compatible, an emergent MRI is the most useful adjunct to the diagnosis; clinical judgment must guide management and determine the potential need for reexploration. This complication may occur even in the presence of normal coagulation parameters and should be anticipated and managed urgently.

Mocco J, Komotar RJ, Ladouceur AK, et al. Radiographic characteristics fail to predict clinical course after subdural electrode placement. *Neurosurgery.* 2006;58(1):120-125; discussion 120. doi: 10.1227/01.NEU.0000192164.32666.77

7. **The answer is C.** Intracerebral hemorrhage (ICH) remote from the site of surgery is an infrequent complication after neurosurgical procedures. Cerebellar hemorrhage after supratentorial craniotomy is the most commonly described pattern of hemorrhage, with an incidence of 0.3% to 0.6%, and it may cause significant neurological morbidity and mortality. RCH most commonly follows supratentorial neurosurgical procedures performed with the patients in the supine position, which involve opening of cerebrospinal fluid (CSF) cisterns or the ventricular system (such as unruptured aneurysm repair or temporal lobectomy). The exact etiology remains unclear, but perioperative hypertension, coagulopathy, preoperative aspirin use, head positioning during surgery, CSF overdrainage, and postoperative epidural drainage are recognized risk factors. Although RCH can cause death or major morbidity, most cases are asymptomatic or exhibit a benign course. Cerebellar "sag," as a result of CSF hypovolemia, causing transient occlusion of superior bridging veins within the posterior fossa, and consequent hemorrhagic venous infarction, is the most likely pathophysiological cause. There is no evidence of subarachnoid hemorrhage (SAH), which may suggest aneurysm rupture; the location of the hemorrhage along the cerebellar folia corresponds to the territory drained by the superior cerebellar veins. Cerebellar hemorrhages related to hypertension are not restricted to the cerebellar folia. Contrast extravasation from the cerebral angiogram would not occur unless there is disruption of the blood–brain barrier or aneurysm rupture.

Friedman JA, Piepgras DG, Duke DA, et al. Remote cerebellar hemorrhage after supratentorial surgery. *Neurosurgery.* 2001;49(6):1327-1340. doi:10.1097/00006123-200112000-00008

Marquardt G, Setzer M, Schick U, et al. Cerebellar hemorrhage after supratentorial craniotomy. *Surg Neurol*. 2002;57(4):241-251; discussion 251. doi:10.1016/S0090-3019(02)00642-0

8. **The answer is A.** The head of the bed should be elevated 30 to 45 degrees postoperatively to diminish edema and to facilitate deep breathing. Antiplatelet therapy is continued without interruption, and the SBP should be kept below 150 mmHg and above 100 mmHg. This may require vasoactive IV medications in the first 24 hours after CEA. The patient is also kept NPO until the first postoperative morning since reexploration is occasionally necessary. Maintenance of IV fluids may be used while the patient in NPO. Hypertension is a common postoperative complication that occurs in approximately 20% of patients who have CEA. Patients who were hypertensive before the operation, especially if poorly controlled, are more likely to have severe postoperative hypertension. The incidence of neurologic deficit and death is significantly higher in these hypertensive patients, necessitating close monitoring of postoperative SBP.

Rasmussen TE, Clouse WD, Tonnessen BH. *Handbook of Patient Care in Vascular Diseases. Great Vessels and Carotid*. 5th ed. Philadelphia, PA: Lippincott Williams & Wilkins; 2008:159-195.

9. **The answer is C.** Although the overall complication rate for elective endovascular treatment of cerebral aneurysms is relatively low, thromboembolic complications remain common and account for more than half of the complications resulting from this procedure. Antiplatelet drugs (aspirin/clopidogrel) administered before and after coil embolization of cerebral aneurysms have been reported to lower the symptomatic thromboembolic complication rate. Intraprocedural anticoagulation using heparin is considered a standard protocol for preventing procedural thromboembolic risks. Oral antiplatelet preparation before stent-assisted aneurysm coiling has also been considered a standard step based on the benefits observed during coronary intervention.

Hwang G, Jung C, Park SQ, et al. Thromboembolic complications of elective coil embolization of unruptured aneurysms: the effect of oral antiplatelet preparation on periprocedural thromboembolic complication. *Neurosurgery*. 2010;67(3):743-748; discussion 748. doi:10.1227/01.NEU.0000374770.09140.FB

10. **The answer is B**. The patient has signs and symptoms of acute hydrocephalus as described by headache, nausea, and vomiting with elevated SBPs. The patient had a colloid cyst removed and acute hydrocephalus can occur in the postoperative period, typically as a result of obstruction of the foramen of Monro by postsurgical blood products. An immediate CT scan of the head should be obtained to assess the cause of the hydrocephalus and emergent external ventricular drainage (EVD) placement should be considered in cases of acute neurological deterioration. The patient does not have any neurologic deficit which makes ICH or damage to the mesencephalon unlikely. The effects of anesthesia usually do not last longer than a few hours following surgery. The signs and symptoms could also be due to diffuse cerebral edema; however, one would also expect altered sensorium.

Greenberg, MS. Colloid cysts. In *Handbook of Neurosurgery*. 7th ed. New York, NY: Thieme Medical Publishers; 2010:665-667.

11. **The answer is C**. The patient has a postoperative fever which is a common occurrence after surgery. The patient needs to have a basic workup. Initiation of antibiotics is not necessary unless a source is identified or a persistent fever exists. For this patient, the likely cause may be atelectasis which could be identified by chest x-rays. The use of incentive spirometry can prevent atelectasis.

Garibaldi RA, Brodine S, Matsumiya S, et al. Evidence for the non-infectious etiology of early postoperative fever. *Infect Control*. 1985;6:273. doi:10.1017/S0195941700061749

12. **The answer is D.** The patient is suffering from postoperative edema following surgical resection of a tumor. The treatment should be to continue steroids or even increase the dosage. There is no need for hypertonic or hyperosmolar therapy. CT demonstrating the peritumoral

edema is sufficient for diagnosis and no further imaging is required; therefore, ordering an MRI would be a costly and unnecessary test. The initiation of D5 with 1/2NS could make the swelling worse and is highly discouraged.

Weingart J, Brem H. Basic principles of cranial surgery for brain tumors. In: Winn R, ed. *Youmans Neurological Surgery*. 6th ed. Philadelphia, PA: Elsevier/Saunders; 2011:1261-1266.

13. **The answer is C.** The patient is displaying signs and symptoms of left-sided ischemic stroke; therefore, a right MCA occlusion or right cerebral hemispheric hemorrhage are incorrect choices. The patient is likely suffering from thrombosis of the bypass. It is important, following surgery, to monitor the superficial temporal artery patency using palpation or dopplers, as blockage could lead to further ischemic injury.

Yu J, Shi L, Guo Y, et al. Progress on complications of direct bypass for moyamoya disease. *Int J Med Sci*. 13(8);2016:578-587. doi:10.7150/ijms.15390

15

Pharmacology and Practical Use of Medications in Neurocritical Care

MONICA LEE, ELIZABETH FRANCO, AND TERESA A. ALLISON

■ QUESTIONS

1. When should antimicrobial therapy be initiated in patients with suspected bacterial meningitis?

   A. As soon as possible after diagnosis
   B. Within 2 hours of diagnosis
   C. Within 4 hours of diagnosis
   D. Within 8 hours of diagnosis

2. Dexamethasone has been shown to be beneficial in treating bacterial meningitis with which organism?

   A. *Neisseria meningitidis*
   B. *Haemophilus influenzae*
   C. *Streptococcus pneumoniae*
   D. *Escherichia coli*

3. What vancomycin trough level concentrations should be achieved for the treatment of bacterial meningitis?

   A. 5 to 10 mcg/mL
   B. 10 to 15 mcg/mL
   C. 15 to 20 mcg/mL
   D. 20 to 25 mcg/mL

4. Why is rifampin recommended for combination therapy only?

   A. Resistance develops when used alone
   B. Rifampin does not penetrate the cerebrospinal fluid (CSF) sufficiently to be used alone
   C. The onset of action with rifampin is delayed
   D. Rifampin's intravenous (IV) fluid activity against common meningeal pathogens is poor

5. What is the initial antimicrobial of choice for *Listeria monocytogenes*?

   A. Ceftriaxone
   B. Ampicillin
   C. Levofloxacin
   D. Trimethoprim–sulfamethoxazole

6. Warfarin is challenging to use in clinical practice for which of the following reasons?

   A. Narrow therapeutic window
   B. Variability in dosing response among individual patients
   C. Interactions with diet and medications
   D. Patient compliance
   E. All of the above

7. Which of the following coagulation factors does warfarin inhibit?

   A. II, VII, IX, and X
   B. II, VIII, IX, and X
   C. II, VIII, X, and XI
   D. II, VII, X, and XI

8. Warfarin has the ability to act as a procoagulant.

   A. True
   B. False

9. Which agent when administered concomitantly with warfarin will prolong the patient's pro-thrombin time (PT) and International Normalized Ratio (INR) response?

   A. Barbiturates
   B. Amiodarone
   C. Rifampin
   D. Carbamazepine

10. When is it not necessary to begin heparin before or at the time of warfarin initiation?

    A. Patient has chronic stable atrial fibrillation poststroke
    B. Patient has a known protein C deficiency
    C. Patient has an acute pulmonary embolism
    D. Patient has a known thrombophilic state

11. For serious and/or life-threatening bleeding, how should vitamin K be administered?

    A. Orally
    B. Subcutaneously
    C. Intravenously by a push
    D. Intravenously by slow infusion

12. What is the dose of protamine for the reversal of intravenous heparin?

    A. 1 mg of protamine neutralizes 50 units of heparin
    B. 1 mg of protamine neutralizes 75 units of heparin
    C. 1 mg of protamine neutralizes 100 units of heparin
    D. 1 mg of protamine neutralizes 125 units of heparin

13. What is the mechanism of action of dabigatran (Pradaxa®)?

    A. Vitamin K antagonist
    B. Direct thrombin inhibitor (DTI)
    C. Factor Xa inhibitor
    D. Factor IIa inhibitor

14. What is the only route of administration available for dabigatran?

    A. Intravenous
    B. Subcutaneous
    C. Oral (including nasogastric and nasojejunal tubes)
    D. Oral (excluding nasogastric and nasojejunal tubes)

15. What is the most effective method of reversing the anticoagulant effects of dabigatran?

    A. Dialysis
    B. Vitamin K
    C. Recombinant activated factor VII (rFVIIa)
    D. Idarucizumab

16. The major use(s) of benzodiazepines is/are to provide

    A. Anxiolysis
    B. Amnesia
    C. Analgesia
    D. A and B
    E. A and C

17. Advantages of benzodiazepines for neurologically injured patients include

    A. Limited effects on cerebral and systemic vascular tone
    B. Anticonvulsant effects
    C. Coupled decreases in cerebral metabolic demand for oxygen and cerebral blood flow
    D. All of the above

18. Which benzodiazepine is best for continuous-infusion short-term sedation but not long-term sedation?

    A. Alprazolam
    B. Midazolam
    C. Lorazepam
    D. Diazepam

19. Which effects of benzodiazepines does flumazenil (Romazicon®) reverse?

    A. Sedation
    B. Respiratory
    C. Sedation and respiratory
    D. None of the above

20. Chest wall muscular rigidity occurs with large intravenous (IV) bolus doses for which agent?

    A. Morphine
    B. Fentanyl
    C. Hydromorphone
    D. Meperidine

21. Potential adverse reactions to the opioid antagonist naloxone (Narcan®) include

    A. Pain
    B. Hypertension
    C. Tachyarrhythmias
    D. All of the above

22. Propofol is available as an emulsion in a phospholipid vehicle. How many kcal/mL from fat should be counted into the daily caloric provisions?

    A. 0.5
    B. 1.1
    C. 1.5
    D. 1.7

23. Which adverse effect of propofol is most concerning and should be monitored for?

    A. Infections
    B. Propofol infusion syndrome
    C. Green urine
    D. Pancreatitis

24. Sodium chloride 23.4% 30 mL intravenously (IV) over 30 minutes can be administered in place of mannitol for the management of elevated intracranial pressure (ICP). Which of the following can be used if the 23.4% concentration is not available?

    A. Sodium chloride 3% 235 mL IV over 30 minutes
    B. Sodium chloride 5% 140 mL IV over 30 minutes
    C. Sodium chloride 14.6% 48 mL IV over 30 minutes
    D. All of the above
    E. None of the above

25. BG is a 22-year-old man (weight: 150 kg, height: 5'6") who presented with headache, neck stiffness, photophobia, and vomiting. On examination, he was febrile with meningismus. Analysis of cerebrospinal fluid (CSF) showed white cells 640×10^6/L (99% lymphocytes), protein 1.6 g/L, and glucose 2.5 mmol/L. No concomitant serum sample was available to report. Polymerase chain reaction (PCR) detected herpes simplex virus-2 (HSV-2) DNA in the CSF, which is consistent with the diagnosis of herpes simplex virus meningitis. The team started him on acyclovir empirically. What is the appropriate dose for acyclovir?

    A. Acyclovir 1,500 mg intravenously (IV) every 8 hours = 10 mg/kg every 8 hours of total body weight
    B. Acyclovir 640 mg IV every 8 hours = 10 mg/kg every 8 hours of ideal body weight (IBW)
    C. Acyclovir 1,000 mg IV every 8 hours = 10 mg/kg every 8 hours of adjusted body weight
    D. Acyclovir 400 mg IV every 12 hours

26. BG was started on 1,500 mg of acyclovir every 8 hours. On day 3 of acyclovir treatment, the nurse informed you that BG's urine output decreased to 20 mL/hr. His creatinine (Cr) and blood urea nitrogen (BUN) increased to 2.5 mg/dL and 46 mg/dL, respectively. Intravenous (IV) fluids were not administered while he was treated with acyclovir. What should you do next?

    A. Acyclovir does not affect renal function. Continue with current dose and start hydrating BG
    B. Discontinue acyclovir and start treating with ganciclovir
    C. Correct the dose of acyclovir per renal function and ideal body weight (IBW), start IV fluid at 100 mL/hour, and continue treatment
    D. None of the above

27. BG's renal function improved and he was discharged home to complete his remaining medication for a total of 2 weeks. Which statement is correct?

    A. Start BG on acyclovir 1,500 mg PO every 8 hours.
    B. IV to PO conversion of acyclovir is a 1:1 ratio; therefore, start on the same dose of acyclovir.

   C. Discharge BG on IV acyclovir since no options are available.

   D. Switch to valacyclovir 1 g PO every 8 hours.

28. Which antiviral medication might require coadministration of probenecid because of the risk of nephrotoxicity?

   A. Acyclovir

   B. Valacyclovir

   C. Cidofovir

   D. Foscarnet

29. Which organism causes the most common nosocomial urinary tract infection (UTI)?

   A. *Escherichia coli*

   B. *Pseudomonas aeruginosa*

   C. *Klebsiella pneumoniae*

   D. *Enterococcus*

30. Which of the following is/are predisposing factor(s) for urinary tract infections (UTIs)?

   A. Female sex

   B. Neurologic dysfunction

   C. Urinary tract instrumentation

   D. All of the above

31. IA is an 80-year-old man who lives in a nursing home. He was transferred to the ICU because of altered mental status (AMS). His medical history includes cerebral vascular disease, hypertension, and diabetes mellitus (DM). On physical examination, he is confused and disoriented with the following vital signs: temperature 102.3°F, heart rate (HR) 110 beats/min, respiratory rate (RR) 17 breaths/min, and blood pressure (BP) 120/65 mmHg. His laboratory values are within normal limits except for increased blood urea nitrogen (BUN) 26 mg/dL, serum creatinine (Cr) 2.1 mg/dL, and white blood cell (WBC) 14,000 (71 polymorphonuclear leukocytes, 8 band neutrophils, 10 lymphocytes, and 5 monocytes). His urinalysis shows turbidity, 2+ glucose, pH 7.0, protein 100 mg/dL, 50 to 100 WBC, + nitrites, 8 red blood cells, and many bacteria and + casts. His preliminary urine culture is positive for Gram-negative rods. Which is the best empiric therapy for IA?

   A. Fluconazole 400 mg intravenously (IV) daily for 5 days

   B. Amoxicillin 500 mg IV daily every 12 hours for 5 days

   C. Gentamicin 150 mg IV every 8 hours for 5 days

   D. Cefepime 500 mg IV every 12 hours for 5 days

32. IA's urine culture is positive for *Proteus mirabilis* (>100,000 bacterial colonies/mL of urine) and is pan-susceptible except for trimethoprim–sulfamethoxazole. What is the best next step?

   A. Continue treatment with broad spectrum antibiotic

   B. Discontinue current therapy and start ceftriaxone 1 g intravenously (IV) daily

   C. Switch to gentamicin 150 mg IV every 8 hours

   D. Add gentamicin to the current regimen

33. AP is a 51-year-old man who has been hospitalized in the neuro-ICU for intracranial hemorrhage for several weeks. His medical history is significant for myocardial infarction, hypertension, and congestive heart failure (CHF). His hospital stay has been complicated by aspiration pneumonia. Today, he has been spiking high temperatures. His blood pressure (BP) is 74/45 mmHg, heart rate (HR) is 120 beats/min, oxygen saturation is down to 88%, white blood cell

(WBC) count is 21,000, and temperature is 103.3°F. A chest x-ray shows infiltrates in the right lower lobe. Which of the following therapies should be initiated next?

A. Norepinephrine 0.2 mcg/kg/min to keep mean arterial pressure (MAP) greater than 65 mmHg
B. Phenylephrine 0.5 mcg/kg/min to keep MAP greater than 65 mmHg
C. Empiric intravenous (IV) antibiotics to start now
D. Normal saline (NS) 500 mL bolus followed by further evaluation of patient's fluid status
E. C and D

34. After appropriate treatment, AP's blood pressure (BP) improved to 125/80 mmHg. His heart rate (HR) continued to rise to the 140s. The decision was made to change to a different vasopressor. He is currently on norepinephrine 0.5 mcg/kg/min to keep his mean arterial pressure (MAP) greater than 65 mmHg. Which vasopressor should you select?

A. Phenylephrine
B. Dopamine
C. Epinephrine
D. Vasopressin

35. Which of the following vasopressors does/do not affect the beta-receptor?

A. Norepinephrine
B. Epinephrine
C. Phenylephrine
D. Vasopressin
E. C and D

36. Two days later, AP became hemodynamically unstable. His urine output was diminished, and his serum creatinine (Cr) rose to 3.2 mg/dL. He was drowsy and confused during morning rounds. He was intubated, and a pulmonary artery catheter (PAC) was placed, which revealed a pulmonary capillary wedge pressure (PCWP) of 25 mmHg, cardiac index of 1.2 L/minute/m^2, and systemic vascular resistance (SVR) of 2,800 dynes/cm^{-5}. What is the next appropriate drug for AP?

A. Initiate milrinone 0.375 mcg/kg/min
B. Add vasopressin 0.03 units/min
C. Start epinephrine and discontinue previous vasopressors
D. All are appropriate options

37. Which of the following is a noncatecholamine, phosphodiesterase inhibitor, and a positive inotrope? The side effect of this drug is vasodilatation and possible arrhythmias.

A. Dopamine
B. Dobutamine
C. Sildenafil
D. Milrinone

38. Which neuromuscular blocker should be avoided in patients with neuromuscular disease (e.g., Guillain–Barré syndrome [GBS])?

A. Rocuronium
B. Vecuronium
C. Succinylcholine
D. Cisatracurium

39. Which of the following neuromuscular blockers is the drug of choice for continuous infusion in patients with severe renal or hepatic dysfunction who require paralysis?

    A. Pancuronium
    B. Rocuronium
    C. Succinylcholine
    D. Cisatracurium

40. JP is a 43-year-old woman admitted to the ICU for traumatic brain injury (TBI). Her medical history includes complex partial seizures for which she was prescribed carbamazepine. Which of the following is true about this drug?

    A. It works by blocking the T-type calcium receptors
    B. It is indicated for absence seizure
    C. It increases the clearance of some drugs and also possesses autoinduction properties
    D. None of the above

41. The advantage of fosphenytoin over phenytoin is:

    A. There are no drug interactions with fosphenytoin, but with phenytoin, there are drug interactions
    B. Higher risk of phlebitis is documented with fosphenytoin
    C. The infusion rate can be up to 150 mg of phenytoin equivalent per minute
    D. The infusion rate can be up to 50 mg of phenytoin equivalent per minute

42. Which of the following antiepileptic drugs can prolong the PR interval and can cause atrioventricular (AV) block?

    A. Lacosamide
    B. Lamotrigine
    C. Benzodiazepines
    D. Levetiracetam

43. A woman was admitted to your unit for an acute-on-chronic subdural hematoma (SDH). She was started on valproic acid (VPA) for better control of her seizure disorder from her initial SDH. This morning her white blood cell (WBC) count was 16,000 and temperature is 102.6°F. Her urine culture and urinalysis came back positive with an extended-spectrum beta-lactamase (ESBL). She was started on meropenem. What would you like to do with her VPA?

    A. Nothing, continue with current dose.
    B. Check the VPA level since meropenem can inhibit the clearance of VPA.
    C. Check the VPA level since meropenem can increase the clearance of VPA.
    D. Change meropenem to cefepime to avoid any possible drug interaction with VPA.

44. The mechanism of action of this drug is by augmenting gamma-aminobutyric acid (GABA) receptors and mediating chloride influx?

    A. Carbamazepine
    B. Diazepam
    C. Lacosamide
    D. Phenytoin

45. Which of the following drugs causes the most prolongation of the QTc interval?

    A. Ziprasidone
    B. Quetiapine

    C. Olanzapine

    D. Haloperidol

46. Among the currently available antipsychotic agents, which drug has the lowest risk for extrapyramidal symptoms (EPS)?

    A. Haloperidol

    B. Fluphenazine

    C. Quetiapine

    D. Olanzapine

47. Which of the following antipsychotic drugs causes the most weight gain with important clinical implications, as this has been linked with the development of impaired glucose tolerance, hyperlipidemia, and increased mortality?

    A. Olanzapine

    B. Ziprasidone

    C. Quetiapine

    D. Lurasidone

48. Which of the following is not a common side effect of atypical antipsychotic drugs?

    A. Renal failure

    B. Anticholinergic effect

    C. QTc prolongation

    D. Hyperprolactinemia

49. AG is a 65-year-old woman with past medical history of atrial fibrillation receiving warfarin therapy, who presented with altered mental status (AMS) and severe headache after tripping and hitting her head on her counter. Noncontrast CT scan revealed a blossoming intracranial hemorrhage. International Normalized Ratio (INR) upon admission was 2.8 and her neurological exam was rapidly declining. Which interventions would **not** be appropriate at this time?

    A. Vitamin K 10 mg intravenously (IV)

    B. Activated charcoal 50 g

    C. 4-factor prothrombin complex concentrate (PCC) (dosing based on weight and INR)

    D. Fresh frozen plasma (FFP) to 5 10 mL/kg IV

50. What would be an appropriate situation to administer idarucizumab?

    A. Low-molecular-weight heparin–associated intracranial hemorrhage or major bleeding

    B. Patient on dabigatran with no evidence of bleeding, but with prolonged prothrombin time (PT)

    C. Dabigatran-associated intracranial hemorrhage in a patient with no evidence of renal dysfunction

    D. Rivaroxaban-associated hemorrhage or major bleeding

51. Four-factor prothrombin complex concentrate (4-PCC) administration for emergent reversal of anticoagulant-associated hemorrhage is recommended for all of the following except:

    A. Vitamin K antagonist

    B. Low-molecular-weight heparin

    C. Direct factor Xa inhibitor

    D. Direct thrombin inhibitor (DTI)

52. Which of the following in **not** an antiepileptic agent that may effectively treat symptoms of myoclonic status epilepticus (MSE)?

    A. Valproic acid (VPA)
    B. Clonazepam
    C. Levetiracetam
    D. Gabapentin

53. What is the expected rise in serum potassium following succinylcholine administration?

    A. 0.0 to 0.3 mEq/L
    B. 0.5 to 1.0 mEq/L
    C. 1.5 to 2.0 mEq/L
    D. 2.5 to 3.0 mEq/L

54. Following coronary revascularization (percutaneous or surgical) in patients with atrial fibrillation and a CHADS2-VASc score of 2 or greater, with a high risk of bleeding, which antithrombotic agent may be omitted from the regimen?

    A. Aspirin
    B. Anticoagulant (warfarin or direct oral anticoagulants)
    C. P2Y12 antagonist
    D. All must be taken for secondary prevention

55. Which of the following are adverse reactions that may be experienced due to brivaracetam?

    A. Dizziness
    B. Somnolence
    C. Irritability
    D. All of the above

56. Clobazam has a Food and Drug Administration (FDA)-approved indication for which of the following conditions?

    A. Dravet syndrome
    B. Lennox–Gastaut syndrome (LGS)
    C. Benign focal epilepsies in infancy
    D. Myoclonic epilepsy of infancy

57. A patient is brought into the ED convulsing. The emergency medical service (EMS) reports that the convulsions have been taking place continuously for the past 10 minutes. You order intravenous (IV) lorazepam 0.1 mg/kg to be given immediately. Which of the following is an acceptable second agent to use?

    A. Fosphenytoin/phenytoin
    B. Valproate sodium
    C. Levetiracetam
    D. All of the above

58. Which is a proposed difference between levetiracetam and brivaracetam?

    A. Dosing frequency
    B. Mechanism of action
    C. Available drug formulations
    D. Side effect profile

59. Which of the following is true for clobazam?

    A. Maximum effects can be seen in 5 to 9 days
    B. Absorption is rapid, extensive and not affected by food
    C. Half-life elimination in adults is 36 to 42 hours
    D. All of the above

60. A 45-year-old female presents to the ED with a 2-week history of altered mental status (AMS) that has been getting progressively worse. She is unable to provide a detailed history but is otherwise alert and oriented to person and time. Upon conducting a thorough examination and gathering all past medical history, you discover that your patient was taking valproic acid (VPA) for generalized seizure disorder. You order a stat ammonia level, VPA level, and liver function tests. The lab values return as: ammonia—123 mcg/dL, VPA—94 mg/L, normal aspart aminotransferase (AST) and alanine aminotransferase (ALT). Which of the following should be done first?

    A. Nothing; the VPA level is within therapeutic range and therefore cannot be the cause of the AMS
    B. Discontinue the medication and get repeat labs every 4 hours to monitor for normalization of ammonia levels
    C. Administer lactulose until at least two soft or loose bowel movements are produced
    D. Treat the patient with L-carnitine 100 mg/kg intravenously (IV) over 30 minutes now due to the severity of the patient's symptoms

61. A patient on clopidogrel for a drug-eluting stent (DES) to the left main artery (placed 2 years ago) presents with a subarachnoid hemorrhage (SAH). Medication compliance is unknown so the team orders a VerifyNow® test. The P2Y12 Reaction Units (PRU) returns as 167. What does this mean in regards to the patient and platelet inhibition due to clopidogrel?

    A. The patient was not taking the medication
    B. There is decreased platelet reactivity
    C. There is no evidence of altered platelet reactivity
    D. The patient is resistant to clopidogrel

62. For hemodynamically unstable patients in atrial fibrillation with rapid ventricular response (RVR), which of the following medications has been shown to be superior for rate lowering effects?

    A. Diltiazem
    B. Amiodarone
    C. Metoprolol
    D. None have been proven to be superior

63. A 55-year-old male with no previous past medical history is diagnosed with intracranial large artery atherosclerosis after experiencing an acute ischemic stroke, attributable to 70% to 99% stenosis. Which of the following interventions is appropriate to initiate?

    A. Intracranial angioplasty and stenting plus risk factor modification
    B. Aspirin plus warfarin with target International Normalized Ratio (INR) of 2 to 3 with risk factor modification
    C. Dual-antiplatelet therapy with aspirin plus clopidogrel for 90 days, followed by long-term aspirin therapy and risk factor modification
    D. Aspirin plus ticagrelor and risk factor modification

64. Which of the following is **false** regarding ticagrelor and clopidogrel?

    A. Clopidogrel is a prodrug that requires hepatic activation
    B. Ticagrelor is an irreversible inhibitor of P2Y12
    C. Ticagrelor results in roughly 20% to 25% greater platelet inhibition when compared to clopidogrel
    D. Clopidogrel can be used in combination with aspirin therapy for secondary stroke prevention

65. What is the recommended systolic blood pressure (SBP) goal for secondary ischemic stroke prevention?

    A. SBP ≤130 mmHg
    B. SBP ≤140 mmHg
    C. SBP ≤150 mmHg
    D. SBP ≤160 mmHg

■ ANSWERS

1. The answer is A. There is no prospective clinical data that correlate the timing of antibiotic administration to clinical outcome in patients with bacterial meningitis. Current literature only examines the duration of symptoms prior to antibiotic administration. However, most would agree the longer the duration of symptoms in patients with bacterial meningitis, the greater the possibility of a poor outcome. Studies have shown that poor outcome is associated with greater amounts of antigen or a large number of microorganisms in cerebrospinal fluid (CSF) samples obtained prior to initiation of antibiotics, and that delayed CSF sterilization after 24 hours of antibiotic administration is a risk factor for subsequent neurological sequelae. The sensible approach is to administer antibiotic therapy as soon as possible after the diagnosis of meningitis is suspected or proven. Two retrospective studies support this thought: one study demonstrated a reduction in mortality with early administration of antibiotics, and the other showed a benefit in neurological outcome and survival in patients who received antibiotic therapy prior to the patient's level of consciousness deteriorating to less than 10 on the Glasgow Coma Scale.

> Tunkel AR, Hartman BJ, Kaplan SL, et al. Practice guidelines for the management of bacterial meningitis. *Clin Infect Dis*. 2004;39(9):1267-1284. doi:10.1086/425368

2. The answer is C. Experimental meningitis studies have demonstrated that outcome is correlated with the severity of the inflammatory response in the subarachnoid space. Steroids have been evaluated as adjunct therapy secondary to their ability to reduce this inflammation. Results from a randomized controlled trial of adjunctive steroid therapy in adults demonstrated that early treatment with dexamethasone improves outcomes. The beneficial effect was most apparent in patients with pneumococcal meningitis. These results were also observed in a systemic review of steroids in adults with acute bacterial meningitis. Treatment with steroids significantly reduced mortality (relative risk = 0.6; 95% confidence interval [CI] 0.4–0.8, p =.002) and neurological sequelae (relative risk = 0.6, 95% CI 0.4–1, p =.05), with a reduction in case fatality of 21% (p =.001) in patients with pneumococcal meningitis. The results were not statistically significant in patients with meningococcal meningitis

> van de Beek D, de Gans J, McIntyre P, et al. Steroids in adults with acute bacterial meningitis: a systematic review. *Lancet Infect Dis*. 2004;4(3):139-143. doi:10.1016/S1473-3099(04)00937-5

3. The answer is C. Based on the potential to improve cerebrospinal fluid (CSF) penetration, optimize therapeutic serum vancomycin concentrations, and improve clinical outcomes, total serum trough vancomycin concentrations of 15 to 20 mcg/mL should be maintained. There is no literature to support higher serum trough concentrations than this will improve patient outcomes.

> Tunkel AR, Hartman BJ, Kaplan SL, et al. Practice guidelines for the management of bacterial meningitis. *Clin Infect Dis*. 2004;39(9):1267-1284. doi:10.1086/425368

4. The answer is A. Rifampin is an excellent agent for the treatment of meningitis secondary to good CSF infection penetration and IV fluid activity against many meningeal pathogens. However, when used alone, resistance rapidly develops; it must be used in combination with other antibiotics.

> Tunkel AR, Hartman BJ, Kaplan SL, et al. Practice guidelines for the management of bacterial meningitis. *Clin Infect Dis*. 2004;39(9):1267-1284. doi:10.1086/425368

5. The answer is B. Ampicillin is the most commonly recommended initial antibiotic for the treatment of meningitis with *Listeria monocytogenes*. Penicillin G may also be used as initial therapy. Addition of an aminoglycoside should be considered to either agent on the basis of the patient's presentation. Owing to poor penetration of the aminoglycosides into the cerebrospinal fluid (CSF) with traditional dosing regimens, *extended* dosing regimens of 7 mg/kg based on ideal or adjusted body weight should be administered *daily*. Alternative agents include trimethoprim–sulfamethoxazole and meropenem.

> Tunkel AR, Hartman BJ, Kaplan SL, et al. Practice guidelines for the management of bacterial meningitis. *Clin Infect Dis*. 2004;39(9):1267-1284. doi:10.1086/425368

6. **The answer is E.** Warfarin is challenging to use in clinical practice for several reasons. Warfarin's therapeutic range is narrow, and it is often difficult to maintain a therapeutic international normalized ratio (INR) for multiple reasons. Patients exhibit considerable variability in dose–response because of genetic differences, concomitant disease states such as congestive heart failure, and daily factors such as the common cold and fever. In addition, warfarin is susceptible to interactions with medications and diets with variations of vitamin K. Patient compliance and missing doses will also alter the INR level and lead to inappropriate dosing changes.

> Ansell J, Hirsh J, Hylek E, et al. Pharmacology and management of the vitamin K antagonists: American College of Chest Physicians evidence-based clinical practice guidelines (8th Edition). *Chest*. 2008;133(suppl 6):S160-S198. doi:10.1378/chest.08-0670

7. **The answer is A.** The vitamin K–dependent coagulation factors are II, VII, IX, and X. These factors require gamma-carboxylation for their procoagulant activity. Administration of warfarin diminishes the amount of vitamin K available for the carboxylation process, which results in the production of undercarboxylated proteins with reduced coagulant activity. The prothrombin time (PT) responds to depletion of factors II, VII, and X at a rate proportional to their respective half-lives. During the first few days, the prolongation of PT is due to reduction of factor VII, which has a half-life of 6 hours. Subsequent effects are due to the depletion of factor X (half-life ~45 hours) and factor II (half-life ~60 hours).

> Ansell J, Hirsh J, Hylek E, et al. Pharmacology and management of the vitamin K antagonists: American College of Chest Physicians evidence-based clinical practice guidelines (8th Edition). *Chest*. 2008;133(suppl 6):S160-S198. doi:10.1378/chest.08-0670

8. **The answer is A.** Warfarin inhibits carboxylation of the regulatory anticoagulant proteins C, S, and Z. It has the ability to be a procoagulant, especially during the initiation period of therapy.

> Ansell J, Hirsh J, Hylek E, et al. Pharmacology and management of the vitamin K antagonists: American College of Chest Physicians evidence-based clinical practice guidelines (8th Edition). *Chest*. 2008;133(suppl 6):S160-S198. doi:10.1378/chest.08-0670

9. **The answer is B.** The S enantiomer of warfarin is five times more potent than the R enantiomer. Drugs that inhibit the clearance of the S enantiomer potentiate the anticoagulant effect. Amiodarone is a potent inhibitor of the metabolic clearance of both the S enantiomer and the R enantiomer, leading to extensive anticoagulation. Rifampin, carbamazepine, and barbiturates each increase hepatic clearance of warfarin, which leads to a decrease of warfarin's anticoagulation effect.

> Ansell J, Hirsh J, Hylek E, et al. Pharmacology and management of the vitamin K antagonists: American College of Chest Physicians evidence-based clinical practice guidelines (8th Edition). *Chest*. 2008(suppl 6);133:S160-S198. doi:10.1378/chest.08-0670

10. **The answer is A.** Unfractionated heparin or low-molecular-weight heparin should be initiated concurrently with warfarin when a rapid anticoagulant effect is required. Early recurrent ischemic stroke occurs in 5% of patients with atrial fibrillation during the initial 2 weeks. Often warfarin will be initiated 2 to 3 days after a stroke to allow for full anticoagulation to occur by day 7 to day 10 and to avoid the period when hemorrhagic transformation is most likely to occur.

> Hart RG, Palacio S, Pearce LA. Atrial fibrillation, stroke, and acute antithrombotic therapy: analysis of randomized clinical trials. *Stroke*. 2002;33:2722-2727. doi:10.1161/01.str.0000035735.49388.4a

11. **The answer is D.** The most concerning adverse effect of vitamin K infusions is anaphylaxis. It is recommended that it be administered orally in patients who are not currently bleeding or at significant risk for bleeding. Oral administration has been shown to more effectively and rapidly reduce the international normalized ratio (INR) than subcutaneous vitamin K

in patients with warfarin-associated coagulopathy. Absorption of subcutaneous vitamin K is often unpredictable and delayed. Anaphylactoid reactions have been reported with other routes of administration; however, they are more prevalent when administered intravenously (IV). The exact mechanism is unknown; however, many believe it to be the dispersants used in the various preparations. One such dispersant, polyethoxylated castor oil (Cremophor EL), which has been used in several agents, was removed from the market because of an alarmingly high rate of anaphylactoid reactions. Intravenous vitamin K should be administered only when a patient is actively bleeding or at a significant risk for bleeding. There is no evidence that lower doses or slower infusion times will reduce the risk of anaphylactoid reactions. However, it is recommended to infuse it no faster than 1 mg/min, while many clinicians will infuse 10 mg over 30 minutes.

Ansell J, Hirsh J, Hylek E, et al. Pharmacology and management of the vitamin K antagonists: American College of Chest Physicians evidence-based clinical practice guidelines (8th Edition). *Chest*. 2008(suppl 6);133:S160-S198. doi:10.1378/chest.08-0670

12. **The answer is C.** The protamine dose is determined by the dose of heparin that was administered and the duration of time since the heparin infusion was discontinued secondary to rapid decreases in heparin serum concentrations. Protamine 1 to 1.5 mg neutralizes approximately 100 units of unfractionated heparin immediately after discontinuation of the infusion. However, if 30 to 60 minutes has elapsed since discontinuation of heparin, the dose will be 0.5 to 0.75 mg for every 100 units of heparin administered. If the time is 2 hours or greater, the protamine dose is 0.25 to 0.375 mg for every 100 units. The dosing is somewhat different for subcutaneous heparin and low-molecular-weight heparin. Following subcutaneous heparin administration, use the same 1 to 1.5 mg protamine for every 100 units of heparin; however, infuse 20 to 25 mg slowly, followed by the remainder of the dose over 8 to 16 hours. The antifactor Xa activity of enoxaparin is neutralized by only 60% to 75%. One milligram of protamine should be administered for each milligram of enoxaparin received. If the partial thromboplastin time (PTT) is prolonged 2 to 4 hours after the first dose, consider giving an additional dose of protamine at 0.5 mg for each milligram of enoxaparin (one-half of the first dose).

Lacy CF, Armstrong LL, Goldman MP, et al. *Drug Information Handbook*. 15th ed. Hudson, OH: Lexi-Comp; 2007:1451-1452.

13. **The answer is B.** Dabigatran (Pradaxa) and its acylglucuronide metabolites are DTIs. Both free and clot-bound thrombin and thrombin-induced platelet aggregations are inhibited by the active moieties.

Pradaxa (dabigatran etexilate) [package insert]. Ridgefield, CT: Boerhinger Ingelheim Pharmaceuticals; November 2015. Available at https://docs.boehringer-ingelheim.com/Prescribing%20Information/PIs/Pradaxa/Pradaxa.pdf

14. **The answer is D.** Dabigatran is a capsule, which must be swallowed whole and intact. It cannot be opened and flushed down a feeding tube. The oral bioavailability of dabigatran increases by 75% when the pellets are removed from the capsule. This may result in a significant increase in the immediate anticoagulation effects of dabigatran.

Pradaxa (dabigatran etexilate) [package insert]. Ridgefield, CT: Boerhinger Ingelheim Pharmaceuticals; November 2015. Available at https://docs.boehringer-ingelheim.com/Prescribing%20Infromation/PIs/Pradaxa/Pradaxa.pdf. Accessed April 9, 2017.

15. **The answer is D.** Idarucizumab is the first and only dabigatran-specific antidote. It is a monoclonal antibody, which binds specifically to dabigatran and its acylglucuronide metabolites with an affinity that is about 350 times greater than thrombin. This neutralizes the anticoagulant effect of dabigatran within minutes. Vitamin K does not reverse nor impact the anticoagulation effects of dabigatran. Idarucizumab is administered as two separate doses of 2.5 g, which should not be given more than 15 minutes apart. Effects can be observed within minutes and hemostasis restored at a median of 11.4 hours. The duration is usually at least

24 hours. The serum half-life of dabigatran is 12 to 14 hours, and given adequate renal function, the plasma concentration is approximately 50% of the maximum concentration at this time. Because the protein binding is low, dialysis may be considered if administration of idarucizumab is not possible; 50% to 60% of the drug is removed over 4 hours of hemodialysis. Although recombinant factor VIIa has not been evaluated in clinical trial, the manufacturer does suggest that is may be considered.

Das A, Liu D. Novel antidotes for target specific oral anticoagulants. *Exp Hematol Oncol.* 2015;4(25):1-5. doi:10.1186/s40164-015-0020-3

Pradaxa (dabigatran etexilate) [package insert]. Ridgefield, CT: Boerhinger Ingelheim Pharmaceuticals; November 2015. Available at https://docs.boehringer-ingelheim.com/Prescribing%20Infromation/PIs/Pradaxa/Pradaxa.pdf. Accessed April 9, 2017.

Stangier J, Clemens A. Pharmacology, pharmacokinetics, and pharmacodynamics of dabigatran etexilate, an oral direct thrombin inhibitor. *Clin Appl Thromb Hemost.* 2009;15:S9-S16. doi: 10.1177/1076029609343004

16. **The answer is D.** Benzodiazepines act principally through potentiation of the central nervous system (CNS) inhibitory neurotransmitter, gamma-aminobutyric acid (GABA). The major use of benzodiazepines is to provide anxiolysis and anterograde amnesia. Additional beneficial effects include sedation and anticonvulsant activity. These agents do not possess any direct analgesic properties.

Mirski MA, Lewin JJ 3rd. Sedation and analgesia in acute neurologic disease. *Curr Opin Crit Care.* 2010;16:81-91. doi:10.1097/MCC.0b013e328337495a

17. **The answer is D.** Advantages of the benzodiazepines for neurologically ill patients include limited disturbance of cerebral and vascular tone, anticonvulsant activity, and a coupled decrease in cerebral metabolic oxygen demand with a decrease in cerebral blood flow.

Mirski MA, Lewin JJ 3rd. Sedation and analgesia in acute neurologic disease. *Curr Opin Crit Care.* 2010;16:81-91. doi:10.1097/MCC.0b013e328337495a

18. **The answer is B.** Midazolam has a rapid onset and short duration of action with single doses, which makes it ideal to treat acutely agitated patients or for short procedures. However, it is recommended that midazolam use be limited to 48 to 72 hours for continuous infusions. Studies directly comparing wake-up times with midazolam and lorazepam show a shorter time to wake up with lorazepam, despite its longer half-life. Prolonged sedative effects may be caused by the accumulation of an active metabolite, alpha 1-hydroxy-midazolam, or its conjugated salt, especially in patients with renal dysfunction. In addition, prolonged sedation has been observed in obese patients or those with low serum albumin levels.

Society of Critical Care Medicine and American Society of Health-System Pharmacists. Clinical practice guidelines for the sustained use of sedatives and analgesics in the critically ill adult. *Am J Health-Syst Pharm.* 2002;59:150-178.

19. **The answer is A.** Flumazenil reverses the sedative effects of benzodiazepines. It does not reverse the respiratory depression, hypoventilation, or cardiac depression effects of benzodiazepines. Note, flumazenil does not reverse the central nervous system (CNS) effects of other agents that affect gamma-aminobutyric acid (GABA)-ergic neurons, such as barbiturates, ethanol, or general anesthetics.

Lacy CF, Armstrong LL, Goldman MP, et al. *Drug Information Handbook.* 15th ed. Hudson, OH: LexiComp; 2007:718-720.

20. **The answer is B.** Fentanyl has some potential advantages over morphine. It has less effect on blood pressure (BP) at sedative doses because it does not promote the release of histamine. Caution is still warranted with IV boluses of high doses. In addition, it tends to reduce heart rate, which is favorable in cardiovascular patients. Fentanyl and fentanyl-containing products are known to cause jaw, abdominal, and chest wall rigidity with administration. This

effect is most commonly associated with either high doses or rapid administration. However, it has also been reported with lower doses. Chest wall rigidity is thought to be an infrequent but serious complication. Respiratory and cardiovascular complications can develop from hypoxemia and hypercarbia, which can lead to significant morbidity or mortality.

Mirski MA, Lewin JJ 3rd. Sedation and analgesia in acute neurologic disease. *Curr Opin Crit Care.* 2010;16:81-91. doi:10.1097/MCC.0b013e328337495a

21. **The answer is D.** Naloxone's effects are due to its action on narcotic reversal, not due to direct effect on opioid receptors. Therefore, adverse events occur secondary to reversal of narcotic analgesia and sedation, which can cause severe reactions. Adverse events that can occur include hyper- or hypotension, tachycardia, ventricular arrhythmias, restlessness, seizures, vomiting, diarrhea, pulmonary edema, pain, and cardiac arrest. Many clinicians will administer 0.4 mg intravenous (IV) push. However, to avoid complications, the 0.4 mg/mL vial should be diluted with 9 mL of sodium chloride 0.9% and administered at 1-mL increments until desired results are achieved.

Lacy CF, Armstrong LL, Goldman MP, et al. *Drug Information Handbook.* 15th ed. Hudson, OH: Lexi-Comp; 2007:1194-1195.

22. **The answer is B.** Propofol is available as an emulsion in a phospholipid vehicle, which provides 1.1 kcal/mL from fat and should be counted as a caloric source. Long-term or high-dose infusions may result in hypertriglyceridemia.

Society of Critical Care Medicine and American Society of Health-System Pharmacists. Clinical practice guidelines for the sustained use of sedatives and analgesics in the critically ill adult. *Am J Health-Syst Pharm.* 2002; 59:150-178.

23. **The answer is B.** A clinically relevant incidence of infections would be suspected because of the phospholipid vehicle. However, this has not been reported. The manufacturers suggest propofol infusions, and tubing should be changed at least every 12 hours. In addition, a preservative has been added to the propofol to decrease the potential for bacterial overgrowth. Propofol, a phenolic derivative, may cause green urine due to a chemical reaction. The green urine is not related to the length of therapy or dose. Elevations of pancreatic enzymes have been reported during prolonged infusion of propofol. However, the most concerning adverse effect of propofol is propofol infusion syndrome. Infusions of high doses (>83 mcg/kg/min) of propofol for more than 48 hours have been associated with lactic acidosis, bradycardia, and an increased risk of cardiac arrest.

Society of Critical Care Medicine and American Society of Health-System Pharmacists. Clinical practice guidelines for the sustained use of sedatives and analgesics in the critically ill adult. *Am J Health-Syst Pharm.* 2002; 59:150-178.

24. **The answer is D.** All of the options provided can be used alternatively to the 23.4% concentration. Thirty milliliters of 23.4% sodium chloride contain 120 mEq of sodium chloride. The volume of the different concentrations should be adjusted to provide 120 mEq sodium chloride. Three percent, 5%, and 14.6% sodium chloride contain 0.51, 0.86, and 2.5 mEq/mL of sodium chloride, respectively. This would provide a final volume of sodium chloride 3% of 235 mL, sodium chloride 5% of 140 mL, and sodium chloride 14.6% of 48 mL.

Lacy CF, Armstrong LL, Goldman MP, et al. *Drug Information Handbook.* 15th ed. Hudson, OH: Lexi-Comp; 2007:1194-1195.

25. **The answer is B.** Acyclovir should be dosed on the basis of the IBW. BG's actual body weight is 150 kg, and his height is 5'6". His IBW is 64 kg. Dosing for a CSF infection is 10 mg/kg/dose (IBW); therefore, his appropriate dose is 640 mg IV every 8 hours (adequate kidney function). Acute renal failure (ARF) has been reported when acyclovir is dosed using actual body weight in obese patients. Absorption, distribution, elimination, and metabolism of the pharmacokinetic parameters of a drug can vary in obese patients. Obese patients have

high levels of lipoproteins, which can bind to serum proteins and decrease the protein bind-ing of drugs. Since acyclovir is poorly protein bound (9%–22%), it is unlikely that drug–drug or drug–disease interactions due to protein binding can happen. Volume of distribution of a drug can also be affected in obese patients. For example, vancomycin has a slightly larger volume of distribution, which requires dosing on the basis of the actual body weight. In comparison, acyclovir has a steady-state volume of distribution, which corresponds to total body water. Therefore, dosing using actual body weight can result in a significant overdose. The package insert recommends using IBW when dosing acyclovir.

Zovirax (acyclovir) [package insert]. Research Triangle Park, NC: GlaxoSmithKlein; June 2005. Available at https://www.accessdata.fda.gov/drugsatfda_docs/label/2005/018828s 030,020089s019,019909s020lbl.pdf. Accessed April 9, 2017.

26. **The answer is C.** The maximum solubility of acyclovir should not exceed 2.5 mg/mL at 37°C in water. If this number is exceeded, acyclovir can precipitate in the renal tubules. High concentrations are achieved in the tubular lumen of the kidneys, as the drug is cleared rapidly through glomerular filtration. The frequency of "acyclovir crystal" is approximately 12% to 48%. Rapid administration of bolus acyclovir can also contribute to precipitation of the drug. Acute renal failure (ARF) can happen within 24 to 48 hours of initiating therapy. BG did not receive any volume resuscitation, and his acyclovir was dosed on the basis of his actual body weight. This explains the reason for his renal failure. If no improvement is seen or renal failure worsens, then acyclovir should be discontinued. Most patients recover renal function after discontinuation of acyclovir and volume resuscitation. The plan is to continue treatment with appropriate dosing and hydration.

Perazella MA. Crystal-induced acute renal failure. *Am J Med*. 1999;106(4):459-465. doi: 10.1016/s0002-9343(99)00041-8

27. **The answer is D.** Oral acyclovir has poor bioavailability (15%–30%). Valacyclovir is a pro-drug, an esterified version of acyclovir that has a greater bioavailability (55%). It is rapidly and nearly completely converted to acyclovir by intestinal and hepatic metabolism. The oral dose for BG will be 1 g every 8 hours since his renal function has returned to normal.

Valtrex (valacyclovir) [package insert]. Research Triangle Park, NC: GlaxoSmithKline; June 2005. Available at http://www.accessdata.fda.gov/drugsatfda_docs/label/2008/020487 s014lbl.pdf. Accessed April 9, 2017.
Zovirax (acyclovir) [package insert]. Research Triangle Park, NC: GlaxoSmithKlein; June 2005. Available at https://www.accessdata.fda.gov/drugsatfda_docs/label/2005/ 018828s030,020089s019,019909s020lbl.pdf. Accessed April 9, 2017.

28. **The answer is C.** Cidofovir is indicated for cytomegalovirus (CMV) retinitis in patients with AIDS. Cidofovir is a last-line agent secondary to nephrotoxicity. The drug must be administered with concomitant probenecid and saline hydration to reduce the potential for nephrotoxicity.

Wolf DL, Rodriguez CA, Mucci M, et al. Pharmacokinetics and renal effects of cidofovir with a reduced dose of probenecid in HIV-infected patients with cytomegalovirus retinitis. *J Clin Pharmacol*. 2003;43(1):43-51. doi:10.1177/0091270002239705

29. **The answer is A.** The highest incidence of nosocomial UTIs is caused by *E. coli*; this accounts for 31%. The incidence of *P. aeruginosa* and other Gram-negative bacilli is approximately 10%, followed by *K. pneumoniae* (9%), *Staphylococcus aureus* (6%), *Proteus mirabilis* (5%), and *Enterococcus* (2%). The incidence of fungal UTIs is about 14%.

Gupta K, Hooton TM, Naber KG, et al. International clinical practice guidelines for the treatment of acute uncomplicated cycstitis and pyelonephritis in women: a 2010 update by the Infectious Diseases Society of America and the European Society for Microbiology and Infectious Diseases. *Clin Infect Dis*. 2011;52(5):e103-e120. doi:10.1093/cid/ciq257

30. **The answer is D.** Predisposing factors for UTI include age, female gender, diabetes mellitus, pregnancy, immunosuppression, urinary tract instrumentation, urinary tract obstruction, renal disease, renal transplant, and neurological dysfunction.

> Gupta K, Hooton TM, Naber KG, et al. International clinical practice guidelines for the treatment of acute uncomplicated cycstitis and pyelonephritis in women: a 2010 update by the Infectious Diseases Society of America and the European Society for Microbiology and Infectious Diseases. *Clin Infect Dis.* 2011;52(5):e103-e120. doi:10.1093/cid/ciq257

31. **The answer is D.** Nosocomial urinary tract infections (UTIs) are the source of up to 15% of all nosocomial bloodstream infections, and the associated mortality rate is approximately 15%. Prevention is crucial, and antibiotic treatment should be started in a timely fashion. Before initiating antibiotics, each hospital should refer to the "antibiogram" to determine current trends in antibiotic susceptibility. The most common cause of nosocomial UTIs are Gram-negative organisms such as *Escherichia coli, Pseudomonas aeruginosa, Proteus, Enterobacter, Serratia,* and *Acinetobacter. E. coli* is still the predominant urinary tract pathogen. However, increased infection rates due to other Gram-negative bacteria have been reported. IA should be empirically started on cefepime for broader coverage until susceptibility is available. Gentamicin is also a drug of choice and should be considered as an option because of the broader Gram-negative bacterial coverage, but the dosing listed for UTI is incorrect. The correct dosing is 1 mg/kg IV every 8 to 12 hours on the basis of kidney function.

> Gupta K, Hooton TM, Naber KG, et al. International clinical practice guidelines for the treatment of acute uncomplicated cycstitis and pyelonephritis in women: a 2010 update by the Infectious Diseases Society of America and the European Society for Microbiology and Infectious Diseases. *Clin Infect Dis.* 2011;52(5):e103-e120. doi:10.1093/cid/ciq257

32. **The answer is B.** There is no need to continue with broader spectrum antibiotics. Once susceptibility has been reported by microbiology, appropriate de-escalation should occur. As explained previously, gentamicin should not be initiated because of the broader coverage.

> Gupta K, Hooton TM, Naber KG, et al. International clinical practice guidelines for the treatment of acute uncomplicated cycstitis and pyelonephritis in women: a 2010 update by the Infectious Diseases Society of America and the European Society for Microbiology and Infectious Diseases. *Clin Infect Dis.* 2011;52(5):e103-e120. doi:10.1093/cid/ciq257

33. **The answer is E.** Early goal-directed therapy should be fluid resuscitation. This can be achieved with crystalloids or colloids, with most treatment algorithms requiring aggressive resuscitation during the first 24 hours of management. There are no clinical outcome differences between crystalloids or colloids; crystalloids require more volume to achieve the same endpoints. Given the patient's chest x-ray, elevated WBC count, and temperature, IV antibiotics should be started empirically within the first hour of recognition of severe sepsis, preferably after appropriate cultures are obtained. Further interventions should be made after a conservative fluid bolus secondary to patient's cardiac history to determine whether patient is in acute cardiogenic shock in addition to septic shock.

> Rhodes A, Evans LE, Alhazzani W, et al. Surviving sepsis campaign: international guidelines for management of sepsis and septic shock: 2016. *Crit Care Med.* 2017;45(3):486-552. doi:10.1007/s00134-017-4683-6

34. **The answer is D.** Vasopressin at a fixed dose of 0.03 units/min would be the next-choice agent in the setting of septic shock and tachycardia from high doses of norepinephrine. Phenylephrine is a pure alpha-adrenergic agonist with minimal cardiac activity. Dopamine stimulates both adrenergic and dopaminergic receptors. Lower doses are mainly dopaminergic stimulating and theorized to produce renal and mesenteric vasodilation, although the clinical significance is yet to be determined. Medium doses are both dopaminergic and beta-1 adrenergic stimulants and produce cardiac stimulation, whereas high doses stimulate alpha-adrenergic

receptors. Epinephrine stimulates alpha, beta-1, and beta-2 receptors resulting in relaxation of smooth muscle of the bronchial tree and increased myocardial oxygen consumption.

Rhodes A, Evans LE, Alhazzani W, et al. Surviving sepsis campaign: international guidelines for management of sepsis and septic shock: 2016. *Crit Care Med.* 2017;45(3):486-552. doi:10.1007/s00134-017-4683-6

35. **The answer is E.** Vasopressin binds to V1, V2, and V3 receptors. V1 receptors are found on vascular smooth muscle, which leads to vasoconstriction. V2 receptors located in the kidney collecting ducts lead to an increase in water permeability and resorption in the distal tubule and collecting ducts. V3 receptors in the pituitary gland lead to an increase in adrenocorticotropic hormone and cortisol production to relieve relative adrenal insufficiency. Phenylephrine is a selective alpha-1 receptor agonist, which leads to vasoconstriction with no direct effect on the beta receptors.

Rhodes A, Evans LE, Alhazzani W, et al. Surviving sepsis campaign: international guidelines for management of sepsis and septic shock: 2016. *Crit Care Med.* 2017;45(3):486-552. doi:10.1007/s00134-017-4683-6

36. **The answer is A.** AP has signs of decreased cardiac output, such as increased serum Cr and decreased mental status. Milrinone is a positive inotropic agent that will increase the cardiac output to maintain perfusion to vital organs. Milrinone works by vasodilating the peripheral vessels to decrease SVR and "unload" the heart.

Yancy CW, Jessup M, Bozkurt B, et al. 2013 ACCF/AHA guideline for the management of heart failure: a report of the American College of Cardiology Foundation/American Heart Association Task Force on Practice Guidelines. *Circulation.* 2013;128:e240-e327. doi: 10.1016/j.jacc.2013.05.019

37. **The answer is D.** Milrinone has dual mechanisms of action and inhibits cyclic adenosine monophosphate (cAMP) breakdown in the heart to increase inotropic activity and cardiac output. In addition, it inhibits cAMP breakdown in vascular smooth muscle to cause peripheral vasodilation and reduce systemic vascular resistance. Hypotension can be one of the concerning side effects of this drug.

Yancy CW, Jessup M, Bozkurt B, et al. 2013 ACCF/AHA guideline for the management of heart failure: a report of the American College of Cardiology Foundation/American Heart Association Task Force on Practice Guidelines. *Circulation.* 2013;128:e240-e327. doi: 10.1016/j.jacc.2013.05.019

38. **The answer is C.** Succinylcholine, the only available depolarizing agent, is used for routine endotracheal intubation and to relax skeletal muscles during surgeries of short duration. It has a rapid onset of action (10–15 seconds) and short duration (10–15 minutes), which makes it the ideal agent for these indications. Depolarization leads to the loss of potassium ions from cells. The serum potassium level typically increases by 0.5 to 1 mEq/L with the administration of succinylcholine. Although it is rare, sudden rises to life-threatening levels of potassium have been reported. Succinylcholine should be used cautiously in patients with insufficient renal function, neuromuscular diseases such as (GBS), myasthenia gravis, and prolonged immobility (e.g., spinal cord injury), as it may trigger severe hyperkalemia. The use of a nondepolarizing agent (atracurium, cisatracurium, rocuronium, and vecuronium) in these patients is recommended despite the slower onset (1–4 minutes) and longer duration of action (20–60 minutes).

McManus MC. Neuromuscular blockers in surgery and intensive care, Part 2. *Am J Health Syst Pharm.* 2001;58(24):2381-2395.

39. **The answer is D.** Many of the neuromuscular blockers can accumulate in patients with renal or hepatic failure. However, any agent can be used with appropriate monitoring. The preferred drug of choice is atracurium or cisatracurium because organ-independent Hofmann elimination and plasma esterases eliminate these agents. Both pancuronium and vecuronium

accumulate in hepatic and renal dysfunction. Rocuronium accumulates in hepatic dysfunction. It is important to adjust the dose on the basis of hepatic and renal function, especially when choosing the initial dose. However, titration of neuromuscular blockers should be based on train-of-four monitoring.

McManus MC. Neuromuscular blockers in surgery and intensive care, Part 2. *Am J Health Syst Pharm*. 2001;58(24):2381-2395.

40. **The answer is C.** Carbamazepine is a potent inducer of the hepatic cytochrome P450 3A4 (CYP3A4) system. The drug is also a substrate for this specific enzyme. Carbamazepine stimulates the metabolism of other CYP3A4 substrates but also autoinduces its own metabolism. This can increase clearance of the drug, requiring higher doses or more frequent dosing. The autoinduction effect usually lasts for approximately 1 month. Carbamazepine works by inhibiting the sodium channel receptors. Indications for carbamazepine include partial seizures with complex symptomatology, generalized tonic–clonic seizures, mixed seizure patterns, and trigeminal neuralgia.

Johannessen SI, Ben-Menacheme. Management of focal-onset seizures: an update on drug treatment. *Drugs*. 2006;66(13):1701-1725. doi:10.2165/00003495-200666130-00004

41. **The answer is C.** Fosphenytoin, a phosphate ester prodrug of phenytoin, is highly water soluble. It can be administered either intramuscularly (IM) or intravenously (IV) with less risk of tissue damage and venous irritation than with parenteral administration of phenytoin. Fosphenytoin is rapidly absorbed and converted to phenytoin by phosphatase enzymes. Phenytoin is associated with infusion-related adverse reactions due to the sodium hydroxide, propylene glycol, and alcohol content of the IV formulation. Venous irritation and tissue damage are most likely to occur when large doses of undiluted phenytoin are administered. Complications such as hypotension and arrhythmias are related to rapid IV administration (>50 mg/min). Caution should be applied to patients with hemodynamic instability or cardiovascular diseases. The rate of infusion when administering fosphenytoin is 150 mg phenytoin equivalent/min. However, phenytoin infusions should not exceed a rate of 50 mg/min. Drug interaction and metabolism effects are similar to those for phenytoin.

Johannessen SI, Ben-Menacheme. Management of focal-onset seizures: an update on drug treatment. *Drugs*. 2006;66(13):1701-1725. doi:10.2165/00003495-200666130-00004

42. **The answer is A.** Lacosamide is indicated for the management of partial onset seizures in combination with other anticonvulsants. Lacosamide should be used cautiously in patients with known cardiac conduction abnormalities. (e.g., marked first-degree AV block, second- or third-degree AV block, and sick sinus syndrome without a pacemaker) or severe cardiovascular disease (e.g., myocardial ischemia and heart failure). The manufacturer recommends obtaining an ECG before initiating lacosamide and after titration to steady state in such patients.

Vimpat (lacosamide) [package insert]. Smyrna, GA: UCB; August 2014. Available at https://www.vimpat.com/vimpat-medication-guide.pdf. Accessed April 16, 2017.

43. **The answer is C.** VPA is a substrate of the hepatic cytochrome P450 system, which can lead to the induction or inhibition of the metabolism of VPA. In addition, VPA can affect the metabolism of other agents by this enzyme system. There are numerous case reports of drug interactions between carbapenems and VAP, although the mechanism of this interaction remains unclear. Coadministration of VAP and meropenem decreases the serum concentration of VAP to subtherapeutic levels, not correctable by increasing the dose of VPA, and is associated with occurrence of seizures.

Bede, P, Lawlor D, Solanki D, et al. Carbapenems and valproate: a consumptive relationship. *Epilepsia Open*. 2017;2(1):107-111. doi:10.1002/epi4.12030

Coves-Orts FJ, Borras-Blasco J, Navarro-Ruiz A, et al. Acute seizures due to a probable interaction between valproic acid and meropenem. *Ann Pharmacother*. 2005;39(3):533-537. doi:10.1345/aph.1E358

44. **The answer is B.** GABA is an inhibitory neurotransmitter. It promotes opening of the post-synaptic receptor, GABA type A (GABA-A). This opening leads to an increased conductance of chloride ions, which results in membrane hyperpolarization and neuronal inhibition. The binding of benzodiazepines to the GABA-A receptor increases the affinity of GABA and its receptor, increasing the frequency of GABA-A receptor firing and potentiating GABA-ergic neurotransmission.

Johannessen SI, Ben-Menacheme. Management of focal-onset seizures: an update on drug treatment. *Drugs*. 2006;66(13):1701-1725. doi:10.2165/00003495-200666130-00004

45. **The answer is A.** All antipsychotic drugs have the potential to prolong the QTc interval to varying degrees. Ziprasidone prolongs the QTc interval longer than haloperidol, risperidone, olanzapine, or quetiapine. The exact point at which QTc prolongation becomes clinically dangerous is unclear. The criterion to define QTc prolongation, which is based on established guidelines from the Committee for Proprietary Medicinal Products, is an increase by greater than 60 milliseconds above baseline—or greater than 450 milliseconds for males and greater than 470 milliseconds for women.

Glassman AH, Bigger JTJr. Antipsychotic drugs: prolonged QTc interval, torsade de pointes, and sudden death. *Am J Psychiatry*. 2001;158(11):1774-1782. doi:10.1176/appi.ajp.158.11.1774

46. **The answer is C.** Acute dystonia, parkinsonism, and akathisia are EPS, which usually occur early after the initiation of treatment, whereas tardive dyskinesia, tardive dystonia, and tardive akathisia have a later onset, usually after years of treatment. In general, the typical agents such as haloperidol and fluphenazine are more likely to cause EPS than atypical agents when used at the current therapeutic doses. Among the currently available atypical agents, quetiapine has the lowest risk for EPS.

Dolder CR, Jeste DV. Incidence of tardive dyskinesia with typical versus atypical antipsychotics in very high risk patients. *Biol Psychiatry*. 2003;53(12):1142-1145. doi:10.1016/S0006-3223(03)00170-7

47. **The answer is A.** Weight gain is documented as one of the most significant side effects and concerns associated with the atypical antipsychotic drugs. The proposed mechanism of action for inducing weight gain can be contributed to the antagonistic effect on the histamine H_1 receptors and serotonin $5-HT_{2c}$ The weight gain is predominantly observed with clozapine and olanzapine; the incidence is lower with ziprasidone and aripiprazole and intermediate with risperidone and quetiapine.

McIntyre RS, Mancini DA, Basile VS. Mechanisms of antipsychotic-induced weight gain. *J Clin Psychiatry*. 2001;62(suppl 23):23-29.

48. **The answer is A.** Renal failure is not a concern with atypical antipsychotic agents. Anticholinergic effects are more significant with the atypical agents. Clinically, patients present with dry mouth, constipation, and urinary retention. Hyperprolactinemia is induced because of the inhibitory effect on the dopamine receptor in the tuberoinfundibular tract, which then elevates serum prolactin. To a lesser extent, risperidone and olanzapine increase prolactin levels; this is dose related. This side effect is more common with the typical antipsychotic agents because of their higher affinity to dopamine receptors.

Wirshing DA, Pierre JM, Erhart SM, et al. Understanding the new and evolving profile of adverse drug effects in schizophrenia. *Psychiatr Clin North Am*. 2003;26:165-190. doi:10.1016/S0193-953X(02)00035-7

49. **The answer is B.** Urgent reversal of vitamin K antagonist–associated intracranial hemorrhage is a strong recommendation. Recommendations for reversal of vitamin K antagonists most often include combinations of vitamin K with either FFP or prothrombin complex concentrates (PCC). The major limitation of vitamin K is the time to reduction of the INR to values less than 1.4. However, vitamin K sustains the anticoagulant activity of other reversal agents and should be dosed as soon as possible. The degree of normalization with FFP depends

on the initial INR as well as the dose. Typical doses range from 10 to 15 mL/kg. However, it should be individualized to the patient based on concomitant disease states and the INR. Prior to the introduction of rVIIa and PCC, FFP was the mainstay of therapy for this indication. However, there are several limitations to FFP including waiting for it thaw, many patients not being able to tolerate the large volumes required, and time to correction. Based on these limitations FFP with vitamin K should be administered when PCC is not available or when adequate INR reversal did not occur with PCC. 4-PCC, which contains factors II, VII, IX, and X, has been shown to more rapidly and completely reverse warfarin compared to FFP. When available 4-PCC with vitamin K 10 mg IV should be given immediately.

Activated charcoal may be considered for use in the reversal of direct factor Xa inhibitors or direct thrombin inhibitors (dabigatran).

Frontera JA, Lewin JJ III, Rabinstein AA, et al. Guideline for reversal of antithrombotics in intracranial hemorrhage: executive summary. A statement for healthcare professionals from Neurocritical Care Society and the Society of Critical Care Medicine. *Crit Care Med.* 2016;44(12):2251-2257. doi:10.1097/CCM.0000000000002057

50. **The answer is C.** Idarucizumab is a monoclonal antibody designed for the reversal of anticoagulant effects of dabigatran, an oral DTI. DTI reversal should be guided primarily by bleeding (major or intracranial), and not primarily by laboratory testing. If DTI ingestion was within 2 hours, administration of activated charcoal (50 g) is recommended in patients with enteral access and/or those at low risk of aspiration. Idarucizumab administration (5 g intravenously [IV] in two divided doses) is recommended if dabigatran was administered within a period of 36 to 60 hours (three to five half-lives) and the patient does not have the evidence of renal failure or if there is renal insufficiency leading to continued drug exposure beyond the normal three to five half-lives. In the event that idarucizumab is not available or contraindicated, hemodialysis is a conditional recommendation.

Frontera JA, Lewin JJ III, Rabinstein AA, et al. Guideline for reversal of antithrombotics in intracranial hemorrhage: executive summary. A statement for healthcare professionals from Neurocritical Care Society and the Society of Critical Care Medicine. *Crit Care Med.* 2016;44(12):2251-2257. doi:10.1097/CCM.0000000000002057

51. **The answer is B.** 4-PCC is recommended as first- or second-line therapy for anticoagulant-associated intracranial hemorrhage and/or major bleeding for all of the stated anticoagulants except for low-molecular-weight heparin. 4-PCC in combination with intravenous (IV) vitamin K is the first-line recommendation for vitamin K antagonist–associated bleeding because it contains factors II, VII, IX, and X as well as protein C and protein S. Reversal of DTI–related bleeding or direct Xa-inhibitor related-bleeding (if idarucizumab is unavailable) should include consideration of last injection and renal function, as well as medication interactions, which may prolong the effects of the agent. Additionally, activated charcoal, dialysis, 4-factor PCC or activated 4-factor PCC 50 units/kg (if hemorrhage occurred within three to five half-lives of drug exposure or in liver failure), or a combination of these should be administered. Reversal of direct factor Xa inhibitor-related bleeding may also include activated charcoal or 4-factor PCC or activated 4-factor PCC. Activated charcoal may be useful if administered within 2 hours of apixaban injection. Due to the high protein binding of these agents hemodialysis is not effective for reversal of these agents. Currently, there is no reversal agent specific for low-molecular-weight heparins. Protamine is used (dose is agent specific); however, it's ability varies significantly. Recombinant factor VIIa may be considered if protamine is contraindicated.

Frontera JA, Lewin JJ III, Rabinstein AA, et al. Guideline for reversal of antithrombotics in intracranial hemorrhage: executive summary. A statement for healthcare professionals from Neurocritical Care Society and the Society of Critical Care Medicine. *Crit Care Med.* 2016;44(12):2251-2257. doi:10.1097/CCM.0000000000002057

52. **The answer is D.** MSE is most commonly observed after cardiac arrest and prolonged hypoxia. Medications used for MSE are mainly for symptom control. The most frequently utilized medications include benzodiazepines, VPA, and levetiracetam. Myoclonus is a known adverse effect associated with gabapentin. The incidence of myoclonus has been reported to be as high as 5% in one case series. Symptoms were usually mild; discontinuation of therapy was not needed in most cases. Gabapentin is cleared completely by renal excretion. The half-life of gabapentin in patients with normal renal function is 5 to 7 hours. However, it has been reported to be as long as 132 hours in patients with end-stage renal disease (ESRD) on nondialysis days, predisposing these patients to toxicity. Myoclonus has been noted in end-stage renal patients receiving gabapentin and dosing adjustments should be made. Patients with ESRD should receive 300 to 400 mg as a loading dose followed by 200 to 300 mg after every 4-hour hemodialysis session.

Asconapé J, Diedrich A, DellaBadia J. Myoclonus associated with the use of gabapentin. *Epilepsia.* 2000;41(4):479-481. doi:10.1111/j.1528-1157.2000.tb00192.x
Kaufman KR, Parikh A, Chan L, et al. Myoclonus in renal failure: two cases of gabapentin toxicity. *Epilepsy Behav Case Rep.* 2014;2:8-10. doi:10.1016/j.ebcr.2013.12.002

53. **The answer is B.** Hyperkalemia is one of the most serious side effects following succinylcholine administration. Patients with acute hyperkalemia secondary to diabetic ketoacidosis or acute renal failure do not have a contraindication to succinylcholine. An increase of 0.5 to 1.0 mEq/L would be expected in these patients. Hyperkalemia usually peaks in 5 minutes after administration and resolves within 15 minutes. Although, sudden-onset, life-threatening hyperkalemia is rare, it can happen in patients with denervated muscle caused by acute upper and lower motor neuron disease. Examples include spinal cord injury, stroke, demyelinating disease, encephalitis, and prolonged immobility with disease. Additionally, it has been reported in severe trauma with muscle injury and burn patients. Serum potassium concentrations may rise by 85%, resulting in peaked T waves, a wide QRS interval, loss of P waves on the ECG, and possible ventricular fibrillation and cardiac arrest. Succinylcholine-associated receptor sensitivity and hyperkalemia has been reported to continue for 2 to 6 months. However, it can last up to 2 years.

McManus MC. Neuromuscular blockers in surgery and intensive care, part 2. *Am J Health-Syst Pharm.* 2001;58:2381-2399.
Succinylcholine [package insert]. Lake Forest, IL: Hospira Pharmaceuticals; September 2010. Available at: http://labeling.pfizer.com/ShowLabeling.aspx?id=4621. Accessed April 16, 2017.

54. **The answer is A.** In patients with atrial fibrillation at high risk of cardioembolic stroke following recent coronary revascularization, the presence of an anticoagulant and a P2Y12 antagonist are recommended for the purpose of preventing stent thrombosis and stroke. In this specific patient population, triple antithrombotic therapy may be necessary (dual-antiplatelet therapy and anticoagulant). Several recent trials suggest that in some low-risk patients, 3 to 6 months of dual-antiplatelet therapy may be adequate due to newer drug-eluting stents (DES) that have less thrombogenic risk. Shorter duration of triple therapy in those treated with newer generation DES may be reasonable and has been recommended, such as 3 months for those with stable ischemic heart disease, and 6 months for those with acute coronary syndrome. Omission of oral anticoagulants could lead to an increased risk of thromboembolic stroke and clopidogrel is essential to prevent stent thrombosis. Therefore, in those at high risk of bleeding and those with atrial fibrillation and acute coronary syndrome who do not undergo coronary stent implantation, dual therapy with warfarin and clopidogrel can be considered in order to reduce bleed risk.

Dewilde WJ, Oirbans T, Verheugt FW, et al. Use of clopidogrel with or without aspirin in patients taking oral anticoagulant therapy and undergoing percutaneous coronary intervention: an open-label, randomised, controlled trial. *Lancet.* 2013;381:1107-1115. doi:10.1016/S0140-6736(12)62177-1
January CT, Wann LS, Alpert JS, et al. 2014 AHA/ACC/HRS guideline for the management of patients with atrial fibrillation: executive summary: a report of the American College of Cardiology/American Heart Association Task Force on Practice Guidelines and the Heart Rhythm Society. *J Am Coll Cardiol.* 2014;64:2246-2280. doi:10.1016/j.jacc.2014.03.021

55. **The answer is D.** The neurological adverse reactions reported with brivaracetam include somnolence, fatigue, dizziness, and disturbance in coordination. Brivaracetam can cause dose-dependent increases in somnolence and fatigue-related adverse events. The risk is greatest at the beginning of therapy; however, it can occur at any time. Psychiatric adverse events, including irritability, have also been reported. Other symptoms, which have been reported include but are not limited to anxiety, nervousness, aggression, agitation, depression, and altered mood.

Briviact (brivaracetam) [prescribing information]. Smyrna, GA: UCB; June 2016. Available at https://www.briviacthcp.com/briviact-PI.pdf. Accessed April 9, 2017.

56. **The answer is B.** In the United States, clobazam is approved by the FDA for the indication of adjunctive treatment of seizures associated with LGS in patients 2 years of age and older. The starting dose is 5 mg daily in patients less than 30 kg and 5 mg twice daily in patients greater than 30 kg. Doses should be titrated according to the patients' tolerability and response. Clobazam is also used for non–FDA-approved indications including tonic–clonic, complex partial, and myoclonic seizures, refractory epilepsies, some types of status epilepticus, as well as anxiety.

Onfi (clobazam) [package insert]. Deerfield, IL: Lundbeck; December 2016. Available at https://www.lundbeck.com/upload/us/files/pdf/Products/ONFI_PI_US_EN.pdf. Accessed April 9, 2017.

57. **The answer is D.** Currently there is no evidence that supports a preferred second therapy of choice. Guidelines recommend the following medications and doses: IV fosphenytoin (20 mg PE/kg,), IV VPA (20–40 mg/kg,) or IV levetiracetam (1000–3000 mg), however, higher doses have been used in clinical practice. The second phase therapy is usually thought to start when seizure duration reaches 20 minutes. However, as soon as it is recognized that an adequate dose of benzodiazepines have been administered with lack of seizure cessation a second agent should be administered. The ongoing study, Established Status Epilepticus Treatment Trial (ESETT), is currently enrolling patients to determine the most effective and/or least effective treatment of benzodiazepine—refractory status epilepticus (SE) comparing fosphenytoin, levetiracetam, and VPA.

Brophy GM, Bell R, Claassen J, et al. Guidelines for the evaluation and management of status epilepticus. *Neurocrit Care.* 2016;17:3-23. doi:10.1007/s12028-012-9695-z
Glauser T, Shinnar S, Gloss D, et al. Evidence-based guideline: treatment of convulsive status epilepticus in children and adults: report of the guideline committee of the American Epilepsy Society. *Epilepsy Currents.* 2016;16(1):48-61. doi:10.5698/1535-7597-16.1.48

58. **The answer is B.** The precise mechanism of action for both brivaracetam and levetiracetam is not known. Levetiracetam's mechanism is suggested to be a combination of inhibition of voltage-dependent N-type calcium channels, facilitation of gamma-aminobutyric acid (GABA)-ergic inhibitory transmission through displacement of negative modulators, and/or binding to synaptic vesicle protein 2A (SV2A) in the brain, which is a synaptic protein that modulates neurotransmitter release and may contribute to the anticonvulsant effects. Brivaracetam, has a high affinity for selectively binding to SV2A; 15 to 30 times greater than levetiracetam. Some of the adverse events experienced by both agents include somnolence, irritability, and dizziness. Both medications are dosed twice daily with the recommended initial dose of 50 mg twice daily for brivaracetam and 500 mg twice daily for levetiracetam. Both are available as a tablet, oral solution, and injection for intravenous use.

Briviact (brivaracetam) [prescribing insert]. Smyrna, GA: UCB; June 2016. Available at https://www.briviacthcp.com/briviact-PI.pdf. Accessed April 9, 2017.
Keppra (levetiracetam) [prescribing insert]. Smyrna. GA: UCB; April 2016. Available at https://www.keppraxr.com/sites/subs/files/pdf/Keppra_IR_Current_COL_10-2017.pdf. Accessed April 9, 2017.

59. **The answer is D.** Clobazam is a benzodiazepine that is indicated for adjunctive treatment for uncontrolled seizures associated with Lennox-Gastauts syndrome (LGS). Clobazam has a bioavailability of approximately 87% to 100% with absorption taking place rapidly. Patients may take this medication with or without food without affecting the absorption. For patients who have difficulty swallowing, tablets may be crushed without compromising the integrity of medication. Clobazam is highly lipophilic with a large volume of distribution. It is extensively metabolized by the liver and produces an active metabolite N-desmethylclobazam which has about 1/5 the potency of the parent drug. The half-life of clobazam and N-desmethylclobazam ranges from 36 to 42 and 72 to 82 hours, respectively. When treatment is initiated, maximum effect should not be expected until 5 to 9 days from the start of therapy.

Onfi (clobazam) [prescribing insert]. Deerfield, IL: Lundbeck; December 2016. Available at https://www.lundbeck.com/upload/us/files/pdf/Products/Onfi_PI_US_EN.pdf. Accessed April 9, 2017.

60. **The answer is B.** Hyperammonemia, an adverse effect associated with the use of VPA, can present as AMS or somnolence. Plasma ammonia concentrations greater than 80 mcg/dL have been described with its use. Hyperammonemia due to VPA, which can occur in acute overdoses or chronic use, may not always be symptomatic. The proposed mechanism for hyperammonemia is due to a VPA metabolite, propionic acid which inhibits mitochondrial carbamoyl phosphate synthetase, an enzyme necessary for the elimination of ammonia. Inhibition of carbamoyl phosphate synthetase can also be seen in states of relative carnitine deficiency, either due to a genetic defect or from VPA-induced carnitine deficiency, where the metabolism of VPA via omega oxidation produces products that inhibit the synthetase. Since this patient's symptoms are rather mild, the appropriate action is to discontinue VPA and monitor the patient for improvement in symptoms and for a decrease in the serum ammonia level. Hyperammonemia often normalizes rapidly once VPA is discontinued. If the patient had presented in a worse condition, or if serum levels do not decrease, then administration of L-carnitine may be considered. Due to the differences in pathophysiology of hyperammonemia by VPA compared to liver failure, lactulose would not be beneficial in this patient population.

Lheureux P, Hantson P. Carnitine in the treatment of valproic acid-induced toxicity. *Clinical Toxicology*. 2009;47(2):101-111. doi:10.1080/15563650902752376

61. **The answer is B.** The VerifyNow test measures the P2Y12 platelet receptor blockade. The reference range for patients who are not experiencing platelet inhibition from a P2Y12 inhibitor is 180 to 376 PRU. A value between 180 and 376 may indicate that the patient was either not taking a P2Y12 inhibitor or may have inadequate response to the medication. A value less than 180 PRU is evidence that a P2Y12 inhibitor is affecting platelet activity.

VerifyNow PRUTest [package insert]. San Diego, CA: Accriva Diagnostics; 2016. Available at https://www.accriva.com/uploads/literature/mvn0005_verifynow_pocket_guide_01.pdf.Accessed April 14, 2017.

62. **The answer is D.** The 2014 American Heart Association (AHA)/American College of Cardiology (ACC) guidelines for atrial fibrillation recommend the use of intravenous (IV) metropolol for hemodynamically stable patients with atrial fibrillation and RVR. However, superior therapy for hemodynamically unstable patients in atrial fibrillation with RVR has not been established. A small study with 60 patients compared diltiazem and amiodarone for rate control in critically ill, hemodynamically unstable adult patients and found that both agents were successful in rapidly controlling the heart rate. Patients in the diltiazem group had significantly better 24-hour rate control, however, had 30% more incidences of hypotension as compared to the amiodarone group. Therefore, amiodarone may be considered for hemodynamically unstable patients, but superiority has yet to be established in a large randomized controlled trial.

Karth GD, Geppert A, Neunteufl T, et al. Amiodarone versus diltiazem fro rate control in critically ill patients with atrial tachyarrhythmias. *Crit Care Med*. 2001;29:1149-1153. doi: 10.1097/00003246-200106000-00011

January CT, Wann LS, Alpert JS, et al. 2014 AHA/ACC/HRS guideline for the management of patients with atrial fibrillation: executive summary: a report of the American College of Cardiology/American Heart Association Task Force on Practice Guidelines and the Heart Rhythm Society. *J Am Coll Cardiol*. 2014; 64: 2246-2280. doi: 10.1016/j.jacc.2014.03.021.

63. **The answer is C.** Intracranial large artery atherosclerosis is one of the most common causes of stroke worldwide and is associated with a high risk of recurrent stroke. Risk factors include hypertension, smoking, diabetes mellitus, and hyperlipidemia; therefore, lifestyle modifications for risk factors are a large portion of secondary prevention. Randomized, controlled trials found that patients with symptomatic large artery stenosis treated with intracranial angioplasty and stenting experienced worse outcomes compared to those treated with maximal medical therapy. For secondary prevention, prospective trials found no statistically significant difference between antiplatelet and anticoagulant therapy; however, warfarin was associated with a higher risk of major hemorrhage and death. Antiplatelet agents are more effective for noncardioembolic ischemic stroke, such as large artery atherosclerosis. One study found that temporary use of dual antiplatelet therapy with aspirin and clopidogrel for the first 90 days was found to contribute to a relatively low rate of combined stroke and death.

Kernan WN, Ovbiagele B, Black HR, et al. 2014 AHA/ASA Guideline: Guidelines for the prevention of stroke in patients with stroke and transient ischemic attack. *Stroke*. 2014;45(7):2160-236. doi: 10.1161/STR.0000000000000024

Wang Y, Wang Y, Zhao X, et al. Clopidogrel with aspirin in acute minor stroke or transient ischemic attack. *N Engl J Med*. 2013;369(1):11-19. doi:10.1056/NEJMoa1215340

64. **The answer is B.** Clopidogrel is an irreversible inhibitor of the P2Y12 component of the adenosine diphosphate (ADP) receptor and prevents ADP binding and activation of platelets. It is a prodrug that requires hepatic activation to form the active drug/metabolite. Clopidogrel, in combination with aspirin, has been shown to be effective for secondary ischemic stroke prevention of noncardioembolic origin for 90 days, followed by long-term aspirin therapy. Ticagrelor reversibly interacts with the P2Y12 ADP-receptor and prevents signal transduction and platelet activation. Ticagrelor, when administered at doses of 100 mg twice daily, was found to cause 88% platelet inhibition compared to clopidogrel 75 mg daily, which resulted in 68% platelet inhibition.

Dobesh PP, Oestreich JH. Ticagrelor: pharmacokinetics, pharmacodynamics, clinical efficacy, and safety. *Pharmacotherapy*. 2014;34(10):1077-1090. doi:10.1002/phar.1477

65. **The answer is B.** The AHA/ASA 2014 stroke guidelines recommend initiation of BP therapy for patients with an ischemic stroke or transient ischemia attack (TIA) who after the first several days have an established SBP ≥140 mmHg or diastolic blood pressure (DBP) ≥90 mmHg. Management of hypertension is considered to be one of the most important interventions for secondary prevention of ischemic stroke. The prevalence of hypertension among patients with a previous stroke is approximately 70%. While the risk of a first stroke has been shown to be directly related to BP, the relationship with recurrent stroke is less clear. A 2009 meta-analysis of 10 randomized control trials confirmed that antihypertensives reduce the risk of recurrent stroke. Larger reductions in SBP tended to be associated with greater reduction in recurrent stroke risk. However, there is limited data specifically assessing the optimal BP target for secondary stroke prevention. A majority of the literature in this area surrounds stroke prevention in high-risk patients with concomitant disease states. It is recommended that though it is reasonable to achieve a SBP goal of less than 140 mmHg, BP goals should be individualized based on the concomitant disease states.

Kernan WN, Ovbiagele B, Black HR, et al. 2014 AHA/ASA guideline: guidelines for the prevention of stroke in patients with stroke and transient ischemic attack. *Stroke*. 2014;45(7):2160-236. doi: 10.1161/STR.0000000000000024

Liu L, Wang Z, Gong L, et al. Blood pressure reduction for the secondary prevention of stroke: a Chinese trial and a systematic review of the literature. *Hypertens Res*. 2009;32:1032-1040. doi:10.1038/hr.2009.139

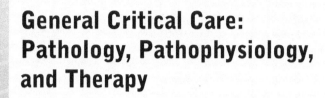

General Critical Care: Pathology, Pathophysiology, and Therapy

16

Cardiovascular Disorders

MEHUL DESAI

QUESTIONS

1. The Food and Drug Administration (FDA)-approved dosage for dabigatran etexilate in patients with severe renal insufficiency is:

   A. 150 mg orally twice daily
   B. 110 mg orally twice daily
   C. 75 mg orally twice daily
   D. 150 mg orally once daily
   E. 110 mg orally once daily

2. A 55-year-old man presents with acute onset of right-sided weakness and aphasia. On subsequent workup, he is found to have a dissection of the ascending thoracic aorta extending into the great arteries of the neck. What is the first step in management of this patient?

   A. Immediate surgery for repair of the aortic dissection
   B. Chest x-ray (CXR)
   C. Start anticoagulation with heparin
   D. Serial check of cardiac enzymes
   E. Medical management of blood pressure (BP) and heart rate (HR)

3. A 57-year-old man is admitted for progressive shortness of breath, chest pain, and palpitations. During his hospital course, he undergoes a diagnostic cardiac catheterization and his tracings are shown as follows. What is the most likely diagnosis for this patient?

   A. Valvular aortic stenosis
   B. Supravalvular aortic stenosis
   C. Hypertrophic obstructive cardiomyopathy (HOCM)
   D. Aortic coarctation
   E. Aortic regurgitation

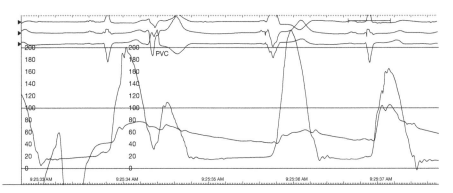

4. A 48-year-old man with a history of hypertension and end-stage renal disease (ESRD) on peritoneal dialysis is hospitalized for acute onset ischemic stroke. Because onset of his symptoms occurred 30 hours prior to presentation in the ED, he is treated conservatively with oral aspirin. On the third day of admission, he develops acute onset shortness of breath, and a CT angiogram of the chest confirms a segmental pulmonary thromboembolus. He loses peripheral intravenous (IV) access, and attempts to reestablish it are unsuccessful. Peripheral blood draws are still possible. What method of anticoagulation is preferable to begin treatment for the pulmonary thromboembolism?

   A. Subcutaneous enoxaparin
   B. Subcutaneous unfractionated heparin
   C. Subcutaneous fondaparinux
   D. Oral warfarin
   E. Oral dabigatran

5. A 58-year-old woman with a significant history of alcohol and substance use is admitted to the ICU after she is discovered obtunded on the street by police. She is profoundly hypotensive and hypoxic. She is intubated for mechanical ventilation, and intravenous (IV) lines are placed for fluid resuscitation. Initial serum chemistries are sent to the laboratory and an ECG and chest x-ray (CXR) are completed. Her CXR is shown here. A pulmonary artery catheter (PAC) is placed to further assess her volume status, and reveals a pulmonary capillary wedge pressure (PCWP) of 10 mmHg. An echocardiogram is also completed, and the results are still pending. Which of the following diagnoses is the least likely to be the cause of the patient's pulmonary edema?

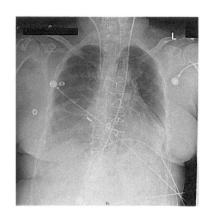

   A. Aspiration pneumonia
   B. Septic shock
   C. Subarachnoid hemorrhage (SAH)
   D. Decompensated congestive heart failure (CHF)
   E. Pancreatitis

6. A 55-year-old man with chronic poorly controlled hypertension presents with a crushing, substernal chest pain radiating to the back. Patient is initially managed medically, with systolic blood pressure (SBP) reduced to less than 120 mmHg. CT angiogram of the chest demonstrates the findings shown as follows. Despite control of blood pressure (BP), patient develops worsening abdominal pain with rising lactic acid. Which is the preferred method of intervention for this patient?

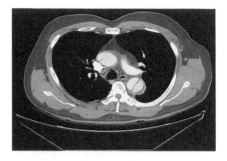

   A. Continue nicardipine infusion with goal reduction SBP to less than 110 mmHg
   B. Emergent surgical intervention
   C. Endovascular stent placement
   D. Start hydralazine for long-term BP control
   E. Continue current management

7. The commonly occurring ECG changes noted in subarachnoid hemorrhage (SAH) include all of the following, **except**:

A. ST-segment elevation
B. ST-segment depression
C. QT_c interval prolongation
D. PR segment prolongation
E. Tall and inverted ("cerebral") T-waves

8. The following parameters are obtained after performing a cardiac catheterization on a 38-year-old woman who presents with shortness of breath: Ao saturation, 97%; PA saturation, 71%; hemoglobin, 14 g/dL; body surface area (BSA), 1.68 m². What is the cardiac output (CO) of this patient using the Fick formula?

A. 3.5 L/min
B. 4.2 L/min
C. 2 L/min
D. 3.9 L/min
E. Cannot be calculated with the given data

9. A 72-year-old man with a history of type II diabetes mellitus (DM) and hypertension presents with hypoxia and right-sided weakness. Spiral CT scan of the chest shows bilateral segmental pulmonary emboli, and MRI of the brain demonstrates a left middle cerebral artery (MCA) occlusion. Echocardiography reveals a large thrombus partially crossing a patent foramen ovale (PFO). Which of the following is **not** a risk factor traditionally associated with paradoxical embolization?

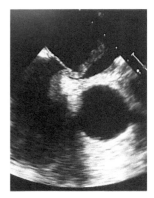

A. Large size of PFO
B. Presence of atrial septal aneurysm
C. Prominent eustachian valve
D. Mitral valve stenosis
E. Pulmonary embolism

10. All of the following are associated with neurogenic pulmonary edema, **except**:

A. Presence of a central nervous system (CNS) insult such as a subarachnoid hemorrhage (SAH), seizure, or stroke
B. Decreased pulmonary capillary permeability
C. Normal left ventricular systolic function
D. Increased sympathetic response after a CNS injury
E. Treatment consists of management of the underlying condition and supportive treatment

11. A 55-year-old woman presents to the ED complaining of worsening occipital headache and confusion. On arrival, her blood pressure (BP) is 220/135 mmHg. On physical examination, she is confused with bilateral papilledema on fundoscopy, and no focal neurological deficit. Laboratory studies demonstrate an elevated creatinine (Cr) of 2.3 mg/dL. ECG shows left ventricular hypertrophy by voltage criteria and nonspecific ST-T wave abnormalities in the lateral leads. CT scan of the head without contrast shows diffuse bilateral white matter changes. Which of the following is the best next step in management?

A. Reduction of the BP to 190/110 over 1 hour using nicardipine infusion
B. Watchful observation in the ED without an acute drop in BP
C. Reduction of the BP to 160/100 over 1 hour using intravenous (IV) labetalol and/or hydralazine
D. Gradual reduction of BP over 24 to 48 hours using oral captopril and long-acting nifedipine
E. Reduction of the BP to 140/90 over 1 hour using nicardipine infusion

12. Tall R wave on 12-lead ECG is noted in the following condition(s):

    A. Duchenne muscular dystrophy
    B. Friedreich's ataxia
    C. Limb girdle muscular dystrophy
    D. Facioscapulohumeral muscular dystrophy
    E. A, B, and C

13. What is the most important laboratory test for diagnosing acute pericarditis?

    A. 2D echocardiogram
    B. ECG
    C. Chest x-ray (CXR)
    D. Cardiac enzymes
    E. Cardiac MRI

14. Which of the following statements does **not** apply to catheter-based reperfusion therapy in acute myocardial infarction (MI) when performed by experienced operators?

    A. Primary stenting compared with angioplasty reduces mortality and recurrent infarction
    B. Primary angioplasty results in lower stroke rates than thrombolysis
    C. Stenting in patients with an acute MI decreases the need for subsequent target vessel revascularization
    D. Primary angioplasty results in higher coronary artery patency rates than thrombolysis
    E. Primary angioplasty results in lower mortality than thrombolysis

15. A 34-year-old woman with a known history of melanoma is admitted for mental status changes due to multiple brain metastases. Restaging is performed and incidentally shows multiple bilateral subsegmental pulmonary emboli. Physical examination is remarkable for left lower extremity pitting edema, and Doppler ultrasound shows a partially occlusive popliteal deep venous thrombosis (DVT) What is the best treatment for her venous thromboembolic disease?

    A. Inferior vena cava filter placement alone
    B. Inferior vena cava filter placement and thrombolytic therapy
    C. Start oral anticoagulation with dabigatran
    D. Systemic anticoagulation and systemic thrombolytic therapy
    E. Start anticoagulation with heparin infusion

16. A 72-year-old man with a history of hypertension, diabetes mellitus (DM) and hyperlipidemia presents to the ED 10 hours after sudden onset of right arm and right leg weakness. He is alert and oriented to time, place, and person. His blood pressure (BP) on presentation is 210/130 mmHg with a mean arterial pressure (MAP) of 157 mmHg. Physical examination demonstrates 2/5 strength in the right upper and lower extremities and 5/5 strength on the left side. No papilledema is seen on fundoscopic examination. Laboratory studies were normal. CT scan of head without contrast shows no evidence of acute hemorrhage. Diffusion-weighted imaged (DWI) from MRI of the brain without contrast is shown here. Which of the following is the best next step in managing this patient's hypertension?

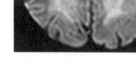

    A. Gradual reduction of MAP by 15% to 20% over 3 hours
    B. Rapid reduction of BP to less than 185/110 mmHg

C. Gradual reduction of MAP by 15% to 20% over 24 hours
D. Watchful observation over 2 to 3 hours to determine whether the BP spontaneously decreases
E. Rapid reduction of BP to less than 180/105 mmHg

17. What is the most sensitive physical finding that suggests cardiac tamponade?

A. Systemic arterial hypotension
B. Elevated jugular venous pressure
C. Pulsus paradoxus
D. Tachycardia
E. Muffled heart sounds

18. Which of the following cardiac biomarkers will provide information about prognosis and help in determining the patient's possible myocardial infarct size?

A. Creatine kinase-muscle/brain fraction.
B. Myoglobin
C. Cardiac troponin T (cTnT)
D. B-natriuretic peptide (BNP)
E. Matrix metalloproteinase (MMP)

19. A 49-year-old woman with multiple sclerosis (MS) is being treated for acute pulmonary thromboembolism with heparin infusion and warfarin. She has a previous history of prophylactic heparin use while inpatient. One day after initiation of therapy, her platelet count has fallen from 230,000 to 45,000. Physical examination reveals dusky areas on several digits as well as edema in the left arm and hand, which was not seen previously. What is the next immediate step in management?

A. Discontinuation of heparin, administration of vitamin K and argatroban
B. Discontinuation of heparin, administration of bivalirudin
C. Discontinuation of heparin, administration of enoxaparin
D. Discontinuation of heparin, continued administration of warfarin to goal International Normalized Ratio (INR) 2.0 to 3.0
E. Continue heparin infusion, consult hematology

20. A healthy 40-year-old man with no medical history travels to east Africa to join a hiking expedition to trek to the top of Mount Kilimanjaro. The group ascends to 3,500 meters in 2 days. On the third day of the expedition, he experiences difficulty breathing, headache, chest tightness, congestion, and cough with pink frothy sputum. One of the guides decides that it is no longer safe for him to continue the climb so together they begin their descent down the mountain. All of the following therapies are beneficial in improving the patient's symptoms immediately **except**:

A. Nifedipine
B. Lasix
C. Supplemental oxygen
D. Hyperbaric treatment
E. Acetazolamide

21. A 60-year-old woman with a history of hypertension, diabetes mellitus (DM), and hyperlipidemia presents to the clinic with the complaint of new onset headache. Her blood pressure (BP) is noted to be 190/125 mmHg. She does not have any altered mental status (AMS) and denies chest pain or shortness of breath. Neurological examination does not show any motor, sensory, or cranial nerve (CN) deficits. No papilledema is seen on fundoscopic examination.

Laboratory workup including chemistries is within normal limits. Which of the following is the most appropriate approach in managing this patient's hypertension?

A. Start oral short-acting antihypertensives under observation
B. Reduction of BP to 155/100 mmHg over 3 to 6 hours using nicardipine infusion
C. Rapid reduction of systolic blood pressure (SBP) to less than 100 mmHg using intravenous (IV) labetalol
D. Reduction of BP to 155/100 mmHg over 24 hours using nicardipine infusion
E. No acute treatment is needed

22. According to current guidelines, in patients with cardiovascular implantable electric devices (CIEDs) needing transcutaneous electrical nerve stimulation (TENS), the correct statement is:

A. TENS units can now be safely used in all patients with devices implanted after 2009
B. Use of TENS units is not recommended because of possible electromagnetic interference
C. TENS units can be safely used in all patients except in the area of the thoracic spine
D. TENS units can be safely used in all patients if the frequency utilized is less than 30 Hz
E. TENS units can only be used with pacemaker (PM) but not defibrillators

23. All the following situations are absolute contraindications to fibrinolytic therapy in acute myocardial infarction (MI) **except**:

A. Suspected aortic dissection
B. Any prior intracranial hemorrhage
C. Known malignant intracranial neoplasm (primary or metastatic)
D. Severe uncontrolled hypertension on presentation (systolic blood pressure [SBP] > 180 mmHg or diastolic blood pressure [DBP] >110 mmHg)
E. Significant closed head or facial trauma within 3 months

24. Cardiogenic shock is defined by the presence of all of the following **except**:

A. Systolic blood pressure (SBP) less than 80 mmHg for more than 30 minutes
B. Decreased cardiac output (CO) resulting in decreased tissue perfusion
C. Pulmonary arterial wedge pressure (PAWP) greater than 15 mmHg
D. Cardiac index (CI) greater than 1.8 L/min/m²
E. Systemic vascular resistance (SVR) is increased

25. In patients being evaluated for cardiac resynchronization therapy, in addition to symptoms of heart failure, the QRS duration on surface ECG should be at least:

A. 100 milliseconds
B. 110 milliseconds
C. 115 milliseconds
D. 200 milliseconds
E. 120 milliseconds

26. What is the leading cause of cardiac tamponade in developed countries?

A. Viral pericarditis
B. Malignant pericardial effusion
C. Radiation-induced pericardial disease
D. Post–myocardial infarction (MI) pericarditis
E. Tuberculosis (TB)

27. A 58-year-old man is admitted to the coronary care unit after a diagnosis of inferior myocardial infarction (MI). The patient did not receive any thrombolytic or catheter-based reperfusion therapy because he was not in the window for reperfusion. The initial ECG showed 1-mm ST elevation and pathologic Q waves in II, III, and aVF. Twenty-four hours after admission, the patient develops mild dyspnea and the chest x-ray (CXR) shows pulmonary vascular redistribution. A faint late systolic murmur is heard at the apex. What is the probable cause of the murmur?

   A. Infarcted posterior papillary muscle
   B. Tricuspid regurgitation
   C. Ventricular septal defect
   D. Aortic stenosis
   E. Ruptured posterior papillary muscle

28. The following have been documented as adverse effects in more than 1% of patients taking amiodarone, **except**:

   A. Peripheral neuropathy
   B. Photosensitivity and halo vision
   C. Worsening of ejection fraction (EF) by less than 5%
   D. Thyroid abnormalities
   E. Interstitial pneumonitis

29. Ventricular tachycardia (VT) ablation should be considered in all of the following scenarios **except**:

   A. A 23-year-old man with congenital heart disease and frequent episodes of syncope related to VT
   B. A 67-year-old woman with coronary artery disease (CAD) and depressed systolic function on optimal medical therapy with symptomatic monomorphic VT
   C. A 56-year-old man with recurrent episodes of polymorphic VT refractory to antiarrhythmic drugs
   D. A 47-year-old man with prior history of CAD, no evidence of systolic dysfunction, and stage I prostate cancer with frequent episodes of symptomatic VT
   E. A 55-year-old woman with episodes of torsade de pointes VT due to prolonged QT in the context of neuroleptic medications

30. Which one of the following is a determinant of cardiac output:

   A. Diastolic time
   B. Heart rate (HR)
   C. Systolic time interval
   D. Arterial pulse–pressure variation
   E. All of the above

31. Complete the following equation: Pressure = _____ × Resistance

   A. Afterload
   B. Volume
   C. Flow
   D. Heart rate (HR)
   E. Impedance

32. The components of the equation for oxygen content of blood (mL O_2/100 mL blood) include:

    A. Partial pressure of O_2 in central venous blood
    B. Oxygen saturation in blood drawn slowly from a pulmonary artery catheter (PAC)
    C. Cardiac output (CO)
    D. Partial pressure of CO_2 in arterial blood
    E. Solubility coefficient of oxygen in blood

33. The partial pressure or percent hemoglobin saturation of oxygen in blood drawn slowly from a pulmonary artery catheter (PAC) is intended to evaluate:

    A. Oxygen consumption by lung tissue
    B. Relationship of oxygen delivered versus consumed by all body tissues
    C. Oxygen absorption across the alveolar–capillary membrane
    D. Oxygen transport (mL O_2/min)
    E. None of the above

34. The ejection fraction (EF) measured by echocardiography primarily evaluates:

    A. Myocardial contractility
    B. Valvular incompetence or stenosis
    C. Cardiac output
    D. Venous preload
    E. Vascular resistance

35. The thermodilution method of cardiac output (CO) measurement by iced-saline injection utilizes all variables listed here, **except**:

    A. Temperature of the pulmonary artery blood
    B. Distance between the injection port and the thermistor
    C. Transpulmonary gas temperature
    D. Volume of saline injected
    E. Temperature of saline injected

36. The normal partial pressure of oxygen in a properly collected mixed venous blood sample is:

    A. 40 mmHg
    B. 65 to 70 mmHg
    C. 100 mmHg
    D. 65% to 70%
    E. None of the above

37. The pulmonary artery "wedge" or occlusion pressure (PAWP) is intended to reflect and direct therapy as a surrogate of:

    A. The ejection fraction (EF)
    B. Left ventricular end-diastolic volume (LVEDV)
    C. Right ventricular end-diastolic pressure
    D. Afterload
    E. None of the above

38. Shunt equation measures the extent that venous blood bypasses (is shunted) oxygenation in the capillaries of the lung. A pulmonary artery catheter (PAC) is required to measure what variable needed to calculate shunt fraction?

    A. End-pulmonary-capillary oxygen content (CcO$_2$)
    B. Arterial oxygen content (CaO$_2$)

C. Cardiac output (CO)
D. Mixed venous oxygen content (C_vO_2)
E. None, a PAC is not needed to measure shunt

39. The arterial pulse pressure variation is used by some cardiac output monitoring devices to guide what intervention?

    A. Preload augmentation
    B. Afterload reduction
    C. Vasopressor (e.g., norepinephrine) administration
    D. Inotropic (e.g., dopamine) support
    E. Resumption of normal sinus rhythm

40. Arterial pressure waveform analysis is used by several commercially available devices to measure cardiac output (CO). These devices calculate the CO after using arterial waveform analysis to define

    A. The dp/dt of left ventricular diastole
    B. Left ventricular ejection time (speed)
    C. Stroke volume (SV)
    D. First derivative of the rate of rise of the first 0.04 seconds of the arterial pressure during systole
    E. The area under the curve of the diastolic relaxation waveform

41. The oxygen saturation in blood drawn from a thoracic central venous catheter (CVC) has been suggested as a clinically satisfactory replacement for what hemodynamic parameter?

    A. Oxygen-carrying capacity of pulmonary blood
    B. Oxygen content of arterial blood
    C. Arteriovenous O_2 difference
    D. Oxygen transport into the systemic circulation
    E. None of the above

42. A 65-year-old man with a recent history of pulmonary embolism on dabigatran presents with a subdural hemorrhage following a fall. CT of head demonstrates midline shift, with rapid deterioration in mental status requiring intubation. What is the preferred reversal agent?

    A. Prothrombin complex concentrates (PCCs) 50 units/kg
    B. Tranexamic acid
    C. Idarucizumab 5 g
    D. Idarucizumab 5 g plus four factor PCC
    E. Fresh frozen plasma (FFP)

43. A 45-year-old healthy woman is admitted to the neuro ICU for management of high-grade aneurysmal subarachnoid hemorrhage (SAH). On monitor, she is noted to have sinus bradycardia with associated hypotension. Atropine is administered and patient is emergently externally paced with resolution of arrhythmia. One hour after the placement of permanent pacemaker (PM), she develops hypotension and becomes confused. What is the next step in diagnosis?

    A. Echocardiography
    B. ECG
    C. CT chest with contrast
    D. CT head
    E. Placement of pulmonary artery catheter (PAC)

44. A 50-year-old man is admitted to the cardiac care unit after cardiac catheterization for ST-elevation myocardial infarction (STEMI) secondary to left anterior descending artery occlusion. Troponin peaks at 75 ng/mL on day 2. On day 5, patient becomes hypotensive and anuric. Serum lactate is increased to 4.2 mmol/L. Mean arterial pressure (MAP) remains 60 mmHg with heart rate (HR) 110 beats per minute (BPM) despite administration of 3 L of normal saline. A pulmonary artery catheter (PAC) is placed while awaiting bedside echocardiography. Initial values include cardiac index (CI) 4.0 L/min/m², pulmonary capillary wedge pressure (PCWP) 13 mmHg, pulmonary arterial pressure (PAP) 29/13 mmHg, residual volume (RV) 28/6 mmHg, systemic vascular resistance (SVR) 640 dynes/sec/cm⁵, S_vO_2 55%, and Hgb 7.4 g/dL, and MAP 58 mmHg. What is the next intervention?

    A. Initiate dobutamine infusion
    B. Initiate milrinone infusion
    C. Initiate norepinephrine infusion
    D. Initiate dopamine infusion
    E. Initiation vasopressin infusion

45. A 35-year-old man presents with status epilepticus (SE). A massive pulmonary aspiration of gastric content occurs during endotracheal intubation in the ED. Over the next 28 hours, the patient develops worsening hypoxemia requiring increased FiO_2 to 100%. Low tidal volume (TV) ventilation protocol is closely followed; however, despite appropriate adjustments in the ventilator setting the patient cannot be oxygenated adequately with PaO_2/FiO_2 ratio persistently below 150. Patient is then paralyzed and undergoes prone positioning. PaO_2/FiO_2 immediately and 3 hours after proning remains less than 50 with pH of 7.15. What intervention should be considered next?

    A. Start inhaled epoprostenol
    B. Recruitment maneuvers with positive end-expiratory pressure (PEEP) of 30 cm H_2O for 30 seconds
    C. Change ventilation mode to airway pressure release ventilation (APRV)
    D. Placement of esophageal balloon
    E. Transfer to extracorporeal membrane oxygenation (ECMO) center for veno–venous (VV) ECMO

46. A 22-year-old woman presents with status epilepticus (SE) secondary to venlafaxine overdose. In the ED, her heart rate (HR) is 115 beats per minute (BPM) with systolic blood pressure (SBP) of 168 mmHg. Four hours after admission to the neuro ICU, patient develops ventricular tachycardia (VA) requiring cardioversion. Despite the administration of antiarrhythmic therapy, patient repeatedly develops VA requiring CPR and multiple cardioversions. Bedside echocardiography after return of spontaneous circulation (ROSC) shows severe biventricular dysfunction with ejection fraction (EF) of approximately 10%, despite initiation of epinephrine and norepinephrine. What is the next best option for cardiac support?

    A. Percutaneous left ventricular assist device (LVAD)
    B. Intra-aortic balloon pump (IABP)
    C. Veno–arterial extracorporeal membrane oxygenation (ECMO)
    D. Veno–venous (VV) ECMO
    E. Cardiac catheterization

47. A 45-year-old man with no past medical history collapses while playing basketball. On arrival, emergency medical service (EMS) finds patient pulseless and initiates CPR. Initial rhythm is ventricular fibrillation; he undergoes cardioversion with return of spontaneous circulation (ROSC). ECG on arrival to the ED demonstrates ST-elevation in the anterolateral leads. Patient is urgently taken to cardiac catheterization and undergoes revascularization with two drug-eluding stents. During the procedure, the patient is noted to be

hypotensive and is started on norepinephrine. Patient's mental status recovers to baseline following the procedure. Upon transfer to the ICU, however, the patient is noted to be on progressively higher doses of norepinephrine. Repeat ECG demonstrates resolution of the ST segment changes and the patient denies chest pain. Echocardiography demonstrates depressed left ventricular function of the anterolateral wall with ejection fraction (EF) of approximately 20%. Nursing notes that urine output has reduced to 10 mL/hr with an increase in lactate to 3.5 mmol/L and blood pressure (BP) of 89/50 mmHg. What is the next best option for providing cardiac support?

A. Increase norepinephrine and consider adding epinephrine to augment cardiac output (CO)
B. Emergent implantable left ventricular assist device (LVAD)
C. Peripherally cannulated extracorporeal membrane oxygenation (ECMO)
D. Percutaneous LVAD
E. Insertion of intra-aortic balloon pump (IABP)

■ ANSWERS

1. **The answer is C.** Dabigatran etexilate is a prodrug that is rapidly converted to the active, reversible, direct thrombin (factor IIa) inhibitor that inhibits both fibrin-bound and free thrombin. This conversion is independent of cytochrome P-450, making drug–drug interactions less likely. Dabigatran etexilate is hydrolyzed to dabigatran by both plasma and hepatic esterases, and is predominantly excreted by kidneys. Dabigatran was evaluated in a large, open-label, randomized trial (RE-LY) in which it was compared with warfarin in 18,113 patients with non-valvular atrial fibrillation. There was no difference in mortality and dabigatran was noninferior to warfarin with respect to the primary efficacy outcome of stroke or systemic embolism. An oral dose of 150 mg twice daily was approved for patients with a creatinine clearance more than 30 mL/min, whereas in patients with severe renal insufficiency (creatinine clearance 15–30 mL/min) the approved dose is 75 mg twice daily. The 110 mg twice-daily dose used in the RE-LY trial did not receive FDA approval.

   Wann LS, Curtis AB, Ellenbogen KA, et al. 2011 ACCF/AHA/HRS focused update on the management of patients with atrial fibrillation (update on dabigatran). A report of the American College of Cardiology Foundation/American Heart Association Task Force on Practice Guidelines. *Heart Rhythm.* 2011;8(3):e1-e8. doi:10.1016/j.hrthm.2011.01.032

2. **The answer is E.** Medical management, specifically, anti-impulse therapy is the first step in the management of aortic dissection. In the absence of contraindications, intravenous (IV) beta-blockade should be initiated and titrated to a target HR of 60 beats/min or less. In patients with clear contraindications to beta-blockade, nondihydropyridine calcium channel–blocking agents should be used as an alternative for rate control. If the systolic blood pressure (SBP) remains greater than 120 mmHg after adequate HR control has been obtained, then first-line vasodilators such as nitroprusside or nicardipine should be administered. In patients with dissections complicated by intracerebral infraction, use of nitroprusside can lead to elevated intracranial pressures (ICPs) and reduced cerebral blood flow. Beta-blockers should be used cautiously in the setting of acute aortic regurgitation because they will block the compensatory tachycardia. Urgent surgical consultation should be obtained for all patients diagnosed with thoracic aortic dissection regardless of the anatomic location (ascending vs. descending) as soon as the diagnosis is made or highly suspected.

   Hiratzka LF, Bakris GL, Beckman JA, et al. 2010 ACCF/AHA guidelines for the diagnosis and management of patients with thoracic aortic disease: executive summary. *Circulation.* 2010;121:1544-1579. doi:10.1161/CIR.0b013e3181d4739e

3. **The answer is C.** The illustrated tracing demonstrates a premature ventricular complex (PVC), and during the beat following the PVC, there is an increase in the gradient between the left ventricle and the aorta, as well as a decrease in the aortic systolic pressure (Brockenbrough–Braunwald–Morrow sign). This finding signifies dynamic outflow tract obstruction. In aortic stenosis and fixed obstruction, in the beat following the PVC, there is an increase in the aortic pressure, whereas in dynamic obstruction, there is a decrease in the aortic pressure and an increase in the left ventricular pressure. This is seen in HOCM and can be observed during physical examination as well.

   Libby P, Bonow RO, Mann DL, et al. *Braunwald's Heart Disease: A Textbook of Cardiovascular Medicine.* 8th ed. Philadelphia, PA: Saunders Elsevier; 2008:1766-1767.

4. **The answer is B.** Although subcutaneous enoxaparin can be dose adjusted for glomerular filtration rates less than 30, its longer half-life compared with unfractionated heparin presents an increased risk for bleeding complications in renal failure. Subcutaneous unfractionated heparin can be monitored by activated partial thromboplastin time (aPTT) in a similar fashion to IV administration. Subcutaneous fondaparinux is contraindicated in renal failure. Both vitamin K antagonist (VKA, warfarin) and non-VKA medications (such as dabigatran, rivaroxaban, apixaban, or edoxaban) are used as long-term anticoagulant therapy for treatment of deep vein thrombosis (DVT) of the leg or pulmonary embolism and no cancer.

However, initial parenteral anticoagulation is given before dabigatran and edoxaban, is not given before rivaroxaban and apixaban, and is overlapped with VKA therapy.

Kearon C, Akl EA, Ornelas J, et al. Antithrombotic therapy for VTE disease: CHEST guideline and expert panel report. *Chest.* 2016;149(2):315-352. doi:10.1016/j.chest.2015.11.026

5. **The answer is D**. It is important to differentiate between cardiogenic and noncardiogenic pulmonary edema as treatment is based upon the underlying pathophysiology. Cardiogenic pulmonary edema occurs as a result of an increase in pulmonary capillary hydrostatic pressure, which causes fluid extravasation into the interstitial space. Noncardiogenic pulmonary edema, in contrast, is a result of increased alveolar–capillary membrane permeability seen in disease states such as acute respiratory distress syndrome (ARDS). Placement of a PAC is one method of distinguishing between the two entities. The PCWP reflects filling pressures on the left side of the heart and indirectly intravascular volume status. PCWP is normally 1 to 5 mmHg less than the pulmonary artery diastolic pressure (6–12 mmHg), and PCWP greater than >18 mmHg, in the context of normal oncotic pressure, suggests left CHF. Since the PCWP is normal in this patient, decompensated CHF is the least likely etiology. The remaining choices are examples of noncardiogenic pulmonary edema and therefore could be present in the patient.

Ware LB, Matthay MA. Clinical practice: acute pulmonary edema. *N Engl J Med.* 2005;353(26):2788-2796. doi:10.1056/NEJMcp052699

6. **The answer is C**. For patients with medical malperfusion syndrome due to an aortic dissection, surgical intervention is the preferred treatment. The stent graft is placed over the intimal flap to seal the entry site of the dissection, inducing thrombosis of the false lumen. Review of data from the International Registry of Acute Aortic Dissection (IRAD) study demonstrates decreased mortality from 32% to 7% in patients managed with endovascular techniques. Complications for the endovascular group were also noted to be less during hospitalization. The Investigation of Stent Grafts in Aortic Dissection (INSTEAD) trial compared medical therapy with goal SBP ≤120/80 mmHg versus medical therapy plus endovascular stenting. Though there was no significant difference in overall survival, the follow-up INSTEAD-XL trial was associated with favorable aorta-specific mortality compared with medical management alone.

Isselbacher EM, Bonaca MP, Di Eusanio M, et al. Recurrent aortic dissection: observations from the international registry of aortic dissection. *Circulation.* 2016;134(14):1013-1024. doi:10.1161/CIRCULATIONAHA.115.019359

7. **The answer is D.** Cardiovascular (CV) changes are extremely common in SAH, especially within the first few days after a high-grade SAH. ECG changes associated with SAH primarily reflect repolarization abnormalities involving the ST-segment, T-wave, U-wave, and QT_c interval. Prolongation of QT_c interval is the most common ECG abnormality seen, and is associated with angiographic vasospasm. Another well-recognized entity is the tall and inverted T-waves, also known as cerebral, neurogenic, or giant T-waves. Because of the combination of ST-segment elevation or depression and abnormal T-wave morphology, myocardial ischemia or infarction is often suspected in patients with SAH. Arrhythmias are a relatively common occurrence as well. Factors that may influence the development of arrhythmias in patients with SAH include cerebral vasospasm, hypoxia, electrolyte imbalance, and sudden increase in intracranial pressure (IP) triggering a sympathetic or vagal discharge due to compression of brain structures. Stress-induced cardiomyopathy occurs at higher rates after SAH compared to ischemic stroke, and can limit the use of vasopressors and induced hypertension for treatment of delayed cerebral ischemia (DCI).

Libby P, Bonow RO, Mann DL, et al. *Braunwald's Heart Disease: A Textbook of Cardiovascular Medicine.* 8th ed. Philadelphia, PA: Saunders Elsevier; 2008:2149-2150.
Tahsili-Fahadan P, Geocadin RG. Heart-Brain axis: effects of neurologic injury on cardiovascular function. *Circ Res.* 2017;120(3):559-572. doi:10.1161/CIRCRESAHA

8. **The answer is B.** CO can be calculated using the Fick formula:

$$CO = V.O_2/C_{a-v}O_2$$

$V.O_2$ represents O_2 consumption and in healthy subjects it is about 125 mL/min/m^2 of BSA for women, 140 mL/min/m^2 of BSA for men, and 110 mL/min/m^2 of BSA for the elderly.

Arteriovenous O_2 difference ($C_{a-v}O_2$) reflects the amount of O_2 taken up by the tissues, and is calculated as ($C_aO_2 - C_vO_2$). The arterial O_2 content (C_aO_2) is measured in oxygenated blood taken from the pulmonary vein or aorta:

$$C_aO_2 = (Hgb \times 1.36 \times S_aO_2) + (P_aO_2 \times .003)$$

The venous O_2 content (C_vO_2) is measured in deoxygenated blood taken from the pulmonary artery:

$$C_vO_2 = (Hgb \times 1.36 \times S_vO_2) + (P_vO_2 \times 0.003)$$

The number 1.36 in these equations represents the fact that each gram of hemoglobin can carry 1.36 mL of O_2; and 0.003 is the solubility coefficient of oxygen in blood.

Placing all of the numbers back into the original formula:

$$CO = V.O_2/C_{a-v}O_2$$

$$CO = (125 \times BSA)/(C_aO_2 - C_vO_2)$$

And to simplify

$$CO = (125 \times BSA)/[(S_aO_2 - S_aO_2) \times Hgb \times 1.36]$$

$$CO = (125\,mL/min/m^2 \times 1.68\,m^2)/[(0.97 - 0.71) \times 14 \times 1.36]$$

$$CO = 210\,mL/min/4.95\,in\,100\,mL\,(1\,dL)\,of\,blood$$

$$CO = 210/(4.95 \times 10) = 4.24\,L/min$$

Willerson JT, Cohn JN, Wellens HJJ, et al. *Cardiovascular Medicine*. 3rd ed. New York, NY: Springer-Verlag; 2007:464.

9. **The answer is D.** Risk factors thought to be associated with increased risk of paradoxical embolism include a large PFO, atrial septal aneurysm, prominent eustachian valve, and conditions that cause elevated right atrial pressure, such as pulmonary embolism or tricuspid regurgitation. Conditions causing increased left atrial pressure, such as mitral valve stenosis, are more likely to decrease shunting across the PFO and decrease risk of paradoxical embolism.

Homma S, Sacco RL. Patent foramen ovale and stroke. *Circulation*. 2005;112(7):1063-1072. doi:10.5853/jos.2015.17.3.229

10. **The answer is B.** Several CNS insults can be complicated by the development of acute pulmonary edema that cannot be otherwise explained. Neurogenic pulmonary edema is a form of noncardiogenic pulmonary edema and these patients have normal left ventricular systolic function. The underlying pathophysiology is not fully understood; the proposed mechanisms include (a) increased permeability of the pulmonary capillaries and (b) a sympathetic surge after a CNS injury. Treatment is supportive.

Bruder N, Rabinstein A. Cardiovascular and pulmonary complications of aneurysmal subarachnoid hemorrhage. *Neurocrit Care*. 2011;15(2):257-269. doi:10.1007/s12028-011-9598-4

Busl KM, Bleck TP. Neurogenic pulmonary edema. *Crit Care Med*. 2015;43(8):1710-1715. doi:10.1097/CCM.0000000000001101

Fein IA, Rackow EC. Neurogenic pulmonary edema. *Chest*. 1982;81(3):318-320. doi:10.1378/chest.81.3.318

11. **The answer is A**. Hypertensive emergencies are characterized by severe elevations in BP (>180/120 mmHg) complicated by evidence of impending or progressive end-organ dysfunction including hypertensive encephalopathy. The initial goal of therapy in hypertensive emergencies is to reduce the mean arterial pressure (MAP) by 15% to 5% over 1 to 2 hours. Rapid and profound reduction in BP may precipitate renal, cerebral, or coronary ischemia. These patients must be managed in the ICU using IV antihypertensive agents for appropriate titration of BP.

Toledano M, Fugate JE. Posterior reversible encephalopathy in the intensive care unit. *Handb Clin Neurol.* 2017;141:467-483. doi:10.1016/B978-0-444-63599-0.00026-0

12. **The answer is E**. ECG abnormalities can be noted in up to 90% of patients with Becker and Duchenne muscular dystrophy. Tall R waves and an increased RS amplitude in V_1 with deep narrow Q waves in the left precordial leads are a characteristic ECG pattern of the posterolateral left ventricular involvement. Incomplete right bundle branch block may also be noted, suggesting right ventricular involvement in these patients. Friedreich's ataxia is commonly associated with concentric hypertrophic cardiomyopathy and at times asymmetric septal hypertrophy. Up to 95% of these patients manifest ECG abnormalities. Surprisingly, ECG manifestations do not always include left ventricular hypertrophy, although echo demonstrates this. Widespread T-wave abnormalities are noted with tall R waves in all leads. Limb-girdle muscular dystrophy is a sarcoglycanopathy and is associated with cardiomyopathy. ECG changes are similar to those seen in Becker and Duchenne muscular dystrophy. Cardiac involvement is rare in facioscapulohumeral muscular dystrophy. Specific cardiac monitoring or treatment has not yet been described.

Libby P, Bonow RO, Mann DL, et al. *Braunwald's Heart Disease: A Textbook of Cardiovascular Medicine.* 8th ed. Philadelphia, PA: Saunders/Elsevier; 2008:2135-2142.

13. **The answer is B**. ECG is the most important laboratory test for diagnosing acute pericarditis. A diagnosis of acute pericarditis should be reserved for patients with an audible pericardial friction rub or chest pain with typical ECG findings. The classic presentation is diffuse, concave upward ST-segment elevation and PR-segment depression. The distinction between acute pericarditis and transmural ischemia is usually not difficult because of more extensive lead involvement in acute pericarditis and the presence of reciprocal ST-segment depression in acute ischemia. An echocardiogram and CXR would be useful in identifying a pericardial effusion or other causes of chest pain, but have otherwise no role in diagnosing pericarditis. A significant fraction of patients with pericarditis have elevated creatine kinase-MB fraction or troponin I values, which suggests concomitant myocarditis.

Lange RA, Hillis LD. Clinical practice: acute pericarditis. *N Engl J Med.* 2004;351(21):2195-2202. doi: 10.1056/NEJMcp041997

14. **The answer is A**. Primary angioplasty in patients with an acute MI, when performed by experienced operators, has shown in large registries and randomized trials to result in higher patency rates (93%–98% vs. 54%) and lower 30-day mortality rates (5% vs. 7%) than thrombolytic therapy. An additional advantage of primary angioplasty over thrombolysis is a significant reduction in bleeding complications and strokes. The superiority of primary angioplasty to thrombolytic therapy is particularly evident in higher-risk patients such as diabetics and the elderly. The use of primary stenting versus primary angioplasty does not result in a mortality advantage, but correlates well with a reduced need for subsequent target vessel revascularization. A meta-analysis of trials comparing primary stenting with angioplasty found little difference in the rates of death (3.7% vs. 3.6%) or recurrent MI (2.1% vs. 2.9%).

Libby P, Bonow RO, Mann DL, et al. *Braunwald's Heart Disease: A Textbook of Cardiovascular Medicine.* 8th ed. Philadelphia, PA: Saunders/Elsevier; 2008:1301-1303, 1308.

15. **The answer is A**. Certain high-risk intracranial carcinomas such as **M**elanoma, **R**enal cell cancer, **C**horiocarcinoma, and **T**hyroid cancer (MR-CT) are contraindications to systemic anti-coagulation and systemic thrombolysis due to high risk of intracranial hemorrhage. Inferior vena cava filter placement is indicated for treatment of pulmonary embolism when anticoagulation is not possible; although anticoagulation in some cases is controversial and should be started once a reversible contraindication has resolved.

   Alvarado G, Noor R, Bassett R, et al. Risk of intracranial hemorrhage with anticoagulation therapy in melanoma patients with brain metastases. *Melanoma Res.* 2012;22:310-315. doi: 10.1097/CMR.0b013e328353efd8

16. **The answer is D**. This patient presented with an acute ischemic stroke. MRI demonstrates a left subcortical ischemic infarct. In such patients, perfusion pressure distal to the obstructed vessel is low, and compensatory vasodilation occurs to maintain adequate blood flow. A high systemic pressure is required to maintain blood flow in these dilated vessels. Therefore, in patients with ischemic stroke, BP should be carefully observed for 1 to 2 hours to see whether it will spontaneously decrease. A persistent elevation in MAP above 130 mmHg or systolic blood pressure (SBP) above 220 mmHg should be carefully treated with an aim to lower the MAP by 15% to 20%. Rapid reduction in BP may compromise the cerebral perfusion and worsen ischemia.

   Lisk DR, Grotta JC, Lamki LM, et al. Should hypertension be treated after acute stroke? A randomized controlled trial using single photon emission computed tomography. *Arch Neurol.* 1993;50:855-862. doi:10.1001/archneur.1993.00540080060015

17. **The answer is C**. Pulsus paradoxus is the most sensitive, although not specific, physical finding that suggests cardiac tamponade. Pulsus paradoxus is not related to pulse rate, and represents a decrease in the systolic blood pressure (SBP) of more than 10 mmHg with inspiration. Pulsus paradoxus can be seen in multiple conditions including tamponade, obstructive lung disease, and chronic sleep apnea. On the other hand, pulsus pardoxus may be absent in patients with chronic hypertension and elevated ventricular diastolic pressures, as well as prior atrial septal defect. Systemic arterial hypotension, elevated jugular venous pressure, muffled heart sounds, and tachycardia are the physical findings associated with cardiac tamponade, but are neither sensitive nor specific.

   Libby P, Bonow RO, Mann DL, et al. *Braunwald's Heart Disease: A Textbook of Cardiovascular Medicine.* 8th ed. Philadelphia, PA: Saunders/Elsevier; 2008:1835-1838.

18. **The answer is C**. Data support the use of cardiac biomarkers to estimate prognosis and infarct size. The GUSTO-III trial of over 12,000 patients showed that 16% of patients with an elevated cardiac TnT had died within 30 days compared with 6% of those without an enzyme leak. A recent meta-analysis of patients with non–ST-segment elevation myocardial infarction (NSTEMI) suggested that patients with elevated cardiac troponins had a greater than three-fold increase of death compared with those with a normal value. Troponins are more specific to cardiac muscle, whereas CK-MB can rise in skeletal muscle damage as well. One-third of patients with acute myocardial infarction (MI) have an elevated cTnT despite a normal CK-MB. Myoglobin, although fast in detecting damage, is not sensitive. BNP and MMP are newer markers correlating with muscle damage and plaque rupture, but will need further studies for determining their effects on prognosis.

   Murphy JG, Lloyd MA. *Mayo Clinic Cardiology: Concise Textbook.* 3rd ed. Boca Raton, FL: Informa Healthcare; 2006:776.

19. **The answer is A**. Onset of heparin-induced thrombocytopenia (HIT) is typically within 24 hours of heparin administration when there is a history of previous heparin exposure, but is otherwise seen in 5 to 14 days when there is no history of previous heparin exposure. Current recommendations from the American College of Chest Physicians (ACCP) for HIT include discontinuation of heparin, avoidance of low-molecular-weight heparin (LMWH), and immediate initiation of an alternative parenteral anticoagulant such as bivalirudin or argatroban.

When warfarin has been coadministered with heparin, the ACCP recommends administration of vitamin K to prevent potential venous limb gangrene associated with protein C deficiency. Coumadin should not be resumed until platelet count has risen to greater than 150,000.

Kearon C, Akl EA, Ornelas J, et al. Antithrombotic therapy for VTE disease: CHEST guideline and expert panel report. *Chest*. 2016;149(2):315-352. doi:10.1016/j.chest.2015.11.026

20. **The answer is B.** The patient is suffering from high-altitude pulmonary edema (HAPE), which is a form of noncardiogenic pulmonary edema. HAPE can result from a rapid ascension in altitude without proper acclimatization. The mainstay of treatment is descent for anything other than mild symptoms. Oxygen is life-saving and should be given at 4 L/min for 4 to 6 hours. In addition to oxygen, nifedipine, acetazolamide, and portable hyperbaric chambers are all beneficial therapies. Nifedipine is thought to work by dilating the pulmonary vasculature, reducing hydrostatic pressures, and subsequent edema in the lungs. Acetazolamide is shown to accelerate acclimatization and acts as a stimulant to induce breathing. Portable hyperbaric chambers are widely used among climbing expeditions and quickly flush carbon dioxide from the system. Diuretics are not advised, or should be used with substantial caution in patients with HAPE since many are already depleted intravascularly and can clinically deteriorate.

Hackett PH, Rennie IDB. High altitude pulmonary edema. *JAMA*. 2002;287(17):2275-2278. doi:10.4103/0019-5278.107066

21. **The answer is A**. This patient has hypertensive urgency. Hypertensive urgency is severe elevation of BP (>180/120 mmHg) without any evidence of end-organ damage. This patient's only symptom is headache; there is no evidence of papilledema and no evidence of cardiac, neurological, or renal complications. In general, hypertensive urgency can be managed using oral antihypertensive agents in an observation setting or outpatient setting with close follow-up. Excessive and rapid reduction in BP should be avoided to prevent hypotension and compromising the cerebral perfusion.

Lipsitz LA, Gagnon M, Vyas M, et al. Antihypertensive therapy increases cerebral blood flow and carotid distensibility in hypertensive elderly subjects. *Hypertension*. 2005;45(2):216-221. doi: 10.1161/01.HYP.0000153094.09615.11
Marik PE, Varon J. Hypertensive crises: challenges and management. *Chest*. 2007;131(6):1949-1962. doi:10.1378/chest.06-2490

22. **The answer is B**. TENS is the use of electric current produced by a device to stimulate the nerves for therapeutic purposes. It covers the complete range of transcutaneously applied currents used for nerve excitation, although more specifically the unit encompasses a stimulator that produces pulses to treat pain. It is usually connected to the skin using two or more electrodes. A typical battery-operated TENS unit is able to modulate pulse width, frequency, and intensity. Generally TENS is applied at high frequency (>50 Hz) with intensity below motor contraction (sensory intensity) or at low frequency (<10 Hz) with intensity that produces motor contraction. According to the Heart Rhythm Society (HRS)/American Society of Anesthesiologists (ASA) Expert Consensus Statement on the Perioperative Management of Patients with Implantable Defibrillators, Pacemakers and Arrhythmia Monitors: Facilities and Patient Management, the use of TENS units is not recommended in patients with CIEDs. TENS can interfere with PM and implantable cardioverter-defibrillator (ICD) function. Adverse responses include inhibition of pacing (or triggering noise reversion mode) and inappropriate ICD therapy due to misinterpreted electrical noise. The transcutaneous impulses could also be misinterpreted as inappropriate supraventricular arrhythmia in atrial tachycardia devices. High-frequency stimulation (>30 Hz) should be maintained at all times. TENS units should be avoided in the thoracic spine, cervical spine, shoulder, upper lumbar, and chest areas because of the proximity of the ICD or PM and lead system. These recommendations generally extend to spinal cord stimulators as well.

Crossley GH, Poole JE, Rozner MA, et al. The Heart Rhythm Society (HRS)/American Society of Anesthesiologists (ASA) Expert Consensus Statement on the perioperative management of patients with implantable defibrillators, pacemakers and arrhythmia monitors: facilities and patient management. *Heart Rhythm*. 2011;8(7):1114-1154. doi:10.1016/j.hrthm.2011.05.010

23. **The answer is D**. Severe uncontrolled hypertension on presentation (SBP >180 mmHg or DBP >110 mmHg) is a relative contraindication for fibrinolytic therapy; however, it could be an absolute contraindication in low-risk patients with MI. Lowering the blood pressure (BP) to levels less than 180/110 mmHg will enable the physician to administer fibrinolytic therapy, but catheter-based reperfusion methods would be preferred if available. All the other choices are absolute contraindications to fibrinolytic therapy, and in addition to those mentioned previously, known structural vascular lesion (e.g., atrioventricular [AV] malformation), ischemic stroke within 3 months except acute ischemic stroke within 4.5 hours, active bleeding, or bleeding diathesis are also contraindications to fibrinolytic therapy.

Willerson J, Cohn JN, Wellens HJJ, et al. *Textbook of Cardiovascular Medicine*. 3rd ed. London, UK: Springer Verlag; 2007:966.

24. **The answer is D**. The CI is derived by dividing the patient's CO by the patient's body surface area (BSA):

$$CI = CO/BSA$$

CO is calculated by multiplying the patient's stroke volume (SV) by the heart rate (HR). Therefore, $CI = (SV \times HR)/BSA$

Normal values for the CI range from 2.6 to 4.2 L/min/m². Cardiogenic shock results in a low CI (<1.8 L/min/m²). The remaining answer choices all define the presence of cardiac shock and provide clinical clues that the patient is unstable and needs additional hemodynamic support.

Libby P, Bonow RO, Mann DL, et al. *Braunwald's Heart Disease: A Textbook of Cardiovascular Medicine*. 8th ed. Philadelphia, PA: Saunders/Elsevier; 2008:1269.
Willerson JT, Cohn JN, Wellens HJJ, et al. *Cardiovascular Medicine*. 3rd ed. New York, NY: Springer-Verlag; 2007:464.

25. **The answer is E**. Approximately 15% to 30% of all patients with heart failure and moderate to severe symptoms have inter- and intraventricular conduction delays with QRS duration greater than 120 milliseconds. This results in mechanical dyssynchrony of right and left ventricular contractions. Furthermore, prolonged conduction has been associated with adverse outcomes. In a large study conducted in Italy involving more than 5,500 patients, a left bundle branch block (LBBB) was associated with an increased 1-year mortality from any cause (hazard ratio, 1.70; 95% confidence interval, 1.41–2.05). LBBB was also associated with an increased 1-year mortality rate from sudden death (hazard ratio, 1.58; 95% confidence interval, 1.21–2.06). Multivariate analysis showed that this increased risk of death due to LBBB was still significant even after adjusting for age, underlying cardiac disease, other indicators of heart failure severity, and prescription of angiotensin-converting enzyme (ACE) inhibitors. A subgroup analysis from the vesnarinone study (VEST) assessed the relationship between QRS duration and mortality. In this analysis, 3,654 resting baseline ECGs of patients with heart failure (New York Heart Association [NYHA] Class II to IV) were digitally scanned. Age, creatinine, left ventricular ejection fraction (LVEF), heart rate, and QRS duration were found to be independent predictors of mortality ($p <.0001$). Patients with wider QRS durations (>200 milliseconds) had a five times greater risk of death than those with narrow QRS durations (<90 milliseconds). On the basis of this finding, the authors concluded that the resting ECG is a powerful, accessible, and inexpensive marker of prognosis in dilated cardiomyopathy.

Saxon LA, DeMarco T, Prystowsky EN, et al. Effects of long-term biventricular stimulation for resynchronization on echocardiographic measures of remodeling. *Circulation*. 2002;105: 1304-1310. doi:10.1161/hc1102.105730

26. **The answer is B**. Malignant pericardial disease is the most common cause of cardiac tamponade in developed countries. Lung carcinoma is the most common, accounting for about 40%

of malignant effusions; breast carcinoma and lymphomas are responsible for about another 40%. In most cancer patients with effusions, it is important that metastatic involvement of the pericardium be confirmed by identification of malignant cells or tumor markers in pericardial fluid.

Little WC, Freeman GL. Pericardial disease. *Circulation.* 2006;113(12):1622-1632. doi:10.1161/CIRCULATIONAHA.105.561514

Spodick DM. Acute cardiac tamponade. *N Engl J Med.* 2003;349:684. doi:10.1056/NEJMra022643

27. **The answer is A**. The posterior papillary muscle is more susceptible to ischemia than the anterior papillary muscle because of the nature of vascularization. The posterior muscle has one blood supply (posterior descending branch of the right coronary artery), whereas the anterior papillary muscle has dual blood supply (diagonal branches of the left anterior descending artery and marginal branches of the circumflex artery). The clinical picture here does not fit a ruptured papillary muscle scenario because the ruptured papillary muscle would cause a graver situation resulting in pulmonary edema. Ventricular septal defect is also a mechanical complication of MI; however, the physical examination findings are not compatible, and a sternal holosystolic murmur would be heard. Tricuspid regurgitation and aortic stenosis are not complications of MI.

Birnbaum Y, Chamoun AJ, Conti VR, et al. Mitral regurgitation following acute myocardial infarction. *Coron Artery Dis.* 2002;13(6):337-344. doi:10.1097/00019501-200209000-00006

28. **The answer is C**. Amiodarone is a complex pharmacological agent with multiple adverse effects on multiple organ systems. Owing to its prolonged half-life (~100 days), organ toxicity is potentially more severe and more difficult to manage. The more common effects include a decrease in the diffusing capacity of the lung for carbon monoxide (DLCO), interstitial pneumonitis, thyroid abnormalities, and photophobia, which can be seen in 15% to 60% of patients. Neurological effects are typically dose dependent. These include ataxia, tremors, and neuropathy with an incidence of 3% to 30%. Adjusting the dose results in resolution of symptoms. Skin effects include photosensitivity and discoloration, which may occur in 75% of patients. These can be managed with reassurance and sun block. Ocular effects such as halo vision and optic neuritis can be noted in up to 5% of cases, with incidence of photophobia being as high as 80%. Reassurance is recommended, although the medication needs to be discontinued if optic neuritis (ON) occurs. Adverse cardiac reactions are uncommon. Although prolongation of QT is expected, torsades de pointes is noted in less than 1% of patients. Ventricular systolic function is not compromised.

Goldschlager N, Epstein AE, Naccarelli GV, et al. A practical guide for clinicians who treat patients with amiodarone: 2007. *Heart Rhythm.* 2007;4(9):1250-1259. doi:10.1016/j.hrthm.2007.07.020

29. **The answer is E**. Selection of catheter ablation for an individual patient should consider risks and benefits that are determined by patient characteristics, as well as the availability of appropriate facilities with technical expertise. In patients with structural heart disease, episodes of sustained VT are a marker for increased mortality; with reduced quality of life in patients who have implanted defibrillators and structural heart disease. Antiarrhythmic medications can reduce the frequency of implantable cardioverter-defibrillator (ICD) therapies, but have disappointing efficacy and side effects. In the past, ablation was often not considered until pharmacological options had been exhausted, often after the patient had suffered substantial morbidity from recurrent episodes of VT and ICD shocks. However, since the release of data of the SMASH-VT trial, the general approach is changing. Contraindications to this procedure include the following:

   i. Presence of a mobile ventricular thrombus (epicardial ablation may be considered)

   ii. Asymptomatic premature ventricular complex (PVC) and/or nonsustained VT that are not suspected of causing or contributing to ventricular dysfunction

   iii. VT due to transient, reversible causes, such as acute ischemia, hyperkalemia, or drug-induced torsade de pointes.

Aliot EM, Stevenson WG, Almendral-Garrote JM, et al. EHRA/HRS Expert Consensus on Catheter Ablation of Ventricular Arrhythmias: developed in a partnership with the European Heart Rhythm Association (EHRA), a registered branch of the European Society of Cardiology (ESC), and the Heart Rhythm Society (HRS); in collaboration with the American College of Cardiology (ACC) and the American Heart Association (AHA). *Heart Rhythm.* 2009;6(6):886-933. doi:10.1016/j.hrthm.2009.04.030

30. **The answer is B.** HR is a clear determinant of COO (CO = HR × stroke volume [SV]) except when myocardial efficiency is altered by various dysrhythmias. The other determinants of CO are the following:

    i. *Afterload (impedance):* usually estimated by the equation for systemic vascular resistance index (SVRI):

    $$SVRI = 80\,(MAP - CVP)/CI$$

    where MAP, mean arterial pressure; CVP, central venous pressure; and CI, cardiac index (CI = CO/BSA)

    ii. *Contractility:* usually measured in the ICU as the ejection fraction (EF) obtained by echocardiography. Other measures such as the dp/dt (defined as rate of rise in left ventricular pressure during systole) may be more accurate, but are not readily available at bedside. Another estimate of contractility is left ventricular stroke work index (LVSWI) as work done during systole. This parameter requires a pulmonary artery catheter (PAC) and is calculated as:

    $$LVSWI = 0.0136\,(MAP - PCWP) \times SVI$$

    where PCWP, pulmonary capillary wedge pressure; and SVI, stroke volume index (=CI/HR)

    iii. *Preload:* the volume of blood returning to the heart per minute, best measured as the left ventricular end-diastolic volume (LVEDV). This volume has traditionally been estimated using the PCWP corresponding to the left atrial pressure and thereby left ventricular end-diastolic pressure (LVEDP). For a pressure to represent a volume, especially when trended overtime, their relationship (DV/DP, LV compliance) must be constant. However, this relationship does not remain constant particularly during sepsis, hypertension, or coronary artery–induced myocardial dysfunction. In addition, changes in intrathoracic pressure that affect venous return during mechanical ventilation make interpretation of these pressures more difficult. Altogether, defining preload is frequently imprecise at bedside.

Kruse JA. Hemodynamic monitoring. In: Kruse JA, Fink MP, Carlson RW, eds. *Saunders Manual of Critical Care.* Philadelphia, PA: Saunders; 2003:774-777.

Oren-Grinberg A, Lerner AB, Talmor D. Echocardiography in the intensive care unit. In: Irwin RS, Rippe JM, eds. *Intensive Care Medicine.* 6th ed. Philadelphia, PA: Wolters Kluwer/Lippincott Williams & Wilkins; 2008:289-302.

31. **The answer is C.** This is a fundamental equation in many aspects of physiology and is modified for cardiovascular physiology as:

    Blood pressure = Cardiac output (L/min) × Systemic vascular resistance

    The equation highlights the interdependency of cardiac output and changes in vascular constriction to maintain blood pressure.

Libby P, Bonow RO, Mann DL, et al. *Braunwald's Heart Disease: A Textbook of Cardiovascular Medicine.* 8th ed. Philadelphia, PA: Saunders/Elsevier; 2008:1269.

32. **The answer is E.** The arterial O_2 content (C_aO_2) is measured in oxygenated blood taken from the pulmonary vein or aorta and is determined by the equation:

    $$C_aC_2 = (\text{Hemoglobin} \times 1.36 \times S_aO_2) + (P_aO_2 \times 0.003)$$

The number 1.36 represents the fact that each gram of hemoglobin can carry 1.36 mL of O_2; 0.003 is the solubility coefficient of oxygen in blood. C_aO_2 is normally 18 to 20 mL O_2/100 mL blood)

Oxygen delivery ($D.O_2$) is the volume of O_2 (ml O_2/dL blood) delivered to the tissue per minute by the cardiac output (CO in L/min):

$$D.O_2 = C_aO_2 \times CO \times 10 \,(\text{Normal}: 900 - 1,100 \text{ mL } O_2/\text{L blood/min})$$

As oxygen is delivered to body tissues, some is consumed and some returns to the right atrium via the superior and inferior venae cavae. The residual venous O_2 in the caval streams do not mix fully until both enter the right ventricle and the pulmonary ("mixed venous O_2"). The O_2 content of the mixed venous blood (C_vO_2) is calculated similar to C_aO_2 from blood aspirated from a pulmonary artery catheter:

$$C_vO_2 = (\text{Hgb} \times 1.36 \times S_vO_2) + (P_vO_2 \times .003)\,(\text{Normal}: \sim 15 \text{ mL/dL})$$

Arteriovenous O_2 difference ($C_{a-v}O_2$) reflects the amount of O_2 taken up by the tissues:

$$C_{a-v}O_2 = C_aO_2 - C_vO_2 \,(\text{Normal}: 3.6 - 5.0 \text{ mL/dL})$$

The amount of oxygen consumed ($V.O_2$) by the whole body can therefore be calculated as the difference between what was delivered (C_aO_2) and what remained in the circulation within mixed venous blood (C_vO_2) adjusted by the CO:

$$V.O_2 = C_{a-v}O_2 \times CO \times 10$$

$$V.O_2 = (C_aO_2 - C_vO_2) \times CO \times 10 \,(\text{Normal}: 200 - 300 \text{ mL/min})$$

To compare patients of different body habitus, the above mentioned values can also be indexed by dividing the parameter by the patient's body surface area (BSA). For instance, normal $D.O_2$ Index is 530 to 600 mL/min/m^2; and $V.O_2$ Index in healthy subjects can be estimated as 125 mL/min/m^2 of BSA in women, 140 mL/min/m^2 of BSA in men, and 110 mL/min/m^2 of BSA in the elderly.

The oxygen extraction ratio (O_2ER) is another important variable that provides perspective on the fraction or percentage of O_2 delivered ($D.O_2$) that is used by the body ($V.O_2$) during normal or stressed metabolism:

$$O_2\text{ER} = V.O_2/D.O_2 = (C_aO_2 - C_vO_2)/C_aO_2 \,(\text{Normal}: 0.22 - 0.28)$$

O_2ER may appear to be reduced by anatomic arteriovenous connections such as in liver disease or may actually be reduced when mitochondrial oxygen uptake is inhibited in sepsis or cyanide poisoning.

During hypoperfusion, blood flow through tissue capillaries becomes slower and allows for increased O_2ER to compensate for reduced delivery. Therefore, as cardiac output falls, more arterial O_2 is removed leading to decreased venous content of O_2 (C_vO_2). This in turn results in decreased S_vO_2. On the other hand, during conditions such as sepsis that reduce oxygen uptake by mitochondria, more O_2 remains in the venous blood resulting in S_vO_2 rise. Similarly, in patients with therapeutic or pathophysiological arteriovenous shunts, S_vO_2 rises. Accordingly trending the S_vO_2 can provide insight into O_2 delivery and consumption.

As explained previously, it is possible and clinically important to compare oxygen supply to oxygen consumed by the entire body. Organ-specific demand/supply relationships would also be important, but are usually difficult to assess unless the specific arteries to and veins from individual organs are cannulated. Because of the unique isolated anatomy of the brain, its supply and consumption have been explored using arterial oxygen delivery and venous return obtained from the jugular vein.

Cheatham ML, Block EFJ, Promes JT, et al. Shock: an overview. In: Irwin RS, Rippe JM, eds. *Intensive Care Medicine*. 6th ed. Philadelphia, PA: Wolters Kluwer/Lippincott Williams & Wilkins; 2008:1831-1842.

33. **The answer is B.** Mixed venous samples are processed via a blood gas analyzer as an arterial specimen. Care must be taken that blood is not drawn too quickly from the PAC, because oxygenated blood may be pulled backward through the capillary and cause an erroneous elevation in the P_vO_2 from which the S_vO_2 is abstracted.

Putterman C. The Swan-Ganz catheter: a decade of hemodynamic monitoring. *J Crit Care.* 1989;4:127. doi:10.1016/0883-9441(89)90128-7

Swan HJ, Ganz W, Forrester J, et al. Catheterization of the heart in man with use of a flow-directed balloon-tipped catheter. *N Engl J Med.* 1970;283:447. doi:10.1056/NEJM197008272830902

34. **The answer is A.** Contractility is one of the four determinants of cardiac output. Left ventricular stroke work has been used as an estimate of contractility and reflects work done by the left ventricle to overcome outflow impedance. Contractility is difficult to quantify in the ICU setting because of its interdependence with preload, afterload, and heart rate (HR). The EF (normal: >55%–60%) obtained by echocardiography is most often used clinically.

Contractility is abnormal in several neurological conditions associated with large amounts of catecholamine release from the brain. "Myocardial stunning" or stress-induced cardiomyopathy, evidenced by decreased contractility, is documented in several central nervous system (CNS) insults such as subarachnoid hemorrhage (SAH) and particularly during the evolution of brain death in some patients. This pattern appears similar to the Takotsubo cardiomyopathy documented in patients with pheochromocytoma and other syndromes associated with high catecholamine release.

Nykamp D, Titak JA. Takotsubo cardiomyopathy, or broken-heart syndrome. *Ann Pharmacother.* 2010;44(3):590-593. doi:10.1345/aph.1M568

35. **The answer is C.** Injection of a known quantity of injectate at a known temperature into a flowing bloodstream also of known temperature induces a temporary temperature change in the pulmonary artery blood as it passes a temperature sensor (thermistor) a known distance from the site of injection. The Stewart–Hamilton equation to determine the cardiac output from this thermodilution method is

$$CO = [60 \times V_i \times C_i \times S_i \times K_{cal} \times K_{cor} \times (T_b - T_i)] / [C_b \times S_b \times \int \Delta Tb\,(t)\,dt]$$

where V_i, injectate volume (mL); C_i and C_b, specific heats of injectate and blood (constants); K_{cal}, calibration constant; S_i and S_b, specific gravity of injectate and blood (constants); K_{cor}, temperature loss constant; T_b and T_i, baseline blood and injectate temperatures; integral term, area under thermal curve of temperature change versus time.

Continuous cardiac output pulmonary artery catheters (PACs) use similar changes in pulmonary blood temperature, but instead generate a burst of heat (not cold) into the bloodstream, and the change in blood temperature is sensed along a thermistor filament within the catheter.

Kruse JA. Hemodynamic monitoring. In: Kruse JA, Fink MP, Carlson RW, eds. *Saunders Manual of Critical Care.* Philadelphia, PA: Saunders; 2003:774-777.

36. **The answer is A.** Normal mixed venous oxygen tension (P_vO_2) is approximately 40 mmHg. Abnormal P_vO_2, either below or above normal, will help evaluate the predominant abnormality in cardiovascular performance or oxygen debt (when O_2 delivery does not meet the demand). Because blood gas analyzers do not directly measure the S_aO_2 or S_vO_2, as does an oximeter or CO-oximeter, it is useful to ensure that the saturation (venous or arterial) presented by the blood gas analyzer is consistent with the measured P_aO_2 or P_vO_2. The extrapolation from partial pressure to saturation is reflection of the oxyhemoglobin dissociation curve. The "30-60-90" guideline is a useful rule of thumb describing Hgb-association parameters: at a P_aO_2 or P_vO_2 of 30 mmHg, there is 60% Hgb saturation, and at P_aO_2 or P_vO_2 of 60 mmHg, Hgb is 90% saturated.

Cheatham ML, Block EFJ, Promes JT, et al. Shock: an overview. In: Irwin RS, Rippe JM, eds. *Intensive Care Medicine.* 6th ed. Philadelphia, PA: Wolters Kluwer/Lippincott Williams & Wilkins; 2008:1831-1842.

37. **The answer is B.** The intention of the pulmonary artery wedge (or occlusion) pressure (PAWP) is used to evaluate cardiac preload. Preload corresponds to the LVEDV but the PAWP corresponds to the left atrial *pressure* and thereby left ventricular end-diastolic pressure (LVEDP). A direct conversion of pressure to volume is not possible. In addition, in order to use the relative trend in their values over time, their relationship (diastolic volume / diastolic pressure or left ventricular compliance) must be constant and normal. However, left ventricular compliance changes over short periods of time. Besides, conditions such as myocardial dysfunction induced by coronary artery disease (CAD), hypertension, diabetes, cardiomyopathies, and sepsis alter diastolic relaxation and compliance of the left ventricle. In this situation, a smaller volume in the stiffer left ventricle leads to an elevated wedge pressure. Therefore, application of PAWP to measure preload in the ICU setting has to be approached cautiously.

Cheatham ML, Block EFJ, Promes JT, et al. Shock: an overview. In: Irwin RS, Rippe JM, eds. *Intensive Care Medicine*. 6th ed. Philadelphia, PA: Wolters Kluwer/Lippincott Williams & Wilkins; 2008:1831-1842.

Mendoza DD, Codella NC, Wang Y, et al. Impact of diastolic dysfunction severity on global left ventricular volumetric filling—assessment by automated segmentation of routine cine cardiovascular magnetic resonance. *J Cardiovasc Magn Reson*. 2010;12:46. doi:10.1186/1532-429X-12-46

Ogunyankin KO. Assessment of left ventricular diastolic function: the power, possibilities, and pitfalls of echocardiographic imaging techniques. *Can J Cardiol*. 2011;27(3):311-318. doi:10.1016/j.cjca.2010.12.042

38. **The answer is D.** Shunt fraction is ratio of the blood "shunted" (Q_s) to the total blood (Q_t or cardiac output) and is calculated using the following formula:

$$Q_s/Q_t = (C_cO_2 - C_aO_2)/(C_cO_2 - C_vO_2)$$

where:

C_cO_2 = End-pulmonary-capillary oxygen content

C_aO_2 = Arterial oxygen content

C_vO_2 = Mixed venous oxygen content

The O_2 content of arterial (C_aO_2) and mixed venous blood (C_vO_2) are measured in blood taken from the pulmonary vein and artery, respectively, using PAC by the following equation:

$$C_aO_2 = (Hemoglobin \times 1.36 \times S_aO_2) + (P_aO_2 \times 0.003)$$

$$C_vO_2 = (Hgb \times 1.36 \times S_vO_2) + (P_vO_2 \times 0.003)$$

The number 1.36 represents the fact that each gram of hemoglobin can carry 1.36 mL of O_2; 0.003 is the solubility coefficient of oxygen in blood.

The C_cO_2 represents the capillary oxygen content of an idealized "perfect" alveolus adjacent to a "perfect" capillary. This value, of course, is not measurable, but utilizes the P_AO_2 in the standard content equation:

$$C_cO_2 = (Hgb \times 1.36 \times S_{PA}O_2) + (0.003 \times P_AO_2)$$

$$Where\ P_AO_2 = (P_BO_2 - 47) \times FiO_2 - (1.25 \times PaCO_2)$$

Normal shunt (QS/QT) is up to 0.08 or 8%.

Cheatham ML, Block EFJ, Promes JT, et al. Shock: an overview. In: Irwin RS, Rippe JM, eds. *Intensive Care Medicine*. 6th ed. Philadelphia, PA: Wolters Kluwer/Lippincott Williams & Wilkins; 2008:1831-1842.

39. **The answer is A.** Variability in the arterial pulse pressure (systolic–diastolic pressure), stroke volume (SV), systolic pressure, and preload are caused by cyclic variation in intrathoracic pressure during mechanical ventilation. Several "minimally invasive" devices (e.g., FloTrac, PiCCO, and LiDCO) derive cardiac output (CO) from arterial pressure waveform contour

and power analysis, and include an analysis of the pulse pressure, SV, and systolic pressure variabilities. When the calculated arterial pulse pressure variability reaches a particular magnitude (10%–13%), the manufacturer recommends rapid fluid administration to improve cardiovascular instability.

Marik PE, Cavallazzi R, Vasu T, et al. Dynamic changes in arterial waveform derived variables and fluid responsiveness in mechanically ventilated patients: a systematic review of the literature. *Crit Care Med*. 2009;37(9):2642-2647. doi:10.1097/CCM.0b013e3181a590da

Powner DJ, Hergenroeder GW. Measurement of cardiac output during adult donor care. *Prog Transplant*. 2011;21(2):144-150. doi:10.1177/152692481102100210

40. **The answer is C.** Characteristics of the arterial pressure waveform are used to derive SV. CO is then calculated from CO = SV × heart rate (HR). The devices (e.g., FloTrac, LiDCO, PiCCO, and others) that utilize this technology and proprietary algorithms calculate CO from the equation:

$$SV = (\int dp/dt)/Z$$

where Z, aortic impedance; $\int dp/dt$, integral of changing pressure over time during systole.

Correlation with thermodilution methods for CO measurement is 0.88 to 0.91, but data are controversial among some patient groups wherein algorithms used in the devices may apply less well.

Cecconi M, Dawson D, Casaretti R, et al. A prospective study of the accuracy and precision of continuous cardiac output monitoring devices as compared to intermittent thermodilution. *Minerva Anestesiol*. 2010;76(12):1010-1017. doi:10.1093/bja/aew461

de Waal EE, Wappler F, Buhre WF. Cardiac output monitoring. *Curr Opin Anaesthesiol*. 2009;22(1):71-77. doi:10.1097/ACO.0b013e32831f44d0

Marik PE, Cavallazzi R, Vasu T, et al. Dynamic changes in arterial waveform derived variables and fluid responsiveness in mechanically ventilated patients: a systematic review of the literature. *Crit Care Med*. 2009;37(9):2642-2647. doi:10.1097/CCM.0b013e3181a590da

Powner DJ, Hergenroeder GW. Measurement of cardiac output during adult donor care. *Prog Transplant*. 2011;21(2):144-150. doi:10.1177/152692481102100210

41. **The answer is E.** Substitution of the percentage oxygen saturation from central venous blood $(S_{cv}O_2)$ for the true mixed venous blood (S_vO_2) from the pulmonary artery was initially proposed within the treatment protocol for septic patients in the ED. Review of this utilization among several patient groups with other diagnoses shows a variable correlation between the two measures. Proponents of the substitution suggest that an $S_{cv}O_2$ above 70% indicates that ongoing treatment is safe and likely meets tissue oxygen delivery needs. Utilization of the $S_{cv}O_2$ during titrated neurocritical care, however, remains poorly defined.

Giraud R, Siegenthaler N, Gayet-Ageron A, et al. ScvO(2) as a marker to define fluid responsiveness. *J Trauma*. 2011;70(4):802-807. doi:10.1097/TA.0b013e3181e7d649

Ho KM, Harding R, Chamberlain J, et al. A comparison of central and mixed venous oxygen saturation in circulatory failure. *J Cardiothorac Vasc Anesth*. 2010;24(3):434-439. doi:10.1053/j.jvca.2007.10.011

Powner DJ, Doshi PB. Central venous oxygen saturation monitoring: role in adult donor care? *Prog Transplant*. 2010;20(4):401-405. doi:10.1177/152692481002000414

Rivers E, Nguyen B, Havstad S, et al. Early goal-directed therapy in the treatment of severe sepsis and septic shock. *N Engl J Med*. 2001;345(19):1368-1377. doi:10.1056/NEJMoa010307

42. **The answer is C.** Idarucizumab is a monoclonal antibody that binds specifically to dabigatran and its metabolites with an affinity of ~350 times greater than thrombin. The use of idarucizumab was examined in the REsynchronization reVErses Remodeling in Systolic Left vEntricular dysfunction (REVERSE) study. In patients at imminent risk of death idarucizumab is the recommended reversal agent. Onset of action is within minutes with duration of effect up to 24 hours. In patients with rebound bleeding a second dose of 5 g can be administered. Combination of idarucizumab with PCC is not recommended due to the increased prothrombotic risk. If idarucizumab is not available then PCC, preferably factor eight inhibitor bypassing activity, at a dose of 50 to 80 units/kg should be administered. Tranexamic acid can be used

for patients with major bleeding; however, it is not the preferred first agent. It can be used in combination with other agents. In cases of potential overdose oral activated charcoal should be administered to remove the unabsorbed drug.

Frontera JA, Lewin JJ, Rabinstein AA, et al. Guideline for reversal of antithrombotics in intracranial hemorrhage: a statement for healthcare professionals from the Neurocritical Care Society and Society of Critical Care Medicine. *Neurocrit Care.* 2016;24:6. doi:10.1007/s12028-015-0222-x

43. **The answer is A:** Bedside echocardiography should be obtained immediately to rule out postoperative complications. Cardiac perforation is a rare complication with incidence of 0.1% to 0.4%. Presence of a pericardial effusion can lead to cardiac chamber collapse during diastole, most commonly the right. Left atrial collapse, if seen, is highly specific for tamponade. Tachycardia and low-voltage ECG can suggest pericardial effusion but is nonspecific. CT chest would demonstrate the effusion; however, it would not identify tamponade.

Adler Y, Charron P, Imazio M, et al. 2015 ESC Guidelines for the diagnosis and management of pericardial diseases: The Task Force for the Diagnosis and Management of Pericardial Diseases of the European Society of Cardiology. *Eur Heart J.* 2015;36(42):2921-2964. doi:10.1093/eurheartj/ehv318

Spodick DH. Acute cardiac tamponade. *N Engl J Med.* 2003;349(7):684-690. doi:10.1056/NEJMra022643

44. **The answer is C.** High normal CI (normal 2.5–4 L/min/m^2), PCWP (normal 6–12 mmHg), and RV pressures suggest preserved cardiac function. Of note, the ability to achieve a higher CI can be blunted by the recent myocardial infarction (MI). Also, a mean PAP of 18 mmHg suggests no underlying pulmonary hypertension (mean PAP >25 mmHg at rest and >30 mmHg with exercise). On the other hand, a low S_vO_2 in conjunction with low SVR is suggestive of distributive (septic) shock.

In patients with septic shock and relatively preserved cardiac function, norepinephrine is the vasopressor drug of choice. Dopamine can be used for treatment of shock if associated with bradycardia; however, in comparison to norepinephrine, dopamine causes more cardiac arrhythmias without a mortality benefit. Milrinone increased cardiac output through inotropy as well as reduction in afterload; patients often develop worsening tachycardia which may be arrhythmogenic in a patient with recent MI. Dobutamine can be considered as an add-on agent if the patient were to develop worsening cardiac output.

De Backer D, Biston P, Devriendt J, et al. Comparison of dopamine and norepinephrine in the treatment of shock. *N Engl J Med.* 2010;362:779-789. doi:10.1056/NEJMoa0907118

45. **The answer is E.** VV ECMO should be considered in patients with severe acute respiratory distress syndrome (ARDS) not responsive to conventional therapy. The CESAR trial demonstrated improved 6-month mortality; however, its results cannot definitively be extrapolated to all healthcare scenarios. A significant portion of patients was noted to not be following conventional ventilator protocols prior to transfer. The authors were able to conclude that referral to an ECMO-capable center resulted in improved 6-month survival without disability. Data regarding the use of inhaled prostaglandins are limited. Though there is some improvement in oxygenation and a reduction in pulmonary artery pressure, a morbidity or mortality benefit has not been shown. Recruitment maneuvers are often used in severe ARDS, with the method and application being variable. A recent study investigated a strategy of escalating PEEP (25 cm H_2O for 1 minute, then 35 cm H_2O for 1 minute, and then 45 cm H_2O for 2 minutes) followed by a gradual reduction in PEEP to the best compliance with an additional 2 cm H_2O of PEEP at this level. The recruitment maneuver group was found to have a higher mortality during the first 7 days (31.9% vs. 25.5%, *p* value .03) with an increased rate of death with barotrauma. Use of APRV has not been shown to reduce morbidity or mortality in large trials, more importantly its use in this patient with severe acidosis is limited as minute ventilation is often reduced in this mode. The use of esophageal balloon can be considered but its use is limited by placement and is not reflective of pressures in all areas of the chest.

Cavalcanti AB, Suzumura ÉA, Laranjeira LN, et al. Effect of lung recruitment and titrated positive end-expiratory pressure (PEEP) vs low PEEP on mortality in patients with acute respiratory distress syndrome: a randomized clinical trial. *JAMA.* 2017;318(14):1335-1345. doi:10.1001/jama.2017.14171

Fuller BM, Mohr NM, Skrupky L, et al. The use of inhaled prostaglandins in patients with ARDS: a systematic review and meta-analysis. *Chest.* 2015;147(6):1510-1522. doi:10.1378/chest. 14-3161

Peek GJ, Mugford M, Tiruvoipati R, et al. Efficacy and economic assessment of conventional ventilatory support versus extracorporeal membrane oxygenation for severe adult respiratory failure (CESAR): a multicentre randomised controlled trial. *Lancet.* 2009;374(9698):1351-1363. doi:10.1016/S0140-6736(09)61069-2

46. **The answer is C.** Cardiogenic shock refractory to vasopressor support can benefit from implementation of mechanical circulatory support. Patients with biventricular failure have limited therapeutic options when inotropic support is inadequate. VA ECMO provides hemodynamic support despite biventricular failure. VV ECMO allows for ventilation/oxygenation support. Cardiac output (CO) can be increased up to 5 L/min with the newer percutaneously inserted ventricular assist devices (such as Impella), but a percutaneous left ventricular assist device (LVAD) requires stable right ventricular function. In addition, limited centers have the ability to place a right-sided ventricular assist device in conjunction with a left-sided assist device. CO with IABP is only up to 0.5 L/min; in addition, use of IABP is also limited by right ventricular failure. Emergent cardiac catheterization in a 22-yeur-old in the absence of prior ST elevation is unlikely to provide improved CO.

Abrams D, Combes A, Brodie D, et al. Extracorporeal membrane oxygenation in cardiopulmonary disease in adults. *J Am Coll Cardiol.* 2014;63:2769-2778. doi:10.1016/j.jacc.2014.03.046

Rihal CS, Naidu SS, Givertz MM, et al. 2015 SCAI/ACC/HFSA/STS clinical expert consensus statement on the use of percutaneous mechanical circulatory support devices in cardiovascular care: endorsed by the American Heart Association, the Cardiological Society of India, and Sociedad Latino Americana de Cardiologia Intervencion; Affirmation of Value by the Canadian Association of Interventional Cardiology-Association Canadienne de Cardiologie d'intervention. *J Am Coll Cardiol.* 2015;65:e1-20. doi:10.1016/j.jacc.2015.03.036

47. **The answer is D.** In patients with acute decompensation post–cardiac catheterization, the current theory is to limit the use of vasopressors and utilize a mechanical support device. The preferred method is a percutaneous LVAD as the patient has primarily left ventricular dysfunction. The use of additional inotropes, specifically epinephrine that provides inotropic and chronotropic support through beta stimulation increases the overall oxygen demand of the heart. An implantable LVAD should only be considered if patient has demonstrated a failure to recover left ventricular function despite optimal therapy. This patient will likely require temporary support. ECMO should be reserved for patients with biventricular failure or an inability to provide adequate support despite use of a percutaneous ventricular assist device. The use of peripheral ECMO as an initial therapy is not preferred in isolated left ventricular failure, as peripheral cannulation will result in increased afterload on the left ventricular. The insertion of an intra-aortic balloon pump (IABP) can provide improved coronary perfusion; however, this patient has undergone revascularization of the culprit lesion. The cardiac output provided by a balloon pump is approximately 0.5-1 L/min which is often inadequate. The balloon pump does provide reduction in the afterload, but since this patient is already hypotensive the benefit is limited. The data from the IABP Shock II trial did not significantly reduce 30-day mortality in patients with cardiogenic shock complicating acute myocardial infarction (AMI) for whom an early revascularization strategy was planned.

Thiele H, Zeymer U, Neumann FJ, et al. Intraaortic balloon support for myocardial infarction with cardiogenic shock. *N Engl J Med.* 2012;367:1287-1296. doi:10.1056/NEJMoa1208410

17

Respiratory Disorders

ADITYA KASARABADA

■ QUESTIONS

1. Which of the following is not standard practice in rapid sequence intubation (RSI)?

    A. Preoxygenate for 5 minutes
    B. Pretreatment with atropine
    C. Sedation
    D. Paralysis
    E. Placement of oral/nasal airway

2. What is the maximum safe dose of lidocaine for topical anesthesia of the airway?

    A. 3 mg/kg
    B. 4.5 mg/kg
    C. 1 mg/kg
    D. 2 mg/kg
    E. There is no toxic dose for topical lidocaine

3. A 57-year-old man is found unresponsive and intubated in the field by emergency medical service (EMS) for airway protection. The initial ventilator settings are respiratory rate (RR) 18 breaths per minute, tidal volume (TV) 500 mL, positive end-expiratory pressure (PEEP) 5 cm H_2O, and FiO_2 0.5. The nurse is concerned that the high-pressure ventilator alarm is being persistently triggered. Upon evaluation the peak inspiratory pressure (PIP) is 70 cm H_2O and the plateau pressure (P_{Plat}) is 20 cm H_2O. All of following can be true in this scenario except:

    A. Patient is biting on the endotracheal tube
    B. The ventilator tubing is compressed between the bed rails
    C. The patient is developing acute respiratory distress syndrome (ARDS)
    D. The respiratory therapist (RT) increased the flow rate from 45 L/min to 120 L/min
    E. There is a mucus plug in the endotracheal tube

4. A 45-year-old man with a past medical history of alcohol abuse presents to the hospital with persistent fever, abdominal pain, nausea and vomiting. His initial vitals are temperature 101°F, heart rate (HR) 110 beats per minute (BPM), respiratory rate (RR) 32 BPM, and blood pressure (BP) 100/72 mmHg. He has mid-epigastric tenderness on exam. While NPO, the patient aspirates. His chest X-ray (CXR) is shown as follows. Labs are arterial blood gas (ABG) = 7.37/35/82 on FiO_2 100%, and white blood cell (WBC) = 18,000. What is the diagnosis?

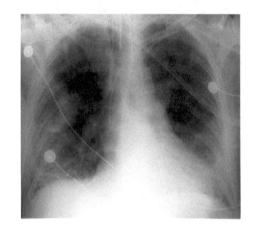

A. Pulmonary edema
B. Aspiration pneumonia
C. Acute respiratory distress syndrome (ARDS)
D. Pleural effusion
E. Pancreatitis

5. The primary determinant of the normal distribution of blood perfusion in the lung is

A. Transthoracic pressure
B. Transpulmonary pressure gradient
C. Cardiac output (CO)
D. Gravity
E. Pulmonary vascular resistance

6. All of the following interfere with bellows function of the chest, **except**:

A. Third-degree chest burn
B. Flail chest
C. Pneumonia
D. Pneumothorax
E. All of the above

7. What are the two key factors that determine the total work of breathing?

A. Compliance and resistance
B. Dead space and pulmonary shunting
C. Tidal volume (TV) and respiratory rate (RR)
D. Respiratory drive and airspace disease
E. Total lung capacity (TLC)

8. Which of the following best describes West zone-3 lung physiology? P_A = alveolar pressure; P_a = arterial pressure, and P_v = venous pressure.

A. $P_a > P_v > P_A$
B. $P_A > P_a > P_v$
C. $P_a > P_A > P_v$
D. $P_{pleural} > P_a > P_v$
E. None of the above

9. What is the proposed physiologic benefit of Heliox© in postextubation stridor?

   A. Reduces airway edema
   B. Provide a low-density high-FiO₂ gas mixture
   C. Lowers the Reynolds number of the airway (airway resistance)
   D. Decreases patient anxiety
   E. Assists with airway irritation and pain

10. Match the following:

A. Inspiratory reserve volume (IRV)	1. The volume of air breathed in and out without conscious effort
B. Total lung capacity (TLC)	2. The additional volume of air that can be inhaled with maximum effort after a normal inspiration
C. Vital capacity (VC)	3. The additional volume of air that can be forcibly exhaled after normal exhalation
D. Expiratory reserve volume (ERV)	4. The total volume of air that can be exhaled after a maximum inhalation
E. Minute ventilation (MV)	5. The volume of air remaining in the lungs after maximum exhalation (the lungs can never be completely emptied)
F. Tidal volume (TV)	6. VC + RV
G. Residual volume (RV)	7. The volume of air breathed in 1 minute

11. All of the following are indications for a chest tube placement in pleural effusions, **except**:

   A. Pus on gross visualization
   B. Loculated pleural effusion
   C. pH less than 7.0
   D. Hemothorax
   E. Pleural fluid glucose greater than 200 g/dL

12. Which of the following neuromuscular disorders is insidious in onset?

   A. Myasthenia gravis
   B. Guillain–Barre syndrome (GBS)
   C. Organophosphate poisoning
   D. Amytrophic lateral sclerosis (ALS)
   E. None of the above

13. What are the key parameters in extubation of patients with neuromuscular disorders?

   A. Rapid shallow breathing index (RSBI) less than 105
   B. Passing a spontaneous breathing trial (SBT)
   C. Vital capacity (VC) greater than 20 mL/kg and negative inspiratory force (NIF) less than −30
   D. Minimal secretions and strong cough
   E. All of the above

14. All of the following are treatments for pulmonary arterial hypertension (PAH), **except**:

   A. Calcium channel blockers
   B. Angiotensin-converting enzyme (ACE) inhibitors
   C. Sildenafil

D. Riociguat

E. Endothelin receptor antagonists

15. A 23-year-old man experienced a generalized tonic–clonic seizure and had a witnessed large volume aspiration of gastric content. He is now on assist control (AC) ventilation. His ventilator settings are as follows: FiO_2 1.0; positive end-expiratory pressure (PEEP) 5 cm H_2O; tidal volume (V_T) 6 mL/kg; and plateau pressure (P_{plat}) 29 cm H_2O with adequate expiratory time. His arterial blood gas (ABG) shows pH 7.18, PCO_2 67 mmHg, PO_2 48 mmHg, and bicarbonate 24 mEq/L. How can his ventilator setting be modified to optimize his clinical picture?

A. Increase PEEP

B. Reduce V_T increase rate

C. Increase PEEP; increase rate

D. Increase PEEP; reduce V_T

E. Increase V_T

16. A 22-year-old man is admitted for asthma exacerbation. Despite treatment with bronchodilators and steroids, his respiratory distress worsens leading to endotracheal intubation. His weight is 85 kg. He is now on assist control (AC) ventilation with a set rate of 10 breaths per minute, tidal volume (TV) of 600 mL, and a positive end-expiratory pressure (PEEP) of 0. Fifteen minutes after intubation, he is noted to be struggling to breathe with a respiratory rate (RR) of 40 and a systolic blood pressure (SBP) of 60 mmHg. What should be the next step?

A. Decrease TV to 500 mL

B. Switch patient to pressure support

C. Temporarily disconnect patient from ventilator

D. Increase PEEP to 10

E. Decrease RR to 8

17. A 38-year-old woman with history of asthma complicated by frequent intubations presents with difficulty breathing, which began earlier in the day. Her vital signs are respiratory rate (RR) 30 breaths per minute, heart rate (HR) 113 BPM, blood pressure (BP) 156/60 mmHg, and SpO_2 96% on room air. Subjectively, she is unable to speak full sentences and is using accessory muscles while sitting upright in a tripod position. Patient has poor air entry bilaterally on auscultation. She is emergently intubated and placed on the following ventilator setting: assist control (AC), set RR 16, tidal volume (TV) 450 mL, positive end-expiratory pressure (PEEP) 5 cm H_2O, and FiO_2 100%. On auscultation postintubation you do not hear wheezing. The ventilator shows a peak pressure of 20 cm H_2O with a plateau pressure (P_{plat}) of 15 cm H_2O. The postintubation arterial blood gas (ABG) is 7.42/36/400/24. What is the most likely diagnosis?

A. Status asthmaticus

B. Vocal cord dysfunction syndrome

C. Acute respiratory distress syndrome (ARDS)

D. Increased intrathoracic pressure

E. Auto-PEEP

18. A 70-year-old man presents to the ED with increasing shortness of breath, purulent productive cough, and a subjective fever for 7 days. On examination, he is in moderate distress with a temperature 102°F, respiratory rate (RR) 26/min, heart rate (HR) 120 beats per minute (BPM), and blood pressure (BP) 80/54 mmHg. He has decreased breath sounds over the right chest. Lab findings are notable for a white blood cell (WBC) count of 21,000/microL with a left shift. Chest x-ray (CXR) shows a right-sided pleural effusion which appears to be loculated on follow-up chest CT scan. Patient is initially resuscitated with intravenous (IV) fluids, followed by a diagnostic thoracentesis. The pleural fluid analysis shows pH 7.1, protein 3.9 gm/dL, lactate dehydrogenase (LDH)

1500 U/L, and glucose 30 mg/dL. In addition to starting patient on antibiotics, what is the most appropriate next step?

A. Repeat imaging
B. Placement of chest tube
C. Decortication
D. Repeat thoracentesis
E. Surgical consultation

19. A 74-year-old woman presents to the hospital with progressive shortness of breath associated with purulent cough and fever for 5 days. Her vital signs are as follows: temperature 38.7°C, heart rate (HR) 106/min, respiratory rate (RR) 32/min, and blood pressure (BP) 98/70. Laboratory findings are significant for white blood cell (WBC) count 3,500/microL and blood urea nitrogen (BUN) 24 mg/dL. Chest x-ray (CXR) shows consolidations in the left upper and lower lobes. She is alert and able to swallow pills. What is the next step in management?

A. Administer intravenous (IV) fluids and observe in the ED
B. Discharge her home with oral antibiotics
C. Admit her to the general medical floor and start antibiotics
D. Check a lactic acid level and decide on desposition
E. Admit her to the ICU

20. A 76-year-old man with a significant history of smoking presents with dizziness and lethargy. In the ED, he is found to be in septic shock secondary to a urinary tract infection (UTI) and is later intubated for airway protection. The chest x-ray (CXR) shows a left upper lobe (LUL) mass. The chest CT scan shows a 5 × 4 cm speculated mass in the LUL along with pleural effusion. There is also another 3.5 × 3 cm mass in the right middle lobe along with enlarged subcarinal lymphadenopathy. The family is unaware of the possibility of lung cancer and asks for the likely stage of the cancer. Based on the available information, the most likely stage of the lung cancer is

A. Stage IIB
B. Stage IIIA
C. Stage IIIB
D. Stage IV
E. Unsure—as there is not enough information to stage

21. Peripheral chemoreceptors sensitive to hypoxemia and its effect on hydrogen ion sensitivity are located in the:

A. Carotid and aortic bodies
B. Pulmonary artery oxygen sensors at the first division of the main pulmonary artery
C. Oxygen sensory center(s) in the medial and lateral dorsal brainstem
D. Left ventricular sensor(s) associated with pro-brain natriuretic peptide (BNP) release sites
E. Neurofibrillary bodies at bifurcation of femoral arteries from the aorta

22. If a normal 20-year-old subject, resting at sea level, is placed on 100% oxygen for about 15 minutes, what would you expect his or her PaO_2 to be about:

A. 100 mmHg
B. 650 mmHg
C. 250 mmHg
D. 800 mmHg
E. 925 mmHg

23. A 25-year-old man with asthma is found to have a FEV_1/FVC ratio (forced exhaled volume in 1 second compared to the full forced vital capacity volume) of less than 50% during pulmonary function testing (PFT). Ten days later the patient presents to the ED with severe respiratory distress and is emergently intubated. The respiratory therapist (RT) asks

for initial ventilator settings. Although all the following parameters are important, based on the patient's baseline lung function, what parameter should you be particularly mindful of?

A. Peak airway pressure
B. Trigger sensitivity
C. Level of pressure support (PS) you order
D. Inhalation time to exhalation time (I:E) ratio
E. Peak:plateau airway pressure ratio

24. The rapid shallow breathing index (RSBI) is a weaning assessment tool. What calculated value is associated with a poor chance of weaning success?

A. Greater than 130
B. Greater than 105
C. Greater than 150
D. Less than 12
E. None of the above

25. A 50-year-old woman with chronic obstructive pulmonary disease (COPD) and pneumonia is intubated for respiratory failure. Initial ventilator settings are as follows: volume control, tidal volume (TV) 500 mL, set rate 24/min, positive end-expiratory pressure (PEEP) 5 cm H_2O, and FiO_2 50%. Over the next few hours patient starts to become increasingly hypotensive and tachycardic. The ventilator graphics with airway pressure versus time, and flow versus time are shown. Which combination of manipulations can be performed to diagnose and ameliorate the condition?

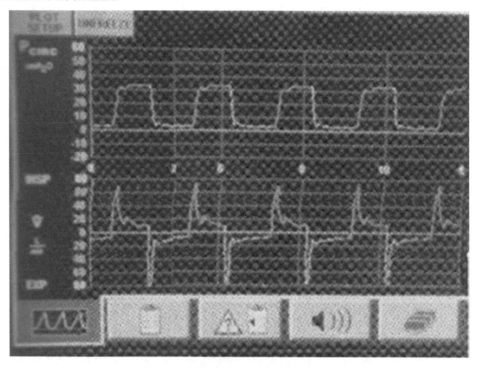

A. Perform an inspiratory pause and increase inspiratory pressure
B. Perform an expiratory pause and increase inspiratory pressure
C. Perform an inspiratory pause and reduce the set rate
D. Perform an expiratory pause and reduce the set rate
E. Do nothing

26. Identify the type of patient-ventilator asynchrony shown in the following ventilator graphics:

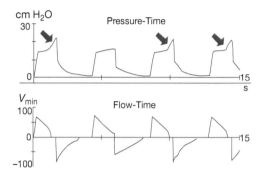

Source: From Nilsestuen JO, Hargett KD. Using ventilator graphics to identify patient-ventilator asynchrony. *Respir care.* 2005;50(2):202-34. With permission.

A. Flow asynchrony
B. Ineffective triggering
C. Double triggering
D. Auto triggering
E. Delayed breath termination

27. Identify the type of patient-ventilator asynchrony shown in the following ventilator graphics:

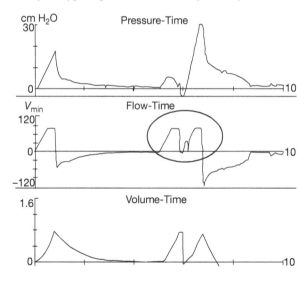

Source: From Nilsestuen JO, Hargett KD. Using ventilator graphics to identify patient-ventilator asynchrony. *Respir care.* 2005;50(2):202-34. With permission.

A. Flow asynchrony
B. Ineffective triggering
C. Double triggering
D. Auto triggering
E. Delayed breath termination

28. Identify the type of patient-ventilator asynchrony shown in the following ventilator graphics:

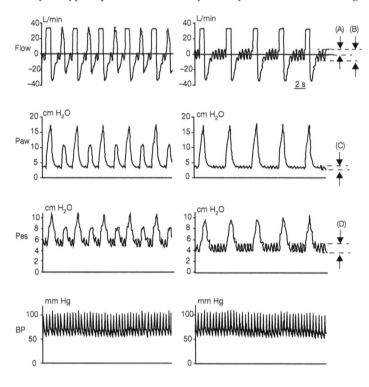

A. Flow asynchrony
B. Ineffective triggering
C. Double triggering
D. Auto triggering
E. Delayed breath termination

29. Identify the type of patient ventilator asynchrony shown in the following ventilator graphics:

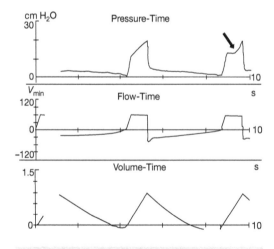

Source: From Nilsestuen JO, Hargett KD. Using ventilator graphics to identify patient-ventilator asynchrony. *Respir care.* 2005;50(2):202-34. With permission.

A. Flow asynchrony
B. Ineffective triggering
C. Double triggering
D. Autotriggering
E. Delayed breath termination

30. A 40-year-old man presents to the ED with worsening shortness of breath over the last 2 days. On exam he appears to be in moderate distress and is tachypneic with a respiratory rate (RR) of 30/min. Chest x-ray (CXR) shows diffuse bilateral infiltrates. Initial arterial blood gas (ABG) shows 7.3/50/60/23 on a 100% nonrebreather mask. Patient is intubated and placed on low tidal volume (TV) lung-protective ventilation strategies. During the course of the first 24 hours, the patient's ventilator settings are adjusted to RR 20/min, tidal volume 350 mL, positive end-expiratory pressure (PEEP) 15 cm H_2O, and FiO_2 100% in order to maintain oxygen saturation of 90%. Repeat ABG after the adjustments shows 7.26/58/70/24. What other interventions have been shown to improve outcomes in this condition?

A. Change ventilator mode to airway pressure release ventilation (APRV)
B. Start patient on inhaled epoprostenolol
C. Continue current ventilator settings and consider prone position ventilation
D. Change to high-frequency oscillation ventilation (HFOV) mode
E. Insert a pulmonary artery catheter (PAC) to guide treatment

■ ANSWERS

1. **The answer is B.** RSI is the preferred method of endotracheal intubation, as it results in the rapid induction of a state of unconsciousness and concurrent neuromuscular blockade (paralysis). This is important in patients who have not fasted and thus are at a much greater risk for vomiting and aspiration. To this end, the goal of RSI is to intubate the trachea without having to use bag-valve-mask (BVM) ventilation, which is often necessary when attempting to achieve intubating conditions with sedative agents alone (e.g., midazolam, diazepam). Instead of titrating to effect, RSI involves administration of weight-based doses of an induction agent (e.g., etomidate) immediately followed by a paralytic agent (e.g. succinylcholine, rocuronium) to render the patient unconscious and paralyzed (usually within 1 minute). This method has been proven safe and effective over the past two decades, and is considered the standard of care. When administered by experienced, well-trained intensivists, use of neuromuscular blocking agents in patients undergoing emergent tracheal intubation is associated with a significant decrease in procedure-related complications. Certain clinical scenarios may call for pretreatment prior to induction/paralysis to optimize physiologic parameters for intubation, such as blunting the sympathetic response to laryngoscopy, preventing upward or downward spikes in blood pressure, avoiding increased intracranial pressure (ICP), and facilitating bronchodilation. These conditions include suspected high ICP (e.g. intracranial hemorrhage or trauma), severe asthma or chronic obstructive pulmonary disease (COPD), hypovolemic shock, and aortic emergencies. Pretreatment with atropine is not a core component of RSI.

   Seder DB, Jagoda A, Riggs B. Emergency neurological life support: airway, ventilation, and sedation. *Neurocrit Care.* 2015;23(suppl 2):S5-22. doi:10.1007/s12028-015-0164-3

2. **The answer is B.** Lidocaine is the most commonly used local anesthetic for a wide range of procedures. Topical anesthetics are partially absorbed into the blood stream. High doses of lidocaine may lead to cardiovascular and neurologic toxicity resulting in arrhythmias and seizures. To avoid the risk of toxic side effects, it is important to limit the volume of topically applied lidocaine to doses well within the safety range. Lidocaine is available in 1%, 2%, and 4% solutions. The maximum dose of lidocaine is 4.5 mg/kg. Lidocaine solution is also available with and without epinephrine (1:100,000). Epinephrine causes local vasoconstriction, which prevents absorption of lidocaine into the bloodstream and allows for more concentrated effect locally. This permits the user to administer a larger dose of drug to be infiltrated without causing systemic toxicity. To calculate the total milliliter permitted: maximum allowable dose (mg/kg) × (weight in kilogram/10) × (1/concentration of local anesthetic) = milliliter lidocaine. Thus, for 1% lidocaine for a 60-kg patient: $4.5 \times 6 \times 1 = 27$ mL of 1% lidocaine.

3. **The answer is C.** In this case the PIP is elevated with a normal (P_{plat}) suggesting that the problem is due to increased transpulmonary resistance. Transpulmonary resistance can be elevated in the case of patient biting the endotracheal tube, the ventilator tubing getting compressed between the bed rails, and a mucus plug in the endotracheal tube. Increasing the inspiratory flow rate will also increase the PIP without changing the compliance and hence the transpulmonary resistance. In the case of ARDS, there is a problem with the lung parenchyma, which results in decreased compliance and thus an increase in the P_{plat}. In this case, the P_{plat} is not elevated.

   Owens W. Chapter 3: troubleshooting. In: Owens W, ed. *The Ventilator Book.* 1st ed. First Draught Press; Lexington, KY: 2012:15-16.

4. **The answer is C.** ARDS is associated with a generalized systemic inflammatory response syndrome (SIRS) and is characterized as the acute onset of hypoxemia within 1 week of known clinical insult or new or worsening respiratory symptoms with bilateral pulmonary infiltrates not fully explained by effusion, lobar lung collapse, or nodules. The respiratory failure cannot be fully explained by cardiac failure or fluid overload and needs objective assessment

(e.g., echocardiography) to exclude hydrostatic edema if no risk factor is present. In addition, the PaO_2/FiO_2 ratio should be less than 300 with a positive end-expiratory pressure (PEEP) or continuous positive airway pressure (CPAP) ≥ 5 cm H_2O. Aspiration pneumonia and pancreatitis are well-established causes for ARDS. This is different from the 1996 consensus definition of the PaO_2/FiO_2 ratio less than 200 mmHg regardless of the level of PEEP with a wedge pressure of less than 18 mmHg. Ventilation is difficult due to poor compliance that results from the protein leak into the lungs. The clinician should be familiar with the ventilator they are using and the mode of ventilation used to facilitate ventilation. Application of PEEP usually improves oxygenation, although this can increase the likelihood of barotrauma. The goal plateau pressure (P_{plat}) should be under 30 cm H_2O, this can be achieved by reducing tidal volume (TV) down to 4 to 6 mL/kg. The goal SaO_2 is greater than 88%. To maintain lower P_{plats}, permissive hypercapnia is tolerated except in acute head or neurologically injured patients. Other possible considerations include sedation, paralysis, prone positioning, and inhaled nitric oxide or inhaled epoprostenol.

Fan E, Brodie D, Slutsky AS. Acute respiratory distress syndrome: advances in diagnosis and treatment. *JAMA*. 2018;319(7):698-710. doi:10.1001/jama.2017.21907

5. **The answer is D.** Under normal circumstances gravity determines the distribution of pulmonary artery blood flow. Therefore, the gravitationally dependent zones of the lung receive more perfusion than nondependent areas. In the supine patient, this is the posterior plane of the lung; standing directs blood flow to the anatomic lung bases, and so on. Because of blood engorgement in the gravitationally dependent lung zones, the gravitationally dependent small airways are slightly smaller than the gravitationally nondependent small airways at the beginning of inhalation. This smaller size reduces small airway surface tension forces and allows those airways to be expanded more easily during normal spontaneous inhalation. During normal conditions, therefore, gas flow is preferentially directed along the path of least resistance, toward the gravitationally dependent airways adjacent to the normally distributed pulmonary blood flow. In this fashion during normal spontaneous breathing, ventilation (V) and perfusion (Q) are mostly matched although not perfectly; with an overall normal V/Q ratio of about 0.85. The accompanying illustration (from standing position) shows those relationships, where "Vol %" is the percentage of tidal volume better distributed to base; "$V_{A/Q}$" is also known as the V/Q ratio, where V_A denotes alveolar ventilation and Q denotes perfusion. Note that the V/Q ratio is lower at the base, indicating increased perfusion at the base.

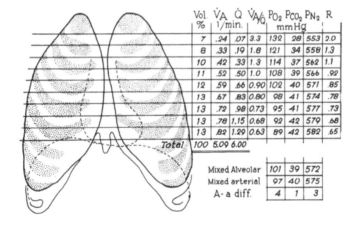

Vol. %	V̇A l/min	Q̇	V̇A/Q	PO₂ mmHg	PCO₂ mmHg	PN₂ mmHg	R
7	.24	.07	3.3	132	28	553	2.0
8	.33	.19	1.8	121	34	558	1.3
10	.42	.33	1.3	114	37	562	1.1
11	.52	.50	1.0	108	39	566	.92
12	.59	.66	0.90	102	40	571	.85
13	.67	.83	0.80	98	41	574	.78
13	.72	.98	0.73	95	41	577	.73
13	.78	1.15	0.68	92	42	579	.68
13	.82	1.29	0.63	89	42	582	.65
Total 100	5.09	6.00					

Mixed Alveolar	101	39	572
Mixed arterial	97	40	575
A-a diff.	4	1	3

Source: Figure printed with permission from West JB. Regional differences in gas exchange in the lung of erect man. *J Appl Physiol.* 1962;17:893-898.

6. **The answer is C.** The chest bellows component of the respiratory system includes the bony thoracic cage that contains the lungs; the diaphragms, which are the major muscles of breathing; and pleural membranes, thin tissues that line both the outside of the lungs and the inside of the thoracic cage. The thoracic or chest cage consists of the ribs that protect the lungs from injury; the muscles and connective tissues that tie the ribs together; and all the nerves that lead into these muscles. The chest bellows is synonymous with the respiratory pump, which is the component of the respiratory system excluding the lungs. Some diseases that impact respiration affect the pump or central nervous system without any direct lung disease.

West JB. *Respiratory Physiology: The Essentials.* 6th ed. Philadelphia, PA: Lippincott Williams & Wilkins; 2000.

7. **The answer is A.** The total work of breathing is the sum of the elastic and resistive work. Resistive work (resistance) decreases with increasing lung volumes and widening airways. Elastic work (compliance) increases at both high and low lung volumes. In obstructive lung disease, resistance increases with no change in compliance. And in restrictive lung disease, compliance decreases with no change in resistance. In the ICU setting, most patients have compliance detriments and increased work of breathing as a result. Mechanical ventilation should be employed in ratio to the degree of decreased work of breathing required to maintain adequate gas exchange while treating the underlying lung disorder.

West JB. *Respiratory Physiology: The Essentials.* 6th ed. Philadelphia, PA: Lippincott Williams & Wilkins; 2000.

8. **The answer is A.** West zones are vertically split zones within the lung (in the upright subject), which explain how alveoli, arterial, and venous pressures differ in each zone and thus affect perfusion and ventilation throughout the lung.

   In zone 1 (the upper zone), the alveolar pressure (P_A) exceeds that of the arterial (P_a) and venous (P_v) pressures ($P_A > P_a > P_v$) resulting in very high ventilation (V) to perfusion (Q) ratio. Zone 1 is not normally seen in healthy human lungs where P_a is greater than P_A throughout the lung. However, under circumstances such as positive pressure ventilation or hemorrhage, P_A exceeds P_a and results in blood vessel collapse, and hence dead space.

   In zone 2 (the middle zone), blood flow is intermittent. Initially, there is no blood flow given obstruction at the venous capillaries. However, as the arterial pressure builds up and exceeds the alveoli pressure ($P_a > P_A > P_v$), blood flow resumes. Accordingly there is an average V/Q in zone 2.

   In zone 3 that comprises the majority of the lungs in a healthy subject both the arterial and venous pressures exceed the alveolar pressure ($P_a > P_v > P_A$), and blood flow is continuous. V/Q is low in zone 3.

West J, Dollery C, Naimark A. Distribution of blood flow in isolated lung; relation to vascular and alveolar pressures. *J Appl Physiol.* 1964;19:713-724. doi:10.1152/jappl.1964.19.4.713

9. **The answer is C.** Upper and total airway resistance may frequently be increased after extubation, resulting in high inspiratory effort, respiratory distress, and airway obstruction in 5% to 16% of patients that may necessitate reintubation. Helium–oxygen (HeO_2) mixture (Heliox©) has a lower density than air and reduces frictional resistance. The resultant decrease in turbulent flow and improved laminar flow (i.e., lower Reynolds number) can decrease the patients' effort to breathe. The benefit of HeO_2 depends on the percentage of helium which reduces the Reynolds number. Potential candidates for its use should require an FiO_2 less than 0.4. While initial studies suggested that HeO_2 could decrease $PaCO_2$, subsequent studies did not show any effect on CO_2.

Letherman J. Mechanical ventilation for severe asthma. *Chest.* 2015;147(6):1671-1680. doi: 10.1378/chest.14-1733

Wittekamp BH, van Mook WN, Tjan DH, et al. Clinical review: post-extubation laryngeal edema and extubationfailure in critically ill adult patients. *Crit Care.* 2009;13(6):233. doi: 10.1186/cc8142

10. **The answers are A→2; B→6; C→4; D→3; E→7; F→1; and G→5.**

    TV is the volume of air breathed in and out without conscious effort. *IRV* is the additional volume of air that can be inhaled with maximum effort after a normal inspiration.

    ERV is the additional volume of air that can be forcibly exhaled after normal exhalation.

    VC is the total volume of air that can be exhaled after a maximum inhalation; therefore, VC = TV + IRV + ERV.

    RV is the volume of air remaining in the lungs after maximum exhalation (the lungs can never be completely emptied).

    $$TLC = VC + RV$$

    MV is the total volume of air breathed in 1 minute.

    Measurements of lung volumes are important to confirm or clarify the nature of lung disorders. Spirometry can measure the total exhaled volume (forced vital capacity or FVC), the forced expiratory volume in 1 second (FEV_1), and their ratio (FEV_1/FVC). The flow-volume loop may indicate an obstructive, restrictive, or obstructive/restrictive pattern, but a further test of lung volume is often necessary for clarification.

    In *obstructive lung disease*, airway obstruction causes an increase in resistance. During normal breathing, the pressure–volume relationship is no different from a normal lung. However, when breathing rapidly, greater pressure is needed to overcome the resistance to flow, and the volume of each breath gets smaller. Increase in the effort to breathe can cause an overdistention of the lungs. The flow-volume loop may show lower than normal FEV_1, but it is not until a lung volume has been determined that an increase in TLC, FRC, and RV can be confirmed. Common obstructive diseases include asthma, bronchitis and emphysema.

    In *restrictive lung disease*, the compliance of the lung is reduced which increases the stiffness of the lung and limits expansion. In these cases, a greater pressure than normal is required to allow the same increase in volume. The flow-volume loop may show lower than normal FVC, but the FEV_1 may only be mildly affected. The lung volume measurement will clearly show a reduction in TLC, functional residual capacity, and RV. Common causes of decreased lung compliance are pulmonary fibrosis, pneumonia, and pulmonary edema. Patients whose respiratory muscles are unable to perform normally because of a neuromuscular disease or paralysis can also show a restrictive pattern.

    Crapo RO. Pulmonary function testing. *N Engl J Med*. 1994;331:25. doi:10.1056/ NEJM199407073310107

    Pellegrino R, Viegi G, Brusasco V, et al. Interpretative strategies for lung function tests. *Eur Respir J*. 2005;26:948. doi:10.1183/09031936.05.00035205

11. **The answer is E.** Pleural effusion fluid can be classified as either transudative or exudative. An effusion is deemed exudative if pleural fluid protein/serum protein ratio is greater than 0.5, or pleural fluid lactate dehydrogenase (LDH)/serum LDH is greater than 0.6, or pleural fluid LDH is greater than 2/3 upper normal limit for serum (Light's criteria). If none of these criteria are met, then the effusion is a transudate and the underlying medical condition is treated. The presence of pus on gross visualization indicates empyema. A pH less than 7.25 indicates that this is likely a complicated parapenumonic effusion which is an indication to place chest tube. If pleural pH cannot be measured then pleural fluid glucose can be measured as a proxy, with glucose levels less than 40 suggesting a pleural cavity infection. Some noninfectious diseases such as rheumatoid arthritis can also reduce pleural fluid glucose. Hemothorax is an indication for chest tube placement.

    Feller-Kopman D, Light R. Pleural disease. *N Engl J Med*. 2018;378(8):740-751. doi:10.1056/ NEJMra1403503

12. **The answer is D.** ALS is more indolent and chronic in its development. ALS is caused by a genetic defect in 10% of cases, the hallmark of the disease is loss of motor neurons (anterior horn cells) which eventually leads to muscles weakening, twitching, and an inability to move the arms, legs, and then torso. When the muscles in the chest area are involved, it becomes

difficult or impossible to breathe on one's own. All of the diseases above (organophosphate poisoning, myasthenia, and GBS) result in some form of neuromuscular blockade and are more acute in onset.

Acute respiratory failure is the most feared complication in patients with neuromuscular diseases. The decision to intubate these patients should be made earlier rather than later, to avoid emergency intubation or cardiorespiratory arrest. Regular assessment for clinical signs of respiratory-muscle fatigue and objective monitoring of vital capacity (VC), inspiratory, and expiratory forces are essential to determine the appropriate timing of intubation and mechanical ventilation. A measure often used in the clinical setting is negative inspiratory force (NIF) which should be less than −40 cmH$_2$O in healthy individuals. A large number of these patients require mechanical ventilation, resulting in high morbidity and mortality including ventilator-associated pneumonia (VAP).

Rabinstein AA. Acute neuromuscular respiratory failure. *Continuum*. 2015;21(5):1324-1345. doi: 10.1212/CON.0000000000000218

13. **The answer C.** In patients with respiratory failure due to neuromuscular diseases, the decision to extubate can be a challenging one, and previous studies have not addressed the topic of weaning and extubation in this patient population. In general, patients should have adequate cough, manageable secretions, and tolerate a low level of pressure support (PS) for an extended period of time without evidence of respiratory fatigue. Objective measures used for extubation typically mirror the measures known to predict intubation including vital capacity (VC) less than 20 mL/kg, NIF less than −30 cmH$_2$O, or greater than 30% reduction in VC.

Rabinstein AA. Acute neuromuscular respiratory failure. *Continuum*. 2015;21(5):1324-1345. doi: 10.1212/CON.0000000000000218

14. **The answer B.** Pulmonary hypertension is defined as a resting mean pulmonary artery pressure (mPAP) of 25 mm Hg or above. Based on the Fifth World Symposium on Pulmonary Hypertension classification, PH is divided in to five groups:

1. Group 1—pulmonary hypertension due to pulmonary vascular disease

2. Group 2—pulmonary hypertension due to left heart disease

3. Group 3—pulmonary hypertension due to lung disease or hypoxia

4. Group 4—pulmonary hypertension due to chronic thromboembolic disease

5. Group 5—a miscellaneous collection of pulmonary hypertension syndromes caused by a variety of disorders (including HIV and sarcoidosis)

PAH refers to group 1 pulmonary hypertension. Calcium channel blockers may be effective in 5% to 10% of PAH patients who respond to acute vasodilatory challenge, defined as a drop in mean pulmonary arterial pressure (mPAP) by 10 mmHg with no decline in cardiac output during right heart catheterization. Riociguat directly stimulates soluble guanylate cyclase independent of nitric oxide, resulting in increased cGMP and pulmonary vasodilation. Endothelin receptor antagonists such as bosentan block endothelin which is a potent vasoconstrictor causing pulmonary vasodilation. PDE5 inhibitors such as sildanafil have been shown to improve PAH.

Thenappan T, Ormiston ML, Ryan JJ, et al. Pulmonary arterial hypertension: pathogenesis and clinical management. *BMJ*. 2018;360:5492. doi:10.1136/bmj.j5492

15. **The answer is C.** The patient had an aspiration event that has resulted in profound hypoxemia with concomitant hypercarbia and acidosis. Based on the concept of permissive hypercapnea, a pH of up to 7.2 is considered acceptable in patients with acute respiratory distress syndrome (ARDS). In the current situation, however, the pH is less than 7.2 due to acute respiratory acidosis. To improve respiratory acidosis, it is necessary to enhance the minute ventilation by increasing either respiratory rate (RR) or V$_T$. However, increasing V$_T$ alone could lead to increased plateau pressures and barotrauma. In addition, there is adequate expiratory time.

Therefore, increasing the respiratory rate is the best way to increase the minute ventilation and improve the acidosis. Furthermore, increasing PEEP will improve oxygenation by recruiting atelectatic lung units, but it will not improve acidosis.

Fan E, Brodie D, Slutsky AS. Acute respiratory distress syndrome: advances in diagnosis and treatment. *JAMA*. 2018;319(7):698-710. doi:10.1001/jama.2017.21907

16. **The answer is C.** The patient has likely developed severe auto-PEEP resulting in poor venous return and reduced cardiac output (CO) leading to hypotension. Auto-PEEP (also known as intrinsic PEEP and dynamic hyperinflation) develops when incomplete expiration prior to the inflation of the next breath results in progressive air trapping and increased alveolar pressure at the end of expiration. It usually occurs due to inadequate expiration time. The expiratory flow waveform does not return to the baseline on the ventilator's screen. In this patient, who is hypotensive, the fastest way to diagnose and relieve the condition would be to disconnect the patient from the ventilator. This allows for complete exhalation and relief of the elevated intrathoracic pressure. The goal of mechanical ventilation in obstructive lung disease, such as asthma, is to support the respiratory muscles while preventing dynamic hyperinflation. To prevent auto-PEEP when the patient is placed back on the ventilator, the settings should be changed to allow for increased exhalation time. This can be achieved by lowering the set rate or the inspiratory time, and provide adequate tidal volume as it usually lowers patient's spontaneous breathing. Of note, a tension pneumothorax is also on the differential and should be considered in this situation.

Parrilla FJ, Moran I, Roche-Campo F, et al. Ventilatory strategies in obstructive lung disease. *Semin Respir Crit Care Med*. 2014;35:431-440. doi:10.1055/s-0034-1382155

17. **The answer is B.** While the patient appears to have all signs and symptoms of status asthmaticus needing intubation, this scenario represents vocal cord dysfunction. Vocal cord dysfunction is an often-missed diagnosis that closely mimics asthma. Classic diagnostic findings on laryngoscopy are inspiratory and expiratory vocal cord adduction with a posterior glottic chink; however, intermittent symptoms make laryngoscopic findings difficult to obtain. Diagnosis should be suspected when signs of status asthmaticus such as wheezing resolve after intubation as seen in this case. In addition, normal airway pressures postintubation suggests that the obstruction was bypassed with intubation as seen in vocal cord dysfunction. In true asthma, the peak pressure would be high due to bronchospasm and increased airway resistance, with normal plateau pressures showing an increase transpulmonary resistance. ABG in this case shows a P/F ratio of 400 inconsistent with ARDS. An increase in intrathoracic pressure would lead to an elevated peak pressure that is not seen here. While no ventilator graphics are shown here, peak pressures are expected to rise with auto-PEEP.

Christopher KL. Understanding vocal cord dysfunction: a step in the right direction with a long road ahead. *Chest*. 2006;129:842-843. doi:10.1378/chest.129.4.842

18. **The answer is B.** The patient is presenting with complicated parapneumonic effusion as evidenced by the exudative nature of the fluid by Light's criteria. The indications for chest tube placement include hemothorax, loculated pleural fluid, pH less than 7.25, and positive Gram stain on pleural fluid and empyema. Expectant waiting with antibiotics and repeat imaging is not recommended as there is no adequate source control. Repeat thoracentesis is also not needed as there are clear indications for chest tube placement. Only patients with persistent pleural infection after multiple attempts at pleural drainage as well as antibiotics should be considered for decortication or surgical consult.

Davis HE, Davis RJ, Davis CW, et al. Management of pleural infection in adults: British Thoracic Society pleural diseases guidelines 2010. *Thorax*. 2010;65(suppl 2):ii41-ii53. doi:10.1136/thx.2010.137000

Feller-Kopman D, Light R. Pleural disease. *N Engl J Med*. 2018;378(8):740-751. doi:10.1056/NEJMra1403503

19. **The answer is E.** According to consensus guidelines on the management of community-acquired pneumonia (CAP) in adults released by Infectious Diseases Society of America

(IDSA) and American Thoracic Society (ATS) in 2007, septic shock requiring vasopressors or acute respiratory failure requiring invasive mechanical ventilation (major criteria) are indications for ICU admission. If the major criteria do not apply, meeting the following three or more minor criteria also warrants admission to an ICU.

RR ≥30 breaths/min

PaO_2/FiO_2 ratio ≤ 250

Multilobar infiltrates

Confusion/disorientation

Uremia (BUN level ≥20 mg/dL)

Leukopenia (WBC count <4,000 cells/mm^3)

Thrombocytopenia (platelet count <100,000 cells/mm^3)

Hypothermia (core temperature <36°C)

Hypotension requiring aggressive fluid resuscitation

This patient meets three minor criteria and requires ICU admission. Of note, IDSA and ATS are updating the guidelines at the time of this publication.

Mandell LA, Wunderink RG, Anzueto A, et al. Infectious Diseases Society of America (IDSA)/American Thoracic Society (ATS) consensus guidelines on the management of community-acquired pneumonia in adults. *Clin Infect Dis.* 2007;44:S27-S72. doi: 10.1086/511159

20. **The answer is D.** Based on the latest edition of the lung cancer staging (2017), the patient's lung cancer would be staged at Stage IVA (T4 N2 M1a). This would carry a 5-year survival of 10%. The latest lung cancer staging system was revised after analyzing data from 94,708 patients treated between 1999 and 2010 across 35 sites in 16 countries. The T component relating to tumor size is subdivided by primary tumor size in 1-cm increments as well as other descriptors of invasion into adjacent structures. The N component is determined by the location of involved lymph nodes. The M component is subdivided into intrathoracic dissemination, a single extrathoracic metastasis, and multiple metastases. These are then used to stage the disease. Accurate staging is essential for selecting appropriate treatment modalities as well as prognostication.

Detterbeck F, Boffa DJ, Kim AW, et al. The eighth edition lung cancer stage classification. *Chest.* 2017;151(1):193-203. doi:10.1016/j.chest.2016.10.010

21. **The answer is A.** Peripheral chemoreceptors for hypoxemia are located in carotid bodies bilaterally at the bifurcation of the common carotid arteries and in aortic bodies in the arch of the aorta. These sensors respond primarily to H^+ ion concentration due to respiratory or metabolic acidosis. Their sensitivity and neural discharges are increased with hypoxemia and are proportional to a PaO_2 less than about 60 torr. The response is made less sensitive by other factors, such as alkalemia, hyperoxia, hypocarbia, anesthetic agents, and older age. The medullary respiratory center is sensitive to CO_2 and regional acidosis.

Prabhakar NR, Peng YJ. Oxygen sensing by the carotid body: past and present. *Adv Exp Med Biol.* 2017;977:3-8. doi:10.1007/978-3-319-55231-6_1

22. **The answer is B.** This question introduces the calculation of the alveolar pressure of oxygen (PAO_2). PAO_2 is the difference between inspired and consumed oxygen.

Inspired O_2 (PIO_2) can be calculated using formula $PIO_2 = (P_B - P_{H_2O}) \times FiO_2$, where P_B = barometric pressure (760 mmHg at sea level) and P_{H_2O} = water vapor pressure (47 mmHg at body temperature). In summary, $PIO_2 = (760 - 47) \times FiO_2 = 713 \times FiO_2$.

Oxygen consumption can be estimated using the respiratory quotient (RQ), which is the ratio of CO_2 produced by the body to O_2 consumed by the body (RQ = $V.CO_2/V.O_2$). Based on this equation, $V.O_2$ roughly equals $PaCO_2/RQ$. RQ depends on the nutritional content (1.0 if primarily using glucose, 0.7 if primarily using fats, and ~0.8 on a mixed diet). To summarize, $V.O_2$ = $PaCO_2 \times 0.8$ = $PaCO_2 \times 1.2$

Therefore, PAO_2 = 713 (FiO_2) − 1.2 ($PaCO_2$). Note that all FiO_2 notations are fractions, not percentages. In the example presented in the question, the PAO_2 = 713 − 40 = 673 mmHg. The alveolar gas equation can be utilized to calculate A-a gradient, which in turn can be used to calculate the shunt fraction or the amount of blood that is getting shunted from the lungs.

West JB. *Respiratory Physiology: The Essentials.* 6th ed. Philadelphia, PA: Lippincott Williams & Wilkins; 2000.

23. **The answer is D.** The FEV_1/FVC ratio is the measure of obstructive pulmonary changes least susceptible to measurement biases and best able to separate patients with normal or restrictive lungs from those with obstructive disease. A normal percentage is above 70%. Patients with obstructive lung disease may depend on a prolonged expiratory time to ensure emptying of their tidal volume. This reflects as an abnormal inhalation time to exhalation time (I:E) ratio during spontaneous breathing (i.e., expiratory component greater than the normal 1:2). A clinical observation of the patient's I:E ratio prior to intubation might have been helpful in choosing the initial ventilator settings. Careful observation of the I:E ratio, calculated by the ventilator, is important to prevent occurrence of auto–positive end-expiratory pressure (PEEP; see Answer 16).

Parrilla FJ, Moran I, Roche-Campo F, et al. Ventilatory strategies in obstructive lung disease. *Semin Respir Crit Care Med.* 2014;35:431-440. doi:10.1055/s-0034-1382155

24. **The answer is B.** The RSBI is a popular test for weaning of mechanical ventilation in the ICU. RSBI is measured during at least 1 minute of spontaneous breathing as the ratio of spontaneous breathing rate to averaged tidal volume (TV) (RSBI = f/V_T). RSBI score greater than 105 is associated with weaning failure while RSBI less than 105 is associated with ~80% chance of successful extubation. RSBI is less accurate in elderly patients and those who have required mechanical ventilation for more than 8 days.

Karthika M, Al Enezi FA, Pillai LV, et al. Rapid shallow breathing index. *Ann Thorac Med.* 2016;11(3):167-176. doi:10.4103/1817-1737.176876

25. **The answer is D.** On the flow–time waveform, the flow does not return to baseline prior to initiation of the next breath suggestive of auto-PEEP. Other methods to determine auto-PEEP would be to perform an expiratory pause or check the frequency dependency of P_{peak} in which you would observe an increase in the peak pressure as the respiratory rate (RR) increases. Adjustments in ventilator setting to prevent or improve auto-PEEP include lowering the RR, tidal volume (TV), or inspiratory time to allow more time for exhalation. Increasing the flow rate will also lower the inspiratory time.

Nilsestuen JO, Hargett KD. Using ventilator graphics to identify patient-ventilator asynchrony. *Respir Care.* 2005;50(2):202-234.
Owens W. Lexington, KY. Chapter 3: troubleshooting. In: Owens W, ed. *The Ventilator Book.* 1st ed. First Draught Press; 2012:15-16.
Parrilla FJ, Moran I, Roche-Campo F, et al. Ventilatory strategies in obstructive lung disease. *Semin Respir Crit Care Med.* 2014;35:431-440. doi:10.1055/s-0034-1382155

26. **The answer is E.** There are essentially two different breaths shown in the pressure–time and flow–time graphs. The second breath consists of normal inspiratory as well as expiratory phase. However, a pressure spike is seen at the end of inspiration in the first, third, and fourth breaths (pointed out with arrows) with a corresponding early cessation of flow suggesting that the patient has transitioned to expiration while the ventilator is still trying to deliver the breath (delayed breath termination). This asynchrony can be fixed by reducing the inspiratory

time on the ventilator to allow the end of the inspiratory breath delivered by the ventilator to coincide with the end of the patient's effort.

Nilsestuen JO, Hargett KD. Using ventilator graphics to identify patient-ventilator asynchrony. *Respir Care*. 2005;50(2):202-234.

27. **The answer is C.** The graphics show double triggering. The first breath shown is normal. In the second breath, the patient initiates breath twice, which makes the ventilator deliver two breaths before an expiratory phase can begin.

Nilsestuen JO, Hargett KD. Using ventilator graphics to identify patient-ventilator asynchrony. *Respir Care*. 2005;50(2):202-234.

28. **The answer is D.** The graphs on the left demonstrate autocycling. Based on the flow–time curve, the patient is on synchronized intermittent-mandatory ventilation mode with pressure support where every other breath is being supported. Note the saw tooth appearance in the esophageal pressure panel corresponding to the heart rate (HR). These changes in intrathoracic pressure are sufficient to trigger the ventilator and initiate a breath. The right-side graphs belong to the same patient after resolution of autocycling by increasing ventilator sensitivities. This asynchrony is seen more commonly in patients after valve replacement procedures or with a bronchopleural fistula and a large volume leak into a chest tube. Occasionally fluid, if present in the tubing connecting the ventilator to the endotracheal tube, can move and trigger the ventilator as well.

Nilsestuen JO, Hargett KD. Using ventilator graphics to identify patient-ventilator asynchrony. *Respir Care*. 2005;50(2):202-234.

29. **The answer is A.** The first breath has normal inspiratory as well as expiratory phases. In the second breath, in comparison to the first breath, the pressure waveform is pulled inward (pointed out with arrow) while the flow returns to baseline and the volume remains unchanged. The pattern suggests that the patient is "sucking in" air faster than the ventilator is providing resulting in a drop in the pressure. The flow asynchrony shown here can be fixed by increasing the flow on the ventilator.

Nilsestuen JO, Hargett KD. Using ventilator graphics to identify patient-ventilator asynchrony. *Respir Care*. 2005;50(2):202-234.

30. **The answer is C.** The clinical scenario is suggestive of acute respiratory distress syndrome (ARDS). The initial ARDSnet trial showed an improved survival with strategies that call for low tidal volume (TV) ventilation in an effort to lower plateau pressures (P_{plat}). It has also been shown that early prone positioning within 12 to 24 hours of developing severe ARDS improves outcomes with a decline in the 28-day mortality from 32.8% (in the supine group) to 16.0% (in the prone group). Other modes of ventilation have also been studied in the management of ARDS. Notably, the trial of HFOV was terminated early at interim analysis due to increased mortality associated with HFOV versus conventional ventilation strategies. APRV has not been shown to result in improved outcomes in ARDS. Inhaled epoprostenolol improves V/Q matching as well as oxygenation; however, it has not been shown to improve outcomes. Pulmonary artery catheter is usually not required for the management of ARDS and is not part of its definition anymore.

Ferguson ND, Cook DJ, Guyatt GH, et al. High-frequency oscillation in early acute respiratory distress syndrome. *N Engl J Med*. 2013;368(9):795-805. doi:10.1056/NEJMoa1215554

Guerin C, Reignier J, Richard JC, et al. Prone positioning in severe acute respiratory distress syndrome. *N Engl J Med*. 2013;368(23):2159-2168. doi:10.1056/NEJMoa1214103

18

Renal Disorders

SUMESKA THAVARAJAH AND DAPHNE H. KNICELY

■ QUESTIONS

1. A 27-year-old-man presents to the ED after a gunshot wound to the chest. Postoperatively, he is in stable condition with blood pressure (BP) 100/80 mmHg, heart rate (HR) 90/min, O_2 saturation 98%, and temperature 98.5°F. He is intubated and sedated on ventilatory support with the following settings: assist control, rate 12, tidal volume (TV) 600 mL, positive end-expiratory pressure (PEEP) 5 cmH$_2$O, and FiO$_2$ 60%. Serum laboratory findings are as follows: Na 150 mEq/L, K 3.5 mEq/L, chloride 100 mEq/L, bicarbonate 30 mEq/L, blood urea nitrogen (BUN) 120 mg/dL, and creatinine (Cr) 1.0 mg/dL. He has been on tube feeds and is tolerating them well. He is noted to be having 3 L of urine output Q8 hours with urine osmolality (UOsm) greater than 300 mOsm/kg. The most likely cause for polyuria and hypernatremia in this patient is:

   A. Polyuria is a result of increasing intravenous (IV) fluids
   B. Hypernatremia is a result of central diabetes insipidus (DI)
   C. Increased osmotic load with high protein intake in tube feeds
   D. Postobstructive diuresis
   E. Hypernatremia as a result of nephrogenic DI

2. A 23-year-old man with a history of obsessive–compulsive disorder (OCD) and heavy tobacco use presents to the ED with pain, fatigue, and 2-day history of nausea with one episode of vomiting. He has been taking paroxetine as prescribed for his OCD symptoms. In the ED, his laboratory findings are as follows: serum Na 114 mEq/L, K 3.5 mEq/L, chloride 90 mEq/L, bicarbonate 23 mEq/L, blood urea nitrogen (BUN) 10 mg/dL, creatinine (Cr) 0.5 mg/dL, and serum osmolality 200 mOsm/kg; urine osmolality (UOsm) 350 mOsm/kg, urine sodium (Una) 70 mEq/L, and urine K 35 mEq/L. Blood pressure (BP) is 130/80 mmHg, orthostatics are negative, and heart rate (HR) is 80/min. The patient is alert and shows no indication of confusion. What is the cause of his hyponatremia?

   A. Water intoxication
   B. Syndrome of inappropriate antidiuretic hormone (SIADH) secretion due to use of selective serotonin reuptake inhibitors (SSRIs)
   C. Diabetes insipidus (DI)
   D. Volume depletion
   E. Solute limited water excretion

3. A 60-year-old woman is admitted with increasing abdominal distention secondary to small bowel obstruction (SBO). A nasogastric tube (NGT) is placed to suction and normal saline (NS) is infused while awaiting surgical consult. Her blood work is as follows: Na 140 mEq/L, K 3.4 mEq/L, chloride 85 mEq/L, bicarbonate 35 mEq/L, blood urea nitrogen (BUN)

40 mg/dL, and creatinine (Cr) 1.4 mg/dL. Arterial blood gas (ABG) shows pH 7.51, $PaCO_2$ 45, and PaO_2 82. Urinary chloride is 8 mEq/L. How would you correct her alkalosis?

A. Increase the intravenous (IV) fluid rate and correct her hypokalemia
B. Discontinue NS and start $NaHCO_3$ infusion
C. Clamp the NGT
D. Start infusing 0.1% HCl via the central line
E. Initiate patient on hemodialysis with low bicarbonate dialysate solution

4. A 70-year-old man with a history of diabetes, hypertension, and chronic obstructive pulmonary disease (COPD) presents to the ED with a COPD exacerbation. He is intubated for severe respiratory distress. His arterial blood gas (ABG) shows pH 7.35, $PaCO_2$ 55 mmHg, and PaO_2 40 mmHg. His respiratory rate (RR) on the ventilator is increased. He is later noted to be unresponsive. Oxygen saturation is greater than 90%. His serum electrolytes are Na 130 mEq/L, K 4.6 mEq/L, chloride 90 mEq/L, bicarbonate 40 mEq/L, blood urea nitrogen (BUN) 30 mg/dL, and creatinine (Cr) 1.5 mg/dL. What is the cause of his neurological decline?

A. Acute stroke
B. Acute correction of his acidosis with intubation and increased RR on ventilator
C. Hyponatremia
D. Pneumothorax
E. Increased oxygen saturations

5. A 30-year-old man presents to the ED with altered mental status (AMS) and combative behavior. His initial serum labs are sodium (Na) 135 mEq/L, K 4.0 mEq/L, chloride 90 mEq/L, bicarbonate 28 mEq/L, blood urea nitrogen (BUN) 28 mg/dL, creatinine (Cr) 1.5 mg/dL, calcium 8.2 mg/dL, and creatine kinase (CK) 300,000. Arterial blood gas (ABG) shows pH 7.53, $PaCO_2$ 35 mmHg, and PaO_2 90 mmHg. Urine drug screen is positive for cocaine and lysergic acid diethylamide (LSD). He has multiple bruises and a fractured femur. How would you most effectively treat this patient's acute kidney injury (AKI)?

A. Start normal saline (NS) infusion 1 to 2 L/hr to maintain urine output of 200 to 300 mL/hr
B. Start D5W with 150 mEq of $NaHCO_3$ infusion
C. Hemodialysis
D. Mannitol infusion
E. Lasix infusion

6. A 40-year-old man with congestive heart failure (CHF) and bipolar affective disorder on lithium presents to the ED with ataxia, tremors, and confusion. Family report a 4-day history of viral illness with poor oral intake. His serum laboratory workup shows lithium level 3.0 mEq/L (normal 0.6–1.0 mEq/L), Na 140 mEq/L, K 3.5 mEq/L, chloride 100 mEq/L, bicarbonate 28 mEq/L, blood urea nitrogen (BUN) 30 mg/dL, and creatinine (Cr) 1.5 mg/dL. What is the next step in management?

A. Normal saline (NS) infusion
B. Mannitol infusion
C. Lasix infusion
D. Administration of activated charcoal
E. Hemodialysis

7. A 70-year-old man presents with urinary retention and abdominal pain for the last week. A Foley catheter is placed in the ED and greater than 1 L of clear urine is drained and continued to flow. Serum labs are as follows: sodium (Na) 140 mEq/L, K 5.0 mEq/L, chloride 100 mEq/L, bicarbonate 20 mEq/L, blood urea nitrogen (BUN) 105 mg/dL, and creatinine (Cr) 10 mg/dL. What is the best step in managing this patient?

A. Keep the Foley catheter and start benign prostatic hypertrophy (BPH) treatment with follow-up with urology in 1 week

B. Infuse 1 to 2 L of normal saline (NS) in the ED and discharge home with follow-up in 1 week with indwelling Foley catheter

C. Instruct patient on intermittent self-catheterization and place on BPH medications with follow-up

D. Admit patient to the hospital and continue to follow urine output closely. Start 0.45% NaCl infusion and adjust fluids as needed with frequent lab checks to ensure electrolyte stability

E. Admit patient to the hospital and start intravenous (IV) fluids containing bicarbonate supplementation

8. A 40-year-old woman with a history of uncontrolled type 2 diabetes (insulin-dependent) and hypertension presents to the ED with a lower extremity ulcer and erythema. She is admitted with a diagnosis of cellulitis and is started on nafcillin with white blood cell (WBC) count decreasing from 35,000 to 15,000 in 2 days. On day 6 of treatment, she is noted to have a rash and fever of 102°F. Her creatinine (Cr) continues to rise, from 1.0 to 6.5 mg/dL in 5 days. What is the cause of her acute kidney injury (AKI), and how would you treat it?

A. Acute tubular necrosis (ATN) secondary to infection and sepsis. Attain cultures and add broader antibiotic coverage.

B. Acute interstitial nephritis (AIN) secondary to nafcillin. Would stop nafcillin now and consider starting steroids if Cr does not improve.

C. Obstruction and urinary retention secondary to her diabetes. Would place Foley now.

D. Postinfectious glomerulonephritis.

E. Immune (idiopathic) thrombocytopenic purpura (ITP) due to nafcillin. Would stop nafcillin and start steroids.

9. A 70-year-old white male with a history of neuroendocrine tumor of unknown origin presents with hypokalemia and metabolic alkalosis. Blood pressure (BP) is elevated at 180/90 mmHg. Serum K 2.4 is mEq/L and serum bicarbonate is 30 mEq/L. How would you manage this patient?

A. Replete potassium and continue to follow up his labs

B. Add aldactone or amiloride and titrate as tolerated to keep potassium within a normal range

C. Start an angiotensin converting enzyme (ACE) inhibitor

D. Start acetazolamide to prevent proximal bicarbonate reabsorption

E. Start HCl infusion

10. A 60-year-old with a history of type 2 diabetes, hypertension, hyperlipidemia, and stage 3 chronic kidney disease (baseline creatinine [Cr] 2.0 mg/dL) presents with chest pain. She is found to have elevated troponins and is diagnosed with a non–ST-elevation myocardial infarction (NSTEMI). Cardiology will take the patient for cardiac catheterization, but needs recommendations for renal protection.

A. Would not recommend cardiac catheterization and follow-up for now

B. Would proceed with cardiac catheterization with infusion of normal saline (NS) or sodium bicarbonate at 1 mL/kg pre- and postprocedure

C. Start N-acetyl cysteine

D. No need for prophylactic measures

E. Hemodialysis to be performed prophylactically after contrast administration

11. A 28-year-old female with a history of heavy alcohol use is found obtunded on the side of the road with a bottle of a sweet-smelling unknown substance. She is tachypneic with a respiratory rate (RR) of 30/min, blood pressure (BP) 80/40 mmHg, temperature 97°F, and heart rate (HR) 110/min. Her serum labs are as follows: Na 135 mEq/L, K 3.5 mEq/L, chloride 100 mEq/L, bicarbonate 10 mEq/L, blood urea nitrogen (BUN) 20 mg/dL, creatinine (Cr)

1.5 mg/dL, glucose 120 mg/dL, and serum osmolality 330 mOsm/kg. Arterial blood gas (ABG) shows a pH 7.23, PaCO$_2$ 25 mmHg, and PaO$_2$ 98 mmHg. Urine microscopy revealed calcium oxalate crystals. What would be your next step?

A. Administer fomepizole and perform emergent hemodialysis
B. Start ethanol (EtOH) infusion
C. Administer fomepizole only
D. Administer activated charcoal
E. Start sodium bicarbonate infusion

12. An 18-year-old who suffered a severe head trauma while riding his motorcycle is admitted to the neuroscience ICU, and found to have a subarachnoid hemorrhage (SAH) with cerebral edema and intracranial pressures (ICPs) measured in the 30s. Over the next few days he has an acute drop in his serum sodium to 112 mEq/L. Other serum laboratory findings are as follows: K 4.0 mEq/L, chloride 74 mEq/L, bicarbonate 25 mEq/L, blood urea nitrogen (BUN) 20 mg/dL, creatinine (Cr) 0.9 mg/dL, and serum osmolality 282 mosmol/kg. Urine studies show: urine osmolality (UOsm) 368 mosmol/kg, urine sodium (Una) 112 mEq/L, and urine K 26 mEq/L. His systolic blood pressures (SBPs) have decreased to the 90s with decreased skin turgor and he has increased urine output of 9 L/24 hr. What is the etiology of patient's polyuria and hyponatremia?

A. Central diabetes insipidus (DI)
B. Physiologic water diuresis in response to hyponatremia
C. Physiological salt diuresis
D. Syndrome of inappropriate antidiuretic hormone (SIADH)
E. Cerebral salt wasting (CSW)

13. A 60-year-old male with a history of type 2 diabetes, hypertension, and bipolar disorder on lithium for years is admitted to the hospital with a diagnosis of small bowel obstruction (SBO). He undergoes nasogastric tube (NGT) placement and is started on normal saline (NS) at 75 mL/hr. He is later noted to be more lethargic. His serum labs are as follows: sodium (Na) 160 mEq/L, K 3.5 mEq/L, chloride 124 mEq/L, bicarbonate 23 mEq/L, blood urea nitrogen (BUN) 32 mg/dL, creatinine (Cr) 1.5 mg/dL, glucose 125 mg/dL, and serum osmolality 331 mOsm/kg. Urine osmolality (UOsm) is 150 mOsm/kg. His urine output is 2 L every 8 hours. What is the cause of his hypernatremia?

A. Central diabetes insipidus (DI)
B. Osmotic diuresis
C. Increased insensible water losses
D. Nephrogenic DI
E. Hypernatremia secondary to NS

14. A 60-year-old patient with a history of type 2 diabetes, hypertension, and stage 3 chronic kidney disease with a glomerular filtration rate (GFR) of 35 mL/min/1.73 m^2 presents with uncontrolled hypertension. There is a concern for renal artery stenosis, and magnetic resonance angiography (MRA) with gadolinium is planned for further evaluation. Would you proceed with MRA?

A. Yes, accepted GFR for gadolinium infusion is greater than 20 mL/min per 1.73 m^2
B. Yes, accepted GFR for gadolinium infusion is greater than 30 mL/min per 1.73 m^2
C. MRA with gadolinium is contraindicated in this patient.
D. Start intravenous (IV) fluids and mucomyst prior to administration of gadolinium
E. Yes, with plans for dialysis following gadolinium administration

15. A 50-year-old male with a history of type 2 diabetes mellitus (DM), hypertension, and congestive heart failure (CHF, ejection fraction [EF] <20%) presents with pulmonary edema and acute respiratory distress. His vital signs are blood pressure (BP) 80/40 mmHg, heart rate (HR)

120/min, O_2 saturation 90% on 100% nonrebreather mask, and respiratory rate (RR) greater than 25/min. Arterial blood gas (ABG): pH 7.57, $PaCO_2$ 25 mmHg, and PaO_2 60 mmHg, serum bicarbonate 22 mEq/L, serum sodium (Na) 140 mEq/L, serum K 2.9 mEq/L, and serum chloride 100 mEq/L. What is the acid–base disturbance?

A. Acute metabolic acidosis
B. Acute respiratory alkalosis
C. Acute respiratory alkalosis with metabolic alkalosis
D. Acute respiratory alkalosis, metabolic acidosis, and metabolic alkalosis
E. Acute respiratory alkalosis and metabolic acidosis

16. A 35-year-old male with a history of alcohol abuse presents to the ED after being found confused on the street. Serum labs are sodium (Na) 133 mEq/L, K 3.2 mEq/L, chloride 86 mEq/L, bicarbonate 14 mEq/L, blood urea nitrogen (BUN) 12 mg/dL, creatinine (Cr) 1.0 mg/dL, albumin 2.0 g/dL; and arterial blood gas (ABG) shows pH 7.38, $PaCO_2$ 20 mmHg, and PaO_2 90 mmHg. What is the patient's acid–base disorder?

A. Metabolic acidosis, metabolic alkalosis, and respiratory alkalosis
B. Metabolic acidosis
C. Hyperchloremic metabolic acidosis
D. Metabolic acidosis and metabolic alkalosis
E. Metabolic acidosis and respiratory acidosis

17. A 70-year-old man with a ruptured abdominal aortic aneurysm is taken to the operating room and requires infusion with multiple units of packed red blood cells (pRBC). Postoperatively, he is in stable condition and his serum labs are as follows: sodium (Na) 135 mEq/L, K 3.5 mEq/L, chloride 110 mEq/dL, bicarbonate 35 mEq/L, blood urea nitrogen (BUN) 30 mg/dL, and creatinine (Cr) 1.5 mg/dL. Arterial blood gas (ABG) shows pH 7.47, $PaCO_2$ 50 mmHg, and PaO_2 90 mmHg. What is the cause of the patient's metabolic alkalosis?

A. Hyperventilation
B. Nasogastric tube (NGT) suctioning
C. Total parenteral nutrition (TPN)
D. Massive pRBC transfusion
E. Ischemia

18. A 25-year-old woman with a history of anorexia nervosa presents to the ED with fatigue and systolic blood pressures (SBPs) in the 80s. Her serum labs are as follows: sodium (Na) 135 mEq/L, K 2.8 mEq/L, chloride 80 mEq/L, bicarbonate 35 mEq/L, blood urea nitrogen (BUN) 30 mg/dL, and creatinine (Cr) 1.0 mg/dL. Urine labs are urine sodium (Una) 30 mEq/L, urine K 35 mEq/L, and urine chloride 42 mEq/L. What is the cause of this patient's metabolic alkalosis?

A. Patient has been taking high quantities of baking soda as a diet regimen
B. Patient has been using diuretics such as lasix
C. Patient has been inducing nausea and vomiting
D. Patient has been using excessive amount of laxatives and has profuse diarrhea
E. Patient has hyperaldosteronism

19. A 30-year-old African American female is admitted for sickle cell crisis. She is noted to have the following serum labs: sodium (Na) 135 mEq/L, K 5.0 mEq/L, bicarbonate 14 mEq/L, chloride 110 mEq/L, blood urea nitrogen (BUN) 15 mg/dL, creatinine (Cr) 1.0 mg/dL. Arterial blood gas (ABG) shows pH 7.31, $PaCO_2$ 29 mmHg, and PaO_2 90 mmHg. Urine pH is greater than 5.5. Patient is started on normal saline (NS) infusion and pain medications. What is the acid–base abnormality and its cause?

A. Metabolic acidosis secondary to increased lactic acid with vaso-occlusive disease
B. Alkalosis due to excess mineralo-corticoid release
C. Hyperkalemia leading to acidosis
D. Non–anion gap (AG) metabolic acidosis secondary to a type 1 renal tubular acidosis
E. Respiratory acidosis due to hyperventilation in the setting of pain

20. A 55-year-old woman with a history of diabetes, hypertension, and coronary artery disease (CAD) is admitted with a ST-elevation myocardial infarction (STEMI). She undergoes emergent cardiac catheterization and stenting of the left anterior descending artery and circumflex arteries, followed by an intra-aortic balloon pump (IABP) placement. On day 2 of admission, her blood urea nitrogen (BUN; mg/dL) and creatinine (Cr; mg/dL) increases from 10 and 1.0 to 30 and 1.5, respectively, with a decrease in urine output. Upon examination, her legs are mottled and ulcerated. What is the cause of her acute kidney injury (AKI)?

A. Cholesterol emboli causing tubular obstruction and acute tubular necrosis (ATN)
B. Ischemic ATN in setting of hemodynamic changes
C. Contrast-induced nephropathy (CIN)
D. Cardio–renal syndrome leading to prerenal azotemia
E. Urinary obstruction

21. A 60-year-old man with chronic obstructive pulmonary disease (COPD), hypertension, type 2 diabetes, stage 3 chronic kidney disease, and morbid obesity is admitted for left lower-leg swelling. Ultrasound shows acute deep vein thrombosis (DVT) and he is started on a therapeutic dose of intravenous (IV) heparin. Two days later, he is noted to have the following serum labs: Sodium (Na) 135 mEq/L, K 6.0 mEq/L, bicarbonate 23 mEq/L, chloride 110 mEq/L, blood urea nitrogen (BUN) 30 mg/dL, and creatinine (Cr) 2.0 mg/dL. What is the cause of the patient's hyperkalemia?

A. Insulin deficiency
B. Renal insufficiency
C. Heparin infusion
D. Dietary intake
E. Distal renal tubular acidosis

22. A 65-year-old woman presents to the ED with a headache over the last week. She has a history of uncontrolled hypertension for more than 10 years. She is currently taking amlodipine 5 mg daily, metoprolol 100 mg BID, and hydrochlorothiazide (HCTZ) 25 mg daily. On physical exam, her blood pressure (BP) is 205/106 mmHg, heart rate (HR) 61/min, and respiratory rate (RR) 12/min. She has the following serum laboratory findings: sodium (Na) 136 mEq/L, K 3.4 mEq/L, blood urea nitrogen (BUN) 18 mg/dL, and creatinine (Cr) 1.1 mg/dL. Renal artery Doppler shows 40% to 50% renal artery stenosis bilaterally. What is the next step in management?

A. Refer for percutaneous renal artery angioplasty
B. Send for magnetic resonance angiography (MRA)
C. Add lisinopril
D. Increase metoprolol
E. Increase amlodipine

23. A 21-year-old woman is brought to the ED by her friends for acting confused. She was previously at a "rave" party, where it is believed she used "Ecstasy" (3,4-Methylenedioxyamphetamine [MDMA]). On physical exam, her blood pressure (BP) is 120/76 mmHg and heart rate (HR) is 92/min. She is confused but arousable. Her laboratory findings show a serum sodium of 119 mEq/dL. Which of the following laboratory findings would be consistent with her clinical situation and hyponatremia?

A. Serum osmolality less than 280 mOsm/kg, urine sodium (Una) greater than 20 mOsm/kg, urine osmolality (UOsm) greater than 250 mOsm/kg

B. Serum osmolality less than 280 mOsm/kg, Una less than 20 mOsm/kg, UOsm less than 100 mOsm/kg

C. Serum osmolality less than 280 mOsm/kg, Una less than 20 mOsm/kg, UOsm greater than 250 mOsm/kg

D. Serum osmolality greater than 285 mOsm/kg, Una greater than 20 mOsm/kg, UOsm less than 100 mOsm/kg

E. Serum osmolality greater than 285 mOsm/kg, Una less than 20 mOsm/kg, UOsm less than 100 mOsm/kg

24. A 45-year-old man is being transferred to a tertiary hospital for the evaluation of multiple myeloma. He is complaining of back pain and fatigue. His vital signs are normal. He has point tenderness along his lumbar spine. His serum laboratory findings are sodium 130 mEq/L, potassium 3.5 mEq/L, chloride 103 mEq/L, bicarbonate 15 mEq/L, glucose 100 mg/dL, blood urea nitrogen (BUN) 20 mg/dL, and creatinine (Cr) 1.3 mg/dL. Arterial blood gas (ABG) shows a pH 7.32, $PaCO_2$ 30 mmHg, and PaO_2 95. Urinalysis shows a pH 5.5 and 2+ glucose. What is the acid–base disturbance?

A. Metabolic alkalosis
B. Non–anion gap (AG) metabolic acidosis
C. AG metabolic acidosis and metabolic alkalosis
D. Respiratory alkalosis, AG metabolic acidosis, and non-AG metabolic acidosis
E. AG metabolic acidosis

25. A 46-year-old woman is found down at her garage in an apparent suicide attempt. She is taken to the ED where she is confused and combative. Vital signs are as follows: blood pressure (BP) 90/46 mmHg, heart rate (HR) 110/min, respiratory rate (RR) 25/min. CT of head shows hypoattenuation bilaterally in the putamen. Laboratory findings are sodium (Na) 143 mEq/L, K 4.5 mEq/L, Cl 111 mEq/L, bicarbonate 5 mEq/L, glucose 120 mg/dL, blood urea nitrogen (BUN) 78 mg/dL, creatinine (Cr) 1.7 mg/dL, lactic acid 2.3 mmol/L, serum osmolality 330 mOsm/kg. Arterial blood gas (ABG) has a pH of 7.18 and $PaCO_2$ of 14. What is the cause of her acid–base disturbance?

A. Isopropyl alcohol ingestion
B. Salicylate overdose
C. Ethylene glycol ingestion
D. Methanol ingestion
E. Acetaminophen overdose

26. A 67-year-old man presents to the ED with worsening shortness of breath and fever for 1 week. His only medication at home is ibuprofen for pain. Initial vital signs are as follows: temperature 102°F, blood pressure (BP) 100/70 mmHg, heart rate (HR) 123/min, and respiratory rate (RR) 20/min. He is noted to have rales bilaterally and a 3/6 murmur at the left lower sternal border. His admission labs show a blood urea nitrogen (BUN) of 18 mg/dL and creatinine (Cr) of 1 mg/dL. A CT scan of the chest with contrast shows multifocal pulmonary infarcts that are suspicious for septic emboli. An echocardiogram shows a vegetation on the tricuspid valve. Blood cultures are drawn, and he is started on broad spectrum antibiotics including gentamicin. On day 7, his Cr increases to 2 mg/dL, and on day 8 to 3.2 mg/dL. Urine microscopy shows muddy brown casts that are too numerous to count. What is the most likely cause of his acute kidney injury (AKI)?

A. Contrast-induced nephropathy (CIN)
B. Acute interstitial nephritis (AIN)
C. Nephrotoxic acute tubular necrosis (ATN)
D. Prerenal AKI
E. Glomerulonephritis

■ ANSWERS

1. **The answer is C.** This is a typical cause of polyuria and hypernatremia in the ICU setting. In osmotic diuresis, nonelectrolyte solutes such as glucose, mannitol, or urea increase the output of urine. A UOsm greater than 300 mOsm/kg signifies an osmotic diuresis versus a water diuresis, which would have a USom less than 250 mOsm/kg. If the urine electrolytes were checked the concentration of sodium plus potassium would be well below the plasma concentration as well illustrating an osmotic diuresis. In this case, the likely high protein load in the tube feeds will need to be reduced, and free water needs to be repleted to meet the patient's current losses. In central or nephrogenic DI the urine is dilute (UOsm <250 mOsm/kg). Polyuria resulting from increased isotonic IV fluids would not cause hypernatremia, so this is incorrect. Postobstructive diuresis can lead to hypernatremia from free water loss, but this would be a water diuresis instead of an osmotic diuresis, and there are no symptoms or signs to suggest obstruction. Hypernatremia in the ICU setting has been associated with higher mortality and prolonged hospitalization.

   Linder G, Funk GC. Hypernatremia in critically ill patients. *J Crit Care.* 2013;28(2):216.e11-20. doi:10.1016/j.jcrc.2012.05.001

2. **The answer is B.** When evaluating hyponatremia, it is essential to assess the volume status of the patient. Normal BP and orthostatics suggest euvolemic hyponatremia. The patient has a state of increased antidiuretic hormone (ADH) as evidenced by concentrated urine (UOsm >100 mOsm/kg) relative to serum. The urine sodium (Una) greater than 20 mEq/L in euvolemic hyponatremia suggests normal dietary intake of sodium. Causes of inappropriate ADH secretion in this clinical situation include nausea/vomiting, pain, and use of SSRIs. All of these factors cause an increase in ADH secretion and, therefore, free water retention. In order to correct this, the patient should be placed on volume restriction, stop SSRIs, suppress nausea and vomiting, and control his pain. Because his vital signs are stable and there is no indication of volume depletion, intravenous (IV) fluids should not be given. If fluids were to be given in this setting, they would worsen the hyponatremia as a result of retention of more free water. Once his increased ADH stimulus is suppressed, he will start urinating more free water, leading to correction of serum sodium. This is where careful monitoring with frequent serum sodium and urine electrolytes should be ordered. Water intoxication would cause a UOsm less than 100 mOsm/kg due to suppression of ADH and Una of less than 20 mEq/L due to urinary dilution. Volume depletion would cause hypovolemia and urine studies would have a Una of less than 20 mEq/L. Solute-limited water excretion would include beer potomania and tea-and-toast diet with large water intake. It would have a similar urinary study profile of water intoxication but with a history suggesting this etiology. DI, either central or nephrogenic, would result in hypernatremia and a UOsm less than 100 mOsm/kg.

   Buffington MA, Abreo K. Hyponatremia: a review. *J Intensive Care Med.* 2016;31(4):223-236. doi: 10.1177/0885066614566794

3. **The answer is A.** The metabolic alkalosis in this patient is likely due to NGT suction, which leads to gastrointestinal (GI) acid loss and volume depletion. The volume depletion increases aldosterone levels, which in turn increases H^+/ATPase transporter activity in the intercalated cells of the collecting tubule of the nephron. This mediates further bicarbonate reabsorption and acid secretion. In the presence of NGT suctioning, there is also loss of HCl. Maintenance of alkalosis can be caused by volume depletion, increased aldosterone, hypokalemia, and chloride depletion. These all lead to increased tubular bicarbonate reabsorption and reduction in bicarbonate excretion by the intercalated cells in the collecting duct. The low tubular concentration of chloride will result in decreased function of the chloride/bicarbonate transporter and will worsen the alkalosis. Hypokalemia can lead to worsening alkalosis due to distal hydrogen secretion mediated by $H^+–K^+$–ATPase exchange pumps in the luminal membrane that actively reabsorb potassium as well as secrete hydrogen. Therefore, to treat this condition, you need to correct the causes that are maintaining the alkalosis, such as repleting the

potassium and giving NS infusion to correct the volume depletion and correct chloride depletion. Clamping the NGT would stop the cause for the alkalosis, but is necessary for managing the SBO.

Galla JH, Gifford JD, Luke RG, et al. Adaptations to chloride depletion alkalosis. *Am J Physiol.* 1991;261(4-Pt2):R771. doi:10.1152/ajpregu.1991.261.4.R771

Soifer JT, Kim HT. Approach to metabolic alkalosis. *Emerg Med Clin North A.* 2014;32(2):453-463. doi:10.1016/j.emc.2014.01.005

4. **The answer is B.** The patient is a chronic retainer of CO_2, and acutely correcting his hypercapnia would lead to metabolic alkalosis. Acute increase in the intracerebral pH can lead to severe brain damage and death. In addition, posthypercapnic alkalemia can decrease cardiac output and cerebral blood flow (CBF) and lead to seizures. Hyponatremia is not severe enough to lead to neurological changes. There is no suggestion of an acute stroke or pneumothorax at this point. Increased oxygen saturations would lead to respiratory depression in a chronic retainer of CO_2 but the ventilator settings have corrected the CO_2 retention.

Dhondup T, Quin Q. Acid base and electrolyte disorders in patients with and without chronic kidney disease: an update. *Kidney Dis.* 2017;3(4):136-148. doi:10.1159/000479968

5. **The answer is A.** Volume expansion is the key to treating severe rhabdomyolysis. Intravenous (IV) isotonic saline should be administered as soon as possible. Initial rate of isotonic saline should be 1 to 2 L/hr. Fluids are titrated to maintain a urine output of 200 to 300 mL/hr. Fluids should be continued until CK levels decrease to less than 5,000 unit/L and continue to trend down. Risk of AKI is lower in patients with a peak CK of less than 5,000 to 10,000 unit/L. Another choice would be $NaHCO_3$ solution to prevent heme pigment–induced AKI. $NaHCO_3$ solution is considered in severe muscle injury with a rising CK or those with severe rhabdomyolysis with CK greater than 5,000 unit/L. It can be given if no hypocalcemia present, pH less than 7.5, and serum bicarbonate less than 30 mEq/L. The infusion of $NaHCO_3$ solution would be 150 mEq of $NaHCO_3$ in D5W at an initial rate of 200 mL/hr with a goal to keep urinary pH above 6.5. This patient has mild hypocalcemia and a pH greater than 7.5. Also there is no clear evidence that alkaline diuresis is more effective than saline diuresis for preventing AKI in rhabdomyolysis. There is no current indication for hemodialysis. Mannitol and furosemide may help in increasing urinary flow and prevent further precipitation of heme-proteins, but there are no data available to establish improved outcomes.

Chavez LO, Leon M, Enov S, et al. Beyond muscle destruction: a systematic review of rhabdomyolysis for clinical practice. *Crit Care.* 2016;20(1):135. doi:10.1186/s13054-016-1314-5

6. **The answer is E.** The patient has lithium toxicity. Hemodialysis should be performed for lithium poisoning if serum lithium is >4 mEq/L regardless of symptoms; or if serum lithium is greater than 2.5 mEq/L and preexisting comorbidities such as congestive heart failure or volume overload limit aggressive intravenous (IV) fluid hydration. Clearance with hemodialysis is about 70 to 170 mL/min. Most require a second session of hemodialysis due to rebound of lithium. This rebound can be avoided if hemodialysis is followed by continuous renal replacement therapy (CRRT). The goal is resolution of symptoms and a serum lithium level less than 1 mEq/L. IV fluids are indicated but will not be effective enough to help the kidney clear such a toxic level. The other modalities have not shown effectiveness in the literature.

Baird-Gunning J, Lea-Henry T, Hoegberg LCG, et al. Lithium poisoning. *J Intensive Care Med.* 2017;32(4):249-263. doi:10.1177/0885066616651582

Mirrakhimov AE, Barbaryan A, Gray A, et al. The role of renal replacement therapy in the management of pharmacologic poisonings. *Int J Nephrol.* 2016;2016:3047329. doi:10.1155/2016/3047329

7. **The answer is D.** The patient likely has BPH and would benefit from keeping the Foley catheter in place. Urology should be consulted and BPH medications started. However, it would not be appropriate to discharge a patient with this level of obstruction and acute kidney

injury (AKI). The patient will develop postobstructive diuresis due to the intrinsic damage to the renal concentrating ability; and therefore, lose free water with consequent hypernatremia. A 0.45% NaCl infusion should be started with close electrolyte monitoring until BUN and Cr improve and polyuria resolves. Down-regulation of aquaporin 2 (AQP-2) channels due to bilateral ureteral obstruction has been shown to be the cause of slow recovery in concentration capacity in rats. Use of IV fluids containing sodium bicarbonate is not indicated.

Kim SW, Cho SH, Oh B, et al. Diminished renal expression of aquaporin water channels in rats with bilateral ureteral obstruction. *J Am Soc Nephrol*. 2001;12(10):2019–2028.

8. **The answer is B.** The patient developed AKI, rash, and fever acutely after a few days of administration of nafcillin, which is more consistent with AIN. The classic triad presentation is fever, rash (erythematous maculopapular rash on trunk and proximal extremities) and peripheral eosinophilia. This triad is an exception rather than a rule and is present in less than 10% of AIN presentations. Urinalysis might show pyuria and WBC casts. Urine eosinophils can be checked, although these are not always present. About 15% of hospitalized patients can have urine eosinophils due to a variety of reasons, including inflammatory disease of the kidney and urinary tract. The appropriate management is to stop the offending agent. Absolute indications for steroids in AIN include Sjogren's syndrome, sarcoidosis, systemic lupus erythematosus interstitial nephritis, tubulointerstitial nephritis and uveitis (TINU), and idiopathic and other granulomatous interstitial nephritis. Relative indications for steroids in AIN include drug-induced with rapid progression of renal failure, diffuse infiltrates on kidney biopsy, impending need for dialysis, and delayed recovery. Usual steroid dosing is methylprednisolone 0.5 to 1 g for 1 to 3 days followed by daily high-dose oral prednisone (1 mg/kg/d). ATN secondary to the infectious process is possible, but the patient has a rash and has been responding to nafcillin with decreasing WBC counts. There are no symptoms or signs of urinary obstruction or features of ITP. Postinfectious glomerulonephritis would not be associated with a fever or the skin rash. The urinalysis would have both red blood cells (RBCs) and WBCs.

Nast CC. Medication induced interstitial nephritis in the 21st century. *Adv Chronic Kidney Dis*. 2017;24(2):72-79. doi:10.1053/j.ackd.2016.11.016

Perazella MA, Markowitz GS. Drug-induced acute interstitial nephritis. *Nat Rev Nephrol*. 2010;6(8):461-470. doi:10.1038/nrneph.2010.71

9. **The answer is B.** A patient with hypokalemia, alkalosis, and hypertension should raise suspicion of hyperaldosteronism. In the setting of malignancy, the tumor is likely secreting an aldosterone-like hormone. Aldosterone acts on the epithelial sodium channel (ENaC) located in the principal cells of the collecting tubule. The increased sodium reabsorption helps in creating a negative electrochemical gradient within the tubule lumen that drives potassium excretion into the lumen via renal outer-medullary potassium (ROMK) channels, promoting hypokalemia. The same lumenal electronegativity from increased sodium reabsorption causes type A intercalated cells in the collecting tubules to increase hydrogen ion excretion leading to alkalosis. Acetazolamide and hydrochloric acid infusions will correct the alkalosis, but this is not the major underlying cause for the hypokalemia. ACE inhibitors will help with BP control and do result in potassium retention, but would not address the hyperaldosterone state. Amiloride would directly block the ENaC channel, correcting hypokalemia and alkalosis. Aldactone is a direct antagonist to aldosterone and would also ameliorate its effects. Repleting potassium alone will not correct the underlying cause.

Vilela LAP, Almeida MQ. Diagnosis and management of primary aldosteronism. *Arch Endocrinol Metab*. 2017;61(3):305-312. doi:10.1590/2359-3997000000274

10. **The answer is B.** The age of the patient and the presence of diabetes and chronic kidney disease are risk factors for contrast-induced nephropathy (CIN). It is important to incorporate prophylactic measures. Data have shown that volume expansion with NS or $NaHCO_3$ has helped prevent contrast-induced acute kidney injury (AKI). Sodium bicarbonate solution might decrease the generation of free radicals but its mechanism remains poorly defined

beyond volume expansion. There is an added burden in preparation and potential for errors. Guidelines recommend either solution for volume expansion and prevention of CIN. There is no standard on the optimal rate or duration of infusion. Some studies suggest 1 to 1.5 mL/kg/hr for at least 6 hours before and after the procedure. Other studies suggested fluids 1 hour prior and continued for 3 to 6 hours after the procedure. Volume of fluid administered needs to be determined after careful evaluation of the patient and their volume status. Mucomyst can be started, although there is no data for definite protection. There is no data supporting prophylactic hemodialysis for preventing AKI.

Sharfuddin AA, Weisbord SD, Palevsky PM, et al. Acute kidney injury. In: Skorecki K, Chertow G, Marsden P, et al. eds. *Brenner and Rector's The Kidney*. 10th ed.Elsevier,PA;2016:3.

Tao SM, Wichmann JL, Schoepf UJ, et al. Contrast induced nephropathy in CT: incidence, risk factors, and strategies for prevention. *Eur Radiol*. 2016;26(9):3310–3318. doi:10.1007/s00330-015-4155-8

11. **The answer is A.** The patient has an anion gap metabolic acidosis with high osmolar gap. The clinical history suggests ethylene glycol ingestion with a bottle of sweet-smelling substance and calcium oxalate crystals on urine microscopy. Treatment begins with inhibiting alcohol dehydrogenase, which converts ethylene glycol to glycolic and oxalic acid. Inhibition can be achieved with giving ethanol or fomepizole. More adverse events occur with ethanol than fomepizole. It is recommended to give a loading dose of fomepizole, then perform hemodialysis if the pH is less than 7.3, serum ethylene glycol concentration is greater than 50 mg/dL (no fomepizole), serum ethylene glycol concentration is greater than 300 mg/dL (after fomepizole), or AKI. This patient has acute kidney injury (AKI), so hemodialysis is indication in addition to fomepizole. She will likely need fomepizole redosed after hemodialysis. The other therapies have proven effective in less severe toxicity. Activated charcoal would be ineffective because ethylene glycol would have been absorbed immediately after ingestion.

Kraut JA, Mullins ME. Toxic alcohols. *N Engl J Med*. 2018;378:270-280. doi:10.1056/NEJMra1615295

12. **The answer is E.** This patient has hypovolemic hyponatremia with polyuria. Elevated UOsm would be present in physiologic salt diuresis, SIADH, and CSW. The distinguishing feature is volume depletion, which is present only in CSW. The clinical history of SAH with cerebral edema and increased ICPs correlates with CSW. Increased ICP leads to increased brain natriuretic peptide (BNP), which is believed to cause salt and water diuresis. Correction requires isotonic or hypertonic saline infusion, which would replete the sodium and volume status and also suppress the high antidiuretic hormone (ADH) state, correcting the hyponatremia.

Spasovski G, Vanholder R, Allollo B, et al. Clinical practice guideline on diagnosis and treatment of hyponatraemia. *Eur J Endocrinol*. 2014;170(3):G1-G47. doi:10.1530/EJE-13-1020

13. **The answer is D.** The patient has nephrogenic DI secondary to chronic exposure to lithium. Lithium enters the epithelial sodium channel (ENaC) in the principal cells of the tubule and interferes with the signaling pathway, inhibiting aquaporin-2 (AQP-2) water channels, resulting in dilute urine and, if not treated, hypernatremia. Nephrogenic DI is treated with thiazide diuretics and/or amiloride. The diuretics lead to hypovolemia that stimulate an increase in proximal sodium and water reabsorption. This results in decreased water delivery to the antidiuretic hormone (ADH)–sensitive sites in the collecting tubules and reducing the urine output. Persistent polyuria can be treated with nonsteroidal anti-inflammatory drugs (NSAIDs), which inhibit prostaglandin production and increase the kidneys' concentrating ability.

Christensen BM, Zuber AM, Loffing J, et al. alphaENaC-mediated lithium absorption promotes nephrogenic diabetes insipidus. *J Am Soc Nephrol*. 2011;22(2):253-261. doi: 10.1681/ASN.2010070734

14. **The answer is B.** The U.S. Food and Drug Administration (FDA) recommends avoiding gadolinium due to the risk of nephrogenic systemic fibrosis (NSF) in patients with a GFR of less than 30 mL/min/1.73 m^2, receiving dialysis, or with acute kidney injury (AKI).

A single hemodialysis session removes about 70% of the administered gadolinium. Two treatments clear 95% and three treatments clear 98%. If the patient has a GFR less than 30 mL/min and gadolinium is necessary, the study can be completed provided that the patient undergoes hemodialysis. Varying guidelines recommend prompt initiation of hemodialysis no later than 2 hours after administration of gadolinium, an additional session within 24 hours of the first session, and a third session is possibly recommended for at least 9 hours of hemodialysis. There are no data yet to confirm this strategy.

Rodby RA. Dialytic therapies to prevent NSF following gadolinium exposure in high-risk patients. *Semin Dial.* 2008;21(2):145-149. doi:10.1111/j.1525-139X.2007.00405.x

15. **The answer is D.** To approach this question, one would first calculate the anion gap (AG): Na − (Cl + HCO_3), which is 18 (normal AG 12 mEq/L +/−4). Therefore, there is an AG metabolic acidosis. Then calculate the change in AG relative to the change in HCO_3 (delta ratio). The change in HCO_3 is 25 − 22 = 3 and AG change is 18 − 12 = 6, with a delta ratio of 2:1 suggests an underlying metabolic alkalosis. Looking at the ABG, the primary disturbance is respiratory alkalosis. A decrease of 10 in $PaCO_2$ causes a decrease of 2 in HCO_3, which is consistent in acute respiratory alkalosis.

Ratnam S, Kaehny W, Shapiro J, et al. Pathogenesis and management of metabolic acidosis and alkalosis. In: Schrier RW, ed. *Renal and Electrolyte Disorders.* 7th ed. Philadelphia, PA: Lippincott Williams & Wilkins; 2010:86-119.

16. **The answer is A.** For every decrease of 1 g/dL of albumin, there is a decrease in anion gap (AG) by 2.5 (corrected AG = AG + [2.5 × (4 − albumin)]). The patient has an AG of 33 corrected for hypo-albuminemia (normal AG 12 mEq/L+/− 4). This is an AG metabolic acidosis. The change in AG is two times greater than the change in bicarbonate (change in AG is 21 and change in bicarbonate is 11), suggesting a metabolic alkalosis. Upon reviewing the ABG, the expected $PaCO_2$ should be 28; however, it is 20 (using Winter's formula $PaCO_2 = [1.5 \times HCO_3]$ + 8), explaining the concomitant respiratory alkalosis component.

Ratnam S, Kaehny W, Shapiro J, et al. Pathogenesis and management of metabolic acidosis and alkalosis. In: Schrier RW, ed. *Renal and Electrolyte Disorders.* 7th ed. Philadelphia, PA: Lippincott Williams & Wilkins; 2010:86-119.

17. **The answer is D.** The patient has received multiple units of pRBCs, which contain citrate. The liver metabolizes citrate to produce 23 mEq of bicarbonate for each unit that is transfused. In the setting of acute kidney injury (AKI), there is decreased clearance of bicarbonate compounding alkalosis. The hypercapnia that occurs as a compensatory measure can further impair the renal correction of the metabolic alkalosis.

Ratnam S, Kaehny W, Shapiro J, et al. Pathogenesis and management of metabolic acidosis and alkalosis. In: Schrier RW, ed. *Renal and Electrolyte Disorders.* 7th ed. Philadelphia, PA: Lippincott Williams & Wilkins; 2010:86-119.

18. **The answer is B.** The patient has hypokalemia, metabolic alkalosis, and volume depletion. In this setting with a high urine chloride, it would suggest current diuretic abuse or Gitelman's syndrome. With her past medical history, there is more of a suspicion of diuretic abuse that can be confirmed by a diuretic screen. For diarrhea or vomiting, the urine chloride would be low. High quantities of baking soda do not explain the volume depletion. Hyperaldosteronism would cause a high urine chloride along with hypokalemia and metabolic alkalosis, but it is considered a volume-expanded state.

Ratnam S, Kaehny W, Shapiro J, et al. Pathogenesis and management of metabolic acidosis and alkalosis. In: Schrier RW, ed. *Renal and Electrolyte Disorders.* 7th ed. Philadelphia, PA: Lippincott Williams & Wilkins; 2010:86-119.

19. **The answer is D.** Sickle cell disease (SCD)–induced hypoxia in the renal medulla results in decreased distal sodium reabsorption. This prevents generation of the gradient need for potassium and hydrogen ion secretion and leads to the development of a non-AG metabolic

acidosis. This patient has a non-AG metabolic acidosis with hyperkalemia and elevated urine pH. Treatment includes replacing bicarbonate at 1 to 2 mEq/kg to offset acid buildup. Hyperventilation would result in a drop in the $PaCO_2$ and respiratory alkalosis. The ABG in this question is not consistent with primary respiratory alkalosis.

Reddy P. Clinical approach to renal tubular acidosis in adult patients. *Int J Clin Pract.* 2011;65(3): 350-360. doi:10.1111/j.1742-1241.2009.02311.x

20. **The answer is A.** The patient's skin findings are consistent with livedo reticularis secondary to cholesterol emboli. She has had vascular manipulation with both cardiac catheterization and an IABP placement. Her AKI is likely due to cholesterol emboli causing ischemic damage to the renal tubules. An inflammatory process with interleukin-5 release by activated T-cells has been described in up to 88% of cases, with some reports of increased survival and renal function improvement with corticosteroids. Ischemic ATN can occur with hemodynamic changes, but would not be associated with the skin changes.

Scolari F, Ravani P. Atheroembolic renal disease. *Lancet.* 2010;375(9726):1650-1660. doi:10.1016/ S0140-6736(09)62073-0

21. **The answer is C.** Heparin causes suppression of aldosterone synthesis by reducing the number and affinity of angiotensin-II receptors in the zona glomerulosa of the adrenal gland. Aldosterone causes increased sodium reabsorption in the principal cells of the collecting tubule and also promotes potassium excretion into the tubular lumen. This uncommon side effect is more common in the elderly, renal insufficiency, and diabetic patients who are unable to compensate the aldosterone reduction with renin increase. The other possibilities are unlikely.

Bengalorka G, Sarala N, Venkatrathnamma PN, et al. Effect of heparin and low-molecular weight heparin on serum potassium and sodium levels. *J Pharmacol Pharmacother.* 2011;2(4):266-269. doi:10.4103/0976-500X.85956

22. **The answer is C.** It is necessary to rule out renal artery stenosis in resistant hypertension. In this case, it is most likely atherosclerotic renal artery stenosis due to age of the patient, rather than nonatherosclerotic renal artery stenosis such as fibromuscular dysplasia as you would see in a young female. Based on several trials, medical management is preferred which includes optimal management of hypertension with an antihypertensive regimen that includes a renin-angiotensin system (RAS) blocker, in addition to low-density lipoprotein cholesterol reduction with a high-intensity statin, smoking cessation, hemoglobin A1c reduction in patients with diabetes mellitus (DM), and antiplatelet therapy. Revascularization is considered in those with refractory hypertension, worsening renal function, and/or intractable heart failure. Further imaging is not necessary with an MRA. Increasing metoprolol would not be recommended at the current HR. Increasing the amlodipine would help the BP but not address the cause of the BP. RAS blockers are indicated in renal artery stenosis.

Whelton PK, Carey RM, Aronow WS, et al. 2017 ACC/AHA/AAPA/ABC/ACPM/AGS/APhA/ ASH/ASPC/NMA/PCNA guideline for the prevention, detection, evaluation, and management of high blood pressure in adults: a report of the American College of Cardiology/American Heart Association Task Force on Clinical Practice Guidelines. *Hypertension.* 2017;71(6):1269-1324. doi:10.1161/HYP.0000000000000066

23. **The answer is A.** MDMA has been associated with hyponatremia. "Ecstasy" leads to secretion of antidiuretic hormone (ADH) and polydipsia due to amphetamines, inducing dry mouth and sensation of thirst. Other factors involved in the pathogenesis of "Ecstasy"-associated hyponatremia include readily available fluids at "rave" parties, encouragement to drink a lot of fluid at these parties, variable solute loss in sweat, absorption of hypotonic fluids from gastrointestinal (GI) tract, and volume depletion from excess sweating/hyperthermia. Serum sodium levels are usually less than 130 mEq/L. Choice A illustrates inappropriate ADH secretion with hypoosmolality, Una greater than 20 mOsm/kg (reflecting dietary intake), and concentrated urine with an osmolality greater than 250 mOsm/kg. Choice B illustrates water intoxication or psychogenic polydipsia with hypoosmolality, Una less than 20 mOsm/kg due

to dilution, and maximally dilute urine. Choice C illustrates volume depleted states or states of decreased effective circulating volume (cirrhosis, heart failure, and nephrosis) with hypoosmolality, decreased Una due to renin–angiotensin–aldosterone system being turned on, and concentrated urine. Choice D illustrates hyperosmotic hyponatremia such as hyperglycemia in the setting of diabetes with Una greater than 20 mOsm/kg due to dietary intake and dilute urine. Choice E would result in hypernatremia.

Campbell GA, Rosner MH. The agony of ecstasy: MDMA (3,4-methylenedioxymethamphetamine) and the kidney. *Clin J Am Soc Neph.* 2008;3(6):1852-1860. doi:10.2215/CJN.02080508

24. **The answer is B.** The patient has a non-AG metabolic acidosis. AG is 12, which is normal. There is respiratory compensation if you check the Winter's formula, which predicts a $PaCO_2$ of 30.5 +/− 2. The patient has multiple myeloma, which might also explain the pseudohyponatremia due to hyperproteinemia in multiple myeloma. The patient likely has Fanconi's syndrome from light chain reabsorption in the proximal tubule. This would explain the urinary glucose in the setting of normal serum glucose. One can develop a type 2 (proximal) renal tubular acidosis due to multiple myeloma.

Gabow PA. Disorders associated with an altered anion gap. *Kidney Int.* 1985;27(2):472-483. doi: 10.1038/ki.1985.34

25. **The answer is D.** There is a high anion gap (AG) metabolic acidosis (AG 27). Osmolar gap is 9, which can occur if most of the toxic alcohol has been metabolized. Based on the CT head findings, methanol ingestion is most likely, which can have characteristic findings in the putamen, optic nerves, and retina. Methanol is converted to formaldehyde and formic acid. Isopropyl alcohol ingestion converts to acetone. Usual findings are somnolence, ketonuria, and normal acid–base findings. Salicylate overdose initially leads to a respiratory alkalosis followed by a mixed respiratory alkalosis and high AG metabolic acidosis. Ethylene glycol ingestion causes a high AG metabolic acidosis similar to methanol but usually does not have findings on CT head affecting the putamen. Acetaminophen overdose can result in increased AG metabolic acidosis but is not associated with the previously-mentioned CT head findings.

Kraut JA, Mullins ME. Toxic alcohols. *N Engl J Med.* 2018;378:270-280. doi:10.1056/NEJMra1615295

26. **The answer is C.** The patient developed AKI on day 7 from admission. This is likely to be nephrotoxic ATN from gentamicin. It usually takes about 7 to 10 days to see aminoglycoside toxicity. Uptake of aminoglycoside in the proximal tubule epithelial cells leads to apoptosis and necrosis of tubular epithelial cells. CIN usually occurs 2 to 3 days after exposure to contrast. Urine microscopy in CIN can also show muddy brown casts since it is a form of ATN. AIN usually has white blood cells (WBCs) (particularly eosinophils) and WBC casts. Prerenal AKI would have a bland urine sediment. The patient was taking nonsteroidal anti-inflammatory drugs (NSAIDs), which can cause minimal change disease and membranous glomerulonephritis, but there is no mention of nephrotic syndrome. He does have endocarditis, which can cause membranoproliferative glomerulonephritis, but there is no mention of dysmorphic red blood cells (RBCs) or RBC casts.

Lopez-Novoa JM, Quiros Y, Vicente L, et al. New Insights into the mechanism of aminoglycoside nephrotoxicity: an integrative point of view. *Kidney Int.* 2011;79(1):33-45. doi: 10.1038/ki.2010.337

19

Endocrine Disorders

FARAH MEAH, MARY ANN EMANUELE,
LILY AGRAWAL, NICHOLAS EMANUELE, AND
ALALEH MAZHARI

■ QUESTIONS

1. Which of the following is **not** a common cause of hypocalcemia in the ICU?

   A. Rhabdomyolysis
   B. Sepsis
   C. Acute pancreatitis
   D. Hypophosphatemia
   E. Osteoblastic metastases

2. What is a cause of tertiary hyperparathyroidism?

   A. Hypocalcemia
   B. Vitamin D deficiency
   C. Hyperphosphatemia
   D. Secondary hyperparathyroidism
   E. All of the above

3. Which isolated clinical findings does **not** constitute initiation of intravenous (IV) calcium therapy?

   A. Altered mental status (AMS)
   B. Cardiovascular (CV) instability
   C. Mood irritability
   D. Seizures
   E. Laryngospasm

4. All of the following are important in the treatment of severe hypocalcemia **except**:

   A. Oral calcium
   B. Calcitriol
   C. Magnesium
   D. Intravenous (IV) calcium
   E. All of the above

5. What is the most common cause of hypercalcemia in the hospital setting?

   A. Primary hyperparathyroidism
   B. Sarcoidosis
   C. Lithium
   D. Hypercalcemia of malignancy
   E. Immobilization

6. In addition to hydration, additional therapy for hypercalcemia in an individual with prostate cancer complicated by skeletal metastases is:

    A. Zoledronic acid
    B. Pamidronate
    C. Denosumab
    D. Calcitonin
    E. Tamoxifen

7. What is the most common cause of hypercalcemia of malignancy?

    A. Myeloma lytic bone metastases
    B. Active vitamin D
    C. Ectopic parathyroid hormone (PTH)
    D. PTH-related peptide (PTHrp)
    E. Vasoactive intestinal peptide (VIP)

8. Which of the following is a common presentation of hypercalcemia?

    A. Perioral numbness
    B. Diplopia
    C. Polyuria
    D. Dysphagia
    E. Shortness of breath

9. What is the most important therapeutic intervention in the management of acute hypercalcemia?

    A. Cinacalcet
    B. Hydration
    C. Recombinant parathyroid hormone (PTH)
    D. Alendronate
    E. Magnesium

10. Pituitary apoplexy is characterized by:

    A. Intermittent dull retroorbital discomfort with increased appetite
    B. Significant antecedent head trauma
    C. Acute hemorrhage or infarction of the pituitary gland
    D. Previous diagnosis of empty sella syndrome with normal endocrine function tests
    E. Family history of pituitary problems

11. Pituitary apoplexy occurs:

    A. Predominantly in women
    B. Predominantly between ages 30 and 40
    C. In uninsured individuals without a primary healthcare provider
    D. All of the above
    E. None of the above

12. Pituitary adenomas are at risk of bleeding and necrosis due to:

    A. Outgrowing their blood supply
    B. Tumor expansion causing infarction by compressing pituitary vessels against the sellar diaphragm
    C. Fragility of tumor blood vessels

D. Increased intrasellar pressure with edema of bordering structures
E. All of the above

13. The most useful tool in the differential diagnosis of pituitary apoplexy is:

A. CT with contrast
B. Formal visual fields
C. MRI
D. Lumbar puncture (LP)
E. Serum electrolytes

14. Predisposing factors for pituitary apoplexy include:

A. Type 2 diabetes
B. Antithrombotic/anticoagulant therapy
C. Hypotension
D. Hypothyroidism
E. Hyperlipidemia

15. Which of the following is correct in regard to pituitary function in apoplexy?

A. Is intact for 5% of patients at presentation
B. Posterior pituitary dysfunction leading to diabetes insipidus (DI) is present in 90% of cases
C. Is associated with decreased intrasellar pressure altering hypothalamic and/or pituitary hormone release
D. Corticotrophic deficiency (secondary adrenal insufficiency) is the most common abnormality
E. Leads to elevated prolactin values

16. All patients with suspected pituitary apoplexy should have immediate labs, including:

A. Electrolytes, renal function, liver function
B. Complete blood count (CBC) and clotting screen
C. Random cortisol, Prolactin, Free T4, Thyroid-stimulating hormone (TSH), Insulin-like growth factor 1 (IGF-1), Growth hormone (GH), Luteinizing hormone (LH), Follicle-stimulating hormone (FSH), and testosterone in men, estradiol in women
D. All of the above
E. None of the above

17. Thyroid storm can present with which of the following signs/symptoms:

A. Agitation
B. Tachycardia
C. Hypothermia
D. Diarrhea
E. A, B, and D

18. Which of the following can be a cardiovascular (CV) manifestation of thyroid storm?

A. Tachycardia
B. Atrial fibrillation
C. Widened pulse pressure
D. CV collapse or shock
E. All of the above

19. Which of the following is not a precipitating factor for thyroid storm?

    A. Starting beta-blocker
    B. Acute illness
    C. Exposure to iodine containing contrast agent
    D. Cessation of thionamide (propylthiouracil [PTU] or methimazole)
    E. Surgery

20. Which one of the following treatment options for thyroid storm does **not** block peripheral T4 to T3 conversion?

    A. Propylthiouracil (PTU)
    B. High-dose propranolol
    C. Methimazole
    D. Corticosteroids
    E. Lugol's solution

21. What are some treatment options that can be considered in refractory cases of hyperthyroidism/thyroid storm?

    A. Lithium
    B. Cholestyramine
    C. Therapeutic plasma exchange
    D. Thyroidectomy
    E. All of the above

22. Which of the following statements regarding treatment of thyroid storm is **false**?

    A. Methimazole and propylthiouracil (PTU) can cause liver dysfunction
    B. It is safe to start saturated solution of potassium iodide (SSKI) or Lugol's solution for treatment of thyroid storm prior to initiation of therapy with methimazole or PTU
    C. In patients with thyroid storm, invasive monitoring may be necessary for patients with heart failure
    D. In patients without enteral access, rectal preparations of methimazole or PTU can be considered
    E. Methimazole and PTU can cause agranulocytosis

23. Myxedema coma can present with which of the following signs/symptoms?

    A. Bradycardia
    B. Diarrhea
    C. Lethargy or coma
    D. Hypothermia
    E. A, C, and D

24. Which of the following lab abnormalities can be seen in the setting of myxedema coma?

    A. Hyponatremia
    B. Hypoglycemia
    C. Anemia
    D. Hyperkalemia
    E. A, B, and C

25. Which if the following can be cardiovascular (CV) manifestions of myxedema coma?

    A. Bradycardia
    B. Low cardiac output (CO)

    C. Narrowed pulse pressure
    D. Pericardial effusion and/or cardiac tamponade
    E. All of the above

26. Which one of the following is **not** a known precipitating factor for myxedema coma?

    A. Infection
    B. Myocardial infarction (MI)
    C. Exposure to hot temperature
    D. Amiodarone
    E. Lithium

27. Which of the following is associated with a higher mortality in patients with myxedema coma?

    A. Lower Glasgow Coma Scale (GCS)
    B. Younger age
    C. Acute Physiologic and Chronic Health Evaluation (APACHE II) score greater than 20
    D. Persistent hypothermia
    E. A, C, and D

28. Treatment of myxedema coma can include:

    A. Intravenous (IV) T4
    B. Admission to ICU for close monitoring
    C. IV liothyronine
    D. Glucocorticoid treatment
    E. All of the above

29. The presentation of acute adrenal crisis includes all the following **except**:

    A. Hypotension
    B. Hypercalcemia
    C. Low eosinophil count
    D. Hyperkalemia
    E. Hyponatremia

30. The causes of adrenal crisis include:

    A. Autoimmune adrenalitis
    B. Adrenal hemorrhage
    C. Sarcoidosis
    D. A and B only
    E. A, B, and C

31. A 35-year-old woman has been on glucocorticoid replacement therapy for a flare-up of an autoimmune condition in the past month and is now being tapered off the glucocorticoid. For how long would the hypothalamic-pituitary-adrenal axis be suppressed and incapable of adequately responding to stress?

    A. One month
    B. Six months
    C. One year
    D. Two years
    E. One to two weeks

32. Clues to the diagnosis of primary adrenal insufficiency from autoimmune adrenalitis are:

    A. Skin hyperpigmentation
    B. Vitiligo
    C. Presence of another autoimmune disease
    D. A, B, and C
    E. None of the above

33. Which set of laboratory values supports the diagnosis of primary adrenal insufficiency?

    A. Low cortisol, low ACTH, low aldosterone, low renin
    B. Low cortisol, high ACTH, low aldosterone, low renin
    C. Low cortisol, low ACTH, low aldosterone, high renin
    D. Low cortisol, high ACTH, low aldosterone, high renin
    E. Low cortisol, high ACTH, high aldosterone, high renin

34. Acute therapy of adrenal insufficiency includes:

    A. Intravenous (IV) hydrocortisone
    B. Oral fludrocortisone
    C. Correction of the underlying condition
    D. IV fluids
    E. All of the above

35. A 26-year-old man is admitted to the ICU for bacterial meningitis and is treated with antibiotics and intravenous (IV) steroids. He has no known history of diabetes mellitus (DM). Random glucose on initial labs is 142 mg/dL. He is monitored with bedside point-of-care (POC) testing and after 4 hours his capillary glucose is 270 mg/dL. Which of the following statements is true?

    A. Hyperglycemia needs to be corrected in the ICU only in patients with known diabetes.
    B. In hospitalized patients, hyperglycemia is not associated with adverse outcomes.
    C. Recent trials in critically ill patients have shown no consistent reduction in mortality from intensive treatment targeting blood glucose 80 to 110 mg/dL versus hyperglycemia management targeting blood glucose less than 180 mg/dL.
    D. Judicious control of hyperglycemia in hospitalized patients is not warranted.
    E. Strict blood glucose control (goal 80–110 mg/dL) in the ICU is associated with better outcomes.

36. Which of the following statements is **false**?

    A. In the ICU, continuous insulin infusion has been shown to be the most effective method for achieving specific glycemic targets.
    B. Once intravenous (IV) insulin therapy has been started, glucose level should be maintained between 140 and 180 mg/dL.
    C. Prolonged therapy with sliding scale insulin as the sole regimen is ineffective in most patients, and may be potentially dangerous in those with type 1 diabetes.
    D. Insulin infusion protocols and standardized computerized treatment algorithms increase the risk of hypoglycemia and are not recommended.
    E. When transitioning to subcutaneous insulin, it should be given 1 to 2 hours before discontinuing IV insulin

37. Clinical situations that can increase the risk of hyper- and hypoglycemia in the hospital include:

    A. Change in clinical status, caloric intake, or medications
    B. Poor coordination of blood glucose testing and timing of insulin administration with meals
    C. Use of long-acting sulfonylureas in older patients, especially those with liver or kidney disease
    D. Inadequate communication during transfer of patient between different care teams
    E. All the above

38. Each of the following is appropriate in the management of patient with diabetic ketoacidosis (DKA) **except**:

    A. Admission to the ICU for monitoring of symptoms, glucose, electrolytes, and fluids
    B. Administration of fixed doses of subcutaneous rapid-acting insulin based on blood glucose every 6 hours
    C. Administration of intravenous (IV) insulin and fluids based on validated protocols
    D. Addition of potassium (20–30 mEq/L) to IV fluids when serum potassium is between 3.3 and 5.3 mmol/L
    E. Transition to subcutaneous insulin once patient can tolerate oral intake and DKA is resolved

39. Initiation of which of the following medicines could exacerbate hyperglycemia or potentially cause diabetic ketoacidosis (DKA)?

    A. Ciprofloxacin (Cipro)
    B. Glucocorticoids (prednisone)
    C. Canagliflozin (Invokana)
    D. Olanzapine (Zyprexa)
    E. B, C, and D

40. Which of the following symptoms may suggest development of cerebral edema due to rapid reduction of osmolality in a patient being treated for DKA/hyperosmotic hyperglycemic non-ketotic state (HHNS)?

    A. Headache
    B. Seizures
    C. Bradycardia
    D. Respiratory arrest
    E. All the above

■ ANSWERS

1. **The answer is D.** There are both parathyroid hormone (PTH)-mediated and non-PTH-mediated causes of hypocalcemia.

   Causes of PTH-mediated hypocalcemia include vitamin D deficiency and pseudohypoparathyroidism. Vitamin D deficiency may be due to decreased dietary intake, decreased exposure to sunlight, malabsorption, or disorders and medications leading to defects in the metabolism and action of vitamin D. Antiresorptives inhibit osteoclast bone resorption and antiepileptic drugs increase vitamin D metabolism leading to hypocalcemia. Both hypomagnesemia and hypermagnesemia alter PTH secretion and lower serum calcium. Calcium chelators such as citrate in blood transfusions and fluoride poisoning can also cause hypocalcemia. Severe vitamin D deficiency can lead to rickets in children and osteomalacia in adults. Pseudohypoparathyroidism is end-organ resistance to PTH action.

   Causes of non-PTH-mediated hypocalcemia include autoimmune (isolated or a part of autoimmune polyglandular syndrome type I also associated with primary adrenal insufficiency and chronic mucocutaneous candidiasis), post-surgical subsequent to thyroid or parathyroid surgery, congenital parathyroid aplasia or hypoplasia (termed DiGeorge syndrome if also associated with craniofacial anomalies and immunodeficiency), infiltrative due to iron (secondary to hemochromatosis or chronic transfusions) or copper deposition (Wilson's disease), and an alteration of the extracellular calcium sensing receptor such that PTH is not released at calcium levels that typically triggers parathyroid hormone release (Autosomal Dominant hypocalcemia). In kidney disease, the kidneys are unable to convert inactive vitamin D (25-hydroxy vitamin D) to active vitamin D (1–25 dihydroxy vitamin D) and calcium-phosphate complexes form in the body due to decreased phosphate excretion, which both lead to hypocalcemia; both these abnormalities lead to a rise in PTH levels by different mechanisms.

   Sepsis or alkalosis can lead to both impaired PTH secretion and resistance. A high-phosphate load (such as in rhabdomyolysis or tumor lysis syndrome) in the setting of acute renal failure (ARF) or calcium precipitation in the abdomen in acute pancreatitis can lead to hypocalcemia. Due to electrolyte shifts, postoperative patients are at risk for hypocalcemia. In aggressive metastatic osteoblastic malignancies such as breast and prostate cancer, the increased bone formation surpasses the extracellular available calcium leading to hypocalcemia.

   Cholst IN, Steinberg SF, Tropper PJ, et al. The influence of hypermagnesemia on serum calcium and parathyroid hormone levels in human subjects. *N Engl J Med.* 1984;310(19):1221-1225. doi:10.1056/nejm198405103101904

   Clarke BL, Brown EM, Collins MT, et al. Epidemiology and diagnosis of hypoparathyroidism. *J Clin Endocrinol Metab.* 2016;101(6):2284-2299. doi:10.1210/jc.2015-3908

   Mantovani G. Clinical review: pseudohypoparathyroidism: diagnosis and treatment. *J Clin Endocrinol Metab.* 2011;96(10):3020-3030. doi:10.1210/jc.2011-1048

   Tong GM, Rude RK. Magnesium deficiency in critical illness. *J Intensive Care Med.* 2005;20(1):3-17. doi:10.1177/0885066604271539

2. **The answer is E.** In primary hyperparathyroidism, a parathyroid adenoma or parathyroid hyperplasia leads to excessive secretion of parathyroid hormone (PTH) causing hypercalcemia and hypercalciuria. Secondary hyperparathyroidism is seen in renal disease whereby hypocalcemia secondary to renal disorders (see Answer 1) leads to a rise in PTH. Prolonged parathyroid gland stimulation as seen in secondary hyperparathyroidism may lead to autonomous parathyroid function and hypercalcemia ("tertiary hyperparathyroidism"). Chronic severe vitamin D deficiency and prolonged hyperphosphatemia can also lead to tertiary hyperparathyroidism.

   Hungry bone syndrome refers to prolonged hypocalcemia greater than 4 days subsequent to parathyroidectomy. Concomitant hypophosphatemia, hypomagnesemia, and hyperkalemia can be seen. Hypocalcemia is a result of increased osteoblast action and bone formation. The rise in alkaline phosphatase may correspond to the decline of calcium level. Risk factors for hungry bone syndrome in dialysis patients include younger age, high-body weight, high-preoperative alkaline phosphatase (ALP) level, and low-preoperative calcium level.

Ho LY, Wong PN, Sin HK, et al. Risk factors and clinical course of hungry bone syndrome after total parathyroidectomy in dialysis patients with secondary hyperparathyroidism. *BMC Nephrol.* 2017;18(1):12. doi:10.1186/s12882-016-0421-5

Jain N, Reilly RF. Hungry bone syndrome. *Curr Opin Nephrol Hypertens.* 2017;26(4):250-255. doi: 10.1097/MNH.0000000000000327

3. **The answer is C.** Hypocalcemia has a prevalence of 15% to 88% in the ICU. Individuals may be asymptomatic or exhibit a broad range of clinical manifestations. Clinical features may be predictive of not only the severity but also the duration of hypocalcemia. Gradual development of hypocalcemia can be asymptomatic or present with relatively few symptoms, such as fatigue and mood changes. Early symptoms of mild neuromuscular irritability include perioral numbness, acral paresthesias, or muscle cramps; and in more severe instances carpopedal spasm, laryngospasm, and seizures. Acute hypocalcemia is more likely to be symptomatic. Carpopedal spasm refers to adduction of the thumb over the palm, flexion of the metacarpophalangeal joints, extension of the interphalangeal joints, and flexion of the wrist and elbow joints. Carpopedal spasms can occur spontaneously in the setting of hypocalcemia or triggered, albeit painfully, by placement of a sphygmomanometer on the upper arm and inflation above systolic blood pressure (SBP) for 3 minutes ("Trosseau sign"). Chvostek's sign refers to contraction of ipsilateral facial muscles upon tapping of the facial nerve anterior to the ipsilateral ear. Tetany is more common in the setting of alkalosis. Tetany is uncommon in those with renal failure and concurrent metabolic acidosis. Other complications include premature cataracts, pseudotumor cerebri, and basal ganglia calcifications.

Guise TA, Mundy GR. Clinical review 69: evaluation of hypocalcemia in children and adults. *J Clin Endocrinol Metab.* 1995;80(5):1473-1478. doi:10.1210/jcem.80.5.7744987

Shoback D. Clinical practice. Hypoparathyroidism. *N Engl J Med.* 2008;359(4):391-403. doi: 10.1056/NEJMcp0803050

Shoback DM, Bilezikian JP, Costa AG, et al. Presentation of hypoparathyroidism: etiologies and clinical features. *J Clin Endocrinol Metab.* 2016;101(6):2300-2312. doi:10.1210/jc.2015-3909

4. **The answer is E.** Therapy of hypocalcemia includes a combination of calcium and vitamin D supplementation in oral or IV formulations depending upon the degree of severity. In the ICU, symptomatic hypocalcemia with neuromuscular irritability (AMS, seizures, laryngospasm), ECG changes (prolonged QT interval), and cardiac failure should be treated with IV therapy. IV calcium injections raise serum calcium transiently thus are typically followed by a continuous infusion with close monitoring of serum calcium to avoid rapid correction. IV calcium is typically administered in two steps: 1–2 ampules (equivalent to 90–180 mg elemental calcium) 10% calcium gluconate in 50 mL 5% dextrose given over 10 to 20 minutes followed by a slower infusion of 0.5 to 1.5 mg/kg/hr calcium gluconate given over 8–10 hours. Magnesium deficiency should be corrected if present. Serum calcium is monitored every 1 to 2 hours until biochemically and clinically stable, at which time frequency can be decreased to every 4 to 6 hours. Oral calcium therapy should be initiated and, if parathyroid hormone (PTH) is low, calcitriol therapy is added as well. The calcium infusion is weaned simultaneously over 24 to 48 hours. Typically if the patient is asymptomatic or has mild symptoms (fatigue and mood changes) and the calcium level is greater than 7.0 mg/dL, oral calcium supplementation may be appropriate. In those with normal PTH, a goal calcium level within the normal range is appropriate. In those with hypoparathyroidism, the calcium goal is typically 8.0 to 8.5 mg/dL. PTH has a stimulatory effect on the renal tubular calcium reabsorption. This is lacking in patients with hypoparathyroidism and therefore they are more prone to hypercalciuria. Since higher serum calcium level can lead to higher urinary calcium excretion, a lower target calcium level is desired in this setting and 24 hour urinary calcium can be measured to avoid hypercalciuria. The use of recombinant PTH (PTH 1–34 and PTH 1–84) in acute hypocalcemia has not been well studied.

Brandi ML, Bilezikian JP, Shoback D, et al. Management of hypoparathyroidism: summary statement and guidelines. *J Clin Endocrinol Metab.* 2016;101(6):2273-2283. doi:10.1210/jc.2015-3907

Shoback D. Clinical practice. Hypoparathyroidism. *N Engl J Med.* 2008;359(4):391-403. doi: 10.1056/NEJMcp0803050

5. **The answer is D.** The incidence of hypercalcemia in hospitalized patients is ~0.5% with hypercalcemia of malignancy representing the most common cause of hypercalcemic crises. The most common causes of hypercalcemia of malignancy include production of parathyroid hormone (PTH)-related protein (as seen in carcinomas), increased production of 1–25 dihydroxy vitamin D (as seen in lymphoma), or destruction of bone by lytic metastatic disease (as seen in myeloma).

   Causes of hypercalcemia can be categorized into parathyroid dependent (PTH-mediated) and parathyroid independent (non-PTH mediated) disorders. Parathyroid dependent causes include primary hyperparathyroidism, familial hypocalciuric hypercalcemia, and lithium-induced hypercalcemia. Parathyroid-independent hypercalcemia encompasses hypercalcemia of malignancy, granulomatous disorders (also sometimes due to increased 1–25 dihydroxy vitamin D), endocrinopathies (most commonly hyperthyroidism), medications (thiazide diuretics, exogenous calcium supplements), and prolonged immobilization. Hypercalcemia occurs by means of increased intestinal absorption and/or bone resorption and/or increased renal reabsorption or decreased renal excretion.

   Carroll R, Matfin G. Endocrine and metabolic emergencies: hypercalcaemia. *Ther Adv Endocrinol Metab*. 2010;1(5):225-234. doi:10.1177/2042018810390260

   Marcocci C, Cetani F. Clinical practice: primary hyperparathyroidism. *New Engl J Med*. 2011; 365(25):2389-2397. doi:10.1056/NEJMcp1106636

   Stewart AF. Clinical practice. Hypercalcemia associated with cancer. *N Engl J Med*. 2005;352(4): 373-379. doi:10.1056/NEJMcp042806

6. **The answer is C.** Denosumab, a human monoclonal antibody against receptor activator of nuclear factor Kappa-B Ligand (RANKL), is more effective in reducing skeletal-related events (SREs) compared to zoledronic acid in the setting of castration-resistant prostate cancer and breast cancer metastatic to bone. Pamidronate, calcitonin, and tamoxifen have not been shown to be superior to denosumab in reducing SREs.

   Fizazi K, Carducci M, Smith M, et al. Denosumab versus zoledronic acid for treatment of bone metastases in men with castration-resistant prostate cancer: a randomised, double-blind study. *Lancet*. 2011;377(9768):813-822. doi:10.1016/S0140-6736(10)62344-6

   Stopeck AT, Lipton A, Body JJ, et al. Denosumab compared with zoledronic acid for the treatment of bone metastases in patients with advanced breast cancer: a randomized, double-blind study. *J Clin Oncol*. 2010;28(35):5132-5139. doi:10.1200/JCO.2010.29.7101

7. **The answer is D.** The most common cause of hypercalcemia of malignancy is tumoral production of PTHrp. In addition, lymphomas can produce active vitamin D and myeloma lytic bone destruction can lead to hypercalcemia. Ectopic PTH production by tumor is rare. The VIPoma syndrome leads to watery diarrhea, hypokalemia, and achlorhydria (WDHA); nearly 50% display laboratory findings of hypercalcemia proposed by various mechanisms including dehydration secondary diarrhea and possible coexisting multiple endocrine neoplasia (MEN) presenting with hyperparathyroidism.

   Carroll R, Matfin G. Endocrine and metabolic emergencies: hypercalcaemia. *Ther Adv Endocrinol Metab*. 2010;1(5):225-234. doi:10.1177/2042018810390260

   Marcocci C, Cetani F. Clinical practice. Primary hyperparathyroidism. *New Engl J Med*. 2011;365(25):2389-2397. doi:10.1056/NEJMcp1106636

   Stewart AF. Clinical practice. Hypercalcemia associated with cancer. *N Engl J Med*. 2005;352(4): 373-379. doi:10.1056/NEJMcp042806

8. **The answer is C.** Duration and severity of symptoms may be predictive of the etiology of hypercalcemia. Early symptoms include fatigue, decreased appetite, polyuria, nausea, emesis, constipation, myopathy, or arthralgia. Hypercalciuria can lead to nephrolithiasis and increased bone resorption may lead to decreased bone mass and increased risk of fracture. Bone pain would be suspicious for bone metastases. Severe abdominal pain may be due to pancreatitis. As hypercalcemia progresses, dehydration (due to nephrogenic diabetes insipidus [DI]), neurologic manifestations (agitation, confusion, drowsiness, altered mental status [AMS]), and cardiovascular instability (bradyarrhythmias, heart block) ensue.

   Carroll R, Matfin G. Endocrine and metabolic emergencies: hypercalcaemia. *Ther Adv Endocrinol Metab*. 2010;1(5):225-234. doi:10.1177/2042018810390260

Fraser WD. Hyperparathyroidism. *Lancet.* 2009;374(9684):145-158. doi:10.1016/S0140-6736(17)31430-7

Marcocci C, Cetani F. Clinical practice. Primary hyperparathyroidism. *New Engl J Med.* 2011;365(25):2389-2397. doi:10.1056/NEJMcp1106636

Minisola S, Pepe J, Piemonte S, et al. The diagnosis and management of hypercalcaemia. *BMJ.* 2015;350:2723. doi:10.1136/bmj.h2723

9. **The answer is B.** In the assessment of calcium disorders, it is always important to follow a corrected calcium for hypoalbuminemia and the ionized calcium especially in the individual with an acid/base imbalance. Mild (<12 mg/dL) or moderate (12–14 mg/dL) hypercalcemia can be treated with hydration. In the setting of neurologic disturbance, cardiovascular instability, or severe (>14 mg/dL) hypercalcemia, it is prudent to treat aggressively with intravenous (IV) hydration. If there is concern for fluid overload, administer a simultaneous loop diuretic so that hydration can be continued. Intramuscular or subcutaneous calcitonin can decrease serum calcium by 1 to 2 mg/dL in the first 4 to 6 hours and is useful in the first 12 to 48 hours of treatment of acute hypercalcemia. Anti-resorptives are given with expectations to lower serum calcium within 2 to 4 days of administration—IV if the creatinine clearance (CrCl) is greater than 35 or denosumab if it is less than 35. Although both IV bisphosphonate and denosumab are associated with postinfusion hypocalcemia, denosumab is associated with a higher risk of hypocalcemia when given to individuals with renal disease; most commonly occurring 5 days after infusion. Severe hypercalcemia refractory to medical therapy may require hemodialysis or surgical resection of the tumor.

Carroll R, Matfin G. Endocrine and metabolic emergencies: hypercalcaemia. *Ther Adv Endocrinol Metab.* 2010;1(5):225-234. doi:10.1177/2042018810390260

Cummings SR, San Martin J, McClung MR, et al. Denosumab for prevention of fractures in postmenopausal women with osteoporosis. *N Engl J Med.* 2009;361(8):756-765. doi:10.1056/NEJMoa0809493

Fraser WD. Hyperparathyroidism. *Lancet.* 2009;374(9684):145-158. doi:10.1016/S0140-6736(17)31430-7

Marcocci C, Cetani F. Clinical practice. Primary hyperparathyroidism. *New Engl J Med.* 2011;365(25):2389-2397. doi:10.1056/NEJMcp1106636

Minisola S, Pepe J, Piemonte S, et al. The diagnosis and management of hypercalcaemia. *BMJ.* 2015;350:2723. doi:10.1136/bmj.h2723

10. **The answer is C.** Pituitary apoplexy is a rare clinical syndrome characterized by an acute hemorrhage or infarction of the pituitary gland. Pituitary apoplexy occurs in a small but significant number of patients who are harboring a pituitary tumor, most often a clinically nonfunctioning macroadenoma. Most series indicate that the incidence of apoplexy in pituitary adenomas is between 2% and 7% when defined on the basis of clinical signs combined with surgical or pathological evidence. Unawareness of a preexisting pituitary adenoma leads to a delay in the diagnosis as other conditions are considered.

The clinical presentation varies depending on the extent of hemorrhage, necrosis, and intracranial pressure (ICP). The symptoms mimic other common neurological emergencies such as subarachnoid hemorrhage (SAH), bacterial meningitis or stroke, leading to delayed or even a missed diagnosis. Therefore, a high degree of clinical suspicion is needed to diagnose pituitary apoplexy, with up to 25% cases presenting at pathological examination without any clinical symptoms (subclinical or silent pituitary tumor apoplexy).

Headache is the most common and initial clinical manifestation of pituitary apoplexy (80%). It is usually sudden and severe, commonly in the retroorbital region but may be bifrontal or diffuse. Sometimes patients may present with a subacute headache. Nausea and vomiting and symptoms of chemical meningitis can be present due to extravasation of blood and necrotic material in the subarachnoid space. Half of the patients may present with visual disturbances, commonly a bitemporal superior quadrant defect (due to compression of the optic chiasm from below), but visual impairment varies depending on the degree of involvement of the surrounding structures. Less commonly, optic tract involvement can cause homonymous hemianopia or optic neuritis (ON). Visual acuity defect and blindness may rarely occur. Compression of the cavernous sinus can involve the cranial nerves (CNs)

III, IV, and VI. CN III is the most commonly involved CN due to its proximity to the sella presenting with mydriasis, ptosis, and inferior and laterally deviated globe. Belschowsky phenomenon is seen in fourth nerve palsy with a vertical diplopia that worsens with the patient gazing toward the opposite direction or downwards and tilting the head toward the direction of the affected eye. The sixth CN is rarely involved. Involvement of the fifth CN may result in facial pain and sensory loss. Damage to the sympathetic nerves may result in Horner's syndrome. Pressure transmitting to the brainstem or hypothalamus may lead to hypotension, fever, cardiac dysrhythmias and impaired levels of consciousness. Compression of the intracavernous carotid artery or vasospasm can lead to symptoms of stroke.

Bi WL, Dunn IF, Laws ER. Pituitary apoplexy. *Endocrine.* 2015;48(1):69-75. doi:10.1007/s12020-014-0359-y

Briet C, Salenave S, Chanson P. Pituitary apoplexy. *Endocrinol Metab Clin North Am.* 2015;44(1):199-209. doi:10.1016/j.ecl.2014.10.016

Giammattei L, Mantovani G, Carrabba G, et al. Pituitary apoplexy: considerations on a single center experience and review of the literature. *J Endocrinol Invest.* 2016;39(7):739-746. doi:10.1007/s40618-015-0424-2

11. **The answer is C.** Apoplexy can occur at all ages but is most frequent in the fifth or sixth decade and shows a slight male preponderance. Pituitary tumor apoplexy patients are statistically more likely to be unmarried, uninsured, and without a primary healthcare provider resulting in a failure to note antecedent warning signs and symptoms until a fulminant presentation results.

Briet C, Salenave S, Chanson P. Pituitary apoplexy. *Endocrinol Metab Clin North Am.* 2015;44(1):199-209. doi:10.1016/j.ecl.2014.10.016

12. **The answer is E.** Pituitary adenomas are at risk of bleeding and necrosis, possibly because they outgrow their blood supply or because tumor expansion causes ischemia with subsequent infarction by compressing pituitary vessels against the sellar diaphragm. The fragility of tumor blood vessels may be responsible for the tendency to hemorrhage. The increase in intrasellar pressure leading to edema of bordering structures may be subtle to pronounced, explaining the wide clinical spectrum from "classic" acute pituitary apoplexy to totally silent necrotic and/or hemorrhagic adenomas found on pathologic examination. The clinical presentation can be either acute or subacute, with slow development of symptoms and signs, and this is largely determined by the extent of hemorrhage, edema, and necrosis. No correlation has been found between the size of the adenomas and occurrence of hemorrhage, according to most authors. Knowing the pituitary gland vascularization may give a better understanding of the pathophysiological mechanisms. Normal pituitary vasculature comprises of the hypophyseal portal system (capillary system) from the hypothalamus via long portal veins and arterial supply, primarily from the inferior hypophyseal arteries originating from branches of the intracavernous internal carotid artery (ICA). Pituitary adenomas have a variable microvasculature with reduced angiogenesis; hence may outgrow their blood supply.

Boellis A, di Napoli A, Romano A, et al. Pituitary apoplexy: an update on clinical and imaging features. *Insights Imaging.* 2014;5(6):753-762. doi:10.1007/s13244-014-0362-0

13. **The answer is C.** MRI is a useful tool in the differential diagnosis of pituitary apoplexy. Many conditions can present with hyperintensity on T1 weighed images (T1WI) in the sellar region, the most frequent MRI feature of pituitary apoplexy. Thus, it is important to use advanced MRI techniques with a careful search for specific radiological findings, such as fluid levels or thickening of the sphenoid mucosa. The posterior lobe of the pituitary gland usually appears as a hyperintense spot on T1WI because of storage of vasopressin; this is a normal finding and should not be confused with a hemorrhage within the gland. In the case of anterior pituitary lobe hyperactivity, the gland may be hyperintense. In these cases, hemorrhage can be easily excluded with the evaluation of T2WI. Another condition to consider for the differential diagnosis is the presence of an aneurysm. Aneurysms arising from the carotid siphon or from the anterior communicating artery usually appear as round hypointense lesions on T2WI because

of flow void. Partially thrombosed aneurysms in the sellar region can show high signal intensity on T1WI. Thus, an imaging study should be completed with magnetic resonance angiography (MRA), preferably with a contrast-enhanced technique, to exclude this possibility. Rathke cleft cysts occur with T1 hyperintensity because of the variable protein content, which can be either intra- or supra-sellar, are usually located along the midline, and do not present a fluid debris level. A hypointense intracystic nodule on T2WI, related to concretion of proteinaceous material within the Rathke cleft cysts, is typical. The variable MRI appearance of Rathke cleft cysts may cause difficulties in the differential diagnosis with pituitary apoplexy. Moreover, a large suprasellar Rathke cleft cyst may mimic pituitary apoplexy even clinically, with acute onset of headache and visual deficit. Craniopharingioma is another pathology that can be difficult to distinguish from pituitary apoplexy. It is usually an intra- or suprasellar lesion with variable solid, cystic, and calcified components. The cystic component may contain a proteinaceous fluid, appearing hyperintense on T1WI, and mimicking hemorrhagic degeneration. Careful evaluation of T2WI together with the acquisition of a CT scan to rule out calcific components can help to obtain the correct diagnosis. Other conditions that can simulate pituitary apoplexy on imaging are lipoma, dermoid cysts, and postoperative changes. Lipoma and dermoid cysts contain fat and can be confirmed with fat-suppressed images. These conditions do not usually occur in the clinical setting of pituitary apoplexy. When the clinical presentation suggests pituitary tumor apoplexy, it is important to consider subarachnoid hemorrhage (SAH), meningitis, encephalitis, pituitary abscess and cavernous sinus thrombosis. Other concerns are a stroke, complex migraine, optic neuritis, sinusitis, and pseudotumor cerebri. Although 20% to 30% of patients may have a prior history of an endocrine problem, 80% of patients have no known pituitary problems. The clinical concern for a potential SAH or bacterial meningitis support the need for a LP, however, the results of an LP may not be helpful in differentiating SAH and bacterial meningitis from apoplexy, which can be associated with a high-red cell count, xanthochromia or pleocytosis, and an increased cerebrospinal fluid (CSF) protein level, particularly when meningeal irritation is present. However, a CSF culture will rule out bacterial meningitis, and LP is thus mandatory if this diagnostic possibility is raised.

Boellis A, di Napoli A, Romano A, et al. Pituitary apoplexy: an update on clinical and imaging features. *Insights Imaging.* 2014;5(6):753-762. doi:10.1007/s13244-014-0362-0

Jho DH, Biller BM, Agarwalla PK, et al. Pituitary apoplexy: large surgical series with grading system. *World Neurosurg.* 2014;82(5):781-790. doi:10.1016/j.wneu.2014.06.005

14. **The answer is B.** Precipitating factors have been identified in up to 40% of cases of pituitary apoplexy. Hypertension was by far the most common (26%) predisposing factor. An acute increase in intracranial pressure (ICP), arterial hypertension, angiographic procedures, and major surgery (particularly cardiac surgery with blood pressure [BP] fluctuations and anticoagulant therapy) are well-known triggers. Anticoagulation therapy, bleeding disorders, medications such as dopamine agonists and high-dose estrogen, radiation therapy, pregnancy, and head trauma also seem to be able to precipitate apoplexy. It also can occur after dynamic endocrine testing (insulin tolerance test and growth hormone-releasing hormone). Pregnancy is associated with apoplexy due to lactotroph hyperplasia increasing pituitary volume, which normalizes 6 months postpartum. Pituitary apoplexy should always be considered in patients who develop headache and neuro-ophthalmic symptoms following major surgery. Pituitary apoplexy has been reported in other intracranial tumors (meningiomas, craniopharyngiomas, malignant tumors, hypothalamic astrocytoma), metastatic prostate, renal cell carcinoma, endometrial, and small cell carcinoma to the pituitary and has been described in patients receiving radiotherapy. It has also rarely been found in hypophysitis, Rathke's cleft cyst, and sellar tuberculoma.

Bujawansa S, Thondam SK, Steele C, et al. Presentation, management and outcomes in acute pituitary apoplexy: a large single-centre experience from the United Kingdom. *Clin Endocrinol.* 2014;80(3):419-424. doi:10.1111/cen.12307

Giammattei L, Mantovani G, Carrabba G, et al. Pituitary apoplexy: considerations on a single center experience and review of the literature. *J Endocrinol Invest.* 2016;39(7):739-746. doi:10.1007/s40618-015-0424-2

15. The answer is D. Endocrine dysfunction, primarily one or more of the anterior pituitary deficiencies, may be prominent with increased intrasellar pressure altering the release of hypothalamic and/or pituitary hormones. Symptoms may present either at the onset of pituitary apoplexy or before the apoplectic event. Corticotrophic deficiency (secondary adrenal insufficiency), occurring in 50% to 80% of the cases, is the most common and the most life-threatening deficit noted in patients with pituitary apoplexy. Patients can have severe hemodynamic compromise with hypotension and hyponatremia. The hyponatremia results either due to the glucocorticoid deficiency per se, versus, rarely, secondary to inappropriate anti-diuretic hormone secretion. Empiric parenteral administration of corticosteroids becomes imperative in these patients, with preferable baseline samples for cortisol and adrenocorticotropic hormone (ACTH); however, treatment should be initiated without waiting for the laboratory results. Other pituitary hormone deficiencies include thyrotrophic (30%–70%) and gonadotrophic (40%–75%) deficiencies. Growth hormone (GH) deficiency is also common. Prolactin levels may be elevated in cases of prolactinomas, with 10%–40% presenting with low prolactin levels. Approximately 5% of cases are associated with posterior pituitary dysfunction leading to DI. It may originally be masked by adrenal insufficiency or hypothyroidism, but becomes evident after steroid or thyroid hormone replacement.

Capatina C, Inder W, Karavitaki N, et al. Management of endocrine disease: pituitary tumour apoplexy. *Eur J Endocrinol.* 2015;172(5):R179-R190. doi:10.1530/EJE-14-0794

16. The answer is D. The outcome of acute apoplexy may vary and remains unpredictable, from rapid deterioration in some cases to spontaneous recovery in some others. Thus, management of an acute apoplexy remains controversial. However, supportive measures should be instituted in addition to intravenous (IV) hydrocortisone after drawing blood samples for random serum cortisol, free T4 and TSH, IGF-1, GH, LH, FSH, and testosterone in men, estradiol in women. Thyroid hormone deficiency should be repleted after correction of hypocortisolemia to prevent excess stimulation of metabolism in an adrenal insufficient patient. Electrolyte imbalance, especially hyponatremia, should also be investigated and anticipated in the acute setting and repleted cautiously.

Rajasekaran S, Vanderpump M, Baldeweg S, et al. UK guidelines for the management of pituitary apoplexy. *Clin Endocrinol.* 2011;74(1):9-20. doi:10.1111/j.1365-2265.2010.03913.x

17. The answer is E. Hyperthyroidism due to excess endogenous production of thyroid hormone can lead to thyroid storm. The main causes of endogenous hyperthyroidism include Graves' disease (autoimmune etiology); toxic nodule or nodules referred to as toxic uninodular or multinodular goiter; as well as extra-thyroidal hormone production including struma ovarii and metastatic differentiated thyroid cancer. Overt hyperthyroidism is defined as elevation of free T3 and/or free T4 with a low to undetectable thyroid-stimulating hormone (TSH). In Graves' disease, which is one of the most common causes of thyroid storm, thyrotropin-receptor antibodies stimulate the TSH receptor, which leads to increased thyroid hormone production. In the setting of toxic thyroid nodule or nodules, there is autonomous function of the nodule(s) that can be caused by somatic activating mutations of genes that control thyroid hormone production.

The exact physiology of progression from compensated hyperthyroidism to thyroid storm is not clearly understood. Thyroid storm is characterized by multisystem involvement and dysregulation of the organ systems involved.

Excess thyroid hormone increases thermogenesis and basal metabolic rate, leading to thermoregulatory dysfunction (fever). It affects the cardiovascular (CV) system and can cause tachycardia, atrial fibrillation, widened pulse pressure (due to peripheral vasodilation), and in severe cases CV collapse and shock. Patients can have central nervous system (CNS) manifestations (agitation) as well as gastrointestinal (diarrhea) and hepatic derangements.

The diagnosis can be challenging given overlap between the signs and symptoms of compensated hyperthyroidism and thyroid storm. Utilizing diagnostic criteria can aid in making the diagnosis of thyroid storm. In 1993, Burch and Wartofsky developed a point scale (BW) to help diagnose thyroid storm. The criteria included in the scale are hyperpyrexia, tachycardia/arrhythmia, heart failure, gastrointestinal/hepatic dysfunction (diarrhea, abdominal pain, nausea/vomiting, jaundice), CNS disturbance (agitation, delirium, psychosis, seizure, coma), and a precipitating factor. A score greater than 45 is very suspicious or suggestive of thyroid storm and a score between 25 and 44 can indicate impending thyroid storm. The Japan Thyroid Association (JTA) has also proposed diagnostic criteria for thyroid storm that is based on clinical features (with an emphasis on CNS manifestations for definite diagnosis of thyroid storm) and presence of thyrotoxicosis. The JTA does not use a point system and it may be less sensitive for the diagnosis of thyroid storm compared to the BW criteria.

Akamizu T, Satoh T, Isozaki O, et al. Diagnostic criteria, clinical features, and incidence of thyroid storm based on nationwide surveys. *Thyroid.* 2012;22(7):661-679. doi:10.1089/thy.2011.0334

Burch HB, Wartofsky L. Life-threatening thyrotoxicosis. Thyroid storm. *Endocrinol Metab Clin North Am.* 1993;22(2):263-277. doi:10.1016/S0889-8529(18)30165-8

Chiha M, Samarasinghe S, Kabaker AS. Thyroid storm: an updated review. *J Intensive Care Med.* 2015;30(3):131-140. doi:10.1177/0885066613498053

Ross DS, Burch HB, Cooper DS, et al. 2016 American Thyroid Association Guidelines for Diagnosis and Management of Hyperthyroidism and Other Causes of Thyrotoxicosis. *Thyroid.* 2016;26(10):1343-1421. doi:10.1089/thy.2016.0229

Swee du S, Chng CL, Lim A. Clinical characteristics and outcome of thyroid storm: a case series and review of neuropsychiatric derangements in thyrotoxicosis. *Endocr Pract.* 2015;21(2):182-189. doi:10.4158/EP14023.OR

18. The answer is E. Cardiovascular effects of thyroid storm inlcude tachycardia, atrial fibrillation, widened pulse pressure (due to peripheral vasodilation), and in severe cases CV collapse and shock.

Chiha M, Samarasinghe S, Kabaker AS. Thyroid storm: an updated review. *J Intensive Care Med.* 2015;30(3):131-140. doi:10.1177/0885066613498053

Ross DS, Burch HB, Cooper DS, et al. 2016 American Thyroid Association Guidelines for Diagnosis and Management of Hyperthyroidism and Other Causes of Thyrotoxicosis. *Thyroid.* 2016;26(10):1343-1421. doi:10.1089/thy.2016.0229

19. The answer is A. Some precipitating factors for thyroid storm include thyroid or nonthyroidal surgery, noncompliance with thionamide or anti-thyroid therapy, infection, trauma, acute iodine load (such as getting iodinated contrast or amiodarone; exposure to iodine containing contrast agent provides substrate for thyroid hormone production and can exacerbate hyperthyroidism and lead to thyroid storm), and parturition. Thyroid storm can also rarely occur after radioactive iodine therapy. Starting a beta-blocker is not a precipitating factor for thyroid storm. Beta-blockers are used for treatment of thyroid storm to control heart rate and at higher doses they can decrease T4 to T3 conversion.

Chiha M, Samarasinghe S, Kabaker AS. Thyroid storm: an updated review. *J Intensive Care Med.* 2015;30(3):131-140. doi:10.1177/0885066613498053

Ross DS, Burch HB, Cooper DS, et al. 2016 American Thyroid Association Guidelines for Diagnosis and Management of Hyperthyroidism and Other Causes of Thyrotoxicosis. *Thyroid.* 2016;26(10):1343-1421. doi:10.1089/thy.2016.0229

20. The answer is C. While thyroid storm is rare, it is a life-threatening condition and timely diagnosis as well as initiation of treatment is crucial given the high mortality (10%–30%) associated with it. The treatment should target thyroid hormone synthesis/release as well as supportive care to treat symptoms and stabilize the patient. Patients with thyroid storm should be admitted to the ICU for close monitoring and aggressive treatment.

Anti-thyroid medications or thianomides including PTU and methimazole are used as one of the main therapies for thyroid storm. Thionamides prevent denovo thyroid hormone synthesis. PTU has the added advantage of also decreasing conversion of T4 to T3 in the periphery. This is important as most of the thyroid hormone effects are mediated through the action of T3 and 80% to 90% of T3 is produced via peripheral conversion of T4 to T3. The doses of PTU and methimazole used in the setting of thyroid storm are higher than that used for treatment of hyperthyroidism and different regimens have been proposed. The American Thyroid Association (ATA) 2016 guidelines recommend PTU 250 mg every 4 hours with the option of administering a loading dose (500–1000 mg) or methimazole 60 to 80 mg/day administered in divided doses.

Beta-blockers are also used for treatment of thyroid storm. Propranolol is the most commonly used beta-blocker and can be given 60 to 80 mg every 4 hours. It is a nonselective beta-blocker and at higher doses it decreases T4 to T3 conversion in the periphery. For more rapid effect, intravenous (IV) beta-blockers can be used. Both propranolol and esmolol can be administered IV.

Corticosteroids are usually administered as part of the treatment of thyroid storm. The 2016 ATA guidelines recommend 300 mg IV loading dose of hydrocortisone followed by 100 mg IV every 8 hours. Corticosteroids can decrease conversion of T4 to T3.

Iodine solution is used as part of the treatment for thyroid storm. Large doses of iodine inhibit the release of preformed thyroid hormone as well as decrease iodine transport and oxidation, which is necessary for thyroid hormone production. However, it is important that iodine solution is administered at least 30 to 60 minutes after initiation of thianomide therapy to avoid iodine being used as a substrate for new thyroid hormone synthesis. The ATA 2016 guidelines recommend treatment with saturated solution of potassium iodide (SSKI) five drops every 6 hours or Lugol's solution eight drops every 6 hours.

Angell TE, Lechner MG, Nguyen CT, et al. Clinical features and hospital outcomes in thyroid storm: a retrospective cohort study. *J Clin Endocrinol Metab*. 2015;100(2):451-459. doi:10.1210/jc.2014-2850

Chiha M, Samarasinghe S, Kabaker AS. Thyroid storm: an updated review. *J Intensive Care Med*. 2015;30(3):131-140. doi:10.1177/0885066613498053

Ross DS, Burch HB, Cooper DS, et al. 2016 American Thyroid Association Guidelines for Diagnosis and Management of Hyperthyroidism and Other Causes of Thyrotoxicosis. *Thyroid*. 2016;26(10):1343-1421. doi:10.1089/thy.2016.0229

Swee du S, Chng CL, Lim A. Clinical characteristics and outcome of thyroid storm: a case series and review of neuropsychiatric derangements in thyrotoxicosis. *Endocr Pract*. 2015;21(2):182-189. doi:10.4158/EP14023.OR

21. **The answer is E.** Lithium can also be used to prevent T3 and T4 synthesis and decrease thyroid hormone release. It can be administered 300 mg orally every 6 to 8 hours and serum lithium levels need to be monitored to avoid toxicity.

Bile acid sequestrants can be used to target recirculation or enterohepatic circulation of thyroid hormone. Cholestyramine can be administered 1 to 4 g twice a day.

In refractory cases of thyroid storm not optimally responding to medical and supportive therapy or adverse effects from treatment (such as leukopenia or agranulocytosis secondary to thionamide use) therapeutic plasma exchange has been utilized to help lower free T3 and free T4. The effect of plasma exchange is transient and it is used in conjunction with medical therapy to stabilize the patient or prior to thyroidectomy. Some side effects associated with therapeutic plasma exchange include coagulopathy, infection, transfusion reaction, respiratory distress, and hypotension, and therefore it needs to be used with caution.

Thyroidectomy can be considered in some patients, including patients with declining clinical status and not responding to medical therapy, patients who experience adverse effects from medical treatment (as noted previously), or patients with underlying medical conditions such as cardiopulmonary failure.

Hagemann E, Arkenau C, Engelmann L, et al. Is there a place for thyroidectomy in older patients with thyrotoxic storm and cardiorespiratory failure? *Thyroid*. 2003;13(10):933-940. doi: 10.1089/105072503322511337

Kaykhaei MA, Shams M, Sadegholvad A, et al. Low doses of cholestyramine in the treatment of hyperthyroidism. *Endocrine*. 2008;34(1-3):52-55. doi:10.1007/s12020-008-9107-5

Schwartz J, Padmanabhan A, Aqui N, et al. Guidelines on the use of therapeutic apheresis in clinical practice-evidence-based approach from the writing committee of the American Society for Apheresis: the seventh special issue. *J Clin Apheresis*. 2016;31(3):149-162. doi: 10.1002/jca.21470

22. **The answer is B.** Iodine is used as a substrate for thyroid hormone production. It is important that thionomide therapy with either PTU or methimazole is initiated prior to initiation of SSKI or Lugol's solution to inhibit thyroid hormone production. PTU and methimazole can be given rectally if enteral access is not available. Both methimazole and PTU can rarely cause liver dysfunction and agranulocytosis. Invasive monitoring may be necessary for patients with heart failure who are experiencing thyroid storm.

Chiha M, Samarasinghe S, Kabaker AS. Thyroid storm: an updated review. *J Intensive Care Med*. 2015;30(3):131-140. doi:10.1177/0885066613498053

Ross DS, Burch HB, Cooper DS, et al. 2016 American Thyroid Association Guidelines for Diagnosis and Management of Hyperthyroidism and Other Causes of Thyrotoxicosis. *Thyroid*. 2016;26(10):1343-1421. doi:10.1089/thy.2016.0229

23. **The answer is E.** Myxedema coma refers to a state of severe or decompensated hypothyroidism resulting in central nervous system (CNS) changes and multiorgan dysfunction. The cause of hypothyroidism can be primary (due to low thyroid hormone production by the thyroid gland) or secondary (due to hypothalamic-pituitary dysfunction). The occurrence of myxedema coma is rare, with a reported incidence of 0.22 per million per year.

Myxedema coma should be suspected in patients with prior history of hypothyroidism, thyroidectomy scar, or history of radioactive iodine treatment. A careful history needs to be taken to identify possible precipitating factor(s) prior to patient's presentation and the medication list needs to be reviewed. Diagnosis of myxedema coma is a clinical one and is made based on history and physical exam.

The laboratory findings will then help provide additional information to support the suspicion for myxedema coma. The thyroid laboratory testing shows elevated thyroid-stimulating hormone (TSH) and decreased T4 and T3. It is important to note that the degree of TSH elevation is not an accurate indicator of the severity of hypothyroidism given the wide range of TSH values that have been reported in the literature.

The CNS symptoms can be variable including lethargy, stupor, cognitive dysfunction, confusion, and coma in severe cases. Psychosis (myxedema madness) and seizures associated with myxedema coma have also been reported.

Hypothermia can be one of the earliest manifestations of myxedema coma (due to decreased thermogenesis and decrease in metabolic rate). Cardiovascular (CV) manifestations include bradycardia, low cardiac output, hypotension, and narrowed pulse pressure. There is impairment of ventilatory drive and response to hypoxia as well as hypercapnia that leads to hypoventilation and respiratory acidosis. This can be further exacerbated by factors such as respiratory muscle weakness, macroglossia, and edema of larynx and nasopharynx. Some patients will require mechanical ventilation. Gastrointestinal (GI) dysfunction (constipation and paralytic ileus) can be present due to decrease in intestinal motility. Diarrhea is usually associated with hyperthyroidism and thyroid storm.

Some of the findings on physical exam can include dry and puffy skin, facial and lower extremity edema (anasarca can also been seen), enlarged tongue, and delayed relaxation of deep tendon reflexes (DTRs).

A diagnostic scoring system has been proposed to aid in the diagnosis of myxedema coma and includes temperature, CNS symptoms, GI dysfunction (abdominal pain, anorexia, constipation, decreased intestinal motility and paralytic ileus), precipitating event, CV dysfunction (bradycardia, ECG changes, pericardial/pleural effusion, pulmonary edema, cardiomegaly and hypotension), and metabolic disturbances (hyponatremia, hypoglycemia, hypoxemia, hypercapnia and decrease in glomerular filtration rate [GFR]). A score of 60 or higher is highly suggestive of myxedema coma, a score of 25 to 59 is suggestive of risk for myxedema coma, and a score below 25 makes myxedema coma unlikely.

Gunatilake SSC, Bulugahapitiya U. Myxedema crisis presenting with seizures: a rare life-threatening presentation—a case report and review of the literature. *Case Rep Endocrinol.* 2017;2017:4285457. doi:10.1155/2017/4285457

Heinrich TW, Grahm G. Hypothyroidism presenting as psychosis: myxedema madness revisited. *J Clinical Psychiat.* 2003;5(6):260-266. doi:10.4088/PCC.v05n0603

Jonklaas J, Bianco AC, Bauer AJ, et al. Guidelines for the treatment of hypothyroidism: prepared by the American thyroid association task force on thyroid hormone replacement. *Thyroid.* 2014;24(12):1670-1751. doi:10.1089/thy.2014.0028

Klubo-Gwiezdzinska J, Wartofsky L. Thyroid emergencies. *Med Clin North Am.* 2012;96(2):385-403. doi:10.1016/j.mcna.2012.01.015

Mathew V, Misgar RA, Ghosh S, et al. Myxedema coma: a new look into an old crisis. *J Thyroid Res.* 2011;2011:493462. doi:10.4061/2011/493462

Popoveniuc G, Chandra T, Sud A, et al. A diagnostic scoring system for myxedema coma. *Endocr Pract.* 2014;20(8):808-817. doi:10.4158/EP13460.OR

24. **The answer is E.** Hyponatremia is a common finding due to altered free water excretion secondary to inappropriate vasopressin secretion or impaired renal function (decreased renal plasma flow). Hypoglycemia can also be present due to hypothyroidism and/or underlying adrenal insufficiency. Anemia in myxedema is secondary to decreased oxygen requirements and erythropoietin. Hyperkalemia is not associated with myxedema coma.

Klubo-Gwiezdzinska J, Wartofsky L. Thyroid emergencies. *Med Clin North Am.* 2012;96(2):385-403. doi:10.1016/j.mcna.2012.01.015

Mathew V, Misgar RA, Ghosh S, et al. Myxedema coma: a new look into an old crisis. *J Thyroid Res.* 2011;2011:493462. doi:10.4061/2011/493462

Popoveniuc G, Chandra T, Sud A, et al. A diagnostic scoring system for myxedema coma. *Endocr Pract.* 2014;20(8):808-817. doi:10.4158/EP13460.OR

25. **The answer is E.** CV manifestations include bradycardia, low CO, hypotension, and narrowed pulse pressure. There can be fluid extravasation due to changes in vascular permeability resulting in nonpitting edema and anasarca. Pericardial effusion may be present. Cardiac tamponade caused by accumulation of mucopolysaccharide-rich fluid can occur. ECG changes can include low voltage, nonspecific ST wave changes, QT prolongation, and rhythm abnormalities.

Klubo-Gwiezdzinska J, Wartofsky L. Thyroid emergencies. *Med Clin North Am.* 2012;96(2):385-403. doi:10.1016/j.mcna.2012.01.015

Majid-Moosa A, Schussler JM, Mora A. Myxedema coma with cardiac tamponade and severe cardiomyopathy. *Proc (Bayl Univ Med Cent).* 2015;28(4):509-511. doi:10.1080/08998280.2015.11929326

Popoveniuc G, Chandra T, Sud A, et al. A diagnostic scoring system for myxedema coma. *Endocr Pract.* 2014;20(8):808-817. doi:10.4158/EP13460.OR

26. **The answer is C.** Myxedema coma can result from longstanding untreated or suboptimally treated hypothyroidism or can be precipitated by a cardiovascular (CV) or cerebrovascular event, trauma, infection, metabolic disturbances, or exposure to cold temperature. It can also occur with use of certain medications such as amiodarone, lithium, sedatives, tyrosine kinase inhibitors, and narcotics. A side effect of immune checkpoint inhibitors (used for treatment of certain types of cancers) is hypothyroidism; and therefore, there is potential for development of myxedema coma if the patient develops severe hypothyroidism and is not treated with thyroid hormone replacement. Myxedema coma has been reported as a result of consumption of large quantities of raw bok choy. Bok choy contains glucosinolates and the breakdown products of glucosinolates can have an inhibitory effect on thyroid hormone production.

Chu M, Seltzer TF. Myxedema coma induced by ingestion of raw bok choy. *N Engl J Med.* 2010;362(20):1945-1946. doi:10.1056/NEJMc0911005

Hassan S, Ayoub W, Hassan M, et al. Amiodarone-induced myxoedema coma. *BMJ Case Rep.* 2014;2014. doi:10.1136/bcr-2013-202338

Lele AV, Clutter S, Price E, et al. Severe hypothyroidism presenting as myxedema coma in the postoperative period in a patient taking Sunitinib: case report and review of literature. *J Clin Anesth.* 2013;25(1):47-51. doi:10.1016/j.jclinane.2012.07.001

Wartofsky L. Myxedema coma. *Endocrinol Metab Clin North Am.* 2006;35(4):687-698, vii-viii. doi:
10.1016/j.ecl.2006.09.003

27. **The answer is E.** Myxedema coma is a medical emergency and is associated with high mortality rate, therefore, timely diagnosis and treatment is crucial. In the past, the mortality rate was reported to be as high as 60% to 70%, but more recently the reported mortality rate dropped to 20% to 25%. Factors reported to be associated with higher mortality rate include lower GCS, APACHE II score greater than 20, Sequential Organ Failure Assessment (SOFA) score greater than 6, older age, persistent hypothermia, and bradycardia.

Dutta P, Bhansali A, Masoodi SR, et al. Predictors of outcome in myxoedema coma: a study from a tertiary care centre. *Crit Care.* 2008;12(1):R1. doi:10.1186/cc6211

Jonklaas J, Bianco AC, Bauer AJ, et al. Guidelines for the treatment of hypothyroidism: prepared by the American thyroid association task force on thyroid hormone replacement. *Thyroid.* 2014;24(12):1670-751. doi:10.1089/thy.2014.0028

Rodriguez I, Fluiters E, Perez-Mendez LF, et al. Factors associated with mortality of patients with myxoedema coma: prospective study in 11 cases treated in a single institution. *J Endocrinol.* 2004;180(2):347-350. doi:10.1677/joe.0.1800347

28. **The answer is E.** The patient should be admitted to the ICU for close monitoring and a multifaceted approach to treatment should be initiated immediately. Given myxedema coma is a rare diagnosis, there is lack of clinical trials comparing the efficacy of different treatment options. Therefore, there is no consensus regarding the type of thyroid hormone utilized for replacement as well as dosing and frequency. The available recommendations are primarily based on expert opinion and case reports. In general, IV administration of thyroid hormone is preferred initially as there may be impaired gastrointestinal (GI) absorption. There is controversy about the use of T4, T3 or both for treatment of myxedema coma. Given concern for reduced conversion of T4 to T3 in sick hypothyroid patients, treatment with T3 in addition to T4 can be considered. Different regimens of loading and maintenance daily doses have been described. Thyroid hormone can be measured every 1 to 2 days to assess response to therapy. There is no specific goal for thyroid-stimulating hormone (TSH) or thyroid hormone level; however, a rise in T4 level and down-trending TSH level is expected. Of note, TSH improvement does take time and lags behind clinical improvement. Subsequent dose adjustments should be made based on clinical and laboratory findings as well as comorbidities (lower doses should be given to older patients or those with a history of coronary artery disease [CAD] or arrhythmias). While there is no consensus on when to stop aggressive treatments, patients can be transitioned from IV thyroid hormone replacement to oral thyroid hormone replacement when there has been improvement in the patient's clinical status.

Given the possibility of underlying adrenal insufficiency, glucocorticoid therapy is recommend prior to administration of thyroid hormone replacement. A baseline cortisol can be measured prior to initiation of therapy. The initial dose of hydrocortisone is 50 to 100 mg every 6 to 8 hours and glucocorticoid treatment can then tapered as tolerated with improvement of the patient's clinical status.

Rodriguez I, Fluiters E, Perez-Mendez LF, et al. Factors associated with mortality of patients with myxoedema coma: prospective study in 11 cases treated in a single institution. *J Endocrinol.* 2004;180(2):347-350. doi:10.1677/joe.0.1800347

29. **The answer is C.** Cortisol has an eosinophil lytic effect. Therefore, eosinophilia rather than low eosinophil count is seen in adrenal crisis. The hypotension is due to the loss of both aldosterone and cortisol. Aldosterone is a salt retainer and the loss of aldosterone results in loss of sodium and accompanying loss of volume. Cortisol deficiency leads to low blood pressure as well since glucocorticoids are required for the vasculature to be fully responsive to circulating vasoconstrictors. The hypercalcemia, which is rare, is due to increased calcium absorption and decreased renal calcium excretion. Hyperkalemia is caused by the loss of the kaliuretic effects of aldosterone. This might be exacerbated by volume contraction and reduced renal perfusion further limiting the elimination of potassium. Hyponatremia is caused by sodium loss from aldosterone insufficiency but perhaps more so because the reduced intravascular

volume leads to an increase in circulating antidiuretic hormone (ADH). In addition, cortisol exerts a negative feedback on ADH and this is lost with the cortisol insufficiency, further increasing ADH and worsening hyponatremia. Borderline hypoglycemia can be attributed to not eating and to the loss of cortisol necessary for hepatic gluconeogenesis. Cortisol physiologically inhibits thyrotropin (TSH). Thus, TSH can be increased at presentation of adrenal insufficiency, but may return to normal with glucocorticoid replacement. Primary adrenal and thyroid insufficiencies can coexist (Schmidt's Syndrome); therefore, if TSH does not normalize with glucocorticoid treatment, the primary hypothyroidism needs to be treated separately. Dehydroepiandrosterone sulfate, DHEA-S, an adrenal androgen from the zona reticularis, is also decreased in primary adrenal insufficiency. Although underlying low DHEA-S levels may cause decreased . . . axillary and pubic hair . . . insufficiency, requiring replacement in a stable outpatient setting, there is no implication for treatment in acute adrenal crisis.

Arlt W, Allolio B. Adrenal insufficiency. *Lancet.* 2003;361(9372):1881-1893. doi:10.1016/S0140-6736(03)13492-7

30. **The answer is E.** There are several causes of hypoadrenalism, both primary (destruction of the adrenal) and secondary (destruction of the hypothalamus and/or anterior pituitary). Autoimmune adrenalitis, infections, adrenal hemorrhage, infiltrative diseases such as cancers, sarcoidosis, amyloidosis, medications, and several genetic diseases can cause adrenal destruction. Hypothalamic-pituitary disease causing secondary adrenal insufficiency is due to any of a large variety of destructive processes of the hypothalamus and/or pituitary. In addition, exogenous glucocorticoid therapy can suppress the hypothalamic-pituitary-adrenal unit and that suppression can continue for some time after the glucocorticoid is stopped.

Bornstein SR. Predisposing factors for adrenal insufficiency. *N Engl J Med.* 2009;360(22):2328-2339. doi:10.1056/NEJMra0804635
Cooper MS, Stewart PM. Corticosteroid insufficiency in acutely ill patients. *N Engl J Med.* 2003;348(8):727-734. doi:10.1056/NEJMra020529

31. **The answer is C.** Exogenous glucocorticoids work at the level of both the hypothalamus and anterior pituitary to inhibit the synthesis and secretion of corticotrophin releasing hormone in the hypothalamus and subsequently of ACTH in the anterior pituitary. The glucocorticoid probably has no direct effect on the adrenal gland. ACTH not only stimulates the synthesis and secretion of adrenal cortisol but it is also a trophic factor for the adrenals. Therefore, a prolonged lack of ACTH can lead to adrenal atrophy. In any case, an individual should be considered to have a suppressed hypothalamic-pituitary-adrenal axis for 1 year after coming off steroids. This may not have significant consequences in day-to-day life, but that individual cannot respond to stress adequately and may require treatment with high-dose glucocorticoids in such situations. In addition, such a patient should have an alert bracelet or necklace indicating that he or she has been on glucocorticoids. He or she should also have oral glucocorticoids at home and know to take double the usual glucocorticoid dose in times of stress. He or she should also know that if the stress involves sickness with vomiting or diarrhea, there should either be injectable glucocorticoid at home or the individual should know to go to a physician immediately.

Cooper MS, Stewart PM. Corticosteroid insufficiency in acutely ill patients. *N Engl J Med.* 2003;348(8):727-734. doi:10.1056/NEJMra020529

32. **The answer is D.** Skin hyperpigmentation is a sign of primary adrenal insufficiency but is not seen in secondary adrenal insufficiency. The skin hyperpigmentation is caused by increased production of proopiomelanocortin (POMC), a pituitary prohormone that is cleaved into the biologically active hormones ACTH, melanocyte stimulating hormone (MSH), and others. MSH leads to increased melanin synthesis in skin and consequent skin hyperpigmentation. MSH is increased because of the loss of negative feedback from reduced cortisol. The diagnosis of autoimmunity causing hypoadrenalism is supported by the presence of another autoimmune disease and vitiligo.

Cooper MS, Stewart PM. Corticosteroid insufficiency in acutely ill patients. *N Engl J Med.* 2003;348(8):727-734. doi:10.1056/NEJMra020529

33. **The answer is D.** One diagnostic approach to primary adrenal insufficiency is to obtain a random cortisol/ACTH pair as well as an aldosterone/renin pair. ACTH and cortisol (as well as aldosterone and renin) work in a closed negative feedback loop. Therefore, low cortisol and aldosterone levels in primary adrenal insufficiency will increase secretion of ACTH and renin.

There is no absolute consensus on what constitutes adequate and normal hormone levels. A random cortisol level of less than 15 µg/dL makes adrenal insufficiency likely. A random cortisol level greater than 34 µg/dL makes adrenal insufficiency unlikely. For cortisol values between 15 and 34 µg/dL, a cosyntropin (a synthetic ACTH) stimulation test is necessary. The results of this test are not significantly affected by diurnal variation and thus can be performed at any time of day. Cosyntropin at 250 µg dose is given IV or intramuscularly (IM); cortisol is measured at baseline, 30 and 60 minutes. A cortisol response of less than 9 µg/dL is compatible with the diagnosis of adrenal insufficiency, whereas a response ≥9 µg/dL speaks against the diagnosis. Dexamethasone 4 mg IV can be given during the test, as a stress dose that does not interfere with cortisol measurement during the test. There are two caveats. First, these targets are somewhat different from those for a normal cosyntropin test done under nonstressed conditions. Second, since cortisol is highly protein bound, clinical situations with very low protein states (albumin can be used as a surrogate) might give falsely low values. In those situations, a free cortisol determination might be appropriate. It should be noted that some authors advocate the use of 1 µg of cosyntropin while others still recommend the 250 µg dose. Aldosterone and renin can be measured as well, but the response is less well defined. Some would consider a doubling of aldosterone as an adequate response.

Some consider the insulin tolerance test a gold standard for testing hypothalamic-pituitary-adrenal function. This is because hypoglycemia is a potent stimulator of the hypothalamic-pituitary unit. However, the cortisol response to hypoglycemia can be well predicted by the cosyntropin stimulation test, which is safer and quicker.

Bornstein SR. Predisposing factors for adrenal insufficiency. *N Engl J Med.* 2009;360(22):2328-2339. doi:10.1056/NEJMra0804635

Bornstein SR, Allolio B, Arlt W, et al. Diagnosis and treatment of primary adrenal insufficiency: an endocrine society clinical practice guideline. *J Clin Endocrinol Metab.* 2016;101(2):364-389. doi:10.1210/jc.2015-1710

34. **The answer is E.** Acute adrenal crisis is a life-threatening emergency. If there is a correctable underlying cause such as infection, it should be corrected. The patient needs intravascular volume (such as glucose/normal saline solution). Hydrocortisone 100 mg IV push should be given immediately. Then the patient should receive IV hydrocortisone 200 to 300 mg per 24 hours with the dose reduced to maintenance as the clinical situation dictates. Fludrocortisone 0.1 to 0.2 mg daily by mouth is needed to replace aldosterone, but this may not be necessary in patients on high-dose glucocorticoid as there is some glucocorticoid "spillover" to the mineralocorticoid receptor. It may be necessary when the patient is transferred to maintenance steroid doses for chronic therapy.

Murad M, Stratakis CA, Torpy DJ. Diagnosis and treatment of primary adrenal insufficiency: an endocrine society clinical practice guideline. *J Clin Endocrinol Metab.* 2016;101(2):364-389. doi:10.1210/jc.2015-1710

35. **The answer is C.** Hyperglycemia is a common problem in hospitalized patients, including in the ICU, and is associated with adverse outcomes and death. Approximately 50% of ICU patients have preexisting diabetes, although many may not be aware of the diagnosis before admission. Even previously normoglycemic patients may become hyperglycemic due to various factors. Stress results in increased release of catecholamines, cortisol, glucagon, and tumor necrosis factor (TNF) alpha. In addition, medicines such as exogenous steroids,

vasopressors, and beta-blockers can lead to hyperglycemia. Supportive treatments such as IV dextrose, enteral and parenteral nutrition (PN) can further worsen hyperglycemia. Patients with known or unknown diabetes but hyperglycemia greater than 140 mg/dL should get a hemoglobin A1c (HbA1c) level if none is available for 2 to 3 months. Patients should be monitored with bedside POC testing, especially since many patients may have undiagnosed DM.

Based on studies in mixed medical/surgical ICUs, strict glycemic control is associated with treatment-related hypoglycemia and increased mortality in critically ill patients. Based on the Normoglycemia in Intensive Care Evaluation–Survival Using Glucose Algorithm Regulation (NICE-SUGAR) trial, current target glycemic goals for the majority of critically and noncritically ill patients are 140 to 180 mg/dL (7.8–10 mmol/L). More stringent goals, such as less than 140 mg/dL (<7.8 mmol/L), may be appropriate for selected patients, if this can be achieved without significant hypoglycemia. Hypoglycemia (<70 mg/dL) and severe hypoglycemia (<40 mg/dL) should be avoided as it may induce cardiac arrhythmias, cognitive deficits, and increased mortality.

Falciglia M, Freyberg RW, Almenoff PL, et al. Hyperglycemia-related mortality in critically ill patients varies with admission diagnosis. *Crit Care Med*. 2009;37(12):3001-3009. doi:10.1097/CCM.0b013e3181b083f7

Inzucchi SE. Management of hyperglycemia in the hospital setting. *N Engl J Med*. 2006;355(18):1903-1911. doi:10.1056/NEJMcp060094

Plummer MP, Bellomo R, Cousins CE, et al. Dysglycaemia in the critically ill and the interaction of chronic and acute glycaemia with mortality. *Intensive Care Med*. 2014;40(7):973-980. doi:10.1007/s00134-014-3287-7

Umpierrez GE, Hellman R, Korytkowski MT, et al. Management of hyperglycemia in hospitalized patients in non-critical care setting: an endocrine society clinical practice guideline. *J Clin Endocrinol Metab*. 2012;97(1):16-38. doi:10.1210/jc.2011-2098

Van den Berghe G, Wouters P, Weekers F, et al. Intensive insulin therapy in critically ill patients. *N Engl J Med*. 2001;345(19):1359-1367. doi:10.1056/NEJMoa011300

Wiener R, Wiener DC, Larson RJ. Benefits and risks of tight glucose control in critically ill adults: a meta-analysis. *JAMA*. 2008;300(8):933-944. doi:10.1001/jama.300.8.933

36. **The answer is D.** In patients hospitalized for an acute illness who have hyperglycemia, insulin is the preferred method for achieving glycemic control. Guidelines recommend that insulin therapy be initiated for treatment of persistent hyperglycemia (starting at a threshold ≥180 mg/dL) as basal-bolus therapy. For lean type 1 diabetes patients, the total daily starting insulin dose is ~0.2 to 0.5 units/kg, and for obese type 2 diabetes patients it is 0.5 to 0.8 units/Kg. This is divided into ~50% basal and ~50 % bolus insulin. Basal insulin provides coverage overnight and between meals and is best delivered as a long-acting insulin analog such as glargine or detemir insulin. Bolus insulin is used before meals and snacks to cover postprandial hyperglycemia. Rapid acting analogs such as lispro, aspart, or glulisine are used for meal coverage. A correction dose of rapid-acting insulin should be added to the scheduled pre-meal insulin regimen for treatment of values above the desired target, according to a pre-specified scale. Prolonged use of sliding scale insulin therapy should be avoided as the sole method for glycemic control in patients with history of diabetes during hospitalization. In critical care settings, continuous IV insulin infusions based on validated protocols provide the best outcomes. Best protocols take into account the prevailing blood glucose, its rate of change, and the current insulin infusion rate. Insulin infusion protocols and standardized computerized treatment algorithms reduce the risk of hypoglycemia and are recommended. At the time of discharge, patients who had acceptable pre-admission glycemic control can be switched back to their home antidiabetic agents or insulin regimen if there is no contraindication to their continued use. This should be done at least one day before discharge to allow assessment of the efficacy and safety of this transition. Diabetes self-management education, including appropriate skills needed after discharge, should be provided.

Umpierrez GE, Smiley D, Zisman A, et al. Randomized study of basal-bolus insulin therapy in the inpatient management of patients with type 2 diabetes (RABBIT 2 trial). *Diabetes Care*. 2007;30(9):2181-2186. doi:10.2337/dc07-0295

37. **The answer is E.** All the above clinical situations can increase the risk of hyper- and hypo-glycemia in the hospital (also see answer 36).

Umpierrez GE, Hellman R, Korytkowski MT, et al. Management of hyperglycemia in hospitalized patients in non-critical care setting: an endocrine society clinical practice guideline. *J Clin Endocrinol Metab.* 2012;97(1):16-38. doi:10.1210/jc.2011-2098

38. **The answer is B.** DKA is a serious complication of diabetes characterized by hyperglycemia (usually between 250 and 800 mg/dL), low arterial pH, high-anion gap (AG) metabolic acidosis (due to accumulation of beta-hydroxybutyric and acetoacetic acids), positive serum and urine ketones, and altered sensorium. Symptoms develop rapidly over 24 hours and include polyuria, polydipsia, lethargy, nausea, vomiting, and abdominal pain. Mortality rate increases substantially with age and concomitant life-threatening illnesses. The underlying mechanism is a reduction in effective insulin concentration and elevation of counter-regulatory hormones (catecholamines, glucagon, cortisol, and growth hormone [GH]). Patients are admitted to an ICU and assessed for vital signs, volume status, cardiorespiratory status, and mental status. Serum electrolytes, blood urea nitrogen (BUN), creatinine (Cr), glucose, blood gas, urine/serum ketones, and urine analysis are obtained. Additional tests may be needed based on clinical condition to rule out infection, pancreatitis, myocardial infarction (MI), and so forth. Leukocytosis can result from increased cortisol and catecholamine secretion in DKA. Patients with white blood cell (WBC) counts greater than 25,000/µL or bands greater than 10% should be evaluated for infection. Serum amylase and lipase may be elevated in patients with DKA who do not have any other clinical or radiological evidence of acute pancreatitis. Correct fluid loss with IV fluids, hyperglycemia with continuous insulin infusion using regular or analog rapid acting insulin and a prespecified protocol, correct electrolyte and acid-based disturbances, and treat any exacerbating factor. If initial serum potassium is less than 3.3 mEq/L, hold insulin and give potassium chloride 20 to 40 mg/h to avoid cardiac arrhythmias and muscle weakness. Continue potassium replacement to maintain serum potassium between 4 and 5 mEq/L. Although administration of subcutaneous rapid-acting insulin every 1 to 2 hours has also been found to be as safe and efficacious as continuous insulin infusion in patients with mild uncomplicated DKA, fixed doses of insulin every 6 hours will not achieve a similar goal. Reaching target glycemic control with minimal hypoglycemia has become more efficient with increasing management of blood glucose through standardized, computerized treatment algorithms that provide a personalized insulin dose recommendation for IV and subcutaneous insulin therapy. Compared to using paper protocols, computerized glucose management systems result in more rapid and tighter glucose control, an increase in the time spent within the target blood glucose concentration, and a decrease in the prevalence of severe hypoglycemia (blood glucose [BG] <40 mg/dL), clinical hypoglycemia (BG <70 mg/dL), and hyperglycemia (BG >180 mg/dL). The hyperglycemic crisis is considered to have resolved once the AG is normalized (<12 mEq/L), serum beta hydroxybutyrate levels are normal, and patient is mentally alert and able to eat. Patient can then be transitioned to scheduled subcutaneous insulin therapy. Give basal insulin dose at least 1–2 hours before discontinuation of insulin infusion to avoid recurrence of hyperglycemia/DKA due to acute reduction in insulin level.

Juneja R, Roudebush CP, Nasraway SA, et al. Computerized intensive insulin dosing can mitigate hypoglycemia and achieve tight glycemic control when glucose measurement is performed frequently and on time. *Crit Care.* 2009;13(5):R163-R163. doi:10.1186/cc8129

Kitabchi AE, Umpierrez GE, Miles JM, et al. Hyperglycemic crises in adult patients with diabetes. *Diabetes Care.* 2009;32(7):1335-1343. doi:10.2337/dc09-9032

Umpierrez GE, Cuervo R, Karabell A, et al. Treatment of diabetic ketoacidosis with subcutaneous insulin aspart. *Diabetes Care.* 2004;27(8):1873-1878. doi:10.2337/diacare.27.8.1873

Umpierrez GE, Jones S, Smiley D, et al. Insulin analogs versus human insulin in the treatment of patients with diabetic ketoacidosis: a randomized controlled trial. *Diabetes Care.* 2009;32(7):1164-1169. doi:10.2337/dc09-0169

39. **The answer is E.** Twenty to 25% of patients with new onset type 1 diabetes may present in DKA. Precipitating factors include noncompliance with insulin treatment, inadequate insulin, insulin pump failure, infection, stroke, myocardial infarction (MI), acute pancreatitis, and certain medications.

    Steroids can induce hyperglycemia or precipitate DKA in patients with previously known, or previously undiagnosed diabetes, due to reduction in insulin mediated glucose uptake and increased hepatic glucose production. Sodium glucose cotransporter-2 inhibitors (such as canagliflozin, dapagliflozin, and empagliflozin) stimulate ketone reabsorption in the kidneys, thus increasing the risk of DKA with mild hyperglycemia. However, if the drug is prescribed in appropriate situations, the risk is negligible in type 2 diabetes mellitus (DM). Atypical antipsychotic agents have been associated with significant hyperglycemia and dyslipidemia that is independent of weight gain. Fluoroquinolones have been associated with severe hypoglycemia. Furosemide may uncommonly cause hyperglycemia but is not associated with DKA.

    Clore J, Thurby-Hay L. Glucocorticoid-induced hyperglycemia. *Endocr Pract.* 2009;15(5):469-474. doi:10.4158/EP08331.RAR

    Monami MB, Nreu S, Zannoni C, et al. Effects of SGLT-2 inhibitors on diabetic ketoacidosis: a meta-analysis of randomised controlled trials. *Diabetes Res Clin Pract.* 2017;130:53-60. doi:10.1016/j.diabres.2017.04.017

    Newcomer JW. Second-generation (atypical) antipsychotics and metabolic effects: a comprehensive literature review. *CNS Drugs.* 2005;19:1-93. doi:10.2165/00023210-200519001-00001

40. **The answer is E.** HHNS is characterized by marked hyperglycemia (often >1,000 mg/dL), elevated serum osmolality (typically >320 mosm/kg), and normal or only mildly reduced serum bicarbonate. Ketones may be present in small quantities. Symptoms are similar to DKA, but develop over a few days. Focal neurological deficits and mental obtundation are more common due to marked hyper osmolality. HHNS may be precipitated by acute infection, stroke, myocardial infarction (MI), acute pancreatitis, endocrinopathies (Cushing's syndrome, thyrotoxicosis, acromegaly), and certain medications (e.g., steroids, beta-blockers, thiazide diuretics, and atypical antipsychotics). Other medical conditions that need to be ruled out include alcoholic ketosis, starvation ketosis, other causes of high-anion gap (AG) metabolic acidosis, and toxic metabolic encephalopathy. Sodium and water deficits should be replaced gradually. Once serum glucose is less than 200 mg/dL, 5 to 10% dextrose is added to the intravenous solution to prevent the serum glucose from falling below 200 mg/dL in DKA (or 250–300 mg/dL in HHNS) and avoid the development of cerebral edema. This is a rare complication of the treatment of DKA/HHNS with a mortality rate 20%–40%, and can present as headache, lethargy, seizures, bradycardia and respiratory arrest.

    Kitabchi AE, Umpierrez GE, Miles JM, et al. Hyperglycemic crises in adult patients with diabetes. *Diabetes Care.* 2009;32(7):1335-1343. doi:10.2337/dc09-9032

20

Infectious Diseases

SALIA FARROKH AND POUYA TAHSILI-FAHADAN

QUESTIONS

1. A 35-year-old man presents to an ED in southern Virginia in July with fever, headaches, confusion, myalgias, and malaise for 5 days. He has been anuric for the past 24 hours. He had been hiking with his friends through the countryside last week. His blood pressure (BP) is 85/45 mmHg, pulse is 133 beats per minute (BPM), and RR is 32 BPM. His skin has petechial lesions over his trunk and extremities with one suspicious necrotic lesion on his thigh. White blood cell (WBC) count is 11,000 cells/mm³ (20% bands) and platelets are 33,000 cells/mm³, with transaminitis (3× normal). He receives all measures of early goal-directed therapy (EGDT) for sepsis. Besides broad-spectrum antibiotic coverage with vancomycin and ceftriaxone, what other antibiotic should you consider?

   A. Linezolid
   B. Doxycycline
   C. Amoxicillin
   D. Bacitracin
   E. Isoniazid

2. A 42-year-old woman with rheumatoid arthritis, on oral prednisone therapy, is brought to the ED with 2 days of fever, headache, severe myalgias, dry cough, dyspnea, and coryza. She is a school teacher, and several kids in her class have been sick with "the flu." Her lungs have scattered crackles in both lung fields, and labs reveal a white blood cell (WBC) count of 13,000 cells/mm³ with 69% lymphocytes. Chest x-ray (CXR) shows bilateral increased interstitial markings. Besides routine supportive and diagnostic measures, what test would you send next?

   A. Urine *Legionella* antigen
   B. Immunofluorescence antibody staining for influenza from blood
   C. Rapid influenza diagnostic test from a urine specimen
   D. Rapid influenza diagnostic test from a throat swab
   E. Viral cell cultures for influenza virus from a throat swab

3. If the rapid influenza test for the patient in Question 2 is positive, which treatment would you institute next? Patient has a normal renal and hepatic function.

   A. Acyclovir 800 mg orally 5 times daily
   B. Ritonavir 600 mg orally 2 times daily
   C. Clarithromycin 500 mg orally 3 times daily
   D. Oseltamivir 75 mg orally 2 times daily
   E. Amantadine 100 mg orally 2 times daily

4. A 59-year-old prison inmate is being evaluated for an abnormal screening chest x-ray (CXR) done during incarceration. He denies any cough, fevers, night sweats, weight loss, or sick contacts. He does endorse receiving a "tuberculosis injection" when he was a young man in Guatemala, which ulcerated and was painful. If his CXR findings are consistent with a remote tuberculosis (TB) infection, which would be the most efficient, sensitive, and specific test for latent TB in this patient?

A. Induced sputum for TB culture
B. Bronchoalveolar lavage for acid-fast stain
C. Tuberculin skin test for induration
D. Quantiferon-TB Gold test
E. Induced sputum for acid-fast stain

5. Which of the following is true regarding the definition of sepsis based on the updated Society of Critical Care Medicine (SCCM) guidelines?

A. Presence of two or more systemic inflammatory response syndrome (SIRS) criteria plus obvious source of infection
B. Life-threatening organ dysfunction caused by a dysregulated host response to infection
C. Hypotension caused by bloodstream infection
D. Hypotension caused by lactate level of greater than 4 mmol/L
E. Reduced cardiac output as a result of anaphyctic reaction

6. Which of the following is true regarding initiation of broad spectrum intravenous (IV) antimicrobials in a patient with suspected septic shock?

A. IV antimicrobials must be initiated as soon as possible after recognition of septic shock and within 1 hour for both sepsis and septic shock
B. IV antimicrobials should only be initiated after adequate fluid resuscitation and initiation vasopressor therapy
C. IV antimicrobials should include agents that cover Gram positive, Gram negative, anaerobes, and atypical organisms for all patients
D. IV antimicrobials must be given only to patients with mean arterial pressure (MAP) <55 mmHg and within 3 hours of recognition of septic shock
E. Patients with a history of penicillin allergy (anaphylaxis) should receive vancomycin and meropenem

7. A 48-year-old man sustaining a 40% total body surface area (TBSA) burn to his left side with likely inhalational injury is admitted to the ICU for mechanical ventilation support. On day 7 of the ICU stay he develops a temperature of 102.1°F (38.9°C) and a white blood cell (WBC) count of 11,000 cells/mm³. He is hemodynamically stable, has a lactate of 1.1 mmol/L, and shows no signs or symptoms of new onset organ dysfunction. He has a Foley catheter in place. Urinalysis shows 5 WBC/hpf, trace red blood cells (RBC), few bacteria, and positive nitrites, and is negative for leukocyte esterase, glucose, protein, ketones, and casts. Patient has no known medication allergies. What is the best next step?

A. Initiate broad spectrum antibiotics with vancomycin and piperacillin/tazobactam for suspected sepsis
B. Initiate ceftriaxone for catheter-associated urinary tract infection (CAUTI)
C. No antibiotic therapy is needed at this point; change the Foley
D. Send for urine culture and then start ceftriaxone
E. Initiate sulfamethaxazole/trimethoprim for CAUTI

8. A 70-year-old woman with a medical history significant for chronic obstructive pulmonary disease (COPD), type 2 diabetes, coronary artery disease (CAD), and a 7-day hospitalization

12 days ago is readmitted to the ICU with respiratory failure requiring intubation secondary to COPD exacerbation. On day 4 of this admission, she develops increased sputum production, temperature of 101.9°F (38.8°C), and worsening oxygenation as well as a new infiltrate in the left lower lung base. Out of suspicion for ventilator-associated pneumonia (VAP), a semiquantitative tracheal aspirate is sent to identify causative pathogen(s). Which empiric antibiotic regimen is best for this patient?

A. Azithromycin plus moxifloxacin
B. Ceftriaxone plus vancomycin
C. Ceftriaxone plus azithromycin
D. Linezolid plus tobramycin
E. Cefepime plus vancomycin

9. A 75-year-old man was admitted from home with a small intracerebral hemorrhage (ICH) after a witnessed fall. Few hours later in the ED, he developed a cough and confusion with new temperature of 102.1°F, respiration rate (RR) 28 BPM, and oxygen saturation of 91% on room air. Rhonchi are auscultated on lung exam, and mild pitting edema is noted in the legs. Labs reveal leukopenia and a blood urea nitrogen (BUN) of 58 mg/dL. Chest x-ray (CXR) reveals a retrocardiac opacity. He is diagnosed with pneumonia. In addition to supplemental oxygen and antipyretics, what is the most appropriate management for this patient?

A. Initiate sulfamethoxazole/trimethoprim, and transfer to the floor
B. Initiate intravenous (IV) piperacillin–tazobactam and vancomycin, and transfer to ICU
C. Administer IV ceftriaxone and azithromycin, and transfer to ICU
D. Obtain blood cultures, administer IV vancomycin within 4 hours, and transfer to ICU
E. Obtain blood cultures and await results prior to initiating antimicrobial therapy

10. A 67-year-old woman is admitted to the ICU for severe metabolic acidosis secondary to diabetic ketoacidosis (DKA). Her ICU stay is complicated by a femoral vein central line-associated bloodstream infection (CLABSI) and related severe sepsis caused by pan-sensitive *E. coli*. Her central line is removed and she receives a 3-day course of empiric piperacillin/tazobactam, followed by 11 days of ceftriaxone as definitive therapy with resolution of sepsis. Starting yesterday, she has had 10 episodes of loose bowel movements. A new leukocytosis of 12,500 cells/mm³ suggests *Clostridium difficile* infection (CDI). She continues to tolerate enteral nutrition. Which is the most appropriate regimen for her suspected CDI?

A. Fidaxomicin 500 mg per feeding tube every 8 hours
B. Metronidazole 500 mg per feeding tube every 12 hours
C. Metronidazole 500 mg intravenously every 8 hours
D. Vancomycin 125 mg per feeding tube every 6 hours
E. Metronidazole 500 mg per feeding tube every 12 hours and fidaxomicin 200 mg per feeding tube every 8 hours

11. Which of the following is a reasonable antibiotic choice for a 28-year-old woman diagnosed with methicillin-resistant *Staphylococcus aureus* (MRSA) pneumonia after being intubated for 5 days and has failed vancomycin therapy evident by clinical worsening? She has normal renal and liver function and no known medication allergies.

A. Stop vancomycin and start daptomycin 6 mg/kg once daily
B. Stop vancomycin and start piperacillin/tazobactam 4.5 gm intravenously (IV) every 6 hours
C. Stop vancomycin and start linezolid 600 mg IV q12h
D. Continue vancomycin but target for a trough goal of 20 to 25 mcg/mL
E. Stop vancomycin and start rifampin 900 mg IV daily

12. A 69-year-old alcoholic man is found unresponsive in an alley, covered in vomit and beer. On arrival to the ED, he is somnolent with temperature 103.5°F, heart rate (HR) 109 beats per minute, and oxygen saturation 89% on room air. He has a severe cough productive of thick, dark red, jellylike sputum. Based on this information, what is the most likely pathogen?

   A. *Aspergillus*
   B. *Mycoplasma pneumonia*
   C. *Mycobacterium tuberculosis*
   D. *Klebsiella pneumonia*
   E. Influenza B

13. A central venous catheter (CVC) is inserted in a patient with traumatic brain injury (TBI) for administration of hypertonic fluids. Which of the following measures has been shown to minimize the risk of central line-associated bloodstream infection (CLABSI)?

   A. Exchanging the CVC over a guidewire every 3 days
   B. Exchanging the CVC over a guidewire every 7 days
   C. Exchanging the CVC with a fresh site every 7 days
   D. Prophylactic daily vancomycin through CVC
   E. None of the above

14. A patient is admitted to the ICU after exposure to poison ivy with a facial rash and edema. He subsequently develops airway obstruction due to tongue swelling and is intubated via the nasal route. Which of the following infectious complications is he at highest risk for?

   A. Urinary tract infection (UTI)
   B. Meningitis
   C. Orbital cellulitis
   D. Maxillary sinusitis
   E. Otitis media

15. Which of the following interventions will significantly reduce the chances of the patient in Question 14 developing the infectious complication?

   A. Prophylactic linezolid intravenously (IV)
   B. Inhaled tobramycin through the endotracheal tube
   C. Clindamycin gel applied to the nasal cavity
   D. Early transfer of endotracheal tube to the oral route
   E. Warmed and humidified air through the endotracheal tube

16. A 62-year-old homeless man is admitted to the ICU with signs of impending respiratory failure. He has a 6-month history of productive cough, progressive weight loss, night sweats, and dyspnea. He progresses to respiratory failure and during intubation the bedside nurse is exposed to his sputum, which later grows acid-fast bacilli. What is the next appropriate plan of action for the nurse?

   A. Offer reassurance that the chances of transmission are extremely low and she needs no further follow-up or care
   B. Order a purified protein derivative (PPD) skin test for tuberculosis (TB)
   C. Order a PPD skin test for TB and order preventive treatment if skin induration is greater than 5 mm
   D. Start preventive therapy with isoniazid, rifampin, and ethambutol
   E. Start preventive therapy with daily isoniazid for 9 months

17. A postal worker is accidentally exposed to a suspicious white powder while handling a package at the post office. He does not report the incident, and a few days later he develops progressive fever, rigors, chills, dry cough, dyspnea, and malaise. His condition worsens to the point of near collapse at work and he is rushed to the hospital. Initial investigation reveals an elevated white blood cell (WBC) count (17,000 cells per mm^3) and bilateral infiltrates and small effusions on chest x-ray (CXR). He progresses to respiratory failure, requiring intubation and mechanical ventilation. Blood cultures grow Gram-positive rods on day 3. What is the most likely diagnosis?

    A. Cat scratch disease
    B. Gastrointestinal (GI) anthrax
    C. Legionnaires' disease
    D. Inhalational anthrax
    E. Cutaneous anthrax

18. Which of the following treatment regimens would be the most appropriate for the patient in Question 17?

    A. Intravenous (IV) ciprofloxacin + IV clindamycin
    B. PO doxycycline
    C. PO ampicillin
    D. IV fluconazole
    E. IV ceftriaxone

19. A 56-year-old man is admitted to the ICU from a nursing home with a large intracerebral hemorrhage (ICH). He is intubated and mechanically ventilated for hypercarbic respiratory failure and airway protection. Which of the following interventions is most likely to reduce his chances of infectious complications of intubation?

    A. Exchanging the ventilator circuit every 3 days
    B. Use of oral antiseptic chlorhexidine swabs
    C. Exchanging the ventilator circuit every 7 days
    D. Use of proton pump inhibitors for gastric acid control
    E. Switching the orotracheal tube to a nasotracheal tube when able

20. A decision is made to start empiric antibiotic therapy for the patient in Question 19, for a clinical diagnosis of ventilator-associated pneumonia (VAP) 4 days after intubation. Which of the following antibiotic regimens would be the most appropriate? Patient has normal renal/hepatic function and a history of penicillin allergy with difficulty breathing.

    A. Intravenous (IV) vancomycin and IV piperacillin/tazobactam
    B. IV vancomycin and IV aztreonam
    C. Oral azithromycin
    D. IV vancomycin and IV ceftriaxone
    E. IV ampicillin/sulbactam

21. For the patient in Question 20, the respiratory culture is finalized as methicillin-sensitive *Staphylococcus aureus* (MSSA). Patient is still febrile with purulent, thick respiratory secretions. What is the best next action?

    A. No change in therapy is needed
    B. Current antibiotics should be stopped. Intravenous (IV) oxacillin should be started after desensitization
    C. Current antibiotics should be stopped. IV sulfamethaxazole/trimethoprim should be started
    D. IV aztreonam should be stopped. IV vancomycin should be continued as monotherapy
    E. Current antibiotics should be stopped. IV doxycycline should be started

22. What is the most appropriate duration of antibiotic therapy for patient in question 21 with methicillin-sensitive Staphylococcus aureus (MSSA) pneumonia (PNA)?

A. 3 days
B. 5 days
C. 7 days
D. 10 days
E. 14 days

23. A 38-year-old man with a history prosthetic mitral valve on warfarin is admitted to the ICU for a 2-week history of progressive fever, chills, anorexia, malaise, myalgias, and night sweats, with significant worsening in the past 24 hours. He admits to intravenous (IV) drug use. At the time of admission, his temperature is 39.9°C, blood pressure (BP) is 94/58 mmHg, heart rate (HR) is 105, and serum white blood cell (WBC) count is 18,000/mm³. Cardiac auscultation reveals a new harsh systolic murmur. Blood cultures reveal growth of *Staphylococcus aureus* in both culture bottles within 12 hours. Sensitivities are pending at this point. Transthoracic echocardiogram shows a 1.2 mm by 8 mm mitral valve vegetation with severe mitral regurgitation. What is the appropriate initial antimicrobial regimen for this patient?

A. IV ampicillin and sulbactam
B. IV vancomycin, rifampin, and gentamycin
C. IV vancomycin and cefepime
D. IV vancomycin, ceftriaxone, and metronidazole
E. IV vancomycin and azithromycin

24. A 28-year-old man with history of traumatic spinal cord injury and recurrent urinary tract infections (UTI) is admitted with sepsis related to UTI. Urine cultures grew *Klebsiella oxytoca* with sensitivities reported as below. What is the best treatment option?

Ampicillin	RESISTANT
Ampicillin/sulbactam	RESISTANT
Ceftazidime	RESISTANT
Ceftriaxone	RESISTANT
Ciprofloxacin	RESISTANT
Ertapenem	SUSCEPTIBLE
Gentamicin	RESISTANT
Piperacillin/tazobactam	SUSCEPTIBLE
Trimethoprim/sulfa	RESISTANT

A. Piperacillin/tazobactam
B. Timethoprim/sulfa
C. Ceftazidime
D. Ertapenem
E. Ciprofloxacin

25. A 23-year-old woman is admitted to the ICU for management of spontaneous intracerebral hemorrhage (ICH) in the context of recent diagnosis of idiopathic thrombocytopenic purpura (ITP). On day 6 of admission, she develops fever (39.5°C) and new purulent discharges and erythema at the insertion site of her central venous catheter (CVC). Initial Gram stain of her blood reveals Gram-positive cocci in clusters. Culture identification and sensitivities will not be available for at least another 24 hours. What is the appropriate antibiotic therapy at this time?

A. Intravenous (IV) linezolid
B. IV penicillin
C. IV oxacillin
D. IV vancomycin and piperacillin/tazobactam
E. IV vancomycin

26. A 32-year-old woman with history of epilepsy and severe penicillin-allergy (anaphylaxis) is admitted to the neuro-ICU for refractory status epilepticus (SE) requiring multiple antiepileptic agents (levetiracetam, lacosamide, valproic acid (VPA), and propofol) and mechanical ventilation. On day 5 of admission she develops high-grade fevers and purulent green endotracheal secretions as well as relapse of her seizures. Initial Gram stain of blood shows Gram-negative rods. During the course of her ICU stay, the neighboring patient has been diagnosed with *Pseudomonas aeruginosa* decubitus ulcers and osteomyelitis (pan sensitive). What is the most appropriate antibiotic therapy at this time?

A. Intravenous (IV) ciprofloxacin
B. IV meropenem
C. IV piperacillin/tazobactam
D. IV vancomycin
E. IV cefotaxime

27. A 32-year-old woman is brought to the ED during the influenza season with traumatic brain injury (TBI) due to a motor vehicle collision. Per patient's mother, she has also had flu-like symptoms for the past 72 hours with severe shortness of breath, rigors, and dizziness. Vital signs in the ED are heart rate (HR) 120, mean arterial pressure (MAP) 60 mmHg, respiratory rate (RR) 24, temperature 102.7°F (39.3°C), and arterial oxygen saturation (SaO$_2$) 85% on room air. She is intubated for hypoxic respiratory failure and airway protection and is admitted to the neuro ICU. A nasal swab is sent for rapid diagnostic testing of suspected influenza infection. What would be the best next step?

A. None; the patient is outside the time window to effectively treat influenza
B. Await rapid diagnostic test results before initiating influenza-specific therapy
C. Start amantadine
D. Start oseltamivir
E. Administer influenza vaccine

28. A 69-year-old woman with a past medical history of congenital hydrocephalus and ventriculoperitoneal shunt who is admitted from home with severe acute abdominal pain in the left lower quadrant. An abdominal CT scan shows free air in the peritoneal cavity and evidence of distal ischemic colitis. She is taken urgently to the operating room, where peritonitis with gross contamination from distal colonic perforation is noted. She is admitted to the neuro ICU for management of septic shock after a partial colectomy with abdominal washout. Which empiric antibiotic regimen would be most appropriate at this point?

A. Ceftriaxone and tobramycin
B. Azithromycin and metronidazole
C. Moxifloxacin
D. Piperacillin/tazobactam
E. Vancomycin

29. A 70-year-old man is admitted to the ICU from the ED with septic shock. He is fluid resuscitated and broad-spectrum antibiotics with piperacillin/tazobactam and vancomycin are administered. On day 3 of admission, the patient remains hemodynamically unstable, requiring escalating doses of norepinephrine. The patient's blood culture is positive for *Enterobacter cloacae*. Which intervention regarding the patient's antimicrobial therapy is most appropriate?

    A. Discontinue vancomycin and change piperacillin/tazobactam to ceftriaxone
    B. Discontinue vancomycin and change piperacillin/tazobactam to ceftazidime
    C. Discontinue vancomycin and continue piperacillin/tazobactam only
    D. Discontinue vancomycin and change piperacillin/tazobactam to meropenem
    E. None of the above, continue the same regimen

30. A 28-year-old man with a history of HIV infection not currently receiving antiretroviral therapy, glucose-6-phosphate dehydrogenase deficiency (G6PD), and sulfa allergy is admitted to the ICU with respiratory distress. He reports a 3-week history of progressively worsening cough and pleuritic chest pain. Chest radiography shows bilateral infiltrates with ground-glass opacities. The patient is intubated for hypoxic respiratory failure receiving 40% fraction of inspired oxygen (FiO$_2$). His relevant laboratory values are white blood cell (WBC) 4×10^3 cells/mm^3, CD4+ count 100/mm^3, serum creatinine 1.0 mg/dL, LDH 550 IU/L, PaO$_2$ 80 mmHg, and PaCO$_2$ 40 mmHg. Which regimen is most appropriate?

    A. Trimethoprim/sulfamethoxazole 15–20 mg/kg intravenously (IV), divided every 6 hours, plus prednisone 40 mg twice daily
    B. Pentamidine 4 mg/kg IV every 24 hours as monotherapy
    C. Primaquine 30 mg orally once daily plus clindamycin 600 mg IV every 8 hours, plus prednisone 40 mg twice daily
    D. Atovaquone 750 mg orally every 12 hours plus prednisone 40 mg twice daily
    E. Trimethoprim/sulfamethoxazole 5 to 10 mg/kg orally divided every 6 hours, plus prednisone 40 mg twice daily

31. A 49-year-old woman presents with respiratory failure due to severe community-acquired pneumonia (CAP) requiring intubation and mechanical ventilation. An internal jugular vein central venous catheter (CVC) is placed in the ED for treatment of septic shock associated with methicilin-sensitive *Staphylococcus aureus* (MSSA) pneumonia. Patient is started on intravenous (IV) oxacillin with resolution of fever and hypotension 72 hours after admission. However, she develops new fever of 101.7°F (38.7°C) with worsening leukocytosis on ICU stay day 5. There is no change on her chest radiograph. Which action would be best to take next?

    A. Initiate broad-spectrum antibiotic therapy for a new sepsis episode
    B. Perform bronchoscopic BAL for suspected ventilator-associated pneumonia (VAP)
    C. Remove the CVC
    D. Send two sets of blood cultures, one from the catheter and one from a peripheral blood sample
    E. No intervention is needed; recovery from MSSA pneumonia can take weeks

32. A 35-year-old man with a history of intravenous (IV) drug use is admitted to the ICU for management of hypercarbic respiratory failure due to opioid overdose. During hospitalization he develops an uncomplicated central line-associated bloodstream infection (CLABSI). The patient has no hardware and no evidence of endocarditis with normal renal and hepatic function. What would be the treatment of choice for his infection?

    A. No antibiotics are needed, this is most likely contamination
    B. Treat with IV piperacillin/tazobactam for 5 to 7 days and keep the catheter
    C. Remove the catheter and treat with IV piperacillin/tazobactam for 7 to 14 days
    D. Remove the catheter and treat with IV piperacillin/tazobactam for 4 to 6 weeks
    E. Remove the catheter and treat with IV moxifloxacin for 5 to 7 days

▪ ANSWERS

1. **The answer is B.** Doxycycline would be an appropriate additional agent for coverage of sus- pected rickettsial and tick-borne infectious diseases. The patient's condition with systemic inflammatory response syndrome (SIRS), petechial rash, necrotic skin lesion, thrombocytope- nia, and transaminitis are all consistent with rickettsial disease.

Walker DH, Raoult D. *Rickettsia rickettsii* and other spotted fever group rickettsiae (Rocky Mountain spotted fever and other spotted fevers). In: Mandell GL, Bennett JE, Dolin R, eds. *Mandell, Douglas, and Bennett's Principles and Practice of Infectious Diseases*. 6th ed. Philadelphia, PA: Churchill Livingstone; 2005:2287-2295.

2. **The answer is D.** Rapid influenza diagnostic test from a throat swab would be the most appro- priate and time-efficient way to confirm the diagnosis in this case. This immunosuppressed patient appears to have been exposed to and developed the flu and therefore would require a diagnostic rapid influenza screen to confirm prior to treatment. A rapid influenza screen and immunofluorescence studies should be checked on nasal secretions and not urine, and viral cell cultures take at least 3 to 5 days for confirmation. There is no historical exposure to *Legionella*, and the diagnostic suspicion is low.

Gavin PJ, Thomson RB. Review of rapid diagnostic tests for influenza. *Clin Appl Immunol Rev.* 2004;4:151-172. doi:10.1016/S1529-1049(03)00064-3

3. **The answer is D.** Although both oseltamivir and amantadine have antiviral activity against influenza, amantadine is no longer recommended therapy due to the high incidence of emerg- ing resistance. Oseltamivir 75 mg twice daily is the correct choice. A macrolide antibiotic, an anti-herpes antiviral, or an antiretroviral agent would not be indicated.

Harper SA, Bradley JS, Englund JA, et al. Seasonal influenza in adults and children—diagnosis, treatment, chemoprophylaxis, and institutional outbreak management: clinical practice guidelines of the Infectious Diseases Society of America. *Clin Infect Dis.* 2009;48:1003-1032. doi:10.1086/598513

4. **The answer is D.** Quantiferon-TB Gold test is the most sensitive and specific screening test for latent TB. Tuberculin skin test is less sensitive and specific and may yield false positive results with a childhood Bacille–Calmette–Guerin (BCG) vaccination, and the other options listed are not appropriate screening tests for latent TB.

Mazurek GH, LoBue PA, Daley CL, et al. Comparison of a whole-blood interferon gamma assay with tuberculin skin testing for detecting latent Mycobacterium tuberculosis infection. *JAMA.* 2001;286:1740-1747. doi:10.1001/jama.286.14.1740

5. **The answer is B.** Based on the 2016 updated definitions, sepsis is defined as life-threatening organ dysfunction caused by a dysregulated host response to infection.

Singer M, Deutschman CS, Seymour CW, et al. The third international consensus definitions for sepsis and septic shock (sepsis-3). *JAMA.* 2016;315:801-810. doi:10.1001/jama.2016.0287

6. **The answer is A.** Based on the 2016 Society of Critical Care Medicine (SCCM) guidelines, IV antimicrobials must be initiated as soon as possible after recognition and within 1 hour for both sepsis and septic shock. IV antimicrobials and fluid resuscitation are often done at the same time. Patients should receive broad-spectrum antibiotics, but anaerobic and atypical coverage are not needed for all patients. Although option E is considered broad-spectrum antimicrobial coverage, patients with anaphylaxis reaction to penicillin should not receive carbapenems due to cross reactivity.

Prescott WA, DePestel DD, Ellis JJ, et al. Incidence of carbapenem-associated allergic-type reactions among patients with versus patients without a reported penicillin allergy. *Clin Infect Dis.* 2004;38:1102-1107. doi:10.1086/382880

Rhodes A, Evans LE, Alhazzani W, et al. Surviving sepsis campaign: international guidelines for management of sepsis and septic shock: 2016. *Intensive Care Medicine.* 2017;43:304-377. doi: 10.1007/s00134-017-4683-6

7. **The answer is C.** CAUTI is defined by the presence of symptoms or signs compatible with a UTI with no other identified source of infection, together with 10^3 CFU/mL or more of one bacterial species in a single catheter urine specimen or in a midstream-voided urine specimen from a patient whose urethral, suprapubic, or condom catheter has been removed within the previous 48 hours. This patient is not showing signs of systemic infection and still has a Foley in place. Foley catheter should be changed and a new urinalysis should be sent.

> Hooton RM, Bradley SF, Cardenas DD, et al. Diagnosis, prevention, and treatment of catheter-associated urinary tract infection in adults: 2009 international clinical practice guidelines from the Infectious Diseases Society of America. *Clin Infect Dis.* 2010;50:625-663. doi: 10.1086/650482

8. **The answer is E.** Although this patient has early-onset ventilator-associated pneumonia (VAP) for the current admission, a history of recent hospitalization is a risk factor for multidrug resistant (MDR) organisms. Empiric antibiotic therapy for VAP in patients with MDR organism risk factors should include agents active against *Pseudomonas aeruginosa* and methicillin-resistant *Staphylococcus aureus* (MRSA). Atypical bacteria coverage is not necessary because their prevalence is low, although consideration should be given if there is a poor response to initial therapy.

> Kalil AC, Metersky ML, Klompas M, et al. Management of adults with hospital-acquired and ventilator-associated pneumonia: 2016 clinical practice guidelines by the Infectious Diseases Society of America and the American Thoracic Society. *Clin Infect Dis.* 2016;63:e61-e111. doi: 10.1093/cid/ciw353

9. **The answer is C.** This is community-acquired pneumonia (CAP) and would best be treated by IV ceftriaxone and azithromycin or a respiratory quinolone. His triage to the ICU is justified by his age, recent brain hemorrhage, confusion, and uremia, which place him at high risk for further complications and decompensation. Various scores (such as the CURB-65) or prognostic scoring systems (Pneumonia Severity Index) can be used to appropriately triage patients with pneumonia.

> Mandell LA, Wunderink RG, Anzueto A, et al. Infectious Diseases Society of America/American Thoracic Society consensus guidelines on the management of community-acquired pneumonia in adults. *Clin Infect Dis.* 2007;44:S27-S72. doi:10.1086/511159

10. **The answer is D.** Based on the new (2017) Infectious Diseases Society of America (IDSA) CDI guidelines, treatment of choice for initial episode, nonsevere CDI (white blood cell [WBC] ≤15,000 cells/mL and serum creatinine [Cr] <1.5 mg/dL) include: vancomycin by mouth 125 mg given 4 times daily for 10 days, **or** fidaxomicin 200 mg given twice daily for 10 days. Alternately, if these agents are unavailable, metronidazole,500 mg three times per day by mouth for 10 days may be used.

> McDonald LC, Gerding DN, Johnson S, et al. Clinical practice guidelines for Clostridium difficile infection in adults and children: 2017 update by the Infectious Diseases Society of America (IDSA) and Society for Healthcare Epidemiology of America (SHEA). *Clin Infect Dis.* 2018;66:e1-e48. doi:10.1093/cid/cix1085

11. **The answer is C.** Drug of choice for MRSA pneumonia that has failed vancomycin therapy is linezolid. Daptomycin is not an option because although it covers MRSA it gets deactivated by the lungs surfactants. Piperacillin/tazobactam does not cover MRSA. Continuation of vancomycin with higher trough levels may lead to toxicity without additional benefit. Rifampin does have activity against MRSA but should not be used as monotherapy.

> Welte T, Pletz MW. Antimicrobial treatment of nosocomial meticillin-resistant Staphylococcus aureus (MRSA) pneumonia: current and future options. *Int J Antimicrob Agents.* 2010;36: 391-400. doi:10.1016/j.ijantimicag.2010.06.045

12. **The answer is D.** *K. pneumonia* is the most likely etiology of pneumonia at the extremes of age, and in immunocompromised and alcoholic patients. Currant red jelly sputum is also

consistent with this pathogen. The other pathogens listed would not be associated with this color of sputum and are less likely in this patient's demographic and clinical picture.

Bennett JE, Raphael D, Martin JB. *Mandell, Douglas, and Bennett's Principles and Practice of Infectious Diseases E-Book*. Philadelphia, PA: Elsevier Health Sciences; 2014.

13. **The answer is E.** None of the measures listed (scheduled catheter exchanges, catheter replacements, or prophylactic antibiotics) have been shown to reduce the incidence of CLABSI.

O'Grady NP, Alexander M, Burns LA, et al. Guidelines for the prevention of intravascular catheter-related infections. *Clin Infect Dis*. 2011:52(9):e162-e1193. doi:10.1093/cid/cir257

14. **The answer is D.** Maxillary sinusitis is highly associated with nasal intubation due to trauma, edema, and obstruction of drainage from the sinus ostia. The incidence of sinusitis can be from 2% to 25%.

Rouby JJ, Laurent P, Gosnach M, et al. Risk factors and clinical relevance of nosocomial maxillary sinusitis in the critically ill. *Am J Respir Crit Care Med*. 1994;150:776-783. doi:10.1164/ajrccm.150.3.8087352

15. **The answer is D.** Early transfer of an endotracheal tube to the oral route will significantly reduce the chances of sinusitis without the unnecessary exposure to antibiotics by any route (local, inhaled, or IV).

Holzapfel L. Nasal vs oral intubation. *Minerva Anestesiol*. 2003;69:348-352.

16. **The answer is E.** Start preventive therapy with daily isoniazid for 9 months. After exposure to *Mycobacterium tuberculosis*, PPD testing may be initially negative and should only be checked after 12 weeks. If exposure to the bacterium is likely, preventive therapy with single-agent therapy (isoniazid daily for 9 months) is indicated. If the PPD is negative at 12 weeks, the preventive therapy can be discontinued. If the bacilli from the index patient are shown to be multidrug-resistant, a more aggressive treatment plan can be pursued.

National Tuberculosis Controllers Association; Centers for Disease Control and Prevention (CDC). Guidelines for the investigation of contacts of persons with infectious tuberculosis. Recommendations from the National Tuberculosis Controllers Association and CDC. *MMWR Recomm Rep*. 2005;54:1-47.

17. **The answer is D.** The patient has a pulmonary infectious etiology with Gram-positive bacteria growing from the blood after exposure to a possible biohazard agent, which is consistent with inhalational anthrax. He does not manifest or report any signs of cutaneous or gastrointestinal disease. Both *Legionella pneumophila* and *Bartonella henselae* (cat scratch disease) are Gram-negative organisms that rarely grow out in blood cultures.

Shafazand S, Doyle R, Ruoss S, et al. Inhalational anthrax: epidemiology, diagnosis, and management. *Chest*. 1999;116:1369-1376. doi:10.1378/chest.116.5.1369

18. **The answer is A.** Ciprofloxacin and doxycycline are both appropriate antimicrobial agents for *Bacillus anthracis*, but in this patient with severe disease (respiratory failure) oral treatment would be inadequate. IV ciprofloxacin coupled with a second agent, IV clindamycin, would be the most appropriate treatment for this severe case of inhalational anthrax. The selection of the second antibiotic is arbitrary. Some favor the use of clindamycin on the basis of its property of inhibiting toxin production in static culture. Ampicillin would be inadequate as a single agent, and ceftriaxone would be an inappropriate choice for *B. anthracis*.

Bartlett JG, Inglesby TV Jr, Borio L. Management of anthrax. *Clin Infect Dis*. 2002;35:851-858. doi: 10.1086/341902

19. **The answer is B.** Large prospective studies have shown that oral antiseptics (like chlorhexidene swabs) reduce the chances of ventilator-associated pneumonia (VAP). Such a benefit has not been demonstrated with scheduled ventilator circuit changes. Both proton pump

inhibitors and nasotracheal intubation have been associated with increased chances for pneumonia and sinusitis.

American Thoracic Society; Infectious Diseases Society of America. Guidelines for the management of adults with hospital-acquired, ventilator-associated, and healthcare-associated pneumonia. *Am J Respir Crit Care Med.* 2005;171:388-416. doi:10.1164/rccm.200405-644ST

20. **The answer is B.** According to the 2016 Infectious Disease Society of America (IDSA) guidelines, broad spectrum antibiotics to cover *Pseudomonas aeruginosa* and methicillin-resistant *Staphylococcus aureus* (MRSA) should be initiated in late VAP. In patients with a history of penicillin allergy, aztreonam is a reasonable Gram-negative coverage.

Kalil AC, Metersky ML, Klompas M, et al. Management of adults with hospital-acquired and ventilator-associated pneumonia: 2016 clinical practice guidelines by the Infectious Diseases Society of America and the American Thoracic Society. *Clin Infect Dis.* 2016;63:e61-e111. doi: 10.1093/cid/ciw353

21. **The answer is B.** The most appropriate antibiotic for methicillin-sensitive staphylococcus aureus (MSSA) coverage is oxacillin. In cases where penicillin (PCN) allergy with anaphylaxis is a concern, desensitization should be done in incremental doses. All other options are inferior to oxacillin for MSSA coverage.

Jones RN. Key considerations in the treatment of complicated staphylococcal infections. *Clin Microbiol Infect.* 2008; 14(suppl 2):3-9. doi:10.1111/j.1469-0691.2008.01923.x

22. **The answer is C.** According to the 2016 Infectious Disease Society of America (IDSA) guidelines, a 7-day course of antimicrobial therapy rather than a longer duration is recommended. Longer duration of therapy should only be considered if clinical, radiologic, and laboratory failure is suspected.

Kalil AC, Metersky ML, Klompas M, et al. Management of adults with hospital-acquired and ventilator-associated pneumonia: 2016 clinical practice guidelines by the Infectious Diseases Society of America and the American Thoracic Society. *Clin Infect Dis.* 2016;63:e61-e111.m doi:10.1093/cid/ciw353

23. **The answer is B.** Current treatment guidelines for infective endocarditis with *S. aureus* suggest combination antimicrobial therapy with vancomycin and rifampin for a minimum of 6 weeks, with the use of gentamicin limited to the first 2 weeks of therapy.

Baddour LM, Wilson WR, Bayer AS, et al. Infective endocarditis in adults: diagnosis, antimicrobial therapy, and management of complications. *Circulation.* 2015;132:1435-1486.

24. **The answer is D.** For patients at high risk of invasive extended spectrum beta-lactamases (ESBL) infections such as this case with urosepsis, early carbapenem therapy should be considered. Bacteremia studies have shown inferiority of piperacillin/tazobactam to carbapenems in cases despite in vitro susceptibility to piperacillin/tazobactam.

Tamma PD, Han JH, Rock C, et al. Carbapenem therapy is associated with improved survival compared with piperacillin-tazobactam for patients with extended-spectrum β-lactamase bacteremia. *Clin Infect Dis.* 2015;60:1319-1325. doi:10.1093/cid/civ003

25. **The answer is E.** IV vancomycin is the most appropriate treatment at this time when the Gram-positive cocci have not been speciated and antibiotic susceptibilities are not known yet. IV linezolid would not be appropriate in a thrombocytopenic patient as it has a high incidence of inducing thrombocytopenia. IV penicillin and oxacillin would be inadequate treatments, and IV piperacillin/tazobactam would be unnecessary in the absence of any Gram-negative organisms.

Liu C, Bayer A, Cosgrove SE, et al. Clinical practice guidelines by the Infectious Diseases Society of America for the treatment of methicillin-resistant Staphylococcus aureus infections in adults and children. *Clin Infect Dis.* 2011;52:e18-e55. doi:10.1093/cid/ciq146

26. The answer is A. IV carbapenems should be avoided in this case due to significant drug–drug interaction and reduction in VPA level (higher risk of seizure). In addition, cross-hypersensitivity has been observed between penicillins and carbapenems. IV piperacillin would not be suitable in a patient with severe allergy to penicillins, and both vancomycin and cefotaxime would be ineffective against suspected pseudomonal infection.

McConnell SA, Penzak SR, Warmack TS, et al. Incidence of imipenem hypersensitivity reactions in febrile neutropenic bone marrow transplant patients with a history of penicillin allergy. *Clin Infect Dis.* 2000;31:1512-1514. doi:10.1086/317507

Park MK, Lim KS, Kim TE, et al. Reduced valproic acid serum concentrations due to drug interactions with carbapenem antibiotics: overview of 6 cases. *Ther Drug Monit.* 2012;34:599-603. doi:10.1097/FTD.0b013e318260f7b3

27. The answer is D. This patient likely has severe influenza due to a local seasonal outbreak. Empiric influenza-specific therapy against influenza A and influenza B strains should be initiated in patients with severe influenza before confirmatory test results are known to avoid a delay in therapy (Answer B is incorrect). Neuraminidase-based therapy is recommended for modern influenza A and B strains (Answer C is incorrect). Even if they are outside 48 hours from symptom onset, patients with severe influenza have benefited from therapy initiated beyond this period (Answer A is incorrect). Influenza vaccine should not be given during active infection (answer E is incorrect).

Harper SA, Bradley JS, Englund JA, et al. Seasonal influenza in adults and children—diagnosis, treatment, chemoprophylaxis, and institutional outbreak management: clinical practice guidelines of the Infectious Diseases Society of America. *Clin Infect Dis.* 2009;48:1003-1032. doi:10.1086/598513

28. The answer is D. The patient suffers from complicated intra-abdominal infection from secondary peritonitis caused by colonic perforation. Although it is community-acquired, the presence of septic shock and hemodynamic instability suggests severe classification increasing the risk of Gram-negative multidrug resistant organism but not methicillin-resistant Staphylococcus aureus (MRSA) (Answers B,C, and E are incorrect). The involvement of the colon also obligates antibiotic therapy active against anaerobes and enterococci (Answer A is incorrect); according to this, piperacillin/tazobactam is the most appropriate agent listed (Answer D is correct).

Marshall JC, Innes M. ICU management of intra-abdominal infection. *Crit Care Med.* 2003;31: 2228-2237. doi:10.1097/01.CCM.0000087326.59341.51

29. The answer is D. *E. cloacae* is an AmpC β-lactamase–producing Enterobacteriaceae. The use of ceftriaxone or extended spectrum penicillins (e.g., piperacillin and ticarcillin) may select out derepressed mutants, which are capable of causing the hyperproduction of AmpC β-lactamases. Derepressed mutants are capable of producing resistance against third-generation cephalosporins, monobactams, and extended-spectrum penicillins (Answers A, B, C, and E are incorrect). This resistance mechanism is adequately treated by a carbapenem. Hence, changing to a carbapenem pending final sensitivities is the most reasonable option in a septic patient (Answer D is correct).

Paterson DL. Resistance in gram-negative bacteria: enterobacteriaceae. *Am J Med.* 2006;119:S20-S28. doi:10.1016/j.amjmed.2006.03.013

30. The answer is B. The patient's history and clinical presentation suggest *Pneumocystis jiroveci* pneumonia. The infection is severe enough to warrant intubation, and the patient has a significant alveolar-arterial (AA) oxygen gradient. The drug of choice for such patients is trimethoprim/sulfamethoxazole; however, this patient has a sulfa allergy (Answers A and E are incorrect). The second-line agent for treatment of severe *P. jiroveci* pneumonia is IV pentamidine (Answer B is correct). Atovaquone and primaquine/clindamycin regimens are usually reserved for patients with milder *P. jiroveci* pneumonia. Furthermore, primaquine should not be administered to someone with a history of G6PD.

Kaplan JE, Benson C, Holmes KK, et al. Guidelines for prevention and treatment opportunistic infections in HIV-infected adults and adolescents; recommendations from CDC, the National Institutes of Health, and the HIV Medicine Association/Infectious Diseases Society of America. *MMWR Recomm Rep.* 2009;58:1-207. doi:10.1093/cid/ciu094

31. **The answer is D.** In the absence of other suspected sources (i.e., no change in chest radiograph), central line-associated bloodstream infection (CLABSI) should be suspected as the cause of new-onset fever and leukocytosis, given the emergency placement and related duration of the CVC (Answer B and E are incorrect). Although catheter removal should strongly be considered, cultures should be obtained before catheter removal for documentation if the patient has a bloodstream infection (Answer C is incorrect). Initiation of broad-spectrum antibiotic may be considered if appropriate, but only after cultures of the suspected source are obtained (Answer D is correct; Answer A is incorrect).

Mermel LA, Allon M, Bouza E, et al. Clinical practice guidelines for the diagnosis and management of intravascular catheter-related infection: 2009 update by the Infectious Diseases Society of America. *Clin Infect Dis.* 2009;49:1-45. doi:10.1086/599376

32. **The answer is C.** Based on the Infectious Diseases Society of America guidelines on Catheter-Related Bloodstream Infection, patients with uncomplicated central venous cather (CVC)-related bloodstream infection (resolution of fever within 72 hours with no hemodynamic instability) with Gram-negative rods and in the absence of hardware and endocarditis should receive 7 to 14 days of appropriate systemic antibiotics after removal of the catheter (answers A, B, and D are incorrect). Answer E is incorrect because moxifloxacin is not appropriate for empiric coverage of Gram-negative rods, as it does not cover *pseudomonas aeruginosa*.

Mermel LA, Allon M, Bouza E, et al. Clinical practice guidelines for the diagnosis and management of intravascular catheter-related infection: 2009 update by the Infectious Diseases Society of America. *Clin Infect Dis.* 2009;49:1-45. doi:10.1086/599376

21

Acute Hematological Disorders

SOO J. PARK AND AARON M. GOODMAN

QUESTIONS

1. A previously healthy 30-year-old woman presents to the ED with new onset of fever, weakness, abdominal pain, and diarrhea. Vital signs on presentation are notable for severe hypertension with a blood pressure (BP) of 180/110 mmHg. Her initial laboratory results are normal except for a mild leukocytosis of $13,000/mm^3$ with predominant neutrophils. Stool cultures and toxin testing are negative. Three days later she develops confusion, new thrombocytopenia with platelet counts down to $32,000/mm^3$, and acute renal failure (ARF) requiring hemodialysis. Peripheral blood smear shows many helmet cells and schistocytes. Which of the following is the most appropriate next step in the management of this patient?

   A. Eculizumab
   B. Rituximab
   C. Steroids
   D. Plasma exchange
   E. Plasma infusion

2. A 31-year-old woman with a new diagnosis of acute lymphoblastic leukemia (ALL) is directly admitted to the hospital to begin chemotherapy for curative intent. She receives pegylated L-asparaginase as part of the standard ALL treatment regimen and after the second dose suffers an episode of focal seizure with left-sided weakness. A MRI scan of the brain showed a superior sagittal sinus thrombosis with a right superior frontal hemorrhagic venous infarct. In addition to therapeutic anticoagulation, what other treatment should be initiated, if any?

   A. Cryoprecipitate
   B. Prothrombin complex concentrate (PCC)
   C. Anticoagulation only
   D. Fresh frozen plasma (FFP)
   E. Antithrombin concentrates

3. A previously healthy 35-year-old woman is admitted to the hospital with a rash over her legs and ankles bilaterally. She first noticed the rash around 3 weeks ago, when it started in her feet and gradually spread up to her knees. She has no other medical history and denies taking any prescription medication. There is no history of trauma or bleeding disorders in her family. Physical examination reveals fine petechiae and purpura around her ankles and lower legs. The rest of the physical examination is unremarkable. Her vital signs are normal. Laboratory studies showed the following values:

Hemoglobin	14.4 g/dL
Mean corpuscular volume	90 fL
Platelet count	16,000/mm^3
Leukocyte count	8,000/mm^3
Segmented neutrophils	60%
Bands	3%
Eosinophils	6%
Lymphocytes	24%
Monocytes	6%
Prothrombin time (PT)	14 seconds
Partial thromboplastin time (PTT)	30 seconds
Plasma fibrinogen	300 mg/dL (200–450 mg/dL)
D-dimer	220 ng/mL (<241 ng/mL)
Sodium (Na)	142 mmol/L
Potassium (K)	3.8 mmol/L
Cardiac index (Cl)	109 mmol/L
Blood urea nitrogen (BUN)	12 mg/dL
Creatinine (Cr)	1.0 mg/dL

Peripheral blood smear is normal. The admitting resident is concerned about the lab results and orders 6 units of random donor platelets for transfusion. The following day, the platelet count drops even further to 10,000/mm^3 and the resident consults the ICU team. Which of the following is the most likely cause of the drop in the platelet count?

A. Disseminated intravascular coagulation (DIC)
B. Thrombotic thrombocytopenic purpura (TTP)
C. Immune thrombocytopenic purpura (ITP)
D. Septicemia
E. Drug-induced thrombocytopenia

4. A patient with acute myeloid leukemia (AML) on chemotherapy has epistaxis that does not stop with pressure. You order a stat complete blood count (CBC), which shows a hemoglobin of 8 g/dL and platelet count of 10,000/mm^3. You decide to transfuse the patient with 6 units of pooled platelets and to repeat the platelet count 1 hour after the transfusion, at which time it was found to be 11,000/mm^3. Which one of the following is the most likely explanation for these findings?

A. This is a normal response
B. You have measured platelet counts too early
C. The patient has antibodies against platelets
D. You have not given enough platelets
E. The patient has disseminated intravascular coagulation (DIC)

5. A 23-year-old male is referred to hematology for new pancytopenia. He is diagnosed with acute promyelocytic leukemia (APL) based on presence of the *PML/RARA* gene fusion on fluorescence in situ hybridization. He is admitted to the hospital to start induction therapy. After 5 days of treatment, he develops a severe headache and a stat CT scan of the head shows a large intracranial hemorrhage. Which one of the following is the most likely cause of the patient's sudden neurologic deterioration?

A. Treatment-induced thrombocytopenia
B. Treatment-induced hyperleukocytosis
C. Disseminated intravascular coagulation (DIC)
D. Differentiation syndrome
E. Pseudotumor cerebri

Questions 6–8 are related to the following vignette:
A 62-year-old woman with a history of hypertension and noncompliance to medications presents with left-sided weakness and headache. She is diagnosed with a right basal ganglia and internal capsule hemorrhage without any evidence of intraventricular hemorrhage (IVH). On hospital day 3, she develops sudden onset of shortness of breath and chest pain, and pulse oximetry shows oxygen saturation of 93% on 4 L of oxygen. A CT angiogram of the chest reveals pulmonary embolism. Her baseline labs are:

Hemoglobin	13.4 g/dL
Hematocrit	39%
Platelet count	310,000/mm^3
Leukocyte count	7,900/mm^3
Prothrombin time (PT)	14 seconds
International Normalized Ratio (INR)	1.06

You start the patient on anticoagulation with unfractionated heparin infusion and warfarin. Her symptoms gradually resolve over the next 5 days. On hospital day 6, she complains of pain and pallor in her left arm. Physical examination reveals a pale and tender distal left arm with diminished pulses. The patient's labs at this time reveal:

Hemoglobin	13.0 g/dL
Hematocrit	38%
Platelet count	48,000/mm^3
Leukocyte count	8,400/mm^3
PT	19 seconds
Partial thromboplastin time (PTT)	60 seconds
INR	1.78

6. Which one of the following is the most likely cause of the patient's condition?

A. Subtherapeutic anticoagulation
B. Heparin-induced thrombocytopenia (HIT)
C. Warfarin-induced skin necrosis
D. Heparin-induced skin necrosis
E. Warfarin-induced thrombocytopenia

7. Which of the following is the most appropriate next step in the management of this patient?

    A. Discontinue warfarin
    B. Discontinue unfractionated heparin
    C. Discontinue warfarin and unfractionated heparin
    D. Discontinue warfarin and unfractionated heparin; initiate low molecular weight heparin (LMWH)
    E. Discontinue warfarin and unfractionated heparin; initiate argatroban

8. Which of the following would have been the most useful strategy in preventing the patient's condition?

    A. Monitor the prothrombin time (PT) frequently
    B. Monitor platelet counts frequently
    C. Substitute low molecular weight heparin (LMWH) for unfractionated heparin
    D. Initiate warfarin after 3 to 5 days of heparin.
    E. Use lower doses of heparin early in the course of treatment

9. A 78-year-old female with a history of atrial fibrillation on warfarin presents to the ED with altered mental status (AMS) and lethargy. Her initial vital signs and blood glucose levels are within normal limits. An electrocardiogram shows atrial fibrillation at 90 beats/minute. A CT scan of the head shows a 5 × 3.8 cm left-sided intracerebral hemorrhage (ICH) without intraventricular extension. Her initial laboratory results shows an International Normalized Ratio (INR) of 4.2 and a platelet count of 320,000/mm^3. Which of the following is the best next step in the management of this patient?

    A. Hold warfarin
    B. Hold warfarin and control the blood pressure (BP)
    C. Hold warfarin and give vitamin K 10 mg intravenously (IV)
    D. Hold warfarin and transfuse platelets
    E. Hold warfarin, give vitamin K 10 mg IV, and give 4-factor prothrombin complex concentrate (4-PCC)

10. A 62-year-old man with a history of hypertension and noncompliance to medication presents to the ED with double vision and imbalance for 2 days. In the ED, his blood pressure (BP) is 220/128 mmHg. A CT scan of the head shows a large cerebellar hemorrhage with effacement of the fourth ventricle. Neurosurgery is consulted and the patient undergoes a suboccipital decompression. His hospital course is complicated by fevers and an elevated white blood cell (WCC) count. Urine culture returns positive and he is started on antibiotics empirically. On hospital day 5, the patient becomes febrile again, with new tachycardia and hypotension. His laboratory results are as follows:

Hemoglobin	11.2 g/dL
Hematocrit	34%
Platelet count	43,000/mm^3
Leukocyte count	15,000/mm^3 (neutrophil predominant)
Partial thromboplastin time (PTT)	72 seconds
Prothrombin time (PT)	26 seconds

The patient is on subcutaneous heparin for prevention of deep vein thrombosis (DVT), which is discontinued and a heparin-induced thrombocytopenia (HIT) immunoassay is sent. Peripheral blood smear shows few schistocytes. Additional labs include:

D-dimer	600 ng/mL (<241 ng/mL)
Fibrinogen	65 mg/dL (200–450 mg/dL)

What is the diagnosis?

A. Disseminated intravascular coagulation (DIC)
B. Thrombotic thrombocytopenic purpura (TTP)
C. Antiplatelet antibodies
D. Septicemia
E. Drug-induced thrombocytopenia

11. A 62-year-old female with a history of *JAK2* positive essential thrombocythemia presents to the ED with an acute onset severe headache. She suffered from a branch retinal artery occlusion in her right eye last year but fully recovered her vision. She admits to noncompliance with hydroxyurea and aspirin. A CT scan of the head shows a large intracranial hemorrhage. Her laboratory results were as follows:

Hemoglobin	8.9 g/dL
Hematocrit	27%
Platelet count	2,000,000/mm^3
Leukocyte count	9,000/mm^3
Partial thromboplastin time (PTT)	43 seconds
Prothrombin time (PT)	14 seconds

Which one of the following is the most likely etiology of her bleeding?

A. Hyperviscosity syndrome
B. Acquired von Willebrand syndrome (AVWS)
C. Acquired factor VIII inhibitor
D. Acquired factor V deficiency
E. Disseminated intravascular coagulation (DIC)

12. A 52-year-old man with a history of congestive heart failure (CHF), diabetes, renal insufficiency, and hypertension develops an intracranial hemorrhage after receiving thrombolytic therapy for an acute ischemic stroke. What is the most appropriate treatment?

A. Protamine sulfate
B. Fresh frozen plasma (FFP)
C. Cryoprecipitate
D. Vitamin K
E. Dialysis

13. You were called to evaluate a patient on a heparin infusion, being bridged to warfarin, who is complaining of a severe headache. The patient was receiving 1,200 units of heparin per hour, and the most current partial thromboplastin time (PTT) and International Normalized Ratio (INR) were 68.7 seconds and 2.04, respectively. Heparin infusion was discontinued and a stat CT scan of the head was obtained that showed a 2 × 3 cm intracerebral hemorrhage (ICH) in the left basal ganglia without any evidence of intraventricular hemorrhage (IVH). Repeat PTT was 110 seconds. Which of the following is the best next step in management?

A. Control the blood pressure (BP), monitor closely, obtain a stat complete blood count (CBC), and if required, order a blood transfusion
B. Give platelets and fresh frozen plasma (FFP) immediately and control the BP
C. Give protamine sulfate 30 mg intravenously (IV) to reverse the heparin
D. Give protamine sulfate 10 mg IV to reverse the heparin
E. Close observation

14. An 82-year-old right-handed woman with a history of nonvalvular atrial fibrillation and previous stroke about 2 years ago without any residual effects is found to be lethargic and less responsive at home by family members. She is brought to the ED and upon arrival her blood pressure (BP) is 188/94 mmHg and pulse rate is 122 beats per minute (BPM); she is minimally responsive, plegic on the right, and flexing on the left. The patient was recently started on dabigatran for atrial fibrillation and took her last dose approximately 4 hours ago. There is no history of fall or head trauma. A stat CT scan of the head shows an intracerebral hemorrhage (ICH) in the left caudate area along with intraventricular hemorrhage (IVH) in the third and lateral ventricles with mild hydrocephalus. Laboratory studies in the ED are as follows:

Hemoglobin	9.4 g/dL
Hematocrit	29%
Platelet count	224,000/mm^3
Prothrombin time (PT)	36 seconds
Partial thromboplastin time (PTT)	94 seconds
International Normalized Ratio (INR)	1.9

What is the best next step in management?

A. Activated charcoal, BP control, and repeat labs as these abnormal values can be due to lab errors
B. BP control, fresh frozen plasma (FFP), and platelet transfusion
C. Airway protection, BP control, and idarucizumab
D. Airway protection, BP control, protamine sulfate, FFP, and platelet transfusion
E. Airway protection, BP control, emergent dialysis, and prothrombin complex concentrate (PCC)

Questions 15 to 16 are related to the following vignette:
A 33-year-old woman with a history of chronic abdominal pain attributed to irritable bowel syndrome presents to the ED with a severe headache and confusion. She vomited twice in the morning. Laboratory studies in the ED are as follows:

Hemoglobin	8.8 g/dL
Hematocrit	26%
Direct antiglobulin test	Negative
Lactate dehydrogenase	500 U/L (25–175 U/L)
Haptoglobin	Undetectable (30–200 mg/dL)
Total bilirubin	3.1 mg/dL
Direct bilirubin	0.3 mg/dL

Peripheral blood smear was notable for polychromatophilia. A CT scan of the abdomen showed a chronic-appearing hepatic vein thrombosis and large hepatic vein collaterals. A MRI scan of the brain showed a superior sagittal sinus thrombosis. The patient was started on a heparin infusion.

15. What is the diagnosis?

   A. Thrombotic thrombocytopenic purpura (TTP)
   B. Pyruvate kinase deficiency
   C. Glucose-6-phosphate dehydrogenase deficiency (G6PD)
   D. Paroxysmal nocturnal hemoglobinuria (PNH)
   E. Autoimmune hemolytic anemia

16. In addition to therapeutic anticoagulation, what other treatment should be initiated?

   A. Steroids
   B. Rituximab
   C. Plasma exchange
   D. Aspirin
   E. Eculizumab

17. You are evaluating a patient in clinic who was referred to you 1 month ago for vertigo. The vertigo has gotten worse and his vision is now blurry. Fundoscopic exam reveals the presence of dilated and segmented retinal veins that look similar to sausage links. You review his chart and discover the patient was seen by hematology 6 months ago for a new diagnosis of Waldenström macroglobulinemia (WM), but he never followed up. You order a stat complete blood count (CBC) which showed a hemoglobin of 8.2 g/dL and platelet count of 90,000/mm^3. Which of the following is the best next step in the management of this patient?

   A. Cryoprecipitate
   B. Red cell transfusion
   C. Platelet transfusion
   D. Plasma exchange
   E. Rituximab

■ ANSWERS

1. The answer is D. The patient has thrombocytopenia, renal failure, and schistocytes on the peripheral blood smear. Based on this, a presumptive diagnosis of thrombotic microangiopathy can be made. Thrombotic thrombocytopenic purpura (TTP) is a medical emergency that is almost always fatal if appropriate treatment is not initiated promptly. In the absence of a known diagnosis of complement-mediated hemolytic uremic syndrome (HUS), plasma exchange therapy should be initiated urgently in all patients presenting with a suspected diagnosis of TTP or complement-mediated HUS.

Nester CM, Thomas CP. Atypical hemolytic uremic syndrome: what is it, how is it diagnosed, and how is it treated? *Hematology Am Soc Hematol Educ Program.* 2012;2012:617-625. doi:10.1182/asheducation-2012.1.617

Rock GA, Shumak KH, Buskard NA, et al. Comparison of plasma exchange with plasma infusion in the treatment of thrombotic thrombocytopenic purpura. Canadian Apheresis Study Group. *N Engl J Med.* 1991;325(6):393-397. doi:10.1056/NEJM199108083250604

Scully M. Thrombocytopenia in hospitalized patients: approach to the patient with thrombotic microangiopathy. *Hematology Am Soc Hematol Educ Program.* 2017;2017(1):651-659. doi:10.1182/asheducation-2017.1.651

Zuber J, Fakhouri F, Roumenina LT, et al. Use of eculizumab for atypical haemolytic uraemic syndrome and C3 glomerulopathies. *Nat Rev Nephrol.* 2012;8(11):643-657. doi:10.1038/nrneph.2012.214

2. The answer is E. The patient developed an intracranial thrombosis after receiving L-asparaginase therapy, which is used as a component of chemotherapy for ALL. Asparaginase induces a hypercoagulable state that can result in venous thrombosis. The most frequent site of thrombosis is intracranial. The mechanism is multifactorial and involves depletion of asparagine, which causes decreased synthesis of plasma proteins including fibrinogen, plasminogen, and antithrombin. Deficiencies of these natural anticoagulants results in impaired inhibition of thrombin. Replacement therapy with antithrombin concentrates may have beneficial effects. Therapeutic anticoagulation is appropriate for patients with venous thrombosis in the setting of asaparaginase.

Caruso V, Iacoviello L, Di Castelnuovo A, et al. Thrombotic complications in childhood acute lymphoblastic leukemia: a meta-analysis of 17 prospective studies comprising 1752 pediatric patients. *Blood.* 2006;108(7):2216-2222. doi:10.1182/blood-2006-04-015511

Goyal G, Bhatt VR. L-asparaginase and venous thromboembolism in acute lymphocytic leukemia. *Future Oncol.* 2015;11(17):2459-2470. doi:10.2217/fon.15.114

Hunault-Berger M, Chevallier P, Delain M, et al. Changes in antithrombin and fibrinogen levels during induction chemotherapy with L-asparaginase in adult patients with acute lymphoblastic leukemia or lymphoblastic lymphoma. Use of supportive coagulation therapy and clinical outcome: the CAPELAL study. *Haematologica.* 2008;93(10):1488-1494. doi:10.3324/haematol.12948

Meister B, Kropshofer G, Klein-Franke A, et al. Comparison of low-molecular-weight heparin and antithrombin versus antithrombin alone for the prevention of symptomatic venous thromboembolism in children with acute lymphoblastic leukemia. *Pediatr Blood Cancer.* 2008;50(2):298-303. doi:10.1002/pbc.21222

Mitchell L, Andrew M, Hanna K, et al. Trend to efficacy and safety using antithrombin concentrate in prevention of thrombosis in children receiving l-asparaginase for acute lymphoblastic leukemia. Results of the PAARKA study. *Thromb Haemost.* 2003;90(2):235-244. doi:10.1160/TH02-11-0283

Nowak-Gottl U, Kenet G, Mitchell LG. Thrombosis in childhood acute lymphoblastic leukaemia: epidemiology, aetiology, diagnosis, prevention and treatment. *Best Pract Res Clin Haematol.* 2009;22(1):103-114. doi:10.1016/j.beha.2009.01.003

Payne JH, Vora AJ. Thrombosis and acute lymphoblastic leukaemia. *Br J Haematol.* 2007;138(4):430-445. doi:10.1111/j.1365-2141.2007.06677.x

3. The answer is C. The patient has isolated thrombocytopenic purpura with no cause identified based on history, physical examination, complete blood count, and peripheral blood smear. Based on this, a presumptive diagnosis of ITP can be made. ITP occurs as a result of platelet destruction by specific autoantibodies. The goal of treatment is to reduce the risk of clinically significant bleeding. Many patients do not require interventions to raise the platelet count. The need for intervention is guided by bleeding symptoms and the severity of thrombocytopenia when severe spontaneous bleeding becomes a concern. Emergent management of symptomatic and life-threatening thrombocytopenia (i.e., massive intracranial hemorrhage, gastrointestinal [GI] hemorrhage, or emergency surgery) includes a combination of high-dose intravenous (IV) corticosteroids, IV immune globulin, romiplostim, and platelet transfusions.

Arnold DM. Bleeding complications in immune thrombocytopenia. *Hematology Am Soc Hematol Educ Program.* 2015;2015:237-242. doi:10.1182/asheducation-2015.1.237

George JN, Woolf SH, Rosko GE, et al. Idiopathic thrombocytopenic purpura: a practice guideline developed by explicit methods for the American Society of Hematology. *Blood.* 1996; 88(1):3-40.

Rodeghiero F, Stasi R, Gernsheimer T, et al. Standardization of terminology, definitions and outcome criteria in immune thrombocytopenic purpura of adults and children: report from an international working group. *Blood.* 2009;113(11):2386-2393. doi:10.1182/blood-2008-07-162503

Toltl LJ, Arnold DM. Pathophysiology and management of chronic immune thrombocytopenia: focusing on what matters. *Br J Haematol.* 2011;152(1):52-60. doi:10.1111/j.1365-2141.2010.08412.x

4. The answer is C. The patient has thrombocytopenia with a platelet count of 10,000/mm^3. Platelets play a critical role in the normal hemostatic mechanism; hence, their deficiency can cause life-threatening hemorrhage. Platelet transfusions are commonly used to prevent or treat acute hemorrhage in patients with thrombocytopenia due to any cause. Post-transfusion platelet counts should be measured 10 to 60 minutes after the completion of transfusion. For an adult with a body surface area of 2.0 m^2, 1 unit of platelet transfusion should immediately raise the platelet count by 5,000/μL. Since this patient received 6 units of platelets, his expected count should be at least 30,000 more than his baseline. If a smaller than expected rise in platelet count is noticed, consider refractoriness to platelet transfusions. Refractoriness to platelet transfusion is defined as an absolute platelet count increment of less than or equal to 5,000/μL per unit of platelet transfusion given to an average-sized adult. Alloimmunization is one of the common and treatable causes, which results from the production of antibodies to human leukocyte antigens (HLA) class-I on the transfused platelets. A platelet count with a normal increment at 1 hour after transfusion, but with a rapid return to baseline within 24 hours, indicates reduced platelet survival in the circulation. This is commonly seen in DIC, sepsis, or active bleeding.

Alcorta I, Pereira A, Ordinas A. Clinical and laboratory factors associated with platelet transfusion refractoriness: a case-control study. *Br J Haematol.* 1996;93(1):220-224. doi:10.1046/j.1365-2141.1996.447982.x

Bishop JF, McGrath K, Wolf MM, et al. Clinical factors influencing the efficacy of pooled platelet transfusions. *Blood.* 1988;71(2):383-387.

Friedberg RC, Donnelly SF, Boyd JC, et al. Clinical and blood bank factors in the management of platelet refractoriness and alloimmunization. *Blood.* 1993;81(12):3428-3434.

Norol F, Kuentz M, Cordonnier C, et al. Influence of clinical status on the efficiency of stored platelet transfusion. *Br J Haematol.* 1994;86(1):125-129. doi:10.1111/j.1365-2141.1994.tb03262.x

Schiffer CA, Anderson KC, Bennett CL, et al. Platelet transfusion for patients with cancer: clinical practice guidelines of the American Society of Clinical Oncology. *J Clin Oncol.* 2001;19(5):1519-1538. doi:10.1200/JCO.2001.19.5.1519

Slichter SJ, Davis K, Enright H, et al. Factors affecting posttransfusion platelet increments, platelet refractoriness, and platelet transfusion intervals in thrombocytopenic patients. *Blood.* 2005;105(10):4106-4114. doi:10.1182/blood-2003-08-2724

Stanworth SJ, Navarrete C, Estcourt L, et al. Platelet refractoriness—practical approaches and ongoing dilemmas in patient management. *Br J Haematol.* 2015;171(3):297-305. doi:10.1111/bjh.13597

5. The answer is C. APL is unique among the acute leukemias for its bleeding diathesis that is secondary to DIC. Coagulopathy associated with APL is either present at diagnosis or occurs soon after the initiation of chemotherapy and constitutes a medical emergency. Untreated APL can cause catastrophic cerebrovascular or pulmonary hemorrhages in up to 65% of patients, resulting in a high rate of early mortality. Since APL is the most frequently curable form of leukemia, with cure rates up to 80%, patients with suspected APL should be started on treatment with all-trans retinoic acid without delay as terminal differentiation of malignant promyelocytes can lead to rapid improvement in the coagulopathy.

de la Serna K, Montesinos P, Vellenga E. Causes and prognostic factors of remission induction failure in patients with acute promyelocytic leukemia treated with all-trans retinoic acid and idarubicin. *Blood*. 2008;111(7):3395-3402. doi:10.1182/blood-2007-07-100669

Mantha S, Tallman MS, Soff GA. What's new in the pathogenesis of the coagulopathy in acute promyelocytic leukemia? *Curr Opin Hematol*. 2016;23(2):121-126. doi:10.1097/MOH.0000000000000221

Sanz MA, Grimwade D, Tallman MS, et al. Management of acute promyeloctic leukemia: recommendations from an expert panel on behalf of the European LeukemiaNet. *Blood*. 2009;113(9):1875-1891. doi:10.1182/blood-2008-04-150250

6. **The answer is B.** After receiving unfractionated heparin, the patient developed arterial thrombosis of the left arm in conjunction with HIT, a well-known complication of heparin therapy. Two forms of HIT have been recognized, depending on the onset, clinical course, and severity:

   a. Type 1 HIT is seen within 1 to 4 days of initiation of heparin therapy, and it is associated with a lesser degree of decline in platelet numbers. The platelet count normalizes in a few days despite heparin continuation, and there are no clinical consequences. Type 1 HIT occurs in 10% to 20% of patients receiving unfractionated heparin.

   b. Type 2 HIT is more serious and is associated with an immune-mediated disorder characterized by the formation of antibodies against heparin-platelet factor 4 complexes. These antibodies bind to the platelet surface, causing platelet activation and aggregation, leading to thrombocytopenia and platelet-rich clots. It typically develops 5 to 10 days after the initiation of heparin therapy. However, in patients with prior exposure to heparin, it may occur earlier. HIT may also occur after heparin is discontinued. Platelet counts can drop in the range of 30,000 to 60,000/mm^3. Spontaneous bleeding is unusual. Immune-mediated HIT is associated with venous and arterial thrombosis. The major manifestations of venous thrombosis are deep venous thrombosis, pulmonary embolism, venous limb gangrene, and cerebral venous sinus thrombosis. Arterial thrombosis can lead to strokes, myocardial infarction (MI), and limb and organ ischemia.

   Warfarin-induced skin necrosis:

   a. Occurs within the first few days of taking high doses of warfarin

   b. *Cause:* High doses of warfarin cause rapid reduction in protein C levels, a natural anticoagulant, resulting in a transient hypercoaguable state

   c. *Lesion location:* Extremities, trunk, and breasts

   d. Not associated with thrombocytopenia

   Heparin-induced skin necrosis:

   a. Complication of unfractionated heparin use

   b. *Lesion location:* Areas rich in fat such as abdomen and distal extremities

   c. *Lesion:* Area of erythema, which quickly progresses to purpura, hemorrhage, and necrosis

   d. Most of these patients do not develop thrombocytopenia

Arepally GM. Heparin-induced thrombocytopenia. *Blood*. 2017;129(21):2864-2872. doi:10.1182/blood-2016-11-709873

Brieger DB, Mak KH, Kottke-Marchant K, et al. Heparin-induced thrombocytopenia. *J Am Coll Cardiol*. 1998;31(7):1449-1459. doi:10.1016/S0735-1097(98)00134-X

Chan YC, Valenti D, Mansfield AO, et al. Warfarin induced skin necrosis. *Br J Surg*. 2000;87(3):266-272. doi:10.1046/j.1365-2168.2000.01352.x

Schindewolf M, Kroll H, Ackermann H, et al. Heparin-induced non-necrotizing skin lesions: rarely associated with heparin-induced thrombocytopenia. *J Thromb Haemost*. 2010;8(7):1486-1491. doi:10.1111/j.1538-7836.2010.03795.x

Schindewolf M, Schwaner S, Wolter M, et al. Incidence and causes of heparin-induced skin lesions. *CMAJ*. 2009;181(8):477-481. doi:10.1503/cmaj.081729

Warkentin TE, Levine MN, Hirsh J, et al. Heparin-induced thrombocytopenia in patients treated with low-molecular-weight heparin or unfractionated heparin. *N Engl J Med*. 1995;332(20):1330-1335. doi:10.1056/NEJM199505183322003

7. **The answer is E.** The first and most important intervention in a patient with suspected or documented heparin-induced thrombocytopenia (HIT) is the immediate cessation of exposure to all heparin products. The patient with HIT still remains at risk for thrombosis, even after the discontinuation of heparin. All such patients need to be anticoagulated with direct thrombin inhibitors (DTIs) like argatroban or bivalirudin. These should be used for prophylaxis and treatment of patients with HIT with or without thrombosis. The choice of agent depends on the co-existing medical conditions. Argatroban is primarily hepatically metabolized and requires dose adjustments in patients with hepatic dysfunction. Bivalirudin has been used in reduced doses in patients with renal failure and combined hepatic and renal failure.

Kiser TH, Fish DN. Evaluation of bivalirudin treatment for heparin-induced thrombocytopenia in critically ill patients with hepartic and/or renal dysfunction. *Pharmacotherapy*. 2006;26(4):452-460. doi:10.1592/phco.26.4.452

Levine RL, Hursting MJ, McCollum D. Argatroban therapy in heparin-induced thrombocytopenia with hepatic dysfunction. *Chest*. 2006;129(5):1167-1175. doi:10.1378/chest.129.5.1167

Linkins LA, Dans AL, Moores LK, et al. Treatment and prevention of heparin-induced thrombocytopenia: antithrombotic therapy and prevention of thrombosis, 9th ed: American College of Chest Physicians Evidence-Based Clinical Practice Guidelines. *Chest*. 2012;141(2 Suppl):e495S-e530S. doi:10.1378/chest.11-2303

Wallis DE, Workman DL, Lewis BE, et al. Failure of early heparin cessation as treatment for heparin-induced thrombocytopenia. *Am J Med*. 1999;106(6):629-635. doi:10.1016/S0002-9343(99)00124-2

Warkentin TE, Kelton JG. A 14-year study of heparin-induced thrombocytopenia. *Am J Med*. 1996;101(5):502-507. doi:10.1016/S0002-9343(96)00258-6

Wisler JW, Washam JB, Becker RC. Evaluation of dose requirments for prolonged bivalirudin administration in patients with renal insufficiency and suspected heparin-induced thrombocytopenia. *J Thromb Thrombolysis*. 2012;33(3):287-295. doi:10.1007/s11239-011-0677-3

8. **The answer is C.** The best way to prevent heparin-induced thrombocytopenia (HIT) is to limit heparin exposure. One way to do this is to use LMWH instead of unfractionated heparin whenever possible. LMWH is associated with a lower incidence of HIT compared to unfractionated heparin. Development of HIT is independent of the dose used and has been reported to occur even with heparin flushes and the use of heparin-coated catheters.

McNulty I, Katz E, Kim KY. Thrombocytopenia following heparin flush. *Prog Cardiovasc Nurs*. 2005;20(4):143-147. doi:10.1111/j.0889-7204.2005.04693.x

Muslimani AA, Ricaurte B, Daw HA. Immune heparin-induced thrombocytopenia resulting from preceding exposure to heparin catheter flushes. *Am J Hematol*. 2007;82(7):652-655. doi:10.1002/ajh.20849

9. **The answer is E.** This patient developed a spontaneous ICH secondary to warfarin-associated coagulopathy. Risk factors for supratherapeutic INR in patients treated with warfarin include comorbidities such as heart failure, impaired liver function, acute illnesses, medication interactions, and daily variations in vitamin K intake.

PCC: Patients with life-threatening intracranial hemorrhage from elevated INR should be treated with vitamin K and 4-PCC. PCC is the preferred treatment for warfarin-associated ICH, if available; otherwise, FFP can be administered. PCC contains coagulation factors VII, IX, X, prothrombin, and proteins C, S, and Z in a concentrated form; unlike FFP, it can be given without waiting for compatibility testing and thawing. The potency of PCC is expressed as factor IX content in international units and varies between preparations.

Treatment of Elevated INR		
INR	Bleeding	Recommendations
Therapeutic to 5	No	Reduce warfarin dose or omit one dose and resume at lower dose when INR is therapeutic
5–9	No	Omit one or two doses and resume at lower dose or omit one dose and give 1 to 2.5 mg of vitamin K if patient is at high risk for hemorrhage*
>9	No	Hold warfarin and give vitamin K 2.5 to 5 mg and resume at lower dose once INR is therapeutic
Any	Yes	Hold warfarin, give vitamin K 10 mg** and 4-PCC. If PCCs are not available, treat with fresh-frozen plasma (FFP)

*Patients at high risk for hemorrhage include patients with a history of hemorrhage and patients with a history of stroke, renal insufficiency, anemia, and hypertension.
** If repeat INR within the first 24–48 h after reversal is still elevated, vitamin K can be redosed at 10 mg IV.

Dose: 50 international units/kg

Volume: 50 to 150 mL depending on the preparation

Caution: Potential to induce thrombosis and disseminated intravascular coagulation (DIC)

FFP: FFP is prepared using apheresis from a single unit of whole blood or plasma, within 8 hours of collection (fresh) and stored at −18 to –30°C (frozen).

Dose: 10 to 15 mL/kg (which corresponds to 3–5 units of FFP)

Volume: One FFP unit is equivalent to 250 mL of volume; 3 to 5 units of FFP corresponds to around 0.75 to 1.25 L of colloid volume

Cautions: (because of large volume): Patients with congestive heart failure (CHF), elderly patients, and children

Alternative: Reduce the rate of infusion to around 1 mL/kg/hour *or* consider cryoprecipitate

Cryoprecipitate: Cryoprecipitate is the precipitate that remains after FFP undergoes a process of centrifugation.

Dose: 1 unit of cryoprecipitate/10 kg body weight

Volume: 250 mL of FFP is equivalent to 10 to 20 mL of cryoprecipitate

Ansell J, Hirsh J, Hylek E, et al. Pharmacology and management of the vitamin K antagonists: American College of Chest Physicians Evidence-Based Clinical Practice Guidelines (8th Edition). *Chest.* 2008;133(6 Suppl):160S-198S. doi:10.1378/chest.08-0670

Garcia, D, Crowther MA, Ageno W. Practical management of coagulopathy associated with warfarin. *BMJ.* 2010;340:c1813. doi:10.1136/bmj.c1813

Penning-van Beest FJ, Geleijnse JM, van Meegen E, et al. Lifestyle and diet as risk factors for over-anticoagulation. *J Clin Epidemiol.* 2002;55(4):411-417. doi:10.1016/S0895-4356(01)00485-1

Penning-van Beest FJ, van Meegen E, Rosendaal FR, et al. Characteristics of anticoagulant therapy and comorbidity related to overanticoagulation. *Thromb Haemost.* 2001;86(2):569-574. doi:10.1055/s-0037-1616088

Penning-van Beest FJ, van Meegen E, Rosendaal FR, et al. Drug interactions as a cause of over-anticoagulation on phenprocoumon or acenocoumarol predominantly concern antibacterial drugs. *Clin Pharmacol Ther.* 2001;69(6):451-457. doi:10.1067/mcp.2001.115723

Treatment Options

Treatment Options	Time to Anticoagulation Reversal	Comments
Stop warfarin	5–14 days	• None
Vitamin K	6–24 hours	• Factor 9 and 10 replacement takes >24 hours • Risk of anaphylaxis with IV injection
FFP	1–12 hours depending on thawing time, volume, and rate of infusion	• Large volume (around 2–4 L) may be needed to normalize INR, depending on degree of coagulopathy
PCC	15 minutes after completion of infusion	• Limited availability • Cost • Variable factor VII content based on manufacturer • Potentially prothrombotic
Factor VIIa concentrate	15 minutes after bolus infusion	• Short half-life • Cost • Uncertain safety • Replaces only factor VII, not other vitamin K–dependent factors

This table is based on the 2008 American College of Chest Physician (ACCP) Guidelines. Pharmacology and management of the vitamin K antagonists: American College of Chest Physicians Evidence-Based Clinical Practice Guidelines (8th ed.). Ansell, *Chest.* 2008;133:160S.

10. **The answer is A.** This patient has thrombocytopenia with an elevated PT, PTT, fibrin degradation products (D-dimer), and reduced fibrinogen levels in the setting of sepsis suggesting the diagnosis of DIC. DIC is a complication of systemic disease causing activation of clotting systems within the blood vessels. This results in consumption of coagulation factors, which leads to thrombocytopenia and elevated PT and PTT leading to bleeding from multiple sites. In addition, these small blood clots can cause multisystem organ failure. Common causes of DIC include:

    A. Malignancy

    B. Sepsis

    C. Massive tissue injury such as trauma and burns

    D. Obstetrical complications

    Treatment: Treat the underlying cause. Patients can be treated symptomatically based on severity. If the patient has severe bleeding, platelets or cryoprecipitate can be transfused, but the underlying problem must be addressed at the same time.

Gando S, Levi M, Toh CH. Disseminated intravascular coagulation. *Nat Rev Dis Primers.* 2016;2:16037. doi:10.1038/nrdp.2016.37

Wada H, Thachil J, Di Nisio M, et al. Guidance for diagnosis and treatment of DIC from harmonization of the recommendations from three guidelines. *J Thromb Haemost.* 2013;11:761-767. doi:10.1111/jth.12155

11. **The answer is B.** Myeloproliferative neoplasms such as essential thrombocythemia and polycythemia vera have been associated with AVWS, particularly when the platelet count is very high and greater than 1 million/μL. Extreme thrombocytosis may promote a hemostatic defect due to the excessive adsorption of large von Willebrand factor multimers to transformed platelets. von Willebrand factor antigen level and ristocetin cofactor activity should be measured in patients with extreme thrombocytosis or any evidence of bleeding. Cytoreductive therapy or plateletpheresis should be considered to reduce the platelet count and correct the hemostatic abnormality. The use of aspirin is contraindicated in AVWS.

Barbui T, Barosi G, Birgegard G, et al. Philadelphia-negative classical myeloproliferative neoplasms: critical concepts and management recommendations from European LeukemiaNet. *J Clin Oncol.* 2011;29(6):761-770. doi:10.1200/JCO.2010.31.8436

Mohri H, Motomura S, Kanamori H, et al. Clinical significance of inhibitors in acquired von Willebrand syndrome. *Blood.* 1998;91(10):3623-3629.

Rottenstreich A, Kleinstern G, Krichevsky S, et al. Factors related to the development of acquired von Willebrand syndrome in patients with essential thrombocythemia and polycythemia vera. *Eur J Intern Med.* 2017;41:49-54. doi:10.1016/j.ejim.2016.11.011

van Genderen PJ, Michiels JJ. Erythromelalgic, thrombotic and haemorrhagic manifestations of thrombocythaemia. *Presse Med.* 1994;23(2):73-77.

12. **The answer is C.** Intracranial hemorrhage is the most devastating complication associated with systemic thrombolytic therapy. American Heart Association/American Stroke Association Stroke Council recommends immediate discontinuation of the thrombolytic infusion and obtain an emergent noncontrast head CT. Laboratory samples to be obtained include complete blood count (CBC), prothrombin time/International Normalized Ratio (PT/INR), partial thromboplastin time (PTT), fibrinogen level, and type and cross-match. Cryoprecipitate contains factor VIII, von Willebrand factor, and fibrinogen. It is suggested to transfuse with 10 units of cryoprecipitate over 10–30 min in patients with thromolytic-associated intracranial hemorrhage who have received a thrombolytic agent in the previous 24 hours (onset in 1 h, peaks in 12 h). Cryoprecipitate can be redosed if fibrinogen level is <200 mg/dL after the first dose. An antifibrinolytic agent such as tranexamic acid (1000 mg IV over 10 min) aminocaproic acid (4–5 g IV over 1 h followed by 1 gr IV) is given until bleeding is controlled. Supportive therapy including management of blood pressure and cerebral perfusion is recommended.

Powers WJ, Rabinstein AA, Ackerson T, et al. 2018 Guidelines for the early management of patients with acute ischemic stroke: a guideline for healthcare professionals from the American Heart Association/American Stroke Association. *Stroke.* 2018;49(3):e46-e110. doi:10.1161/STR.0000000000000158

13. **The answer is C.** Urgent reversal of heparin with protamine sulfate is indicated for this patient with intracerebral bleeding. The dose of protamine sulfate is calculated based on the dose of heparin administered in the past 2 hours and the time elapsed since the last heparin dose. Full neutralization of heparin is achieved with 1 mg of protamine sulfate per 100 units of heparin. Because the half-life of heparin is approximately 30–60 minutes, the dose of protamine sulfate is calculated by estimating the amount of heparin remaining in the plasma at the time that reversal is required. This patient received 2,400 units of heparin in the 2 hours prior to need for reversal and thus would require about 25–30 mg of protamine sulfate.

Frontera JA, Lewin JJ III, Rabinstein AA, et al. Guideline for reversal of antithrombotics in intracranial hemorrhage: a statement for healthcare professionals from the Neurocritical Care Society and Society of Critical Care Medicine. *Neurocrit Care.* 2016;24:6-46. doi:10.1007/s12028-015-0222-x

14. **The answer is C.** Dabigatran is an oral anticoagulant that works as a direct thrombin inhibitor (DTI). Peak plasma concentration is reached 1 to 2 hours after ingestion. Anticoagulant effects decrease by 50% at 12 hours after administration. However, in patients with renal insufficiency, the half-life can be substantially longer. The anticoagulant effect is through direct inhibition of thrombin, thus making replacement of clotting factors ineffective. Idarucizumab is a

humanized monoclonal antibody fragment that can be used for emergency reversal of dabigatran's anticoagulant effect. As dabigatran is primarily excreted renally, hemodialysis may also be used to remove active medication from the circulation. Hemodialysis may be effective in removing approximately 50% of the drug.

Getta B, Muller N, Motum P, et al. Intermittent haemodialysis and continuous veno-venous dialysis are effective in mitigating major bleeding due to dabigatran. *Br J Haematol.* 2015;169(4): 603-604. doi:10.1111/bjh.13236

Khadzhynov D, Wagner F, Formella S, et al. Effective elimination of dabigatran by haemodialysis. A phase I single-centre study in patients with end-stage renal disease. *Thromb Haemost.* 2013;109(4):596-605. doi:10.1160/TH12-08-0573

Pollack CV Jr, Reilly PA, Eikelboom J, et al. Idarucizumab for dabigatran reversal. *N Engl J Med.* 2015;373(6):511-520. doi:10.1056/NEJMoa1502000

Pollack CV Jr, Reilly PA, van Ryn J, et al. Idarucizumab for dabigatran reversal—full cohort analysis. *N Engl J Med.* 2017;377(5):431-441. doi:10.1056/NEJMoa1707278

Wanek MR, Horn ET, Elapavaluru S, et al. Safe use of hemodialysis for dabigatran removal before cardiac surgery. *Ann Pharmacother.* 2012;46(9):e21. doi:10.1345/aph.1R081

15. **The answer is D.** The patient's laboratory testing and peripheral blood smear suggest a diagnosis of nonautoimmune hemolytic anemia. Her clinical presentation is notable for thromboses in atypical locations. PNH is a rare acquired hematopoietic stem cell disorder characterized by inactivating mutations in *PIGA* resulting in uncontrolled complement activity leading to a wide range of clinical findings, primarily through intravascular hemolysis and platelet activation. The PIGA protein is involved in the first step in the synthesis of the glycosylphosphatidylinositol anchor which prevents complement-mediated intravascular hemolysis. Thrombosis is the most frequent complication of PNH and the leading cause of death in these patients. The cerebral venous system is the second most frequent location of thrombosis after the intra-abdominal vasculature.

Hill A, DeZern AE, Kinoshita T, et al. Paroxysmal nocturnal haemoglobinuria. *Nat Rev Dis Primers.* 2017;3:17028. doi:10.1038/nrdp.2017.28

Hill A, Kelly RJ, Hillmen P. Thrombosis in paroxysmal nocturnal hemoglobinuria. *Blood.* 2013;121(25):4985-4996. doi:10.1182/blood-2012-09-311381

Poulou LS, Vakrinos G, Pomoni A, et al. Stroke in paroxysmal nocturnal haemoglobinuria: patterns of disease and outcome. *Thromb Haemost.* 2007;98(3):699-701. doi:10.1160/TH07-04-0316

Ziakas PD, Poulou LS, Pomoni A. Thrombosis in paroxysmal nocturnal hemoglobinuria at a glance: a clinical review. *Curr Vasc Pharmacol.* 2008;6(4):347-353. doi:10.2174/157016108785909742

16. **The answer is E.** Optimal management of acute thrombotic events requires therapeutic anticoagulation and initiation of eculizumab. Eculizumab is a humanized monoclonal antibody that reduces complement-mediated hemolysis by inhibiting formation of the membrane attack complex. Eculizumab is the only therapy that has been shown to prevent thrombosis in patients with paroxysmal nocturnal hemoglobinuria (PNH). Eculizumab carries a black box warning for increased risk of meningococcal disease. The warning includes a recommendation to administer meningococcal vaccines to patients receiving eculizumab at least 2 weeks prior to administration of the first dose, if possible. Daily oral antibiotic prophylaxis may also be considered.

Hillmen P, Muus P, Duhrsen U, et al. Effect of the complement inhibitor eculizumab on thromboembolism in patients with paroxysmal nocturnal hemoglobinuria. *Blood.* 2007;110(12): 4123-4128. doi:10.1182/blood-2007-06-095646

Hillmen P, Muus P, Roth A, et al. Long-term safety and efficacy of sustained eculizumab treatment in patients with paroxysmal nocturnal haemoglobinuria. *Br J Haematol.* 2013;162(1):62-73. doi:10.1111/bjh.12347

Parker C. Eculizumab for paroxysmal nocturnal haemoglobinuria. *Lancet.* 2009;373(9665):759-767. doi:10.1016/S0140-6736(09)60001-5

17. **The answer is D.** WM is a B-cell neoplasm that results from the accumulation of clonal lymphoplasmacytic cells secreting a monoclonal IgM protein. Hyperviscosity syndrome is a medical emergency that arises from high serum IgM levels and requires emergent plasma exchange. The pentameric configuration of the IgM molecules increases serum viscosity and

slows the passage of blood through capillaries which can lead to severe neurologic impairment and oronasal bleeding. Red cell transfusions and treatment with rituximab may further increase whole blood viscosity and should be avoided prior to plasma exchange.

Dimopoulos MA, Kastritis E, Owen RG, et al. Treatment recommendations for patients with Waldenstrom macroglobulinemia (WM) and related disorders: IWWM-7 consensus. *Blood.* 2014;124(9):1404-1411. doi:10.1182/blood-2014-03-565135

Gertz MA, Kyle RA. Hyperviscosity syndrome. *J Intensive Care Med.* 1995;10(3):128-141. doi:10.1177/088506669501000304

Oza A, Rajkumar SV. Waldenstrom macroglobulinemia: prognosis and management. *Blood Cancer J.* 2016;6:e391. doi :10.1038/bcj.2015.42

22

Acute Gastrointestinal and Genitourinary Disorders

PHILIP M. SOMMER AND ASAD LATIF

QUESTIONS

1. A 65-year-old woman with a known history of duodenal ulcer presents to the ED with a major upper gastrointestinal (UGI) hemorrhage. At home she was being treated with diet modification and acid-suppressive therapy. She is resuscitated with intravenous (IV) fluids and packed red blood cells (pRBC). Her heart rate (HR) and blood pressure (BP) have stabilized after appropriate resuscitation. Which of the following is the most appropriate next step?

   A. Begin bismuth, tetracycline, and metronidazole
   B. Start a pantoprazole infusion
   C. Endoscopy with coagulation of the bleeding vessel
   D. Immediate laparotomy and repair of the bleeding vessel
   E. Placement of nasogastric tube (NGT) and lavage with saline

2. A 34-year-old man is brought to the ED by his friends early in the morning, complaining of hematemesis. He admits that he had been drinking heavily the night before and had vomited multiple times. On physical examination, his clothes are stained with blood and he is complaining of mild abdominal pain. His vital signs are stable other than tachycardia in the low 100s and his physical exam is largely unremarkable. The most appropriate statement regarding his primary complaint is:

   A. It is a complication of gastroesophageal (GE) reflux
   B. It involves esophageal rupture near the GE junction
   C. Profuse hemorrhage is the most common manifestation
   D. Bleeding can generally be managed medically
   E. Vagotomy is indicated for patients requiring surgery

3. A 54-year-old woman with a 20-year history of substantial alcohol use presents to the ED with fevers and hypotension. She has a history of ascites and had a large-volume paracentesis several months ago. She is diagnosed with spontaneous bacterial peritonitis (SBP), admitted to the ICU, and treated with appropriate antibiotics. During her hospitalization, she also undergoes upper endoscopy and is found to have several large esophageal varices. Which of the following decreases this patients' risk of an initial upper gastrointestinal (UGI) hemorrhage from her varices?

   A. Transjugular intrahepatic porto-systemic shunt
   B. Sclerotherapy
   C. Splenorenal shunt
   D. Beta-blockade
   E. Proton pump inhibitors

4. A 55-year-old man fell off a 10-foot scaffolding two days ago. At the time he refused medical care, but has been having significant back and chest wall pain since the fall. He has been medicating himself with acetaminophen. He presents to the ED this morning with an acute onset of fever, right-sided abdominal aching, and jaundice. His family mentions that he has also been more confused during the past 24 hours. He admits to taking more than 24 pills of Extra-Strength (500 mg) Tylenol since his injury. His examination is significant for right upper quadrant (RUQ) tenderness. His labs show elevated transaminases, an International Normalized Ratio (INR) of 2.5, and a venous pH of 7.38. All of the following are components of the King's College criteria for acute liver failure (ALF), **except**:

A. INR
B. Serum creatinine
C. Arterial pH
D. Serum transaminases
E. Hepatic encephalopathy

5. For the patient in Question 4, which of the following would be an appropriate next step in his treatment?

A. Gastric lavage
B. List for liver transplantation
C. Administration of N-acetylcysteine
D. Fluid resuscitation and stabilization
E. Monitor for 2 hours and follow up in clinic

6. An 88-year-old paraplegic woman presents to the ED with new onset of abdominal pain and distention. She was at the nursing home in her usual state when these symptoms began. On examination she is afebrile and her abdomen is distended but not tender. She has no obvious previous surgical scars, and upon questioning states that she has been passing scant watery stools. Abdominal x-ray shows dilated loops of large and small bowel without any clear sign of obstruction. Her diagnosis could be associated with all of the following, **except**:

A. Malignant infiltration of the celiac plexus
B. Neuroleptic medications
C. Opiate usage
D. Excess parasympathetic tone
E. Scleroderma

7. Which of the following statements is true regarding plain radiographs in small bowel obstruction (SBO)?

A. Gas within the small bowel is distinguished from gas within the colon by luminal lines perpendicular to the bowel wall. The small bowel lines partially cross the lumen, whereas the colonic lines completely cross the lumen
B. Ileus may be difficult to distinguish from SBO on abdominal x-ray, since both conditions can produce gaseous distention of the bowel with air fluid levels
C. The "string of pearls" sign refers to a series of radiolucent images in the small bowel representing the gallstones of gallstone ileus
D. A gasless abdomen seen on plain film rules out a SBO
E. Abdominal x-ray can rule out SBO

8. A 66-year-old man with a known history of sigmoid diverticulosis presents to the ED with an acute onset of fever, chills, and severe left lower quadrant pain. On examination, the patient has a temperature of 39°C, heart rate (HR) 120/min, and a blood pressure (BP) of 90/40 mmHg. He demonstrates peritoneal signs on abdominal examination. CT scan of the abdomen demonstrates evidence of pneumo-peritoneum and mesenteric stranding around the sigmoid colon. Which of the following is the correct treatment for this patient?

   A. ICU admission, fluid resuscitation, intravenous (IV) antibiotics within 30 minutes, and laparotomy
   B. ICU admission, fluid resuscitation, IV antibiotics within 30 minutes, and percutaneous drainage
   C. Admission to the surgical floor, fluid resuscitation, and IV antibiotics on call to the OR for laparotomy
   D. Admission to the surgical floor and wait for operating room availability
   E. Directly to operating room for emergent laparotomy

9. A 37-year-old investment banker presents to the ED with an acute onset of abdominal pain. On history, he admits to a high-stress work environment, frequently taking antacids. He denies taking any nonsteroidal anti-inflammatory drugs (NSAIDs). On examination, the patient does not appear toxic, but has significant epigastric tenderness without obvious peritonitis. A plain abdominal radiograph demonstrates free air. A follow-up CT scan confirms this finding along with a significant amount of fat stranding surrounding the first portion of the duodenum. Which of the following is not associated with the patient's condition?

   A. Excessive NSAID use
   B. Acid hypersecretory state
   C. *Helicobacter pylori* infection
   D. Need for operative intervention
   E. Patient has to receive acid suppressive therapy

10. Which of the following statements accurately characterizes acute occlusion of the superior mesenteric artery (SMA)?

   A. The right and left colon are generally spared as a result of sparing of the middle colic artery
   B. Emboli most commonly arise from atheromatous plaques within the aorta
   C. Acute occlusion of the SMA usually results in complete foregut infarction
   D. Sudden complete occlusion is most often caused by embolism rather than by thrombosis
   E. Abdominal radiograph can be diagnostic in diagnosis of mesenteric ischemia.

11. A 76-year-old woman is incidentally found to have a 7-cm infrarenal aortic aneurysm. She elects to have open repair of her aneurysm and undergoes the surgery without any complications. During the operation, her vascular surgeon is able to place the aortic cross clamp below the renal arteries, and does not reimplant any vessels. On her first postoperative day, she complains of severe abdominal pain and has an episode of bloody diarrhea. Which of the following is true regarding her probable condition?

   A. The most common symptoms of ischemic colitis are lower abdominal pain and bleeding
   B. Occlusion of major mesenteric vessels is responsible for producing ischemia in most cases
   C. Nonoperative management is not justified, because in a significant percentage of such cases perforation and peritonitis eventually develop
   D. The cecum and rectum are the most commonly involved areas
   E. A diagnosis is best made with an abdominal x-ray

12. An 80-year-old woman is seen in the ED with abdominal pain and constipation. On examination, she is afebrile and mildly tachycardic, with a stable blood pressure and no respiratory distress. Her abdomen is distended and tympanic, but there are no peritoneal signs. Abdominal x-ray shows a significantly distended loop of bowel pointing to the right upper quadrant (RUQ). The first step in her management should be:

   A. Administration of laxatives and cleansing enemas
   B. Barium enema
   C. Rigid sigmoidoscopy
   D. Sigmoid resection
   E. Empiric antibiotics

13. A 54-year-old male presents to the ED with a 1-day history of cramping abdominal pain, multiple episodes of emesis, and inability to pass flatus or have a bowel movement in 48 hours. The patient is otherwise healthy, but has a history of a previous open appendectomy at the age of 23. On examination, he is afebrile with mild tachycardia. His abdominal exam is tender, distended, but without evidence of peritonitis. Which of the following is the best confirmatory test for his diagnosis?

   A. Abdominal radiographs
   B. Upper gastrointestinal (UGI) series with small bowel follow-through
   C. CT scan without contrast
   D. MRI
   E. Barium enema

14. A 66-year-old male presents to the ED with a 3-hour history of abdominal pain, nausea, and vomiting. The patient states that the onset of pain was sudden and is radiating to the back. On examination, he is tachycardic and has tenderness to palpation in the epigastrium. Hyperamylasemia is diagnostic of acute pancreatitis when associated with which of the following laboratory findings?

   A. Hyperlipasemia
   B. Increased urinary amylase levels
   C. Hypocalcemia
   D. Transaminitis
   E. None of the above

15. Routine initial management of a patient with alcoholic pancreatitis and five Ranson's criteria should include which of the following measures?

   A. Intravenous (IV) resuscitation, admission to the floor, and clear liquid diet
   B. Admission to an ICU, aggressive fluid resuscitation, and gastric decompression
   C. Peritoneal lavage
   D. Octreotide
   E. Admission to the hospital for scheduled surgical exploration

16. An alcoholic patient has acute pancreatitis with five of Ranson's criteria. He gradually improves over the course of a couple of weeks but then develops tachycardia with a heart rate (HR) of 120 and a temperature of 39°C, along with abdominal distention. A CT scan is obtained that demonstrates a large amount of air within the pancreas. After initial stabilization in the ICU, which of the following is the most appropriate next step?

   A. Percutaneous catheter drainage
   B. Peritoneal lavage
   C. Laparoscopy
   D. Operative drainage
   E. Observation

17. A 65-year-old man is unable to void after an abdominoperineal resection. Postvoid residuals have been 600 to 800 mL. The treatment of choice in this patient is:

A. Chronic Foley catheterization
B. Transurethral prostatectomy
C. Clean intermittent catheterization
D. Transurethral sphincterotomy
E. Alpha-blockers alone

18. A 74-year-old male with a significant history of tobacco and alcohol use presents to the ED with the chief complaint of "blood in my urine." He denies fevers, abdominal pain, or nausea. His examination is essentially unremarkable. The evaluation of gross or microscopic hematuria involves all the following except:

A. Upper tract imaging with intravenous pyelogram (IVP), ultrasound imaging, or CT scanning
B. Cystoscopic studies
C. Serum tumor markers
D. Pelvic examination
E. Repeat urinalysis

19. A 27-year-old otherwise healthy male is brought to the ED after a motor vehicle collision trauma. He is initially hemodynamically unstable and has a positive focused assessment with sonography in trauma (FAST) exam for blood in the abdomen. He is taken to the operating room, where a splenic avulsion is diagnosed and a splenectomy is performed. The anesthesiologist informs the surgeon that there is gross blood in the Foley bag. Which of the following is most likely true about the patient's condition?

A. Rupture is usually extraperitoneal when associated with pelvic trauma
B. A single-view retrograde cystogram in the ED demonstrates most significant bladder injuries
C. Primary closure is generally indicated for extraperitoneal ruptures
D. Intraoperative injury usually requires repair with a suprapubic cystostomy
E. It is most likely related to traumatic urinary catheterization in the ED

20. A 21-year-old woman presents to the emergency room with abdominal pain. She describes that she has been having mild lower abdominal and pelvic pain for about two weeks, but it has now acutely worsened over the last couple of days to involve the right upper quadrant (RUQ) pain radiating to her right shoulder. Her vitals are stable other than a mild fever, and laboratory results show a white blood cell (WBC) count of 16 and mildly elevated transaminases, but are otherwise unremarkable. Her presentation is most consistent with:

A. Asherman syndrome
B. Fitz-Hugh-Curtis syndrome
C. Meigs syndrome
D. Sheehan syndrome

21. A 63-year-old woman with alcoholic cirrhosis is admitted with altered mental status (AMS) including slurred speech secondary to hepatic encephalopathy. On exam, she has a protuberant abdomen, jaundice, spider angiomas, and asterixis. A head CT scan is negative for any acute abnormalities or lesions. A hepatology consult is called and she is started on treatment with lactulose and rifaximin. What acid–base abnormality is this patient most likely to develop in the next week?

A. Anion gap (AG) metabolic acidosis
B. Metabolic alkalosis
C. Normal AG metabolic acidosis

D. Respiratory acidosis
E. Respiratory alkalosis

22. A 30-year-old man is admitted to the ICU following a motorcycle accident where he sustained an open-book pelvic fracture and a small subarachnoid hemorrhage (SAH). He undergoes surgical fixation of his pelvis on day 2. His SAH has remained stable. On day 4, he develops episodic vomiting. His nasogastric tube output has been clear yellow and steady at about 2 liters a day. On exam, his blood pressure (BP) is 93/64 mmHg, heart rate (HR) is 113/min, respiratory rate (RR) is 8/min, and he does not have any noticeable bowel sounds. What is the most appropriate management for this patient?

A. Administer acetazolamide and 80 mEq of ammonium chloride
B. Bolus 500 mL of 5% albumin and start an infusion of lactated Ringer solution at 150 mL/hr
C. Perform emergency dialysis
D. Bolus a liter of normal saline with 20 mEq KCL/L and start an infusion at 150 mL/hr
E. Bolus a liter of lactated Ringer

23. A 56-year-old man with a history of hepatitis C cirrhosis is admitted to the ICU with altered mental status (AMS), fever, nausea, and vomiting, and increasing abdominal discomfort without rebound or guarding on physical exam. Serum laboratory data on admission to the ICU shows white blood cell (WBC) 12.2 K/mm^3, hemoglobin 9.6 g/dL, platelets 57 K/mm^3, creatinine (Cr) 1.8 mg/dL (baseline 0.9 mg/dL), and blood urea nitrogen (BUN) 56 mg/dL. A noncontrast CT scan of the abdomen and pelvis reveals an umbilical hernia and ascites. An abdominal paracentesis was performed which revealed the following: clear straw colored fluid; red blood cell (RBC) 70/μL, WBC 610/μL (neutrophils: 50%; lymphocytes: 23%; and monocytes: 27%), and glucose: 72 mg/dL. Blood pressure (BP) is 92/52 mmHg, heart rate (HR) is 108 beats per minute (BPM), and respiratory rate (RR) is 20 breaths/min. Which of the following steps is indicated in the treatment of this patient?

A. Exploratory laparotomy
B. CT scan with intravenous (IV) contrast
C. Starting vancomycin, cefepime, and metronidazole
D. IV albumin
E. Clinical observation

■ ANSWERS

1. **The answer is C**. In the presence of an acute hemorrhage, none of the listed drug regimens provide immediate control of the bleeding. Beginning bismuth, tetracycline, and metronidazole would be a treatment option for patients with *Helicobacter pylori* infection. While *H. pylori* infection is commonly found in patients with duodenal ulcers, treatment does not address the acute hemorrhage. Pantoprazole infusions may be of benefit in patients with bleeding gastric ulcers; however, there is no convincing evidence that they are beneficial in patients with duodenal ulcer hemorrhage. Therapy in this patient, after appropriate resuscitation, is endoscopic visualization and control of the bleeding vessel. If endoscopy fails to control the bleeding, or if the bleeding recurs, then immediate laparotomy with oversewing of the bleeding vessel is often necessary. After control of the bleeding, the patient should be tested for *H. pylori* and continued on antacid therapy.

   Klein A, Gralnek IM. Acute, nonvariceal upper gastrointestinal bleeding. *Curr Opin Crit Care*. 2015;21(2):154-162. doi:10.1097/MCC.0000000000000185

2. **The answer is D**. Mallory–Weiss syndrome refers to a tear of the mucosa and submucosa near the GE junction that occurs as a result of retching. The tear is usually on the gastric side of the GE junction and on the lesser curvature. In only about 10% of cases is there profuse hemorrhage. Bleeding often stops spontaneously and can often be managed nonoperatively. If not, an attempt at endoscopic clipping can be performed. The definitive treatment is laparotomy with simple oversewing of the bleeding mucosal tear. Boerhaave syndrome is a transmural perforation of the esophagus as opposed to Mallory-Weiss, although both are associated with vomiting and retching. Patients with Boerhaave syndrome will classically have crepitus and intense retrosternal pain.

   Feinman M, Haut ER. Upper gastrointestinal bleeding. *Surg Clin North Am*. 2014;94(1):43-53. doi:10.1016/j.suc.2013.10.004

3. **The answer is D**. Esophageal varices are the most common cause of massive bleeding in a patient with cirrhosis and typically result from the shunting of blood from the mesenteric circulation through the coronary vein to the esophageal submucosal venous plexus. When the pressure in the varices rises above 12 mmHg, spontaneous rupture will occur in 30% of patients. In addition to variceal hypertension, mucosal ulceration can also predispose to rupture. Beta blockade is the most effective way to prevent the first bleeding episode. Sclerotherapy, transjugular intrahepatic portosystemic shunt, and surgical shunts have not been associated with a reduction in first bleeding events in patients with alcoholic cirrhosis. Prophylaxis is of utmost importance because variceal bleeding in cirrhotic patients carries a 1-year mortality rate of 70%. Child's Class C patients with variceal bleeding have a 70% mortality rate at 6 weeks. Both nadolol and propranolol are nonselective beta blockers that have been approved for prophylaxis against variceal hemorrhage.

   Brunner F, Berzigotti A, Bosch J. Prevention and treatment of variceal hemorrhage in 2017. *Liver Int*. 2017;37(suppl 1):104-115. doi:10.1111/liv.13277

4. **The answer is D**. The King's College criteria were first developed in 1989, based on the observations of 588 patients with ALF who presented to the King's College Hospital between 1973 and 1985. These patients were retrospectively studied to determine if there were certain clinical factors that predicted a worse prognosis. These criteria were further subdivided for acetaminophen and nonacetaminophen causes of acute liver failure. For ALF as a result of acetaminophen toxicity, the criteria include an arterial pH <7.3, INR >6.5, serum creatinine >300 µmol/L, and Grade III/IV encephalopathy. The specificity and sensitivity of these criteria are 90% and 69%, respectively. As a result, the American Society for the Study of Liver Disease has recommended that the criteria be used as an early parameter in ascertaining the need for liver transplantation in these patients.

   Yoon E, Babar A, Choudhary M, et al. Acetaminophen-induced hepatotoxicity: a comprehensive update. *J Clin Transl Hepatol*. 2016;4(2):131-142. doi:10.14218/JCTH.2015.00052

5. **The answer is C**. Gastric lavage and activated charcoal have proven benefit only if the ingestion was recent, more specifically within 30 minutes. Liver transplantation is an option in certain patients with acute liver failure (ALF); however, our patient does not meet any of the King's College criteria; as a result his prognosis is fairly good and liver transplantation would not be an option in him at this time. Acetylcysteine replenishes the stores of glutathione, which is important in the inactivation of the toxic metabolite of acetaminophen, NAPQI. It is important to start the acetylcysteine within 8 hours of ingestion, because after 8 hours, irreversible liver damage has started to occur. The recommended adult dosage regimen for the intravenous (IV) formulation is a loading dose of 150 mg/kg in 200 mL of 5% dextrose given over 15 to 30 minutes. This is followed by a maintenance dose at 50 mg/kg in 500 mL of 5% dextrose given IV over 4 hours and then 100 mg/kg in 1,000 mL of 5% dextrose given IV over 16 hours. Adjustments are required for children and patients at risk for fluid overload. Fluid overload can potentially cause hepatic congestion and worsen failure.

Chiew AL, Gluud C, Brok J, et al. Interventions for paracetamol (acetaminophen) overdose. *Cochrane Database Syst Rev.* 2018;2:CD003328. doi:10.1002/14651858.CD003328.pub3

6. **The answer is D**. Ogilvie first described a profound colonic ileus in the absence of bowel pathology. His patients had suffered from malignant infiltration of the celiac plexus. Ogilvie's syndrome most often appears as a complication of other clinical conditions. It is typically characterized by massive colonic distention in the absence of a mechanical obstruction. Neuroleptic medications, opiate usage, and severe metabolic disease have produced a similar clinical picture. The exact cause of colonic ileus has not been identified; a presumed mechanism is excessive sympathetic tone, resulting in a loss of normal colonic peristalsis. It appears that the typical at-risk patient is elderly and bedridden. Associated medical conditions include hypothyroidism, diabetes, chronic renal failure, scleroderma, multiple sclerosis, and electrolyte disturbances. It may also be seen in the setting of severe trauma. Ogilvie's syndrome is of concern due to the risk of colonic perforation, the cecum being the area of the colon most at risk, especially when the cecal diameter exceeds 12 cm. Patients typically present with a distended, tender abdomen. Unlike mechanical bowel obstructions, the pain is usually not colicky. Abdominal x-rays and CT scans can be used as adjuncts and typically demonstrate a diffusely dilated colon without evidence of a mechanical cause. Therapy aims at correcting electrolyte abnormalities and ruling out a mechanical cause of obstruction. Treatment of underlying medical disorders is mandatory. Colonic decompression can be accomplished with neostigmine, endoscopic decompression, or surgical decompression. Of note, patients receiving neostigmine should be kept in a monitored setting secondary to the risk of bradycardia. Typically, surgical therapy is reserved for refractory distention and/or complications such as colonic perforation.

Pereira P, Djeudji F, Leduc P, et al. Ogilvie's syndrome-acute colonic pseudo-onstruction. *J Visc Surg.* 2015;152(2):99-105. doi:10.1016/j.jviscsurg.2015.02.004

Valle RG, Godoy FL. Neostigmine for acute colonic pseudo-obstruction: a meta-analysis. *Ann Med Surg (Lond).* 2014;3(3):60-64. doi:10.1016/j.amsu.2014.04.002

7. **The answer is B**. Plain radiographs of the abdomen are useful in evaluating patients with suspected SBO. Gas-filled loops of small bowel are typically seen in the central portion of the abdomen. The presence of both normal and dilated small bowel loops is typical of SBO. The small bowel is recognized radiographically by the vavulae conniventes that are visible as lines that completely cross the intestinal lumen. Colonic gas is typically located peripherally and the colon is identified by lines that partially cross the colonic lumen (plicae semilunaris). Air–fluid levels can be seen in both ileus and small bowel obstruction, and typically are seen only on upright or decubitus films. A gasless abdomen can be seen in SBO and typically results from proximal decompression by emesis or by completely fluid-filled loops of small bowel. It is important to distinguish between partial and complete SBO. In partial obstruction, gas is usually seen in decompressed loops of small bowel distal to the point of obstruction. In contrast, a complete obstruction presents with obstipation and a paucity of gas in the distal decompressed small bowel.

Harvey CJ, Allen S, O'Regan D. Interpretation of the abdominal radiograph. *Br J Hosp Med (Lond)*. 2005;66(11):M66-M69. doi:10.12968/hmed.2005.66.Sup4.20038

8. **The answer is A**. The patient in this scenario likely has a free perforation from acute diverticulitis. He is not a candidate for percutaneous therapy because he has peritonitis and a drainable collection is unlikely to form this early, nor was evident on the CT scan. This patient will require operative exploration in an expedited fashion. However, the first priority is to start antibiotics (covering Gram-negative organisms and anaerobes) and resuscitate the patient with IV fluid. Since the patient is exhibiting signs of shock given his tachycardia and hypotension, the best disposition for this patient is in the ICU.

O'Leary DP, Lynch N, Clancy C, et al. International, expert-based, consensus statement regarding the management of acute diverticulitis. *JAMA Surg*. 2015;150(9):899-904. doi:10.1001/jamasurg.2015.1675

9. **The answer is A**. By history and by the CT scan results, this patient likely has a type II peptic ulcer. Type I ulcers are found in the lesser curve of the stomach, type II are duodenal, type III are prepyloric, type IV are located on the lesser curve close to the gastroesophageal (GE) junction, and type V are located anywhere in the stomach and are associated with NSAID use. Types II and III are classically associated with acid hypersecretion, while any of the types with the exception of type V are associated with *H. pylori* infection. Treatment priorities in this patient include intravenous (IV) antibiotics and operative closure of the perforation. Type I ulcers are usually treated with distal gastrectomy with a Billroth I or II to remove the ulcer. Type II and III can be treated with vagotomy and antrectomy. Type IV has a number of possibilities for surgical correction depending on the extent of the ulceration. Testing for *H. pylori* should also be done, and the patient should be treated if the test is positive.

Laine L. Upper gastrointestinal bleeding due to a peptic ulcer. *N Engl J Med*. 2016;374:2367-2376. doi:10.1056/NEJMcp1514257

10. **The answer is D**. Arterial emboli are the most common cause of acute occlusion of the SMA. The SMA is most commonly occluded because of its large caliber and narrow takeoff. These emboli most frequently arise from the heart, either from a mural thrombus after myocardial infarction (MI) or from the atria in patients with atrial fibrillation. Paradoxical embolism through a patent foramen ovale may also be a cause of arterial occlusion. The initial abdominal pain is severe and often out of proportion to the physical findings. The physical findings of peritonitis imply transmural ischemia and thus represent a late stage in the evolution of the process. Acute occlusion of the SMA does not result in complete foregut infarction because the proximal jejunum is typically spared in the case of embolic disease due to most emboli lodging 3 to 10 cm distal to the origin of the SMA. CT scan of the abdomen with IV contrast is very helpful in early diagnosis of acute mesenteric ischemia

Acosta S. Mesenteric ischemia. *Curr Opin Crit Care*. 2015;21(2):171-178. doi:10.1097/MCC.0000000000000189

11. **The answer is A**. Ischemic colitis should be considered in the differential diagnosis of any patient with lower abdominal pain and bright red blood per rectum, especially after an aortic aneurysm repair where the inferior mesenteric artery is usually sacrificed. It is most common in elderly patients, but can be found in patients of any age who also have polyarteritis nodosa, lupus, rheumatoid arthritis, scleroderma, or polycythemia vera. The severity of clinical presentation varies with the extent and duration of vascular occlusion, the adequacy of collateral circulation, and the extent of septic complications. Mild or moderate ischemia is compensated for by collateral circulation, and the mucosal sloughing usually heals in 2 to 3 days. Transmural ischemia may lead to future stricture development and ultimately may progress to full-thickness gangrene leading to perforation and peritonitis. In ischemic colitis, the vascular insult appears to be confined to small arterioles, sparing the major colonic vessels. Although the ischemia can affect any part of the colon, it is more common in the splenic

flexure and distal sigmoid colon. These areas have been traditionally referred to as "watershed" areas that rely on the marginal artery of Drummond for perfusion. Diagnosis is typically made via endoscopy, which usually reveals pale/edematous mucosa that may be covered by an exudative membrane. Barium enema is also often used for diagnosis, demonstrating classic thumb printing of the bowel wall. If perforation is suspected, these diagnostic modalities are contraindicated, and urgent laparotomy is the diagnostic and therapeutic modality of choice. Management is usually nonoperative, as the ischemia typically improves over several days with appropriate hydration and medical comorbidity optimization. Surgical therapy remains the mainstay of therapy for peritonitis and stricture development.

Trotter JM, Hunt L, Peter MB. Ischaemic colitis. *BMJ.* 2016;355:i6600. doi:10.1136/bmj.i6600

12. **The answer is C.** This patient has sigmoid volvulus. The first and foremost management principle is to ensure that the patient is nontoxic; that is, there is no peritonitis or shock. Maintenance of end-organ perfusion should be ensured with urine output monitoring and fluid resuscitation, as needed. For sigmoid volvulus without perforation, there is no need for the routine administration of antibiotics. Passing a sigmoidoscope past the point of obstruction allows immediate decompression of the dilated and gas-filled colonic segment. The likelihood of recurrence after sigmoidoscopic decompression is very high, and an elective sigmoid resection should be planned in the medically fit patient. Laxatives, cleansing enemas, and barium enemas are dangerous and can lead to colonic perforation. There is no role for decompressive transverse colostomy.

Kapadia MR. Volvulus of the small bowel and colon. *Clin Colon Rectal Surg.* 2017;30(1):40-45. doi:10.1055/s-2008-1075856

13. **The answer is C.** Among the answer choices, CT scan of the abdomen would be the best imaging modality to diagnose and distinguish between partial and complete bowel obstructions. It also provides additional information regarding the etiology of the obstruction. In the clinical scenario presented in the question, the most likely etiology is adhesive disease, although other causes are certainly possible. Addition of oral contrast, although helpful in identifying the transition point in cases of low-grade obstructions, is not mandatory. Many radiology protocols in tertiary care centers have abandoned the routine use of oral contrast for the diagnosis of bowel obstruction. It is important to appreciate that high-grade bowel obstructions can be associated with large fluid losses, both from vomiting and secondary to sequestration within the bowel wall and lumen. This may lead to profound hypovolemia with compromised end-organ perfusion. It is of utmost importance to ensure adequate volume status and electrolyte repletion. Elderly patients with multiple comorbidities may require ICU monitoring. Routine use of antibiotics is not recommended in cases of bowel obstruction without intestinal perforation.

Köstenbauer J, Truskett PG. Current management of adhesive small bowel obstruction. *ANZ J Surg.* May 14, 2018. doi:10.1111/ans.14556

14. **The answer is D.** The diagnosis of acute pancreatitis is based on the clinical presentation and supported by biochemical data and morphological findings on CT scan. There is no biochemical finding that is pathognomonic for pancreatitis. None of the other answer choices are specific or sensitive for the diagnosis of pancreatitis; they can occur in patients with other abdominal and extra-abdominal disorders. These other conditions include acute cholecystitis, intestinal infarction, and perforated peptic ulcer. In addition, severe pancreatitis can occur even without marked elevations in these serum enzymes. The mortality from pancreatitis can be predicted with Ranson's criteria that includes age, white blood cell (WBC), glucose, aspartate aminotransferase (AST), and lactate dehydrogenase (LDH). Reassessment at 48 hours includes the following variables: calcium, Hematocrit, PaO₂, blood urea nitrogen (BUN), base deficit, and sequestration of fluids.

Forsmark CE, Vege SS, Wilcox CM. Acute pancreatitis. *N Engl J Med.* 2016;375(20):1972-1981. doi:10.1056/NEJMra1505202

15. **The answer is B**. The diagnosis of pancreatitis is usually a presumptive one. Patients presenting with an acute onset of abdominal pain need a thorough workup to exclude other causes of abdominal pain for which immediate laparotomy may be indicated. In a patient with acute pancreatitis, the initial management is nonoperative and focuses on fluid resuscitation and prevention of complications. These patients are usually best managed in an intensive care setting. Gastric decompression is often indicated because of the associated paralytic ileus and delayed gastric emptying. Controlled studies have consistently demonstrated no benefit from empiric antibiotics in patients with pancreatitis. If there is evidence of pancreatic necrosis with superimposed infection, then antibiotics are definitely recommended. Planned surgical exploration in patients with acute pancreatitis is associated with a significantly higher rate of complications. Operation is therefore delayed until complications such as hemorrhage or infection arise.

Forsmark CE, Vege SS, Wilcox CM. Acute pancreatitis. *N Engl J Med*. 2016;375(20):1972-1981. doi:10.1056/NEJMra1505202

16. **The answer is D**. Pancreatic infection complicating acute pancreatitis should be suspected in any patient who fails to improve with supportive medical therapy or who initially improves but then deteriorates clinically. Pancreatic infection occasionally occurs early in the course of the disease, but typically presents later as in the clinical scenario presented in the question. CT scanning is the best method for pancreatic imaging and should be used frequently in patients with severe pancreatitis. When pancreatic infection is present, operative drainage and debridement are the gold standard for treatment. While some specialized centers have had success with laparoscopic or endoscopic drainage techniques, these modalities should be reserved for practitioners with significant experience with these techniques. Commonly, these infections are caused by gut bacteria such as *E. coli, Pseudomonas, Klebsiella*, and *Enterococcus*. Empiric antibiotics when initiated should consist of a carbapenem, or a quinolone, ceftazidime, or cefepime combined with metronidazole for anaerobic coverage.

Werge M, Novovic S, Schmidt PN, et al. Infection increases mortality in necrotizing pancreatitis: a systemic review and meta-analysis. *Pancreatology*. 2016;16(5):698-707. doi:10.1016/j.pan.2016.07.004

17. **The answer is C**. Bladder dysfunction has been reported in up to 50% of patients after abdominoperineal resection and/or other major pelvic surgery. The type of voiding dysfunction that occurs depends on the specific nerve involved and the degree of injury. The majority of patients are best treated by clean intermittent catheterization. Most patients (80%) will have resolution of their symptoms in 3 to 6 months. The use of a chronic catheter is of benefit in some patients; however, chronic catheterization carries a higher risk of infection. The use of alpha-blockers alone or transurethral resection of the prostate is likely to be unsuccessful. Transurethral sphincterotomy does not treat the underlying problem and may actually lead to incontinence.

Prieto JA, Murphy C, Moore KN, et al. Intermittent catheterisation for long-term bladder management (abridged cochrane review). *Neurourol Urodyn*. 2015;34(7):648-653. doi:10.1002/nau.22792

18. **The answer is C**. All patients with gross hematuria and all patients with microscopic hematuria on two separate urinalyses require some sort of evaluation. Patients should undergo upper-tract imaging, cystoscopic studies, bladder washings, and a pelvic examination. It is important to evaluate the urinalyses for signs of infection and proteinuria. The differential diagnosis consists of nephrolithiasis, renal or bladder cancer, urinary tract infection, bleeding disorders, trauma, benign or essential hematuria, or prostatic disorders (in men).

Cohen RA, Brown RS. Clinical practice. Microscopic hematuria. *N Engl J Med*. 2003;348(23): 2330-2338. doi:10.1056/NEJMcp012694

19. **The answer is A**. Bladder injury may occur from blunt or penetrating trauma or during pelvic surgery. When associated with pelvic fractures, the injury is usually to the extraperitoneal

bladder, caused by the shearing force of the pelvic fracture. Isolated extraperitoneal bladder rupture is treated with 7 to 10 days of Foley drainage. Blunt injury without pelvic fracture is associated with intraperitoneal bladder rupture, particularly if the bladder is full and the injury occurs at the dome of the distended bladder. Bladder trauma should be suspected in any patient with lower abdominal trauma if there is hematuria or the patient is unable to void. Single-view cystographic studies will likely miss a significant injury. The treatment for an intraperitoneal bladder injury typically requires operative repair with a two-layer closure. Intraoperative injury typically does not require a suprapubic cystostomy, but does require suture repair with several days of bladder drainage with a Foley catheter. It is mandatory to be vigilant that the Foley catheter does not become obstructed, as this could lead to bladder distention and breakdown of the repair.

Pereira BM, de Campos CC, Calderan TR, et al. Bladder injuries after external trauma: 20 years experience report in a population-based cross-sectional view. *World J Urol.* 2013;31(4): 913-917. doi:10.1007/s00345-012-0871-8

20. **The answer is B**. Pelvic inflammatory disease can encompass a wide spectrum of clinical presentations, which can range from mild, vague pelvic symptoms to fatal intra-abdominal sepsis. In certain cases, the inflammation can extend to the liver capsule, causing acute perihepatitis or Fitz-Hugh-Curtis syndrome, a localized inflammation marked by a purulent or fibrinous exudate affecting the surface of the liver (Glisson capsule), which can cause referred pain from the adjacent diaphragm. Clinical presentation is usually characterized by acute onset of severe RUQ which can be confusing for acute cholecystitis. Chlamydia trachomatis is the most common organism. Associated signs and symptoms include fever, leukocytosis, abdominal pain, cervicitis, and mildly elevated transaminases. Asherman syndrome is the presence of intrauterine adhesions, usually associated with endometrial curettage that presents due to secondary amenorrhea. Meigs syndrome consists of a benign ovarian tumor with associated ascites and pleural effusion. Sheehan syndrome is a functional hypopituitarism that occurs due to ischemic necrosis of the pituitary gland secondary to peripartum hypotension, usually due to excessive hemorrhage and shock.

Brunham RC, Gottlieb SL, Paavonen J. Pelvic inflammatory disease. *N Engl J Med.* 2015;372(21): 2039-2048. doi:10.1056/NEJMra1411426

21. **The answer is C**. Lactulose is a synthetic disaccharide that is not absorbed in the gastrointestinal (GI) track, and is metabolized by colonic flora to short-chain fatty acids like lactate. This causes a significant decrease in pH, allowing the trapping of ammonia for excretion with stool, and thereby decreasing plasma ammonia concentrations. Lactulose also causes an osmotic diarrhea, which can lead to the loss of a large amount of bicarbonate and organic acid anions. The dose of lactulose needs to be titrated to achieve two to three soft stools per day.

Wijdicks EF. Hepatic encephalopathy. *N Engl J Med.* 2016;375(17):1660-1670. doi:10.1056/ NEJMra1600561

22. **The answer is D**. The patient has hypochloremic metabolic alkalosis secondary to the loss of H^+ and Cl^- in the gastric acid via his nasogratric tube (NGT) and vomiting outputs. This leads to an overall positive bicarbonate balance in the body. The normal renal compensatory mechanism of bicarbonate excretion requires sodium as a cotransport ion, and is impaired in the setting of overall dehydration, resulting in a metabolic alkalosis. The respiratory system tries to compensate by hypoventilation to increase carbon dioxide retention to buffer the alkalosis via carbonic anhydrase.

Normal saline (NS) has the highest sodium and chloride content of the isotonic resuscitative fluids that is required to facilitate the excretion of bicarbonate by the kidneys and should be administered to the patient. Each liter contains 154 mEq of sodium, compared with 130 mEq in lactated Ringer, and 140 mEq in Plasma-Lyte A. Chloride is needed as the replacement anion. Treatment also benefits from inclusion of potassium in patients with adequate renal function. Acetazolamide can be considered for treatment in patients who are not intravascular volume depleted. Careful administration of acids, such as hydrochloric acid, ammonium chloride, arginine hydrochloride, and lysine hydrochloride, can be used in patients with severe metabolic alkalosis with renal insufficiency.

Soifer JT, Kim HT. Approach to metabolic alkalosis. *Emerg Med Clin North Am*. 2014; 32(2): 453-463. doi:10.1016/j.emc.2014.01.005

23. **The answer is D**. This patient is presenting with spontaneous bacterial peritonitis (SBP). Common presenting signs and symptoms are increasing abdominal distention, worsening pain, nausea and vomiting, low-grade fevers, AMS, diarrhea, and or ileus. CT scan is often unremarkable except for ascites in the abdomen. Ultrasound of the abdomen can also be useful to diagnose ascites as well as for assistance with paracentesis. Laboratory abnormalities often include a leukocytosis and possibly an increase in BUN and creatinine due to an onset of hepatorenal syndrome (HRS).

Indications for paracentesis include clinical deterioration including hypotension, worsening mental status, acidosis, leukocytosis, and worsening renal function. The diagnostic criteria for SBP by paracentesis includes an ascitic fluid polymorphonuclear cell count of at least 250/mL, a positive ascitic fluid culture, and absence of secondary causes of peritonitis.

Treatment of SBP begins after the diagnosis is made by paracentesis. Antibiotics are a mainstay of treatment and choice of antibiotics should be made with local resistance patterns taken into consideration. Most SBP is caused by *E. coli* or *Klebsiella*, with smaller numbers coming from streptococcal and staphylococcal species. Initial treatment should begin with a third-generation cephalosporin such as ceftriaxone, cefpodoxime, cefdinir, or cefotaxime. Fluoroquinolones can also be used in the initial treatment of SBP. Antibiotic resistance is a large problem in this population, so the antibiotic regimen should be narrowed as culture data becomes available.

Renal failure is a major concern in patients who develop SBP. About 30% to 40% of patients who develop SBP will have some form of renal failure. The development of renal failure is attributed to the activation of the renal-angiotensin system and an effective decrease in intravascular volume. Studies have shown that patients who are started on albumin replacement therapy (1.5 gm/kg on day 1 and 1.0 gm/kg on day 3) have significantly reduced incidence of renal impairment and a decreased mortality.

Koulaouzidis A, Bhat S, Saeed AA. Spontaneous bacterial peritonitis. *World J Gastroenterol*. 2009; 15(9): 1042-109. doi:10.3748/wjg.15.1042

23

Diagnosis of Brain Death

SUBHASHINI RAMESH

▨ QUESTIONS

1. The committee recognized in the United States as attempting to first define brain death was:

   A. The Minnesota Code of brain death
   B. The Joint Committee of the Royal College of Physicians
   C. The Ad Hoc Committee of the Harvard Medical School to Examine the Definition of Brain Death
   D. The Mayo Committee for the determination of irreversible coma

2. The 2010 American Academy of Neurology (AAN) guidelines for determining brain death in adults noted:

   A. Recoveries in adults have been reported since the adoption of the AAN 1995 guidelines
   B. The apnea test is safe using the apnea oxygenation method
   C. Confirmatory tests are reliable and useful
   D. There is evidence to support a minimally acceptable observation period to ensure neurologic functions have ceased irreversibly.

3. The act that led to determining death based on neurological criteria was:

   A. U.S. Collaborative Study of Cerebral Death Act
   B. The Uniform Determination of Death Act (UDDA)
   C. The Snyder Act
   D. The Wagner National Health Act

4. Ancillary tests are not mandatory to make a diagnosis of brain death in:

   A. United States
   B. Poland
   C. Germany
   D. Ireland

5. The term used to describe the neuropathological findings in brain death is:

   A. Respirator brain
   B. Asphyxial encephalopathy
   C. Neuritic plaques
   D. Subcortical leukoencephalopathy

6. Caution should be used in performing brain death testing in a patient:

    A. Who was recently treated with moderate hypothermia
    B. In whom neuroimaging explains coma
    C. With no acid base disturbance
    D. With absent brainstem reflexes

7. The technique of the commonly used apnea test is called:

    A. Apneic oxygenation diffusion test
    B. Continuous oxygen supplementation technique
    C. Intermittent positive pressure ventilation
    D. Extracorporeal respiratory support

8. Motor responses during the exam:

    A. Are common
    B. Are uncommon
    C. Suggest faulty technique
    D. Argue against brain death

9. What level of hypernatremia is acceptable in brain death?

    A. 175
    B. 160
    C. 200
    D. Only normonatremia is acceptable

10. How can breathing drive be differentiated from ventilator auto cycling?

    A. Increasing the tidal volume
    B. Decreasing trigger sensitivity
    C. Reducing the respiratory rate (RR)
    D. Raising the positive end-expiratory pressure (PEEP)

11. The following are believed to be mimics of brain death, except:

    A. Guillain-Barre syndrome (GBS)
    B. Baclofen overdose
    C. Delayed vecuronium clearance
    D. Barbiturate overdose
    E. Hyperthermia

12. Pupillary reactivity in a brain dead person shows:

    A. Midpoint 4 to 6 mm and absent light reflex
    B. Divergent eyes with normal size and reflex
    C. Convergent eyes with normal size and reflex
    D. Midpoint or pinpoint, with absent light reflex

13. All these ancillary tests measure blood flow in brain death, except:

    A. EEG
    B. Transcranial Doppler (TCD)
    C. Four-vessel cerebral angiogram
    D. Nuclear perfusion scan

14. After the declaration of brain death, who meets with the family to request organ donation?

    A. The attending physician
    B. The attending physician in the presence of the organ procurement organization (OPO) coordinator
    C. The transplant surgeon
    D. The OPO coordinator

15. After a patient is declared brain dead, no civil or criminal liability will result from removing the body from life support in all but which of these two states, where physicians are required to honor the family's religious obligations?

    A. Georgia and South Carolina
    B. California and Wisconsin
    C. New York and New Jersey
    D. Montana and Utah

16. Brain-death criteria may include an ancillary atropine test. The response that supports the diagnosis of brain death is:

    A. Constriction of pupils
    B. Heart rate (HR) acceleration at least 10 beats per minute (BPM) above the baseline
    C. Absent bowel sounds and decreased urine output
    D. HR acceleration less than 5 BPM above the patient's baseline

17. Which statement(s) is correct in regard to donation after cardiac death (DCD)?

    A. Anticipates that cardiac arrest will occur within 3 hours
    B. May provide kidney, liver, and lung for transplantation
    C. Requires that asystole or pulselessness be sustained for more than 10 minutes before cardiac death is declared
    D. Excludes members of a recipient's transplantation team from determining the time of death
    E. Both B and D are correct

■ ANSWERS

1. **The answer is C.** In the United States, the initial attempt to determine death based on neurologic criteria is often attributed to the 1968 Harvard criteria. However, the first steps toward using loss of cerebral function to define death actually began a decade earlier in France, where physicians Mollaret and Goulon published an article "Le Coma depasse," often considered the signature piece in the development of clinical criteria of death by neurologic standards. The Harvard criteria were published in the *Journal of the American Medical Association* (*JAMA*) on August 5, 1968. It was titled "A definition of irreversible coma." The criteria included "unreceptivity and unresponsivity no movements or breathing, absent brainstem reflexes, and a flat electroencephalogram." All of the above tests were repeated after at least 24 hours of no change or hypothermia (below 32.2°C). Central nervous system depressants had to be excluded. A lot of our knowledge about brain death has since changed and the current criteria used in the United States were specified by the quality standards subcommittee of the American Academy of Neurology Practice Parameters for determining brain death in adults; initially published in 1995 and subsequently updated in 2010.

   A definition of irreversible coma. Report of the Ad Hoc Committee of the Harvard Medical School to examine the definition of brain death. *JAMA*. 1968;205:337-340. doi: 10.1001/jama.1968.03140320031009

2. **The answer is B.** The new 2010 AAN guidelines separated evidence-based data from opinion based data. These guidelines noted that:

   • No recoveries in adults have been reported since the adoption of the AAN 1995 guidelines.

   • The apnea test is safe using the apnea oxygenation method.

   • Confirmatory tests are less reliable and useful than has been suggested and should be sparingly used.

   • Adequate documentation may be facilitated with checklist.

   • There is insufficient evidence to determine the minimally acceptable observation period to ensure that neurologic functions have ceased irreversibly.

   Wijdicks EFM, Varelas PN, Gronseth GS, et al. Evidence based guideline update: determining brain death in adults. Report of the quality Standards Subcommittee of the American Academy of Neurology. *Neurology*. 2010;74:1911-1918. doi:10.1212/WNL.0b013e3181e242a8

3. **The answer is B.** The President's Commission for the Study of Ethical Problems in Medicine and Biomedical and Behavioral Research published guidelines in 1981 defining brain death as an irreversible cessation of all clinically ascertainable functions of the entire brain including the brainstem. This was to be demonstrated by unreceptivity, unresponsivity, absent brainstem reflexes, and apnea. The report specifically indicated that true decerebrate or decorticate posturing or seizures was inconsistent with a diagnosis of brain death. This report led to the UDDA, whereby an individual who has sustained either (1) irreversible cessation of circulatory or respiratory function or (2) irreversible cessation of all function of the entire brain including the brainstem, could be pronounced deceased. A determination of death must be made in accordance with accepted medical standards.

   President's Commission for the Study of Ethical Problems in Medicine and Biomedical and Behavioral Research. *Defining Death: A Report on the Medical Legal and Ethical Issues in the Determination of Death*. Washington, DC: Government Printing Office; 1981.

4. **The answer is A.** In the earlier days of refining criteria in the diagnosis of brain death there was a desire to show additional absent electrical function or absent blood flow to the brain. In the United States, the EEG became a part of the clinical determination of brain death after the publication of the Harvard criteria. The American Neurological Association stated in 1977 that the EEG was a valuable confirmatory indicator of brain death and its use was strongly

recommended. However, as we have gained more knowledge and experience in the determination of death by neurological criteria, the latest 2010 American Academy of Neurology (AAN) guideline argues against the routine use of ancillary tests, specifically stating that confirmatory tests are less reliable and useful than has been suggested and should be used sparingly. The tests can be divided into those that evaluate neuronal function and those that assess blood flow. In Europe, there is fairly uniform agreement on the criteria for evaluation of brain death, but there remains considerable variation in use of ancillary tests. In a recent survey of 25 countries, 11 required confirmatory tests, including Poland, Ireland, and Germany.

Wijdicks EFM. The case against confirmatory tests for determining brain death in adults. *Neurology.* 2010;75:77-83. doi:10.1212/WNL.0b013e3181e62194

5. **The answer is A.** The extent of neuropathologic findings varies in brain death. The typical finding of a "respirator brain," where there is complete necrosis with a musky brain and disintegration when the cerebrum is removed from the skull, is now uncommon. Respirator brain occured due to prolonged support of a poorly or nonperfused brain. The most recognizable finding is a herniated swollen brain with autolysis of herniated cerebellar tonsils. In some cases the tonsils can displace into the intrathecal space and widespread ischemic neuronal changes are found. The microscopic abnormalities surprisingly spare vulnerable areas such as the hippocampus.

Leestma J, Hughes J, Diamond E. Temporal correlates in brain death. EEG and clinical relationships to the respirator brain. *Arch Neurol.* 1984;41:147-152. doi:10.1001/archneur. 1984.04050140045021

6. **The answer is A.** The presence of a central nervous system (CNS)-depressing drug effect may be excluded by history, drug screen, and calculation of clearance using 5 times the drug's half-life, assuming normal renal and hepatic function. If possible, drug plasma levels should be drawn. The half-life of commonly used sedative medications can be prolonged in patients who have received therapeutic hypothermia. Doubling the "five half-lives" rule may be inadequate and caution should be exercised in evaluating such patients. It may be prudent to wait several days prior to proceeding with formal brain death testing.

Webb A, Samuels O. Reversible brain death following cardiopulmonary arrest. *Crit Care Med.* 2010;38(suppl):723.

7. **The answer is A.** Apneic oxygenation diffusion is the most commonly used technique to demonstrate lack of ventilatory drive. The 2010 American Academy of Neurology (AAN) guideline recognized that the apnea test, using the apneic oxygenation method, is safe. This diagnostic tool involves placement of a source of 100% oxygen in the trachea with subsequent convection resulting in lung oxygenation. Pre-oxygenation to a PaO_2 >200 mmHg results in elimination of nitrogen stores and facilitates oxygen transfer. An oxygen insulation catheter proving O_2 at a rate of 6 L/min is usually placed 1 cm beyond the tip of the endotracheal tube after the patient is disconnected from the ventilator. A target $PaCO_2$ of 60 mmHg has been proposed as the level at which the respiratory centers are maximally stimulated. Absence of breathing during this time period suggests a positive apnea test. Hypotension is the most common complication and the patient should be reconnected to the ventilator when systolic blood pressure (SBP) drops below 70 mmHg. The 2010 AAN guidelines state that that there is insufficient evidence to determine the comparative safety of techniques used for apnea testing.

Jumah M, McLean DR, Rajesh S, et al. Bulk diffusion apnea test in the diagnosis of brain death. *Crit Care Med.* 1992;20:1564-1567. doi:10.1097/00003246-199211000-00014

Wijdicks EFM, Varelas PN, Gronseth GS, et al. Evidence based guideline update: determining brain death in adults. Report of the quality Standards Subcommittee of the American Academy of Neurology. *Neurology.* 2010;74:1911-1918. doi:10.1212/WNL.0b013e3181e242a8

8. **The answer is A.** Noxious stimuli should produce no motor response other than spinal-mediated reflexes. Careful note should be made to ensure that absent motor responses are not due to a severed cervical cord. Motor responses may occur spontaneously, after stimulation or during the apnea test, especially when hypoxemia or hypotension occurs. These spinal responses can include slow movements in the upper limbs, flexion of the fingers, or fine finger tremors, but should not integrate into decerebrate or decorticate responses. Ocular micro tremors, slow head turning to one side, and the Lazarus sign have been reported but are rare. These movements extinguish with repeated stimulation.

Bueri JA, Saposnik G, Maurino J, et al. Lazarus' sign in brain death. *Mov Disord*. 2000;15:583-586. doi:10.1002/1531-8257(200005)15:3<583:AID-MDS1026>3.0.CO;2-Y

9. **The answer is B.** Of all the electrolyte abnormalities, hypernatremia is most common in brain death and considered a confounding factor. It is usually due to net water loss from diabetes insipidus (DI), or from iatrogenic administration of hyperosmolar therapy like mannitol and hypertonic saline prior to the diagnosis of brain death. The level at which hypernatremia may confound the clinical exam is defined as 160 mmol/L or more. However, plasma osmolality may be better correlated with drowsiness than an absolute value of sodium, and the cutoff is believed to be about 350 mosm/L. Treatment usually consists of correction of water deficits using D5W. The rate can be calculated using the Adrogue Madias formula.

Aiyagari V, Deibert E, Diringer MN. Hypernatremia in the neurologic intensive care unit: how high is too high? *J Crit Care*. 2006;21:163-172. doi:10.1016/j.jcrc.2005.10.002

10. **The answer is B.** It is indeed alarming when a brain dead patient appears to be triggering the ventilator. This phenomenon may indicate ventilator auto-cycling and is fairly common. Flow triggered mode is susceptible to noise and auto triggering can occur from leaks in the circuit. "Breaths" usually trigger if sensitivity is set at a high-level and decreasing the trigger sensitivity level will cause these breaths to disappear. Ventilator auto-cycling can also be due to pericardial movements.

Harboe S, Hjalmarsson S, Soreide E. Autocycling and increase in intrinsic positive end expiratory pressure during mechanical ventilation. *Acta Anaesthesiol Scand*. 2001;45:1295-1297. doi:10.1034/j.1399-6576.2001.451021.x

11. **The answer is E.** There are no reports in peer-reviewed medical journals of conditions mimicking brain death that have described a complete brain death exam. Several studies have, however, claimed brain death can be mimicked by GBS, baclofen overdose, barbiturate overdose, and delayed vecuronium clearance. Any intoxication with sedative medications can mimic brain death, but pupillary responses will remain intact. Another major mimicking condition is hypothermia, which is also a manifestation of brain death, but temperatures rarely fall below 35°C. Moreover, Osborne waves are never seen on ECG and, if present, point toward severe accidental hypothermia.

Joshi MC, Azim A, Gupta GL, et al. Guillain Barre syndrome with absent brainstem reflexes-a report of two cases. *Anaesth Intensive Care*. 2008;36:867-869.

12. **The answer is A.** The response to bright light should be absent in both eyes. Round, oval, or irregularly shaped pupils may be seen. Most are midpoint, 4 to 6 mm in size. Many drugs can influence pupil size but light response remains intact. In conventional doses, atropine has no influence on pupillary size in a brain-dead individual. Preexisting anatomic abnormalities to the iris or effects of previous surgery should be excluded.

Shulgman D, Parulekar M, Elston JS, et al. Abnormal pupillary activity in a brainstem dead patient. *Br J Anaesth*. 2001;86:717-720. doi:10.1093/bja/86.5.717

13. **The answer is A.** The American Academy of Neurology (AAN) in 1977 stated that the EEG was a "valuable indicator of brain death and its use is strongly recommended." In fact, the EEG became a part of the clinical examination of these patients after the publication of the

Harvard report. During the years since that report, additional ancillary tests have been introduced. These can be divided into those that tests neuronal function and those that assess cerebral blood flow. Electrophysiologic tests include EEG and auditory and sensory evoked potentials, while tests of brain flow include four vessel angiography, TCD, CT angiogram (CTA), magnetic resonance angiogram (MRA), and nuclear medicine studies. The determination of brain death is a clinical assessment. In the United States, ancillary tests are helpful when they do what they are supposed to: confirm the clinical diagnosis of brain death. The most common indication for ancillary tests in suspected brain death is the inability to perform or complete the apnea test.

Wijdicks EFM. The case against confirmatory tests for determining brain death in adults. *Neurology*. 2010;75:77-83. doi:10.1212/WNL.0b013e3181e62194

14. **The answer is D.** Hospitals must report all deaths to the OPO in a timely manner. The OPO determines medical suitability and only an OPO staff member may approach the family of a potential donor for consent for organ, tissue, or eye donation. The Uniform Anatomical Gift Act (UAGA) grants individuals the power to donate organs and tissue. The OPO may request that life-sustaining interventions continue so as to preserve organs.

Iltis AS, Rie MA, Wall A. Organ donation, patient's rights, and medical responsibilities at the end of life. *Crit Care Med*. 2009;37:310-315. doi:10.1097/CCM.0b013e3181928ff8

15. **The answer is C.** The main consequence of Uniform Declaration of Death Act (UDDA) is that a patient that has been declared brain dead will be declared deceased, and wills and insurance proceedings become active. No civil or criminal liability will arise from removing the body from life support. In New York and New Jersey, however, devout Orthodox Jewish families may demand that support be continued due to a law that was enacted by the two states to provide this exception.

Uniform Determination of Death Act, 12 uniform laws annotated 589 (West 1993 & West supp 1997).

16. **The answer is D.** When required, the dose of atropine specified by the hospital policy is given intravenously. Loss of vagal response to atropine eliminates the expected tachycardia and hence an accelerated heart rate would negate the diagnosis of brain death because of a responsive vagal effect.

Hutterman E, Schelenze C, Sakka SG, et al. Atropine test and circulatory arrest in the posterior fossa assessed by transcranial Doppler. *Intensive Care Med*. 2000;26:422-425. doi:10.1007/s001340051176

17. **The answer is E.** DCD organ donation anticipates rapid progress to cardiac arrest after life-sustaining measures are withdrawn. This rapidity intends to minimize "warm ischemic time" of diminishing organ perfusion during a prolonged period of decreasing blood pressure (BP), oxygenation, and so on. While no regulations specify the duration of tolerable warm ischemic time, the customary time permitted is about 1 hour. Usually if cardiac arrest has not occurred during that time, organ removal is canceled and the patient is moved from the operating room to another patient unit. Either asystole or an absent pulse waveform during intravascular monitoring or to palpation initiates a waiting time before pronouncement of cardiac death and organ procurement. National recommendations and common practice (no regulations, only individual hospital policy) use either 3 or 5 minutes of sustained asystole or pulselessness before organs may be removed. Individual policies address the response if recovery of cardiac function occurs after initial pulselessness or asystole, but before pronouncement of cardiac death. Kidneys and the liver are commonly removed for donation, and with increasing frequency one or both lungs are being recovered. Most policies eclipsed members of the recipient transplant team from any function until the patient has been declared deceased by the physician in attendance with that responsibility.

Frontera JA. How I manage the adult potential organ donor: donation after cardiac death (Part 2). *Neurocrit Care*. 2010;12:111-116. doi:10.1007/s12028-009-9294-9

24

General Trauma and Burns

SASHA D. ADAMS, NORI L. BRADLEY, AND
AMY R. ALGER

▨ QUESTIONS

1. For evaluation of the cervical spine after trauma:

   A. Cervical collar can be removed from an awake patient with a painful femur fracture who does not complain of neck pain
   B. Cervical spine should be evaluated by three-view cervical spine series supplemented by swimmer's views as needed
   C. Flexion/extension radiography should not be performed on an obtunded patient
   D. All penetrating cranial injuries must be stabilized with a cervical collar
   E. Isolated severe blunt traumatic brain injury (TBI) is rarely associated with cervical spine injury

2. Angiographic evaluation of the neck for vascular injury is warranted in all of the following situations, **except**:

   A. Blunt trauma with neurologic deficit and no closed head injury
   B. C3 vertebral body fracture through the foramen transversarium
   C. Seat belt abrasion on the anterio-lateral neck
   D. Hyperextension or hyperflexion mechanism of injury
   E. Orbital wall fracture

3. Which of the following is **not** a risk factor for coagulopathy following multisystem trauma?

   A. Resuscitation with 6 L crystalloid, 10 units of packed red blood cells (RBCs) and 10 units of fresh-frozen plasma (FFP)
   B. Prolonged exposure and hypothermia
   C. Traumatic brain injury (TBI)
   D. Metabolic alkalosis
   E. 75-year-old patient with coronary artery disease (CAD)

4. A healthy 30-year-old multisystem trauma patient is in the ICU for resuscitation. He has a known pelvic fracture, traumatic subarachnoid hemorrhage (tSAH), and multiple extremity fractures. Hct = 17, pulmonary artery catheter (PAC) shows cardiac index of 1.8, systemic vascular resistance (SVR) = 3,000, and wedge pressure is 5. Urine output is 10 mL/hour. The most appropriate initial treatment would be:

   A. Start levophed drip, goal mean arterial pressure (MAP) >60 mmHg
   B. Give 3% hypertonic saline bolus
   C. Renal dose dopamine
   D. Lasix 40 mg intravenous (IV) × 1
   E. Blood transfusion

5. After emergent craniotomy for a large epidural hemorrhage, a 21-year-old ejected unrestrained passenger of a motor vehicle collision (MVC) is brought to the ICU for the remainder of his workup. On examination of an open humeral fracture, which of the following signs does not require immediate vascular operative intervention?

   A. Pulsatile bleeding
   B. Expanding hematoma
   C. Proximity of wound or injury to artery
   D. Absent or diminished distal pulse
   E. Cold blue hand

6. A 21-year-old man is admitted to the ICU after being involved in a motorcycle collision (MCC) in which he was thrown 20 feet. He is intubated with a closed head injury, and although he initially responded to 2 L crystalloid resuscitation, is now hypotensive in the ICU. His pelvic x-ray revealed a fractured pelvis with anterolateral compression, and CT scan did not find any intra-abdominal injury or contrast extravasation near fracture sites. The next step in management should be:

   A. Angioembolization of active hemorrhage
   B. Placement of pelvic binder
   C. Give 2 L of crystalloid fluid
   D. Start epinephrine drip
   E. Exploratory laparotomy

7. An 18-year-old woman is involved in a motorcycle collision and is admitted with bilateral femoral fractures and closed head injury. She is intubated and taken to the ICU for monitoring. On hospital day 2 she is taken to the OR for bilateral femur fixation with placement of intramedullary rods. She receives 1 unit of packed red blood cells (RBCs) in the operating room (OR). Postoperatively, she is increasingly hypoxic, is refractory to conventional ventilation, has bilateral pulmonary infiltrates on chest x-ray (CXR), and worsening altered mental status (AMS). All the following are possible causes of hypoxia, **except**:

   A. Fat embolism syndrome (FES)
   B. Aspiration
   C. Transfusion-related acute lung injury (TRALI)
   D. Pulmonary contusion
   E. Bronchial injury

8. If the diagnosis for the patient in Question 7 is fat embolism syndrome (FES):

   A. Without ventilator support, FES can be fatal
   B. There are strict diagnostic criteria for FES
   C. She should be started immediately on steroids and heparin
   D. Respiratory symptoms are typically of short duration
   E. Delayed femur fixation would have decreased her risk of symptoms

9. A 54-year-old man is in the ICU for serial neurological exams following a low-speed motor vehicle collision (MVC) with traumatic subarachnoid hemorrhage (tSAH) and a right tibial-plateau fracture. He has been stable over the past 10 hours, but is complaining of increasing pain in his leg. He states he cannot move his toes, and he describes a tingling sensation near his first toe. On physical exam, his right leg is swollen and tense, with palpable dorsalis pedis/posterior tibial (DP/PT) pulses. The next step in management should be:

   A. Elevate the leg
   B. Check an ankle brachial index
   C. Call the surgeon

D. Elastic compression bandage

E. Electromyography (EMG)

10. A 67-year-old homeless man jumps off a bridge and lands on his feet. He has altered mental status (AMS) due to alcohol intoxication. What injury pattern is typically seen with this mechanism?

A. Calcaneal fracture

B. Rib fractures

C. Lumbar spine fracture

D. A and C

E. All of the above

11. A 19-year-old man was unrestrained and ejected following a high-speed motor vehicle collision (MVC). His injuries include multiple rib fractures on the right and a hemopneumothorax for which a right-sided chest tube is placed. Of the following choices, which indicates a need for immediate surgical intervention?

A. Persistent pneumothorax on chest radiograph

B. Initial 900 mL of sanguineous output following tube placement

C. 200 mL/hour of sanguineous drainage for 4 hours

D. SaO_2 of 86% and pulmonary contusion on chest CT scan

12. A 25-year-old woman involved in a high-speed motorcycle accident is admitted to the ICU with a grade IV liver laceration, multiple right-sided rib fractures and associated pulmonary contusion, left femur fracture, and facial trauma. She is intubated and on mechanical ventilation. Over the first 24 hours, she has received 6 units of packed red blood cells (pRBC), 6 units of fresh-frozen plasma (FFP), a platelet 6-pack, and 6 L of crystalloid, after which she stabilized. On ICU day 3, she becomes hypotensive to 96/54 mmHg, plateau airway pressures are 34 mmHg, and pCO_2 is 55 mmHg. Urine output has decreased over the past 6 hours to 10 mL/hour. Blood draw reveals a creatinine of 2.8 g/dL, up from 1.0 on admission, and hemoglobin is stable from ICU day 2 at 9.8 mg/dL. Central venous pressure (CVP) is 18. Bladder pressure is measured at 32 mmHg. The next intervention is:

A. Angiography for liver embolization

B. Operative abdominal decompression

C. Continuous venovenous hemofiltration (CVVH)

D. PRBC and FFP transfusion

E. Bronchoscopy

13. A 45-year-old man was thrown from a horse. He presented to the ED hypotensive at 90/50, but responded to a fluid bolus and has remained normotensive since. Imaging revealed a small subdural hematoma (SDH) for which he is being observed, right 10–11 rib fractures, and a grade III liver laceration.

A. Nonoperative management of liver lacerations results in increased length of hospital stay

B. If liver lacerations are managed nonoperatively, the patient should remain on bed rest for 1 week

C. Nonoperative management is appropriate for grades I and II liver laceration, but grades III and IV require either operation or angioembolization

D. Nonoperative management can be used for select cases of penetrating trauma with isolated liver injury

E. The CT scan should be repeated prior to discharge to ensure healing of the liver laceration

14. A 38-year-old man is admitted to the ICU after being involved in a motor vehicle collision (MVC) as an unrestrained driver. Among other injuries, he has significant bruising to his chest from the steering wheel, and there is a sternal fracture and several left-sided rib fractures on his chest x-ray (CXR). You are concerned about blunt cardiac injury (BCI).

    A. Normal ECG, enzymes, and blood pressure (BP) rule out BCI
    B. Angiography should be performed immediately to look for injury
    C. Cardiac enzymes, specifically creatine kinase MB isoenzyme (CK-MB), should be checked three times at 8-hour intervals and, if elevated, further workup for cardiac injury is warranted
    D. His sternum should be operatively stabilized
    E. An echocardiogram should be done on all patients with blunt chest trauma

15. A 37-year-old woman was brought to the ICU after assault, with injuries including blunt head trauma and stab wounds to the arm and anterior midabdomen. The only studies obtained were a CT scan of the head and plain films of the chest and abdomen. On local wound exploration, her stab wounds did not appear to violate the fascia, and she was followed with serial exams. On ICU day 2 she is hypotensive, oliguric, and on exam has increased abdominal distension. What is your next step in management?

    A. Obtain upright kidney–ureter–bladder (KUB) x-ray
    B. Start dopamine infusion, mean arterial pressure (MAP) >60 mmHg
    C. Hold tube feeds for 1 hour, then restart
    D. Give lasix 20 mg intravenous (IV) × 1
    E. 3% hypertonic saline bolus

16. A patient with third-degree burns on 5% of his lower extremities is being treated with topical agents. Concerns include:

    A. Mafenide acetate is painful when applied
    B. Silver nitrate has good penetrance of eschar
    C. Pseudomonas is best treated with silver sulfadiazine
    D. Silver sulfadiazine is associated with significant electrolyte abnormalities
    E. Metabolic acidosis is seen following silver nitrate treatment

17. A 26-year-old with electrical burns is brought to the ED after grabbing a high-voltage power line with both hands at work. He fell out of a bucket approximately 25 feet to the ground and was unconscious. He has third-degree burns over a 3% body surface area (BSA) and weighs 75 kg. He has been intubated and taken to the operating room emergently for bilateral upper extremity fasciotomies and muscle debridement. The most appropriate management would be:

    A. Intravenous (IV) fluids titrated for urine output of at least 100 mL/hour
    B. IV fluid resuscitation as per the Parkland formula
    C. Avoid tetanus toxoid since he has no open wounds
    D. Delay operative intervention until fully resuscitated
    E. Start high-volume fluid resuscitation only if he shows laboratory signs of rhabdomyolysis

18. In addition to the treatment in Question 17, the patient should be closely monitored and examined for:

    A. Cardiac arrhythmia
    B. Myoglobinemia
    C. Traumatic injuries to spine and extremities
    D. Compartment syndrome of both forearms
    E. All of the above

19. A 76-year-old woman is found in her burning home by firefighters after apparently falling asleep with a heater on in her bedroom. She has first-degree burns to both arms and chest and 3% second-degree burns to her right arm. She is breathing spontaneously but has a raspy voice, and has soot around her nose with singed nasal hair.

A. If her oxygen saturation (SaO$_2$) is greater than 97%, she does not require intubation
B. She should be placed on a nonrebreather face mask with 100% O$_2$
C. Burns should be treated topically, and then she should be prescribed pain medicine and discharged to home under her son's care
D. Resuscitate her with intrevenous (IV) hydration at 2 mL LR × body weight (kg) × % total body surface area (BSA) burn
E. She should be urgently intubated for airway protection

20. A 42-year-old man was trapped in a house fire and rescued by firefighters from his basement meth lab. He is brought to the ICU with 80% third-degree burns, sparing only both feet and lower legs. He is started on Parkland formula resuscitation with adequate urine output. Four hours into resuscitation, the respiratory therapist (RT) reports that he is becoming difficult to ventilate and has elevated airway pressures. Your next step should be:

A. Increase positive end-expiratory pressure (PEEP)
B. Perform immediate chest escharotomies
C. Switch to oscillator ventilation
D. Give nebulizer treatments
E. Initiate veno-venous (VV) extracorporeal membranous oxygenation

21. A 28-year-old male was brought to ICU after motorcycle crash. He sustained severe traumatic brain injury (TBI) requiring intracranial pressure (ICP) monitor, pelvic fracture, left humerus fracture, and Grade 2 splenic laceration, managed nonoperatively. By postadmit day 8, his orthopedic wounds have been stabilized, his bolt has been removed, but his Glasgow Coma Scale (GCS) remains 6T. He undergoes percutaneous tracheostomy at the bedside. The procedure was uneventful and tracheostomy location was confirmed via direct bronchoscopy postinsertion. Twenty minutes later, he becomes hypoxic, tachypneic, and tachycardic with decreased breath sounds on the right side. His blood pressure (BP) is stable. The most useful diagnostic test is:

A. Stat arterial blood gas (ABG)
B. Stat complete blood count (CBC)
C. Stat chest x-ray (CXR)
D. Stat bronchoscopy
E. Needle decompression in the 2nd intercostal space, mid-clavicular line

22. Two weeks later, the patient in question 21 has a percutaneous endoscopic gastrostomy (PEG) tube placed in the endoscopy suite. The procedure was uncomplicated. Four hours later, he becomes tachycardic and hypotensive. He is cold peripherally. The most appropriate next step in management is:

A. Stat kidney–ureter–bladder (KUB) to assess for free air
B. Empiric broad-spectrum antibiotics for presumed perforation
C. Stat sinogram/tube contrast study assess tube position
D. ECG and troponins to rule out myocardial infarction (MI)
E. Fluid bolus and stat complete blood count (CBC) to assess for bleeding

23. A 52-year-old male was brought in by emergency medical service (EMS) after being pulled from home garage fire. He had stridor, carbonaceous sputum, singed nares, and was intubated at the scene for airway protection and hypoxia. He had 22% second-degree burns to his

face, neck, arms, and torso. No other traumatic injuries were identified on primary survey, secondary survey, or full trauma CT scans. However, he remains hypoxic with O_2 saturations 80% to 85% on 100% FiO_2, intermittent runs of nonsustained ventricular tachycardia (VT) and systolic blood pressure (SBP) in the low 90s. Arterial blood gas (ABG) shows severe metabolic acidosis (pH 7.17) with PO_2 of 54 and lactate of 14. What is the most appropriate next step?

A. Double his previously calculated burn resuscitation hourly fluid rate.
B. Obtain cardiac troponins and stat echocardiogram
C. Initiate veno-venous (VV) extracorporeal membranous oxygenation
D. Administer hydroxycobalamin
E. Start urgent dialysis

24. A 36-year-old female presents after an all-terrain vehicle rollover in a field. She is neurologically intact but imaging reveals significant pulmonary contusions, multiple rib fractures, a grade IV liver injury without active extravasation, and a Gustillo IIIB open tibial fracture. She receives 1 u packed red blood cells (pRBC) and 1 u fresh-frozen plasma (FFP) and stabilizes hemodynamically. She receives cefazolin for open fracture and is taken to the operating room for wound debridement and placement of an external fixator. Postop day 1, she becomes tachycardic and hypotensive. Her hemoglobin has dropped from 9 to 8.5 g/dL. Her white blood cell (WBC) count is 32,000. The wound is red, exquisitely tender, and has crepitus. She is diaphoretic with clammy extremities. The most appropriate next step is:

A. Add gentamicin for high-risk open fracture
B. X-ray of the leg to assess for gas in the subcutaneous tissues
C. CT scan of the leg to assess for gas in the subcutaneous tissues
D. Call surgery for stat wound debridement
E. CT angiography (CTA) of the abdomen to rule out bleeding from liver injury

25. A 46-year-old female is involved in a high-speed motor vehicle collision (MVC). She is hemodynamically stable. Secondary survey reveals a prominent seat belt sign, abdominal tenderness, and decreased sensation in her legs. CT scans show a L1 burst fracture with cord compression. No intraabdominal injuries were identified. She goes to the operating room for urgent spinal decompression and fixation. Postop day 2, she has tachycardia and tachypneic with increasing abdominal distention and significant tenderness. White blood cell (WBC) count is 18,000. The most likely diagnosis is:

A. Postoperative ileus
B. Missed small bowel injury
C. Aspiration pneumonia
D. Spinal surgical wound infection
E. Meningitis

■ ANSWERS

1. **The answer is C.** CT scan evaluation of the cervical spine following trauma has supplanted plain radiography as the primary screening modality following trauma. CT scan is more accurate, is both time- and cost-effective, and does not require additional films that may delay final diagnosis. Clinical clearance remains the standard in awake, alert trauma patients who have no neck pain or tenderness with full range of motion; however, clinical exam is unreliable in those with neurologic deficit or a distracting painful injury such as a long-bone fracture, in which case collars should be maintained until CT clearance is obtained. Flexion extension films in an obtunded patient are minimally useful for identification of ligamentous injury and may cause further harm. Immobilization in a cervical collar after penetrating trauma to the neck or brain is not necessary unless the trajectory suggests direct injury to the cervical spine or the physical exam is consistent with a neurological deficit. Many of these patients will require emergent airway management, and spine immobilization may complicate airway access.

   Como JJ, Diaz JJ, Dunham CM, et al. Practice management guidelines for identification of cervical spine injuries following trauma: update from the eastern association for the surgery of trauma practice management guidelines committee. *J Trauma*. 2009;67(3):651-659. doi:10.1097/TA.0b013e3181ae583b

2. **The answer is E.** Blunt injury to the carotid or vertebral vessels (blunt cerebro-vascular injury [BCVI]) was historically diagnosed after the development of neurological symptoms, with significant resultant neurologic morbidity. With increased screening of asymptomatic patients, BCVI has been diagnosed in 1% of all blunt trauma patients, allowing for treatment and prevention of related morbidity and mortality.

   Bromberg WJ, Collier BC, Diebel LN, et al. Blunt cerebrovascular injury practice management guidelines: the Eastern Association for the Surgery of Trauma. *J Trauma*. 2010;68(2):471-477. doi:10.1097/TA.0b013e3181cb43da

3. **The answer is D.** Hemostasis is the primary goal in a bleeding trauma patient, and following surgical and endovascular therapies, detection and aggressive correction of systemic coagulopathy remain critical. The coagulopathy in trauma is multifactorial in origin, not uncommon, and an independent predictor of mortality. Massive hemorrhagic loss includes coagulation factors and platelets, which are then further diluted with crystalloid resuscitation. FFP transfusion replenishes most coagulation factors; however, platelet transfusion is necessary to correct thrombocytopenia. In a massive hemorrhage setting, 1 unit platelet transfusion is given with every 6 units of packed RBCs and FFP. Hypothermia and acidosis both impede the function of coagulation factors by interfering with necessary enzyme reactions. TBI can cause thromboplastin exposure, which results in a consumptive disseminated intravascular coagulopathy. Elderly patients with comorbidities are more likely to be on antiplatelet therapy or anticoagulant agents prior to the trauma.

   Rhee P, Inaba K. Coagulopathy in the trauma patient. In: Cameron JL, ed. *Current Surgical Therapy*. 9th ed. Philadelphia, PA: Mosby/Elsevier; 2008:940-944.

4. **The answer is E.** This patient is in hemorrhagic shock, as evidenced by the low central venous pressure (CVP), low cardiac index, and high SVR. The severity of shock correlates with the amount of blood loss, and cardiac output (CO) starts to decline after 20% to 40% of blood volume is lost. When more than 40% blood volume is lost, the resultant shock is imminently life-threatening. SVR is elevated due to the body's vasoconstriction response to hypovolemia. The most important interventions are replacement of blood volume and control of ongoing hemorrhage through operative intervention or correction of coagulopathy.

   Cinat ME, Hoyt DB. Hemorrhagic shock. In: Gabrielli A, Layon AJ, Yu M, eds. *Civetta, Taylor & Kirby's Critical Care*. 4th ed. Philadelphia, PA: Wolters Kluwer; 2009:893-923.

Mullins RJ. Management of shock. In: Moore EE, Mattox KL, Feliciano DV, eds. *Trauma Manual.* 4th ed. New York, NY: McGraw-Hill; 2003:chap 7, 71-83

Moreno PL. *The ICU Book.* 2nd ed. Philadelphia, PA: Lippincott Williams & Wilkins; 1998:154-165.

5. **The answer is C.** Attention to physical exam findings is essential to the diagnosis of peripheral vascular injury. Patients with hard signs of peripheral vascular injury need immediate operative intervention. Hard signs include absent or diminished pulses, pulsatile bleeding, palpable thrill or bruit, expanding or pulsatile hematoma, or signs of distal ischemia, pain, pallor, paresthesia, paralysis, and coolness. Soft signs of injury warrant further investigation with arteriography. Soft signs include a wound in proximity to the path of the artery, a small nonpulsatile hematoma, neurologic deficit in the extremity, and prehospital arterial bleeding.

Zarzaur BL, Croce MA. The management of vascular trauma. In: Cameron JL, ed. *Current Surgical Therapy.* 9th ed. Philadelphia, PA: Mosby/Elsevier; 2008:1028-1032.

6. **The answer is B.** Pelvic fractures are estimated to occur in about 9% of all blunt injury patients, and 9% of these are severe with substantial deformation and displacement. Hemorrhage can be significant from arterial and/or venous injury, and pelvic fractures are the third leading cause of death in MVCs. Concerning physical exam findings include pain with pelvic movement, perineal and/or scrotal bruising, vaginal bleeding, and blood at the urethral meatus. Pelvic fractures represent a hidden source of hemorrhage into the retroperitoneum. Finding of a "blush" extravasation of contrast on CT scan represents active arterial hemorrhage which requires interventional radiology embolization. Rapid control of pelvic hemorrhage is obtained by external compression with a pelvic binder. This maneuver is the most effective option for control of venous hemorrhage. After infusion of 2 L of crystalloid, the next resuscitative fluid should be blood.

Cryer HG. Pelvic fractures. In: Cameron JL, ed. *Current Surgical Therapy.* 9th ed. Philadelphia, PA: Mosby/Elsevier; 2008:1037-1042.

Winfield RD, Lottenberg L. Secondary and tertiary triage of the trauma patient. In: Gabrielli A, Layon AJ, Yu M, eds. *Civetta, Taylor & Kirby's Critical Care.* 4th ed. Philadelphia, PA: Wolters Kluwer; 2009:1109-1128.

7. **The answer is E.** FES is estimated to occur in 19% of patients with major trauma, although this may be underreported. There is no universal definition for FES, so diagnosis requires a high degree of suspicion and is a diagnosis of exclusion. The classic triad of symptoms is respiratory insufficiency, AMS, and upper extremity and thoracic petechiae, although all three are seldom seen together. Major signs present within 24 hours in 65% of patients. TRALI symptoms include dyspnea, hypotension, pulmonary edema, and fever. Symptoms must be of acute onset with bilateral infiltrates that usually occur within 6 hours of transfusion. Pulmonary contusion is a direct bruise of the lung parenchyma, followed by alveolar hemorrhage and edema. In moderate-to-severe contusions, ventilator management is critical to minimize barotrauma. Bronchial injury is unlikely without a pneumothorax.

Meredith JW. Injury to the esophagus, trachea and bronchus. In: Moore EE, Mattox KL, Feliciano DV, eds. *Trauma Manual.* 4th ed. New York, NY: McGraw-Hill; 2003:chap 20, 178-187.

Richardson JD. Injury to the lung and pleura. In: Moore EE, Mattox KL, Feliciano DV, eds. *Trauma Manual.* 4th ed. New York, NY: McGraw-Hill; 2003:chap 21, 188-194.

Stern D, Pollack A, Scalea TM. Orthopedic critical care. In: Gabrielli A, Layon AJ, Yu M, eds. *Civetta, Taylor & Kirby's Critical Care.* 4th ed. Philadelphia, PA: Wolters Kluwer; 2009:1279-1289.

Sungur M, Uzun K. Other embolic syndromes (air, fat, amniotic fluid). In: Gabrielli A, Layon AJ, Yu M, eds. *Civetta, Taylor & Kirby's Critical Care.* 4th ed. Philadelphia, PA: Wolters Kluwer; 2009:2159-2170.

8. **The answer is A.** There are no specific treatments for FES. Previous treatments with heparin, dextran, and corticosteroids have not been shown to reduce morbidity or mortality. Treatment is largely supportive with ventilator strategies similar to acute respiratory distress syndrome (ARDS) treatment, maximizing recruitment and gas exchange while minimizing ventilator-associated lung injury. With supportive treatment, mortality is usually less than 10%, with

complete resolution of pulmonary and neurologic abnormalities. If the emboli pass through pulmonary vasculature, they can cause brain and kidney injury. Early long-bone fixation has resulted in a nearly 5-fold decrease in resultant FES.

Meredith JW. Injury to the esophagus, trachea and bronchus. In: Moore EE, Mattox KL, Feliciano DV, eds. *Trauma Manual*. 4th ed. New York, NY: McGraw-Hill; 2003:chap 20, 178-187.

Moore EE, Mattox KL, Feliciano DV. Injury to the lung and pleura. In: *Trauma Manual*. 4th ed. New York, NY: McGraw-Hill; 2003:188-194.

Stern D, Pollack A, Scalea TM. Orthopedic critical care. In: Gabrielli A, Layon AJ, Yu M, eds. *Civetta, Taylor & Kirby's Critical Care*. 4th ed. Philadelphia, PA: Wolters Kluwer; 2009:1279-1289.

Sungur M, Uzun K. Other embolic syndromes (air, fat, amniotic fluid). In: Gabrielli A, Layon AJ, Yu M, eds. *Civetta, Taylor & Kirby's Critical Care*. 4th ed. Philadelphia, PA: Wolters Kluwer; 2009:2159-2170.

9. **The answer is C.** This patient has compartment syndrome of his extremity, which is a surgical emergency. Compartment syndrome results from increased content within a closed musculofascial compartment. This can be due to edematous structures within the compartment (e.g., crushed muscle) or hemorrhage into or around these structures. Delay in treatment can result in severe ischemia and tissue loss. Typical symptoms are pain out of proportion to exam findings, numbness or tingling of the extremity, pain with passive dorsiflexion, and sensory deficit. Arterial pressure is significantly higher than the elevated compartment pressure, so distal pulses are present unless there is concomitant arterial injury. Normal pressure is up to 8 mmHg. A pressure greater than 30 mmHg is consistent with impaired tissue perfusion.

Feliciano DV. The management of extremity compartment syndrome. In: Cameron JL, ed. *Current Surgical Therapy*. 9th ed. Philadelphia, PA: Mosby/Elsevier; 2008:1032-1037.

10. **The answer is D.** The so-called lover's triad is what can occur after jumping from an upper-floor window. The typical triad consists of calcaneous fractures, lumbar vertebral spine compression fracture, and forearm fractures. Any mechanism involving an axial load warrants a search for these injuries.

Scaletta TA, Schaider JJ. *Emergent Management of Trauma*. 2nd ed. New York, NY: McGraw-Hill; 2001:336.

11. **The answer is C.** Acute massive hemothorax following trauma is an indication for an early thoracotomy to control intrathoracic hemorrhage. Indications include initial chest tube output exceeding 1,500 mL, lack of resolution of hemothorax after chest tube placement, or a continued hourly output of greater than 200 mL for 4 consecutive hours. Delay in intervention is associated with a higher mortality due to the volume of blood loss. The source of bleeding can be lung parenchyma, heart, or any of the great vessels. Residual pneumothorax on chest radiograph may indicate a need for an additional chest tube. Pulmonary contusion on imaging associated with desaturation may indicate a need for optimization with nonconventional mechanical ventilation.

Gruen RL, Jurkovich GJ. Hemothorax. In: Cameron JL, ed. *Current Surgical Therapy*. 9th ed. Philadelphia, PA: Mosby Elsevier; 2008:705-708.

12. **The answer is B.** This patient has abdominal compartment syndrome (ACS). Intraabdominal hypertension is defined by intraabdominal pressure (IAP) greater than 12 mmHg, and ACS is defined as IAP >20 mmHg associated with new onset single or multiple system organ failure. Treatment of ACS is emergent decompressive laparotomy, and further delay could lead to complete cardiovascular collapse. Angiography would be appropriate if there were ongoing transfusion requirements; however, her hemoglobin is stable and further transfusion is not necessary. CVVH would improve creatinine; however, the renal failure is due to decreased renal perfusion, and once the abdominal pressure is relieved, the kidneys will again be well perfused and will return to normal function. Increased plateau airway pressures are secondary to elevated abdominal pressures. There is no role for bronchoscopy.

Hojman J, Rabinovici R. Abdominal compartment syndrome. In: Cameron JL, ed. *Current Surgical Therapy*. 9th ed. Philadelphia: Mosby/Elsevier; 2008:970-975.

Winfield RD, Lottenberg L. Secondary and tertiary triage of the trauma patient. In: Gabrielli A, Layon AJ, Yu M, eds. *Civetta, Taylor & Kirby's Critical Care*. 4th ed. Philadelphia, PA: Wolters Kluwer; 2009:1109-1128.

13. **The answer is D.** Nonoperative management of blunt adult hepatic and splenic injuries is the treatment modality of choice in hemodynamically stable patients, irrespective of the grade of injury. This is associated with a low overall morbidity and mortality and does not result in increased lengths of stay, transfusion requirement, or bleeding complications when compared to operative management. Neither grade of injury nor degree of hemoperitoneum on CT scan predicts the outcome of nonoperative management. The hemodynamic status is the most reliable criterion. The presence of a contrast blush on the vascular phase of the CT scan may portend failure of nonoperative management. In this situation, angiography and embolization may be used to successfully control ongoing hemorrhage in the hemodynamically stable patient. There is no evidence to support the practice of keeping a clinically stable patient on bed rest. There is no evidence that serial abdominal CT scans are needed to follow up the injury in a clinically stable patient without other reasons for a scan. Selective cases of penetrating injury without peritoneal signs and CT evaluation of trajectory indicating no additional injuries can be managed nonoperatively with either endovascular or percutaneous interventions to facilitate management.

Como JJ, Bokhari F, Chiu WC, et al. Practice management guidelines for selective nonoperative management of penetrating abdominal trauma. *J Trauma*. 2010;68(3):721-733. doi:10.1097/TA.0b013e3181cf7d07

Demetriades D, Hadjizacharia P, Constantinou C, et al. Selective nonoperative management of penetrating abdominal solid organ injuries. *Ann Surg*. 2006;244(4):620-628. doi:10.1097/01.sla.0000237743.22633.01

14. **The answer is A.** An estimated 20% of trauma patients who die in the prehospital setting are thought to have sustained significant cardiac injury. Of those who arrive to the hospital alive, BCI is suspected in those with a high-energy mechanism and is often seen in conjunction with multiple injuries. In a conscious patient, complaints of chest pain should raise suspicion. In an obtunded patient, worrisome signs include refractory hypotension, muffled heart sounds, and jugular venous distension. Associated injury patterns include chest bruising, multiple rib fractures, and sternul fracture. A focused assessment with sonography for trauma (FAST) exam can evaluate the pericardium for fluid. An ECG should be obtained. A normal ECG and normal troponin I level are associated with a negative workup, and no further tests are indicated.

Haut ER. Blunt cardiac injury. In: Cameron JL, ed. *Current Surgical Therapy*. 9th ed. Philadelphia, PA: Mosby/Elsevier; 2008:1063-1066.

Winfield RD, Lottenberg L. Secondary and tertiary triage of the trauma patient. In: Gabrielli A, Layon AJ, Yu M, eds. *Civetta, Taylor & Kirby's Critical Care*. 4th ed. Philadelphia, PA: Wolters Kluwer; 2009:1109-1128.

15. **The answer is A.** This patient is septic from a missed bowel injury. An upright KUB should demonstrate free air underneath the diaphragm. The only appropriate intervention at this time is exploratory laparotomy and resection of the bowel injury. This patient had previously been managed nonoperatively, which is an acceptable management plan in select stab wounds without fascial penetration on local exploration and no peritoneal signs on exam. One large study reported a 2.9% rate of missed injuries that required subsequent surgery. Some delayed diagnoses do not add significant morbidity, but bowel injuries can occasionally lead to major septic complications.

Fabian TC. Injury to the lung and pleura. In: Moore EE, Mattox KL, Feliciano DV, eds. *Trauma Manual*. 4th ed. New York, NY: McGraw-Hill; 2003:214-230.

16. **The answer is A.** Mafenide acetate, silver sulfadiazine, and silver nitrate are the three most common topical antimicrobials used in burn wounds treatment. Mafenide acetate (Sulfamylon) has good eschar penetration, but is quite painful. It is highly effective against Gram-negative organisms, including most *Pseudomonas* species. It is an inhibitor of carbonic anhydrase and, therefore, can cause significant metabolic acidosis. Silver sulfadiazine (Silvadene) has limited eschar penetration but is painless. It occasionally induces neutropenia via bone marrow suppression. Silver nitrate also does not have good eschar penetrance and is therefore painless. Due to leaching of electrolytes across the eschar, it can cause significant electrolyte abnormalities.

Richards WT, Mozingo DW. Burn injury: thermal and electrical. In: Gabrielli A, Layon AJ, Yu M, eds. *Civetta, Taylor & Kirby's Critical Care*, 4th ed. Philadelphia, PA: Wolters Kluwer; 2009: 1313-1324.

17. **The answer is A.** High-voltage burns have a very different treatment regimen than do thermal burns. Resuscitation requirements are often twice those of the Parkland formula recommendation for thermal burns, and renal failure from myoglobinemia is a significant danger. Prevention of acute renal failure (ARF) requires prompt aggressive fluid resuscitation and maintenance of polyuria greater than or equal to 1.5 to 2 mL/kg/hour. Some authors also advocate urine alkalinization to a goal pH greater than 6.5; however, this recommendation is not consistent. All patients with burns should receive tetanus toxoid, plus tetanus immunoglobulin if the last booster is unknown or greater than 10 years old.

Bagshaw SM, Bellomo R. Acute renal failure. In: Gabrielli A, Layon AJ, Yu M, eds. *Civetta, Taylor & Kirby's Critical Care*. 4th ed. Philadelphia, PA: Wolters Kluwer; 2009:2381-2392.

Mlcak RP, Buffalo MC. Pre-hospital management, transportation, and emergency care. In: Herndon DN, ed. *Total Burn Care*. 3rd ed. Philadelphia, PA: Saunders; 2007:81-92.

Spence RJ. Electrical and lightning injuries. In: Cameron JL, ed. *Current Surgical Therapy*. 9th ed. Philadelphia, PA: Mosby/Elsevier; 2008:1079-1083.

18. **The answer is E.** In addition to elevated myoglobin from rhabdomyolysis, patients with electrical burns have significant risk for cardiac arrhythmias, and therefore require continuous cardiac monitoring. Due to muscle damage and resultant edema with aggressive resuscitation, this patient will most likely develop compartment syndrome of both forearms requiring operative fasciotomies. This patient fell 25 feet and therefore is at a significant risk for extremity and spine fractures.

Purdue GF, Arnoldo BD, Hunt JL. Electrical injuries. In: Herndon DN, ed. *Total Burn Care*. 3rd ed. Philadelphia, PA: Saunders; 2007:513-520.

Spence RJ. Electrical and lightning injuries. In: Cameron JL, ed. *Current Surgical Therapy*. 9th ed. Philadelphia, PA: Mosby/Elsevier; 2008:1079-1083.

19. **The answer is B.** Inhalation injury is one of the most critical types of thermal injury. Inhalation injury occurs with prolonged smoke exposure in an enclosed space and not usually with flash burns such as experienced by this patient. Head and neck cutaneous burns can cause swelling that endangers the airway; however, the patient has minimal facial burns. It is important to follow the carboxyhemoglobin level because both partial pressure of oxygen and oxygen saturations may be normal despite oxygen displacement by carbon monoxide. The correct Parkland formula is 4 ml fluid x body weight (kg) x % total BSA burn.

Nugent N, Herndon DN. Diagnosis and treatment of inhalation injury. In: Herndon DN, ed. *Total Burn Care*. 3rd ed. Philadelphia, PA: Saunders, 2007:262-272.

20. **The answer is B.** In circumferential torso burns, escharotomies may be necessary to relieve chest wall restriction and improve ventilation. This procedure can be performed bedside with intravenous (IV) sedation and electrocautery.

Gamelli RL, Silver GM. Burn wound management. In: Cameron JL, ed. *Current Surgical Therapy*. 9th ed. Philadelphia, PA: Mosby/Elsevier; 2008:1066-1071.

21. **The answer is C.** Pneumothorax is an immediate complication following percutaneous tracheostomy. It is generally reported in ~1% of cases, but has been reported up to 17%. An ABG would confirm hypoxia but not the underlying cause. A CBC may help if hemothorax is suspected but a drop in hemoglobin would unlikely be immediately apparent. CXR is mostly likely to differentiate between pneumothorax, hemothorax, or mucus plug. Bronchoscopy would confirm false passage or pulmonary hemorrhage, but position was already confirmed by bronchoscopy, and CXR has higher diagnostic yield in this setting. Needle decompression may diagnose a pneumothorax, but can fail in 25% to 95% of cases (depending on body mass index). Lack of air release would fail to differentiate pneumothorax from mucus plug. New recommendations now support emergent decompression in the 4th intercostal space, anterior axillary line.

American College of Surgeons. *Advanced Trauma Life Support Student Course Manual.* 10th ed. Chicago, IL: American College of Surgons; 2018.
Powers WF, Clancy TV, Adams A, et al. Proper catheter selection for needle thoracostomy: a height and weight based selection criteria. *Injury.* 2014;45:107-111. doi:10.1016/j.injury.2013.08.026
Rashid AO, Islam S. Percutaneous tracheostomy: a comprehensive review. *J Thoacr Dis.* 2017;9(Suppl 10):S1128-S1138. doi:10.21037/jtd.2017.09.33

22. **The answer is E.** Hypotension, tachycardia, and cold extremities postprocedure is consistent with hemorrhagic shock. A KUB will almost always have free air after a PEG, and is unhelpful in ruling in or out perforation in the immediate postprocedure period. Four hours is very early for sepsis, even in the unlikely even of a bowel perforation or gastric spillage from tube malposition. If the tube is at the appropriate skin position from the procedure, a tube study is also unlikely to be helpful immediately postprocedure, and usually takes more time to organize than would be appropriate for a patient in shock. An MI is unlikely in a young patient, especially in the setting of a low-risk procedure.

Blumenstein I, Shastri YM, Stein J. Gastroenteric tube feeding: techniques, problems and solutions. *World J Gastroenterol.* 2014;20(26):8505-8524. doi:10.3748/wjg.v20.i26.8505

23. **The answer is D.** Smoke inhalation is the most common cause of cyanide toxicity, reported in up to 76% of with smoke inhalation injury. Cyanide binds the ferric ions in cytochrome c oxidase, disrupting the mitochondrial electron transport chain and blocking aerobic metabolism. The mechanism of injury, hypoxia with arrhythmia, metabolic acidosis, and lactate greater than 9 are suggestive of cyanide poisoning. First-line treatment is hydroxycobalamin, for presumed or confirmed cyanide toxicity. It binds cyanide by substituting a hydroxyl group for CN to form cyanocobalamin. It has a low side-effect profile. It has faster onset of action than sodium thiosulfate, and does not worsen potential carbon monoxide poisoning like sodium or amyl nitrite.

MacLennan L, Moiemen N. Management of cyanide toxicity in patients with burns. *Burns.* 2015;41(1):18-24. doi:10.1016/j.burns.2014.06.001

24. **The answer is D.** The clinical scenario, physical exam, and investigations are consistent with necrotizing fasciitis. Gentamicin is appropriate for high-risk open fractures, but should be started at presentation; it would be inadequate treatment for this change in clinical status. Palpation of crepitus precludes the need for imaging to confirm gas. Delayed bleeding from a blunt liver injury is possible, but would unlikely to be accompanied by the elevated WBC and extremities would expected to be cold. Emergent surgical debridement is the appropriate treatment for necrotizing skin and soft tissue infections.

Bulger, E. Necrotizing skin and soft tissue infections. In: Cameron JL, ed. *Current Surgical Therapy.* 10th ed. Philadelphia, PA: Mosby/Elsevier; 2011:662-665.

25. **The answer is B.** Small bowel perforation is an uncommon complication of blunt trauma. However, the presence of a seat belt sign (ecchymoses along the chest or abdominal wall) increases likelihood of small bowel perforation. After MVC, a seat belt sign is associated with a 4.7 fold increase in the relative risk of small bowel perforation. Even higher rates of small

bowel injury are seen in the presence of with lumbar fractures and seat belt sign, prompting the term "seat belt syndrome." Postoperative ileus is unlikely to be tender or associated with an elevated WBC. Aspiration pneumonia can have tachycardia, tachypnea, and elevated WBC, but not abdominal pain. Surgical site infection or meningitis would be unlikely to present on post-operative day 2, and should not be accompanied by abdominal tenderness.

Vercruysse GA, Rhee P. Stomach and small bowel. In: Moore EE, Feliciano EV, Mattox KL, eds. *Trauma*. 8th ed. New York, NY: McGraw-Hill; 2017:597-620.

Ethical and Legal Aspects of Critical Care Medicine

NASIYA AHMED

QUESTIONS

1. Which one of the following is **not** one of the four ethical principles used to balance decision making in a difficult situation?

    A. Beneficence (do good)
    B. Justice (fairness)
    C. Respect (for moral and religious values)
    D. Autonomy (the right to self-determination)
    E. Nonmaleficence (do no harm)

2. A 61-year-old woman with a past medical history of hypertension, hyperlipidemia, diabetes, and chronic kidney disease presented to the ED with a subarachnoid hemorrhage (SAH) and acute renal failure (ARF) that has worsened during the course of her hospitalization. While she has been cooperative with procedures up until this point, she is adamantly refusing dialysis. What should you do next?

    A. Sign a two-physician consent for emergent dialysis
    B. Ask the family to consent for dialysis
    C. Assess her decision-making capacity
    D. Consult hospice services
    E. Continue your current plan of care and call an ethics consult

3. A 75-year-old nursing home resident with a past medical history of hypertension and hyperlipidemia has been admitted with a stroke that has resulted in left upper extremity weakness and difficulty swallowing. On physical exam, he is extremely cachectic. However, the patient is alert, oriented, and able to make his own decisions. On morning rounds, you discuss placing a feeding tube to help him eat and he adamantly refuses. Which ethical principle is he using?

    A. Beneficence
    B. Justice
    C. Respect
    D. Autonomy
    E. Nonmaleficence

4. Which of the following statements about informed consent is/are **incorrect**?

    A. Double framing allows patients to see the risk–benefit analysis from both perspectives
    B. Informed consent is not needed in emergency circumstances
    C. During the process of informed consent, the physician should disclose to the patient the diagnosis and the risks and benefits of the various treatment options

D. Informed consent is required for all human-subject research
E. The key to informed consent is communicating and establishing a relationship with the patient

5. Which of the following statements about decision makers is/are correct?

   A. A durable power of attorney is appointed by the patient and/or close family members to make decisions for him or her in the event that the patient is unable to do so
   B. Spouse, parents, children, and siblings, in this order, can become surrogate decision makers
   C. In many cultures, the family retains decision-making authority for a sick patient who has intact decision-making capacity, and physicians should respect this tradition
   D. Advance directives or living wills allow physicians to make decisions for the patient without permission from the durable power of attorney
   E. Patients for whom a surrogate decision maker cannot be found will require a court-appointed guardian to make decisions on his or her behalf

6. Which situation best describes substituted judgment?

   A. The medical power of attorney is unable to make a decision and appoints someone to do it on his or her behalf
   B. A person does not have an advance directive, so the family is asked to make decisions based on his religious, personal, or moral values
   C. A patient does not have a surrogate decision maker and cannot have a court-appointed guardian due to illegal immigration status, so the physician is required to make decisions for the patient
   D. A patient has replaced his written advance directives with a recently created oral advance directive heard by only a few family members, who must carry out his wishes

7. Which statement about futility is **incorrect**?

   A. Futile interventions often increase the patient's pain and discomfort in the final days of life
   B. While patients have autonomy and the right to decide their plan of care, it is the physician's responsibility to not offer futile treatment options
   C. Deeming a treatment futile should be based on solid research and evidence-based medicine
   D. Occasionally, futile interventions may be continued to help the family come to terms with the situation
   E. A treatment that confers a physiological benefit on a patient is not futile

8. Which of the following statements about terminal extubation is **incorrect**?

   A. In terminal extubation, the positive end-expiratory pressure (PEEP) and the respiratory rate (RR) are weaned to normal, prior to removing the tube and placing the patient on oxygen
   B. After a patient is extubated he or she may live anywhere from minutes to days
   C. Terminal extubation is an acceptable form of euthanasia
   D. Low-dose paralytics can be used to prevent respiratory distress and agitation during extubation process
   E. Symptom control with opiates and benzodiazepines should be initiated prior to extubation unless the patient is comatose

9. Mrs. Smith is a 79-year-old white woman who has been in the neurocritical care unit for 2 weeks after a hemorrhagic stroke. After a lengthy discussion with the family, they agree to terminal extubation. The nurse starts morphine at a rate of 1 mg/hour and extubates the

patient. The family complains that the patient is having difficulty breathing. Which of the following medications will **not** help improve her breathing?

A. Glycopyrolate 0.25 mg subcutaneous injection
B. Scopolamine patch
C. Ativan 0.5 mg IV
D. Morphine 2 mg IV
E. Lasix 40 mg IV

10. Palliative care:

A. Is the total care of patients, controlling pain and other symptoms while minimizing emotional, social, and spiritual issues in a hospice setting
B. Maintains quality of life, but may hasten death
C. Is available to patients with AIDS or end-stage cardiac, renal, pulmonary, and neurologic disease, regardless of how long they have to live
D. Is mostly done in the ambulatory setting, usually when there are no additional treatment options available for the patient

11. Which of the following is **not** a part of the signs and symptoms of an actively dying patient?

A. Fever
B. Delirium
C. Respiratory distress
D. Skin changes
E. Nausea and vomiting

12. Which one of the following is **not** one of the six steps used in communicating bad news?

A. Preparation
B. Apologizing prior to telling bad news
C. Determining what the patient would like to know
D. Responding to the patient's feelings
E. Discussing treatment options

13. Sources of conflict in a family meeting include which of the following?

A. Inadequate or incorrect information
B. Emotions, especially guilt and anger
C. Family dynamics
D. Physician mistrust
E. All of the above

14. The United States spends the most per capita on healthcare of any developed country. If this trend continues, then Medicare will no longer be able to provide care for its members. Methods to prevent this include:

A. Rationing
B. Healthcare tax
C. Cost containment
D. Increasing Medicaid funding

15. Rationing care violates which one of the four ethical principles?

A. Beneficence (do good)
B. Justice (fairness)

    C. Autonomy (the right to self-determination)

    D. Nonmaleficence (do no harm)

16. If a patient (or patient's family) request treatment that is futile, what should the physician do?

    A. The patient (and/or family) has autonomy and the physician should provide the requested treatment

    B. The physician should transfer patient care to a physician who is comfortable with carrying out the patient/family's request

    C. The physician should ask the patient/family to request a second opinion from another physician

    D. The physician should request the hospital ethics committee or a palliative care physician to help him/her negotiate an acceptable treatment plan with the family

    E. The physician should explain to the family that carrying out their requested treatment is contrary to his belief of nonmaleficence and he/she is unable to perform such a request

17. Which of the following statements is incorrect?

    A. Physicians can use the practice of "slow codes" in an emergency situation to help the family come to terms with their loved one's critical situation and impending death while not prolonging futile care

    B. Patient/family members may remain uncomfortable with being asked to withdraw treatment, but may understand the limits of therapeutic interventions and be willing to sign a Do Not Escalate Treatment (DNET) form

    C. Detailed prognostication calculations may help a physician make more accurate end of life decisions

    D. Critically ill patients can reduce the chance of unwanted treatments by completing a Physician's Orders for Life Sustaining Treatment (POLST) form

18. Voluntary active euthanasia is legal in which states?

    A. New York

    B. Colorado

    C. Texas

    D. California

    E. None of the above

19. Which of the following statements regarding physician-assisted death (PAD) is correct?

    A. A family member or surrogate decision maker should be involved in the decision-making process

    B. Palliative sedation, hospice, refraining from food and drink, and refusing life-sustaining therapy are other options to PAD

    C. Depression/hopelessness and fear of becoming a burden at the end of life are associated with increased likelihood of PAD

    D. Elderly, widowed, Caucasian females are the largest socioeconomic group requesting PAD

    E. Approximately 60% of patients requesting prescriptions for PAD complete the process

■ ANSWERS

1. **The answer is C.** The four principles, adapted from the Belmont report, do not include respect. These four principles help highlight difficult aspects of a case. Determining the role of each of the four principles from the physician's perspective as well as from the patient's perspective helps highlight difficult aspects of a case. Oftentimes, there is a conflict not only between these principles but also within one of the principles.

   Watson M, Lucas C, Hoy A, et al. *Oxford Handbook of Palliative Care.* 2nd ed. New York, NY: Oxford University Press; 2009.

2. **The answer is C.** Decisional capacity refers to the patient's ability to make a decision. In order to have decision-making capacity, a patient must be able to describe the medical situation, describe the risks and benefits of various treatment options, and arrive at a logical and consistent decision. Depending on patients' cognitive status, they may not have decisional capacity to make all their decisions; for example, the patient may be able to consent to an arterial line being placed, but not fully understand the concept and the need for dialysis to be able to consent to it. The family cannot consent to dialysis if the patient has decision-making capacity. There is no indication that the dialysis is emergent, requiring a two-physician consent or withholding informed consent. There is no indication that the need for dialysis is permanent; therefore, the patient would be unlikely to meet hospice criteria for end-stage renal disease (ESRD). Although you should continue your plan of care while the dialysis issue is sorted out, the only reason for an ethics consult is if other treatments are futile without dialysis.

   Watson M, Lucas C, Hoy A, et al. *Oxford Handbook of Palliative Care.* 2nd ed. New York, NY: Oxford University Press; 2009.

3. **The answer is D.** This is based on the principle of autonomy. If the patient has decision-making capacity, providers have a duty to respect his or her decision.

   Watson M, Lucas C, Hoy A, et al. *Oxford Handbook of Palliative Care.* 2nd ed. New York, NY: Oxford University Press; 2009.

4. **The answer is D.** Informed consent is required for all procedures, and to perform a procedure without informed consent is considered battery, regardless of the outcome. The goal of informed consent is to educate the patient (inform the patient) so that he or she can make a voluntary and intelligent decision. The physician should disclose the patient's medical condition, the risks and benefits of the treatment option, as well as the risks and benefits of other treatment/nontreatment options. The risks and benefits should be based on sound medical research. The framing of information can significantly affect decision making, and framing bias should be minimized using double framing; for example, the physician explains that there is a 70% chance that surgery will benefit the patient, which means there is a 30% chance that there will be no benefit from surgery. Not all human-subject research requires informed consent.

   Watson M, Lucas C, Hoy A, et al. *Oxford Handbook of Palliative Care.* 2nd ed. New York, NY: Oxford University Press; 2009.

5. **The answer is E.** Advance directives and living wills allow the patient to carry out his/her treatment wishes in the event that he or she is not able to do so; in essence, advance directives allow patients to preserve their autonomy. These documents can be simple, stating that the patient does not want to have CPR or intubation, to extremely complex situations such as when artificial nutrition and dialysis may be permitted; laws differ from state to state on what can be stated in an advance directive. Some laws also allow for oral advance directives with witnesses present; an oral advance directive can replace a previously written advance directive. A durable or medical power of attorney is a person who is legally appointed by the patient to make medical decisions for him or her in the event that he or she is unable to do so. If the patient has both a medical power of attorney and an advance directive, the medical power of attorney should follow the advance directive when making decisions for

the patient, but this often does not happen, as the medical power of attorney does have the right to make the final decision. If there is no legal medical power of attorney, a surrogate decision maker is chosen from the family; the hierarchy for selecting a surrogate is spouse, children, parents, siblings, and religious clergy (some states allow for other relatives prior to using religious clergy). If there is more than one child or sibling, it is best to reach a consensus or majority agreement. Not all states recognize same sex partners or common law partners as spouses. If there is no family available, then a court-appointed guardian must be chosen as a surrogate decision maker. Oftentimes, guardianship takes time and a two-physician consent or religious clergy is used for more emergent procedures. Finally, there are many cultures in which the family prefers to make decisions for the patient; it is the physician's duty to ask the patient how much he or she would like to be involved in the decision-making process.

Watson M, Lucas C, Hoy A, et al. *Oxford Handbook of Palliative Care.* 2nd ed. New York, NY: Oxford University Press; 2009.

6. **The answer is B.** Often patients do not have advance directives, especially if they are young. The family should then make a decision in the best interest of the patient, based on his or her religious, moral, and personal values. This is called substituted judgment.

Watson M, Lucas C, Hoy A, et al. *Oxford Handbook of Palliative Care.* 2nd ed. New York, NY: Oxford University Press; 2009.

7. **The answer is E.** The physician's goal is to care for sick people. While patients have autonomy in deciding their plan of treatment, a physician should only offer the patient options that can improve the patient's clinical state or quality of life and not futile interventions. A procedure that may improve a patient physiologically but does not provide a noticeable benefit to the patient is futile. Futility should be based on sound research and standard of care practices. Futile interventions often increase the patient's pain and discomfort in the final days of life. Oftentimes family will request procedures that are futile; in such situations, the physician should communicate openly with the family and discuss why certain treatment options were withheld because of futility. Occasionally, futile interventions may be continued to help the family come to terms with the situation; for example, patients in a comatose or vegetative state may be kept on a ventilator for a few days in hopes of improvement.

Watson M, Lucas C, Hoy A, et al. *Oxford Handbook of Palliative Care.* 2nd ed. New York, NY: Oxford University Press; 2009.

8. **The answer is D.** The physician and the family must jointly agree that the ventilator has become a futile intervention for the patient and that ventilator withdrawal or terminal extubation is a better option; this agreement should be documented in the chart. It is the physician's job to explain in detail the extubation procedure as well as the types of treatment that will be initiated for symptom management. The physician should encourage the family to choose a time for all to be present and make arrangements for religious and cultural rituals. Furthermore, the physician must explain to the family that the patient may not pass away immediately. The time between extubation and death is a difficult time for the family and they often doubt their decision; the physician should be supportive during this period. Two methods for terminal extubation have been described. The first, immediate extubation, involves removing the endotracheal tube and replacing it with humidified oxygen, while the second, terminal weaning, involves tapering the RR, oxygen saturation, and PEEP over time and removing the endotracheal tube if the patient survives the weaning process; the choice is determined by the patient's clinical presentation and the healthcare team's preferences. All life-sustaining treatment, including nutrition, hydration, paralytics, and blood pressure support, should be stopped prior to extubation. Symptom control with morphine and midazolam or propofol should be initiated prior to extubation, even if the patient is comatose.

Watson M, Lucas C, Hoy A, et al. *Oxford Handbook of Palliative Care.* 2nd ed. New York, NY: Oxford University Press; 2009.

9. **The answer is E.** Both scopolamine and glycopyrolate will help dry out secretions. Morphine will decrease the perceived work of breathing, allowing the patient to breathe at a normal rate and pattern. Benzodiazepines will help minimize anxiety that may cause an increased respiratory rate. Lasix will benefit only if there is pulmonary edema, which is not mentioned in this case. Depending on the patient's cognitive and functional status, nonpharmacologic means of treating shortness of breath include elevating the head of the bed and using a fan.

Watson M, Lucas C, Hoy A, et al. *Oxford Handbook of Palliative Care.* 2nd ed. New York, NY: Oxford University Press; 2009.

10. **The answer is C.** The definition of palliative care is the total care of patients, controlling pain and other symptoms while minimizing emotional, social, and spiritual issues, whether at home or in a clinic, hospital, or hospice. Palliative care maintains quality of life while neither hastening nor postponing death. It is available to patients with AIDS and end-stage cardiac, renal, pulmonary, and neurologic disease, regardless of how long they have to live. Most hospitals have palliative care consult services; there are also palliative care clinics and home visit physicians. In the hospital palliative care, physicians should be consulted early on; they will help determine goals of care and provide pain and symptom management recommendations that will improve the patient's intervention and treatment experience. While palliative care physicians can follow patients in hospice and eventually death, not all patients needing palliative care are hospice patients.

Watson M, Lucas C, Hoy A, et al. *Oxford Handbook of Palliative Care.* 2nd ed. New York, NY: Oxford University Press; 2009.

11. **The answer is E.** Fever often occurs with pneumonia or other infections at the end of life; it also occurs with liver infiltration due to malignancy. Terminal delirium is the agitation that may occur as death approaches; it can be due to pain, constipation, urinary retention, side effects of medication, or simply anxiety associated with the impending death. Respiratory distress, Cheyne–Stokes breathing, or gurgling (often called the death rattle) also occurs as death nears. Breathing becomes apneic and the body is no longer able to clear secretions in a normal manner. As death approaches, a patient's skin will become cold and take on a bluish, cyanotic tinge.

12. **The answer is B.** The SPIKES protocol is a systematic approach to breaking bad news to the family. S stands for settings or, where the conversation will take place; make sure it is a quiet room with no distractions, that all family members involved are present, and that you, the physician, are calm, well versed in the details of the case, and ready to listen. P stands for perception; always ask first what the patient and his or her family know about the medical situation. I stands for invitation; ask the patient how much information he or she would like to know and how much he or she would like to participate in making treatment decisions. K stands for knowledge; always preface your bad news with a warning, such as "Unfortunately, I have some bad news." Do not use technical language, and give the information in repetitive small bits. E stands for empathy; listen and validate the patient's emotions. S stands for summary; summarize the main points that were discussed and the plan of care.

Watson M, Lucas C, Hoy A, et al. *Oxford Handbook of Palliative Care.* 2nd ed. New York, NY: Oxford University Press; 2009.

13. **The answer is E.** Before leading a family meeting, a physician should decide the goals of the meeting. The first step to leading a family meeting is to determine if everyone present understands the current medical situation; the explanatory model can be used for this. It is important for the physician to give information in small pieces, acknowledge the family members' emotions as they speak, and summarize the diagnosis and treatment plan at the end of the meeting. Gaps in information occur when the family doesn't understand the patient's situation or they are confused by conversations with multiple physicians and advice from well-meaning friends. Emotions, especially grief and fear due to the impending loss, guilt from having neglected their loved one, and hope, often contribute to the conflict. Different

family members, with differing value systems, complicate the situation. Last, if the family does not trust the physician, they are apt to disagree with the physician's treatment plan. All of these factors play a role in the medical plan of care; these emotions are often grouped under denial, but when you can tease out the different factors, it helps to improve the situation as a whole.

Watson M, Lucas C, Hoy A, et al. *Oxford Handbook of Palliative Care*. 2nd ed. New York, NY: Oxford University Press; 2009.

14. The answer is C. Cost containment and the Patient Protection and Affordable Care Act signed by President Obama propose to decrease or reallot Medicare reimbursements as well as streamline insurance processes to save money and offer better healthcare to more people.

Watson M, Lucas C, Hoy A, et al. *Oxford Handbook of Palliative Care*. 2nd ed. New York, NY: Oxford University Press; 2009.

15. The answer is B. Rationing care, where two patients with the same medical diagnosis receive different levels of interventions, violates the principle of justice. If, however, the intervention is futile in one patient but not futile in another patient, then withholding a futile intervention is not rationing care.

Watson M, Lucas C, Hoy A, et al. *Oxford Handbook of Palliative Care*. 2nd ed. New York, NY: Oxford University Press; 2009.

16. The answer is D. A joint policy statement released by the Society of Critical Care Medicine (SCCM) has outlined a process for conflict resolution. The physician should maintain an open and communicative relationship with the family throughout this process and should request the hospital ethics committee or palliative care physician for help in redirecting the patient's goals of care. The physician is under no obligation to provide futile care as this would contradict his or her own belief of beneficence. Oftentimes the line between clinically acceptable and futile treatment is not clearly delineated; in such a situation a clinician can transfer care of the patient. In such a situation, the physician can also request a second opinion, but he or she should not put the responsibility of finding a second physician on the patient and/or family.

Watson M, Lucas C, Hoy A, et al. *Oxford Handbook of Palliative Care*. 2nd ed. New York, NY: Oxford University Press; 2009.

17. The answer is A. The practice of slow codes is misleading and unethical. A DNET form can be used when families are not willing to withdraw care, but the physician is trying to limit futile care. A POLST form is completed by a patient with a physician for a patient undergoing a specific critical event; such forms allow physicians to develop a more pertinent treatment plan. Because these forms are signed by a physician they are considered medical orders and transferrable with the patient. While prognostication may provide added information to a physician, most studies using prognostication to help determine which patients will benefit from treatment in a critical care setting have been inaccurate in predicting patient mortality.

Watson M, Lucas C, Hoy A, et al. *Oxford Handbook of Palliative Care*. 2nd ed. New York, NY: Oxford University Press; 2009.

18. The answer is E. Voluntary active euthanasia is when a physician administers an intravenous (IV) form of a medication resulting in death and is illegal in the United States. Physician-assisted death (PAD) is when a physician provides a patient with a prescription for a lethal dose of medication; it is legal in Oregon, Washington, Vermont, Montana, California, Colorado, and the District of Columbia. In states where PAD is legal, a physician should have a second physician (preferably a palliative care physician) evaluate the patient to make sure there are not financial issues, depression, or pain motivating the desire to die and the patient has an intact decision-making capacity. There is also a waiting period from the date that the physician writes the prescription to the date the patient is allowed to fill the prescription. The dose is usually 10g to 15 g of phenobarbital

(100–150 pills), that are dissolved in a liquid or pudding and ingested in a span of 1 minute; this is usually accompanied by an anti-emetic.

Quill TE, Battin MP. Physician-assisted dying: understanding, evaluating, and responding to requests for medical aid in dying. Available at: www.uptodate.com/contents/physician-assisted-dying-understanding-evaluating-and-responding-to-requests-for-medical-aid-in-dying.

19. **The answer is B.** A patient carrying out PAD does not need to inform anyone of his or her decision. While psychiatric and emotional stressors as well as a fear of becoming a burden at the end of life are associated with increased likelihood of asking a physician about PAD, these factors are not associated with an increased likelihood of completing the process. Patients requesting PAD are usually Caucasian, well-educated, upper middle class, married, insured males who suffer from cancer or amytrophic lateral sclerosis (ALS). In the United States (most of our data comes from Oregon), only 1/300 patients asking about PAD actually die from PAD.

Quill TE, Battin MP. Physician-assisted dying: understanding, evaluating, and responding to requests for medical aid in dying. Available at: www.uptodate.com/contents/physician-assisted-dying-understanding-evaluating-and-responding-to-requests-for-medical-aid-in-dying.

26 Principles of Research in Critical Care

SUUR BILICILER AND JUSTIN KWAN

QUESTIONS

1. A study is conducted to determine the dose limiting toxicity of a drug for treatment of acute hemorrhagic stroke. This is an example of what type of trial?

   A. Preclinical testing
   B. Phase I trial
   C. Phase II trial
   D. Phase III trial
   E. Phase IV trial

2. What is the main benefit of the randomization process in a clinical trial?

   A. It always results in equal numbers of patients in each treatment arm
   B. It allows the clinical investigator to assign the patients to treatment arms based on current practice guidelines
   C. It always assigns the same number of men and women to each treatment arm.
   D. It reduces the chance of bias in a study
   E. It results in a representative sample

3. A noninferiority trial:

   A. Provides evidence that two treatments are completely identical
   B. Is an example of a placebo-controlled study
   C. Requires a smaller sample size than a superiority trial
   D. Determines whether the experimental therapy is equal or noninferior to the standard therapy
   E. Shows that an experimental treatment is better than a standard treatment

4. Which of the following National Institutes of Health (NIH) funded grants do not have training as a significant component of the grant?

   A. K99/R00
   B. K08
   C. R01
   D. K23
   E. T32

5. The Health Insurance Portability and Accountability Act (HIPAA):

   A. Allows researchers to enroll patients in studies without their knowledge
   B. Allows researchers to share identifiable data from patients without their consent
   C. Is governed by the Privacy Rule to protect an individual's medical information

    D. Provides funding for all National Institutes of Health (NIH) sponsored research

    E. Allows researchers to share clinical data nationwide

6. What is expedited Institutional Review Board (IRB) review?

    A. The review of a protocol with minimal risk as defined by U.S. Department of Health and Human Services and by a single reviewer

    B. The same as routine IRB review except it is performed in less than an hour

    C. A review of research protocols performed in life-threatening conditions

    D. A review of research protocols that have a high probability of death

    E. To make a determination that the research meets the criteria for exemption

7. A study of the benefits of hypothermia in stroke compared the outcomes of 17 patients admitted with acute stroke and treated with hypothermic therapy with 56 age-, gender-, stroke severity-, and body temperature-matched patients from the stroke database. This is an example of what type of study?

    A. Cohort study

    B. Randomized controlled study

    C. Cross sectional study

    D. Case control study

    E. Systematic review

8. In the 2 × 2 table below, positive and negative test results are compared with the gold standard determining the presence and absence of disease. What does a/(a+c) represent?

	Disease	No Disease
Positive	a	b
Negative	c	d

    A. Positive predictive value

    B. Negative predictive value

    C. Sensitivity

    D. Specificity

    E. Negative likelihood ratio

9. In the above 2 X 2 table, what does d/(c+d) represent?

    A. Positive predictive value

    B. Negative predictive value

    C. Sensitivity

    D. Specificity

    E. Positive likelihood ratio

10. In the Stenting versus Endarterectomy for Treatment of Carotid-Artery Stenosis study, the absolute difference in the percentage of patient who had a stroke of any type in the two interventions during the peri-procedure period was 1.8 with a 95% confidence interval of 0.4 to 3.2. What is the most appropriate interpretation of this data?

    A. The average difference in the percentage of strokes between the two treatments is 1.8 in 95 out of 100 patients if both interventions were used in secondary stroke prevention.

    B. In 95% of patients treated with stenting, there was a 1.8% increase in strokes.

    C. There is 95% confidence that the actual difference in the percentage of stroke in the two treatments was 1.8 and the standard deviation is between 0.4 and 3.2.

D. The absolute difference in the percentage of stroke in the two treatments in this study was 1.8. If the same study using the same methods was carried out in many independent samples of patients, the difference in the percentage of stroke between the two treatments will be between 0.4 to 3.2 in 95% of the samples, but will be outside this range in 5% of the time.
E. The absolute difference in the percentage of stroke is less than 0.4 in 5% and more than 3.2 in 5% of the sample.

11. What is alpha or type 1 error?

A. Failure to reject the null hypothesis when the null hypothesis is false
B. Failure to reject the null hypothesis when the null hypothesis is true
C. Reject the null hypothesis when the null hypothesis is false
D. Reject the null hypothesis when the null hypothesis is true
E. Error due to nonrandomization

12. What is the consequence of setting a small p value in a study?

A. The probability of type 2 error will decrease
B. The probability of type 1 error will increase
C. The probability of false positive will decrease
D. The probability of false negative will decrease
E. The probability of false positive will increase

13. Two doses of a novel agent were used compared to placebo in a randomized controlled trial for the treatment of acute intracranial hemorrhage with the p value for statistical significance set at 0.05. Both doses of the novel agent showed lower mortality at 3 months compared with placebo. The p value for the lower dose was 0.02 and the p value for the higher dose was 0.01. How can these results be interpreted?

A. The higher dose is twice as effective as the lower dose
B. The high dose is more effective in preventing mortality
C. The results are not statistically significant because the p value for this study was set at 0.05
D. The lower dose is twice as effective as the higher dose
E. Both drugs are effective treatments

14. A subject participating in a study of the effectiveness of a new antiplatelet agent for secondary prevention of cerebral ischemia has a gastrointestinal bleed requiring hospitalization during the study. What is the responsibility of the site investigator to report this event?

A. The site investigator does not need to report this event because she is not the principal investigator.
B. The site investigator should wait until the end of the study to report the event.
C. The site investigator should immediately report the event to the institutional review board (IRB) and sponsor.
D. The site investigator should report the event to the chief of the stroke division.
E. The site investigator should only report the events leading to worse neurological outcomes.

15. A neurocritical care fellow would like to evaluate the effects of vasoconstrictors on cerebral blood flow. What does she need to do to conduct this study?

A. Submit a protocol to the institutional review board (IRB) and wait for the IRB to approve the protocol before starting any aspect of the study
B. Proceed with data collection by reviewing patient medical records before submitting a protocol to the IRB
C. Proceed with data collection after getting written permission from the critical care attending while the IRB reviews the protocol
D. Ask the medical student to start reviewing the chart while she writes the protocol to submit to the IRB
E. Submit a protocol to the IRB prior to publication of the final results

16. A study has been approved as an emergency research study and granted emergency research waiver. In which of the following scenarios can a subject be enrolled in this study?

A. A medically stable subject evaluated in the emergency room who can be admitted to the general medical floor without monitoring

B. A medically unstable and unconscious subject who has a life-threatening condition and no family members or legally authorized representative could not be reach by the study team

C. A medically unstable subject evaluated in the emergency room who is awake and refuses to provide consent for the study

D. A medically unstable subject who is intubated in the emergency room and the patient's family at the bedside decline to participate in the study

E. A medically stable patient who does not speak English

17. Which of the following is an ethical principle that guides human research?

A. Justice
B. Loyalty
C. Altruism
D. Truth
E. Cost-effectiveness

18. A study examining the effectiveness of a new drug on intracerebral blood flow randomizes the subjects to start either with the control period followed by the active treatment or with the active treatment then switch to control. What type of study design is used?

A. Crossover design
B. Washout design
C. Time-series design
D. Learning design
E. Factorial design

19. Which of the following is the most appropriate statistical test to determine whether the mean values of a continuous variable significantly differ in two different groups?

A. Chi-squared test
B. Sign test
C. Z-test
D. T-test
E. ANOVA

20. An investigator records all clinical, laboratory, and quantitative imaging data on hospital day one of all patients admitted to the neurointensive care unit who have intracerebral hemorrhage due to cerebral amyloid angiopathy to determine the effect of anti-platelet therapy use on the size of the hemorrhage. What type of study is this?

A. Case control study
B. Cross sectional study
C. Cohort study
D. Equivalence study
E. Randomized clinical trial

■ ANSWERS

1. **The answer is B.** The goal of a phase I clinical trial is to determine the highest dose of a drug that can be administered with an acceptable level of toxicity. The goal of phase II and III trials is to establish the efficacy of a drug. Phase IV, also known as postmarketing surveillance, trial is conducted after a device or drug is approved. Preclinical testing is the evaluation of candidate drugs in relevant animal species to establish the safety and biological activity of the drug prior to use of the agent in human studies.

   Kelly WK, Halabi S. *Oncology Clinical Trials: Successful Design, Conduct, and Analysis*. New York, NY: Demos Medical;2010:chaps 4 and 6.

2. **The answer is D.** The goals of the randomization process in a clinical trial are to assign patients to treatment arms while reducing the likelihood of introducing bias in the study.

   Kelly WK, Halabi S. *Oncology Clinical Trials: Successful Design, Conduct, and Analysis*. New York, NY: Demos Medical;2010:chap 10.

3. **The answer is D.** The goal of a noninferiority trial is to determine whether or not a novel treatment is no worse than the standard treatment. It is often used to establish new treatments that have fewer side effects, are easier to administer, are less invasive, or cost less. The noninferiority margin or difference in efficacy between the treatment arms is established in advance so that the new treatment is preferred if the difference in efficacy is less than the pre-specified noninferiority margin. Noninferiority studies require larger sample sizes than superiority studies due to the statistical design. An infinite sample size is required to establish two treatments as truly identical and this type of study is not feasible.

   Kelly WK, Halabi S. *Oncology Clinical Trials: Successful Design, Conduct, and Analysis*. New York, NY: Demos Medical;2010:chap 13.

4. **The answer is C.** The K99/R00 is the NIH Pathway to Independence Award. The K99/R00 award provides 5 years of support in two separate phases. The first phase is a 2-year mentor phase for investigators who have not had more than 5 years of postdoctoral research training experience at the time of initial application or resubmissions. In the second phase, the investigator is an independent scientist at an extramural sponsoring institution in which the grant recipient has a tenure-track full-time faculty position. The K08 is a Mentored Clinical Scientist Research Career Development Award. The K23 is a Mentored Patient-Oriented Research Career Development Award. The difference between the K08 and K23 is the type of research the individual is conducting. The T32 enables institutions to make national research service awards to individuals selected by them for pre- and postdoctoral research training in specified shortage areas. The R01 is the NIH Research Project Grant Program to support a specific project performed by an independent investigator.

   Office of Extramural Research, NIH. www.grants.nih.gov. Published December 12, 2008. Accessed October 10, 2018.

5. **The answer is C.** HIPAA requires all researchers to obtain permission from patients before using identifiable medical data for research. The U.S. Department of Health and Human Services uses the Privacy Rule to set the standard for the use and disclosure of patient medical information.

   U.S. Department of Health and Human Services. www.hhs.gov. Published August 14, 2002. Accessed October 10, 2018.

6. **The answer is A.** An IRB-expedited review is a review of a study protocol that can be performed by a single reviewer without the entire IRB committee for studies that have minimal risk to the participants as defined by the Department of Health and Human Services.

   Hulley SB. *Designing Clinical Research: An Epidemiologic Approach*. 2nd ed. Philadephia, PA: Lippincott Williams and Wilkins;2001:chap 14.

7. **The answer is D.** A case control study is a study comparing a group of subjects treated with a new intervention with a group of subjects who are not treated with the new intervention. The allocation of subjects to the treatment arms is not random. A cohort study is a study of a group of subjects followed over time. A randomized control study is one in which an intervention group is compared to a control group in which the subject assignment is determined by a formal randomization procedure. A cross sectional study is a study in which the clinical measures of interest are all obtained at the same time or within a short period of time.

Kammersgaard LP, Rasmussen BH, Jørgensen HS, et al. Feasibility and safety of inducing modest hypothermia in awake patients with acute stroke through surface cooling: a case-control study: the Copenhagen Stroke Study. *Stroke.* 2000;31(9):2251-2256. doi: 10.1161/01.STR.31.9.2251

8. **The answer is C.** Sensitivity is the proportion of subjects who test positive for the disease when the disease is present. Specificity is the proportion of subjects who test negative when the disease is absent. Positive predictive value is the proportion of subjects who test positive for the disease when the disease is present. Negative predictive value is the proportion of subjects who test negative for the disease when the disease is absent.

Hulley SB. *Designing Clinical Research: An Epidemiologic Approach.* 2nd ed. Philadephia, PA: Lippincott Williams and Wilkins;2001:chap 12.

9. **The answer is B.** Sensitivity is the proportion of subjects who test positive for the disease when the disease is present. Specificity is the proportion of subjects who test negative when the disease is absent. Positive predictive value is the proportion of subjects who test positive for the disease when the disease is present. Negative predictive value is the proportion of subjects who test negative for the disease when the disease is absent.

Hulley SB. *Designing Clinical Research: An Epidemiologic Approach.* 2nd ed. Philadephia, PA: Lippincott Williams and Wilkins;2001:chap 12.

10. **The answer is D.** The confidence interval gives a range of values that reflects the precision of a sample estimate. A 95% confidence interval of an estimate provides the range of values such that if the experiment is repeated in multiple independent samples, the estimate will fall in the confidence interval in 95% of the samples.

Brott TG, Hobson RW 2nd, Howard G, et al. Stenting versus endarterectomy for treatment of carotid-artery stenosis. *N Engl J Med.* 2010;363(1):11-23. doi: 10.1056/NEJMoa0912321
Motulsky H. *Intuitive Biostatistics: A Nonmathematical Guide to Statistical Thinking.* 2nd ed. New York, NY: Oxford University Press;2010:chap 12.

11. **The answer is D.** Type 1 error is when an investigator rejects a null hypothesis when the null hypothesis is in fact true in the population.

Motulsky H. *Intuitive Biostatistics: A Nonmathematical Guide to Statistical Thinking.* 2nd ed. New York, NY: Oxford University Press;2010:chap 16.

12. **The answer is C.** The *p* value represents the probability that the finding will occur by chance if the null hypothesis was actually true. A lower *p* value will results in a low probability of making a type 1 error but increase the probability of making a type 2 error.

Motulsky H. *Intuitive Biostatistics: A Nonmathematical Guide to Statistical Thinking.* 2nd ed. New York, NY: Oxford University Press;2010:chap 16.

13. **The answer is E.** The *p* value represents the probability that the finding will occur by chance if the null hypothesis was actually true. The *p* value has no information regarding the treatment effect.

Hulley SB. *Designing Clinical Research: An Epidemiologic Approach.* 2nd ed. Philadephia, PA: Lippincott Williams and Wilkins;2001:chap 5.

14. **The answer is C.** It is the responsibility of the site investigator to report all serious adverse events to the IRB and sponsor.

Motulsky H. *Intuitive Biostatistics: A Nonmathematical Guide to Statistical Thinking*. 2nd ed. New York, NY: Oxford University Press;2010:chap 12.

15. **The answer is A.** It is federal regulation that all human research be approved by an IRB.

Hulley SB. *Designing Clinical Research: An Epidemiologic Approach*. 2nd ed. Philadelphia, PA: Lippincott Williams and Wilkins;2001:chap 14.

16. **The answer is B.** In order for research studies to qualify for Emergency Research Consent Waiver, the subject's condition must be life-threatening, available treatments are unproven or unsatisfactory, obtaining the informed consent from the subject is not feasible, participating in the study may directly benefit the subject, the research study cannot be carried out without the consent waiver, and the study protocol defines the length of the therapeutic window based on scientific evidence, IRB review and approval, and additional protections of the rights and welfare of the subjects as outlined in the Federal Register, Vol 61, pp. 51531-51533.

U.S. Department of Health and Human Services. www.hhs.gov. Informed Consent Requirement in Emergency Research [OPRR Letter, 1996], Number 97-01, Human Subjects Protections, October 31, 1996.

17. **The answer is A**. The three ethical principles of human research are respect for person, beneficence, and justice.

Hulley SB. *Designing Clinical Research: An Epidemiologic Approach*. 2nd ed. Philadephia, PA: Lippincott Williams and Wilkins;2001:chap 14.

18. **The answer is A.** This is an example of a crossover design that has features of within-group and between-group designs.

Hulley SB. *Designing Clinical Research: An Epidemiologic Approach*. 2nd ed. Philadephia, PA: Lippincott Williams and Wilkins;2001:chap 11.

19. **The answer is D.** The *t*-test (or Student's *t*-test) is the best test to determine whether the mean value of a continuous variable differs in two independent groups. The Chi-square test is used to test the association of two categorical variables.

Hulley SB. *Designing Clinical Research: An Epidemiologic Approach*. 2nd ed. Philadephia, PA: Lippincott Williams and Wilkins;2001:chap 6.

20. **The answer is B.** In a cross-sectional study, the investigator records all measures at a single time point or within a very short period of time. In a case control study, the investigator evaluates a predictor variable in one group with an outcome and compares it with another group without the outcome. In a cohort, an investigator measures the variables that may predict an outcome of interest in a group of subjects and follows up on the subjects over time to measure the outcome.

Hulley SB. *Designing Clinical Research: An Epidemiologic Approach*. 2nd ed. Philadephia, PA: Lippincott Williams and Wilkins;2001:chap 8.

27

Procedural Skills and Monitoring

JING WANG, GEORGE W. WILLIAMS, AND LAITH ALTAWEEL

■ QUESTIONS

1. A patient with severe peripheral vascular disease has a forehead pulse oximeter placed secondary to poor signal quality in his extremities. This oximeter operates primarily via which of the following principles?

   A. Absorption spectrophotometry
   B. Photoelectric spectrophotometry
   C. Mixed spectrophotometry
   D. Reflectance spectrophotometry

2. A 65-year-old male, status post motor vehicle collision (MVC) with bifrontal cerebral contusions, presents with a tense abdomen on examination. Which of the following could be used to assess gut perfusion?

   A. Femoral central line
   B. Foley catheter
   C. Ventilator driving pressure
   D. Arterial waveform

3. A bedside RN calls you to address significant variability in a patient's blood pressure (BP). On assessment, you observe a clinical technician holding the patient's arm still in order to facilitate acquisition of a BP reading. Which of the following would explain the variable results in this case?

   A. False arterial pulsations from the arm-restraining clinical technician
   B. False Korotkoff sounds from the arm-restraining clinical technician
   C. Random oscillations from the arm-restraining clinical technician
   D. Agitation associated with significant variability in BP

4. During an application of the Advanced Cardiac Life Support protocol on an unstable patient, the medical student suggests that the pulse oximeter is inaccurate because the patient is hypotensive. Which is the lowest blood pressure at which a pulse oximeter is reliably accurate?

   A. 50 mmHg
   B. 40 mmHg
   C. 30 mmHg
   D. 30 mmHg, as long as there is no arterial line in the measured extremity

5. While placing a right subclavian central venous catheter (CVC), a lead can be removed while still maintaining the most sensitivity for arrhythmias during Seldinger wire placement. Which of the vector-based leads would meet this criterion?

   A. Right upper lead
   B. Left upper lead
   C. Left lower lead
   D. All of the above leads must be present

6. In order to maximize detection of left ventricular ischemia, what is the ideal position of the precordial lead monitored in the ICU?

   A. Midclavicular line, fifth intercostal space
   B. Anterior axillary line, fifth intercostal space
   C. Along left sternum, fourth intercostal space
   D. Along right sternum, fourth intercostal space

7. Hemodialysis catheters are generally 2-fold larger bore than comparable triple-lumen catheters. The primary rationale for this is to:

   A. Minimize the risk of venous stenosis following removal of the catheter
   B. Ensure a catheter flow rate of at least 100 mL/min
   C. Increase blood flow by 16-fold
   D. Prevent luminal thrombus

8. A pulmonary arterial catheter (PAC) is placed under sterile conditions in a nonemergent setting. The following waveforms are noted on the monitor as the PAC is advanced. Which of the following is the most appropriate next step?

   A. Administer beta blockade
   B. Withdraw PAC
   C. Deflate and inflate balloon
   D. Administer fluid bolus

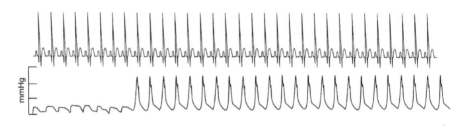

Source: Image created by George Williams, MD.

9. Trendelenburg positioning is recommended while placing an internal jugular or subclavian central line primarily due to which of the following reasons?

   A. Ease of practitioner access to landmarks/ natomical structures
   B. To facilitate engorgement of target veins
   C. Reduction of ectopy/arrhythmia risks because of increased myocardial preload
   D. To reduce the complications of air embolisms

10. You are caring for a patient with a medical history significant for pulmonary hypertension and decide to place a pulmonary arterial catheter (PAC) to measure pulmonary systolic/diastolic pressures and pulmonary arterial wedge pressure (PAWP). The accompanying chest x-ray (CXR) demonstrates the PAC placement (upright) with different directions that the catheter could potentially point as labeled. Which of the following statements is true?

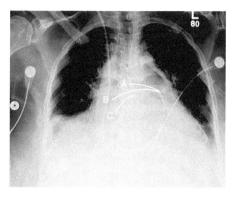

A. The pressure waveform on line A would reflect left atrial pressure most accurately
B. The pressure waveform on line B would reflect left atrial pressure most accurately
C. The pressure waveform on line C would reflect left atrial pressure most accurately
D. There are no significant differences among the lines shown
E. The PAC waveform cannot be accurate because of the right lower lobe pneumonia

11. A patient with a history of systolic heart failure is placed on mechanical ventilation. Which of the following is an effect of adequate mechanical ventilation on the cardiovascular (CV) system?

A. Increased preload
B. Decreased afterload
C. Decreased dead space
D. Tachycardia

12. A standard thermometer probe placed in a patient's bladder functions by which of the following mechanisms?

A. Conductance
B. Magnetic induction
C. Compliance
D. Photon absorption

13. A patient with a spinal abscess is admitted to the ICU in septic shock and requires pressors. Which of the following agents would be most efficacious for increasing cardiac output (CO) while increasing mean arterial pressure (MAP)?

A. Dopamine
B. Phenylephrine
C. Epinephrine
D. Norepinephrine

14. Which of the following factors does **not** affect systemic vascular resistance (SVR)?

A. Mean arterial pressure (MAP)
B. Left ventricular end systolic volume
C. Cardiac output (CO)
D. Central venous pressure (CVP)

15. Which of the following techniques may be used to prevent interference to an EEG recording?

    A. Use lighter electrodes
    B. Apply rigid electrode leads
    C. Use electrodes in which the metallic surface is as close to the skin as possible
    D. Minimize the volume of conducting jelly

16. You are called to the bedside of a patient who has an intracranial pressure (ICP) reading of 23 mmHg. The patient's blood pressure (BP) is 99/78. A CT scan from 2 hours ago demonstrated diffuse cerebral edema. The accompanying waveform is shown on the monitor. What is the most appropriate next step in management?

    A. Administer mannitol 0.75 g/kg
    B. Elevate the head of the bed to 60°
    C. Repeat CT scan in 4 hours
    D. Increase sedation with fentanyl infusion

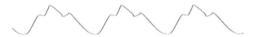

17. A patient (status post left basal ganglia hemorrhagic stroke 2 days ago) has been on nasal cannula since admission, but now appears to be in respiratory distress. The patient has an arterial blood gas (ABG) that reveals pH 7.39, PaCO2 41, PaO2 54, base excess −2. Which of the following would be the most appropriate choice for management of this patient?

    A. Amantadine
    B. Nasal tracheal suctioning
    C. Continuous positive airway pressure (CPAP)
    D. Bilevel positive airway pressure (BiPAP)

18. A 63-year-old patient with a Fisher grade 3 subarachnoid hemorrhage (SAH) has an external ventricular drain (EVD) in place that is reporting an intracranial pressure (ICP) of 54 mmHg. Her blood pressure (BP) is 109/61. You look at the EVD and realize that the pressure transducer is mechanically fixed 20 cm below the level of the circle of Willis. Which of the following most accurately reflects the most appropriate interpretation of this EVD reading?

    A. The ICP is actually much higher
    B. The ICP is actually much lower and no intervention is necessary
    C. The ICP is actually much lower, but the patient's cerebral perfusion pressure (CPP) remains less than 60 mmHg
    D. No accurate conclusion can be drawn since the transducer is not level

19. You are notified of a patient having severe hypotension and diaphoresis secondary to hemorrhagic shock requiring intubation. The patient has an oxygen saturation of 93% on 4 L/minute nasal cannula, blood pressure (BP) of 74/30, and body mass index of 26 kg/m². Which of the following would be the most appropriate order to proceed?

    A. Preoxygenate for 1 minute, perform a rapid sequence intubation (RSI)
    B. Preoxygenate for 3 minutes, perform a normal sequence intubation
    C. Preoxygenate for 5 minutes, perform a normal sequence intubation
    D. Preoxygenate for 7 minutes, insert a nasogastric tube (NGT), perform an RSI

20. During an emergent intubation, you have performed direct laryngoscopy two times, with each attempt resulting in an esophageal intubation. Long-acting muscle relaxation has already been

administered, and you are able to bag-mask the patient, although it is difficult. You were able to improve visualization of the glottis on the second attempt with towel rolls and cricoid pressure. Which of the following best describes the most appropriate next step?

A. Perform a fiberoptic intubation
B. Use a bougie
C. Place a laryngeal mask airway (LMA)
D. Call for help

21. You are performing a conscious sedation with benzodiazepines on a patient having an external ventricular drain (EVD) placed. The patient's oxygen saturation remains in the mid-90s but the patient is not responding to commands. You measure nasal cannula end-tidal carbon dioxide (ETCO$_2$) to assess the patient's status; the ETCO$_2$ is 16 mmHg and a respiratory rate (RR) of 12 breaths/minute. What does this result signify?

A. The patient is likely appropriately sedated
B. The patient should receive flumazenil
C. The patient is likely having a pulmonary embolism
D. The patient should receive further sedation

22. A 34-year-old male (status post blunt head trauma 6 hours ago) has a poor neurologic examination. A jugular venous bulb catheter is placed. Which of the following best describes the most accurate technique for acquiring jugular venous bulb oxygen saturation (SjvO$_2$)?

A. Right internal jugular
B. Left internal jugular
C. Use of a fiber-optic catheter for continuous recording
D. None of the above

23. You are caring for a trauma patient who has significant bilateral contusions apparent on a recent head CT scan. The overnight team placed a jugular venous bulb oxygen saturation monitor and the value is elevated. Which of the following is the least likely cause of this elevation?

A. Focal cerebral ischemia with surrounding hyperemia
B. Decreased oxygen delivery
C. Extracerebral contamination
D. Blood draw rate of 0.2 mL/second

24. A 55-year-old male with a history of hypertension is now post-bleed day 5 following a Fisher grade 3 subarachnoid hemorrhage (SAH). Transcranial Dopplers (TCDs) are ordered to determine the likelihood of vasospasm. Which of the following is not a factor or application that increases the clinical utility of TCDs?

A. Lindegaard index
B. High frequencies (10–12 Hz)
C. Acoustic windows
D. Brain-death pattern

25. A patient who has been admitted for 11 days, undergoing intermittent endovascular therapy for vasospasm following a moderate-grade subarachnoid hemorrhage, has been cleared by neurosurgery to have the external ventricular drain (EVD) weaned with the goal of removal. The EVD is currently at 10 cm H$_2$O and open. Which of the following is the safest and most expeditious method of weaning this EVD (with the EVD being reopened in the event of intracranial hypertension or hydrocephalus)?

A. Clamp now, check a CT scan tomorrow

B. Raise by 5 cm now and every day until 25 cm, then clamp, then perform a CT scan 24 hours later

C. Raise to 20 cm now, clamp tomorrow, perform a CT scan 24 hours later only if patient has symptoms

D. Raise to 20 cm now, clamp tomorrow, then perform a CT scan 24 hours later

26. In preventing meningitis in patients with external ventricular drains (EVDs), which of the following is most accurate?

   A. Catheter tunneling reduces long-term infection rates
   B. There is no correlation between catheter irrigation and infection rates
   C. Changing catheters every 5 days reduces infection rates
   D. Protocol development for insertion reduces infection rates

27. A patient returns from a procedure in the operating room (OR) under general anesthesia and you attempt to acquire a postprocedure examination. Which of the following factors does not potentiate the drugs commonly given during anesthesia?

   A. Hypomagnesaemia
   B. Hypothermia
   C. Chronic renal insufficiency
   D. Gentamycin
   E. Hypernatremia

28. Which of the following factors most affects the respiratory quotient?

   A. Fraction of inspired oxygen (FiO_2)
   B. Partial pressure of carbon dioxide in arterial blood (PaCO2)
   C. Partial pressure of H2O
   D. Consumption of oxygen
   E. Nutritional status

29. A 29-year-old traumatic brain injury (TBI) patient on day 3 of his hospitalization has a Glasgow Coma Scale (GCS) of 4 on pressure regulated volume control (PRVC) with 50% FiO_2, positive end-expiratory pressure (PEEP) 5, and good ventilator synchrony. PaO2 is 120 mmHg on arterial blood gas (ABG) with a mean arterial pressure (MAP) of 120 mmHg, intracranial pressure (ICP) of 11 mmHg, Hgb of 11 g/dL, and brain tissue oxygen partial pressure (PbtO2) of 2 mmHg, down from 25 mmHg, 24 hours earlier. What is the next appropriate step in this patient's management?

   A. Increase vasopressor dose to achieve a MAP increase of 20 mmHg
   B. Transfuse 1 unit packed red blood cells (pRBC)
   C. Initiate a 100% FiO_2 challenge
   D. Administer paralytics
   E. Obtain a head CT

30. A 68-year-old male, on warfarin for atrial fibrillation, presents to the ED after being found down at home. Initial Glasgow Coma Scale (GCS) was 8 with reactive pupils. He was intubated and paralyzed for transport. CT head shows a 30 mL left basal ganglia intracerebral hemorrhage (ICH). After CT, measurement of optic nerve sheath diameter (ONSD) was obtained (see following ultrasound image). What is the next step?

   A. Send for hemicraniectomy
   B. Administer hyperosmolar agent

C. Place an intracranial pressure (ICP) monitor
D. Repeat CT brain
E. Request ophthalmology consult

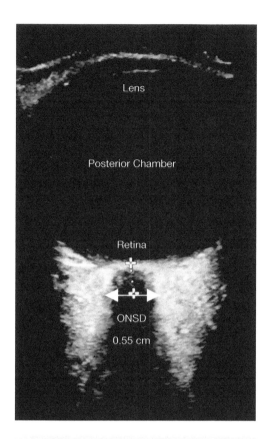

Transverse B-mode ultrasonography demonstrating
the left optic nerve sheath diameter (ONSD) of
0.55 mm, measured 3 mm posterior to the retina.

31. A 45-year-old female is intubated after presenting with a high-grade ruptured middle cerebral
artery (MCA) aneurysmal subarachnoid hemorrhage (SAH). A left subclavian central line is
placed and follow up ultrasound of the left lung reveals no lung sliding, loss of B-lines, and a
notable lung point; chest X-ray confirms a left sided pneumothorax (see following radiograph
image). Plateau pressure 16, blood pressure is 120/75, heart rate is 95/min, and oxygen saturation is 99% on 40% FiO_2. Intracranial pressure (ICP) is 12 mmHg. What is the appropriate
next step in the management of this patient?

A. Transfer patient to operating room to clip the aneurysm
B. Place thoracostomy tube
C. Needle decompression followed by placement of thoracostomy tube
D. Proceed with spontaneous breathing trial (SBT) with intent to extubate
E. Lower positive end-expiratory pressure (PEEP) to 5

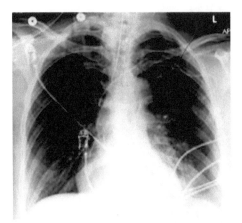

32. A 69-year-old female presents to the hospital after being found unresponsive, with Glasgow Coma Scale (GCS) of 7 and reactive pupils. CT head reveals as diffuse subarachnoid hemorrhage (SAH) and a right posterior communicating artery aneurysm, which is eventually coiled to occlusion. A left frontal extraventricular drain, as well as, microdialysis and brain tissue oxygen partial pressure (PbtO2) catheters are placed. On post hemorrhage day 6, she develops dense left hemiparesis. Transcranial Doppler (TCD) velocities are elevated on the right middle cerebral artery (MCA). Cerebral perfusion pressure (CPP) range from 80 to 110 mmHg. On arterial blood gas (ABG), PaO_2 is 88 mmHg. Hgb is 10 g/dL. $PbtO_2$ is 25 mmHg cerebral glucose and pyruvate are normal but the lactate to pyruvate ratio (LPR) is greater than 40. What is the most likely etiology for the abnormalities noted in the microdialysis values?

    A. Reduced cerebral blood flow (CBF)
    B. Hypoxia
    C. Mitochondrial dysfunction
    D. Anemia
    E. Raised intracranial pressure (ICP) with reduced CPP

33. A 55-year-old man, admitted with a Hunt and Hess grade 4 aneurysmal subarachnoid hemorrhage (SAH), is now post bleed day 5 with increasing Transcranial Doppler (TCD) velocities. Mean arterial pressure (MAP) is 76 mmHg on norepinephrine 12 mcg/min, up from 5 mcg/min 24 hours earlier, intracranial pressure (ICP) is 12 mmHg, and heart rate (HR) is 110/min with sinus rhythm. He is febrile to 38°C. He is spontaneously breathing on volume control mechanical ventilation receiving 7 mL/kg tidal volume (TV) with positive end-expiratory pressure (PEEP) of 10 mmHg. Arterial blood gas (ABG) reveals a PaO2/FiO2 ratio of 250. White blood cell (WBC) count is 11,000 with a new infiltrate on chest x-ray (CXR); and serum creatinine has increased to 1.5 mg/dL. Fluid balance over the past 24 hours is 2 L positive with good urine output. In addition to sending blood cultures, lactate, and starting antibiotics, how can volume status be assessed to determine whether additional fluid is needed for adequate resuscitation?

    A. Bolus 2 L normal saline (NS) over 2 hours and assess change in vasopressor requirement.
    B. Perform a straight leg raise and assess for change in cardiac output (CO).
    C. Place a Swan-Ganz catheter given the presence of shock and evidence of fluid overload.
    D. Measure inferior vena cava size change during inspiration and expiration.
    E. Insert arterial line and measure pulse pressure or stroke volume (SV) variability.

■ ANSWERS

1. **The answer is D.** This question is assessing knowledge of the mechanism by which pulse oximetry operates; this mechanism is spectrophotometry. Spectrophotometry allows transmission of light through a medium to determine its molecular composition (using the Lambert–Beer law). The most common type of pulse oximeter that is applied to a patient's finger operates based on absorption spectrophotometry (light transmitted through a medium), whereas forehead pulse oximeters utilize reflectance spectrophotometry. Answers B and C are distracters and have no clinical relevance.

   Marino PL, Sutin KM, eds. Oximetry and capnography. In: *ICU Book*. 3rd ed. Philadelphia, PA: Lippincott Williams & Wilkins; 2007: chap 20, 385-402.

2. **The answer is B.** Abdominal compartment syndrome (ACS) is a surgical emergency that should always be considered in a patient presenting with neurological trauma, especially when the patient is unable to express clinical distress secondary to neurological injury. Furthermore, ACS can serve to increase intracranial pressure (ICP) and impede venous return from the brain. Measuring intraabdominal pressure (IAP) via the inferior vena cava is well described, but is invasive and not preferred; nonetheless, a femoral central line would not facilitate measurement of this value. Instilling as little as 20 mL of saline in an empty bladder with a Foley catheter in place can allow the intensivist to measure IAP accurately and is the most common means of measuring this variable. Ventilator driving pressure can be expected to increase with ACS, though it is not a reliable means to measure IAP or determine the severity of ACS. While ACS impedes venous return to the heart, there is not a pathognomonic change appreciable on an arterial waveform.

   Balogh ZJ, Moore FA. Abdominal compartment syndrome. In: Vincent JL, Abraham E, Moore FA, et al., eds. *Textbook of Critical Care*. 7th ed. Philadelphia, PA: Elsevier; 2017: chap 163, 1143-1146.

3. **The answer is C.** Modern automated BP cuffs do not utilize Korotkoff sounds, but oscillometry. Auscultatory BP measurements have many downsides, including limited usefulness in the setting of shock or limited flow secondary to vasopressor administration, and lack of automation. With this system, the point of maximum oscillation reflects the mean arterial pressure (MAP; see the accompanying figure). If there is an aberrant oscillation (from pressing on the cuff) during the deflation cycle, the software that calculates the MAP will potentially make errors in the calculation of the MAP, as well as systolic and diastolic BPs (see accompanying image). While agitation may result in increased BP, it is not frequently associated with a high-degree of BP variability without pharmacologic intervention from sedative drugs.

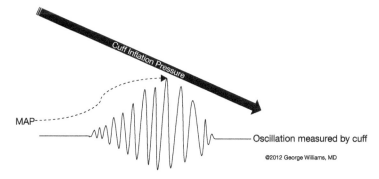

MAP

Oscillation measured by cuff

©2012 George Williams, MD

   Marino PL, Sutin KM, eds. Oximetry and capnography. In: *ICU Book*. 3rd ed. Philadelphia, PA: Lippincott Williams & Wilkins; 2007: chap 20, 385-402.

4. **The answer is C.** Pulse oximeters have been demonstrated to be accurate to a pressure of 30 mmHg (normal accuracy is within 3% of the actual SpO_2). This accuracy is maintained even when taken distal to a cannulated radial artery.

Marino PL, Sutin KM, eds. Arterial blood pressure. In: *ICU Book*. 3rd ed. Philadelphia, PA: Lippincott Williams & Wilkins; 2007: chap 8, 151-162.

5. **The answer is B.** The optimal lead for monitoring signal propagation through the cardiac conduction system is lead II, which best follows the natural course of this signal. Lead II is generated from the vector between the right upper and left lower leads, and the left upper lead is therefore not required to generate it. The accompanying illustration shows a schematic outlining of Einthoven's triangle, demonstrating the relative vector direction in association with cardiac conduction system anatomy.

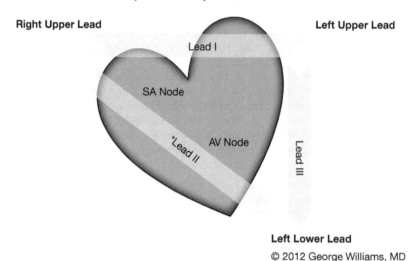

© 2012 George Williams, MD

Goldberger AL, et al. ECG leads. In: Goldberger AL, Goldberger ZD, Shvilkin A, eds. *Clinical Electrocardiography: A Simplified Approach*. 9th ed. Philadelphia, PA Elsevier; 2006: chap 4, 21-31.

6. **The answer is B.** All of the answers relate to positioning of the precordial leads; the leads listed include V1, V2, V4, and V5. V5 is the most sensitive lead for ventricular ischemia of the leads listed. The following list outlines the position of each precordial lead.

   Lead V1: along right sternum, fourth intercostal space

   Lead V2: left sternum, fourth intercostal space

   Lead V3: a line midway between V2 and V4

   Lead V4: midclavicular line, fifth intercostal space

   Lead V5: anterior axillary line, fifth intercostal space

   Lead V6: midaxillary line, fifth intercostal space

It is important to note that each of these leads reflects different components of the myocardium. Lead V5 demonstrates inferior, posterior, and a significant portion of the anterior wall's vascular territory. Many monitors default to a V5 label on the precordial lead for this purpose, though there are several that generically label the precordial lead as V1.

Goldberger AL, et al. ECG leads. In: Goldberger AL, Goldberger ZD, Shvilkin A, eds. *Clinical Electrocardiography: A Simplified Approach*. 9th ed.Philadelphia, PA Elsevier; 2006: chap 4, 21-31.

7. **The answer is C.** The large-bore catheters used for hemodialysis should be able to support blood flow between 200 and 300 mL/minute; the dialysate fluid (opposite side of membrane)

flows at 500 to 800 mL/minute. The primary reason for the 2-fold increase in size of the catheter, when compared to a triple lumen catheter, is the 16-fold increase in flow that is achieved (recall the Hagan–Poiseuille equation).

- Resistance = $(8 \times \mu \times L) \div (\pi \times r^4)$, where L is the length of tubing, μ is the fluid viscosity, and r is the tubing radius.

Venous stenosis is correlated with the insertion site: subclavian insertion has the highest incidence of stenosis, reducing the eventual option of placing chronic access distal to the vein. The femoral vein has a higher rate of thrombosis when compared to the internal jugular vein, but patient comfort or cooperation frequently limits the option of placing internal jugular access; catheter maintenance (periodic flushing, etc.) is more important than catheter bore size in determining rates of thrombosis. It is important to note that increasing length will reduce flow through the catheter as well.

Marino PL, Sutin KM, eds. Oliguria and acute renal failure. In: *ICU Book*. 3rd ed. Philadelphia, PA: Lippincott Williams & Wilkins; 2007: chap 31, 579-594.

8. **The answer is B.** The waveform shown demonstrates a PAC being floated that is remaining in the right ventricle. The graph appears tachycardic from a resolution standpoint, but does not actually indicate an elevated heart rate (HR). Deflating and reinflating the balloon cannot be expected to reliably aid in advancing the catheter. Administering a fluid bolus would help increase preload, but would not likely result in prompt movement of the catheter forward in the cardiac circulation; additionally, a bolus would take a relatively significant amount of time and could precipitate arrhythmias. The most appropriate action is to withdraw the PAC and reattempt insertion.

Rosen M, Latto P, Ng WS, et al., eds. Practical aspects of technique. In: *Handbook of Percutaneous Central Venous Catheterisation*. 2nd ed. Philadelphia, PA: W.B. Saunders Company; 1992: chap 3, 45-52.

9. **The answer is D.** Normal Trendelenburg positioning is achieved at 10° to 30° tilt; however, factors such as moving unnecessary equipment, tilting the head, and shoulder rolls actually improve the visualization of anatomical landmarks. Engorgement of the target veins is a clear benefit of the Trendelenburg position; however, it is not the primary reason for this positioning from a patient safety perspective. The central venous line placement is highly risky for sudden cardiac death because of potential arrhythmias caused by irritation of the cardiac conduction system from the guide wire used to place the line; this is particularly important in patients with left bundle branch block (LBBB) since the wire could precipitate a right bundle branch block, causing a complete heart block. Nonetheless, increased preload from Trendelenburg positioning has not been demonstrated to reduce the risk of ectopy. Air embolism may easily result from central line placement; a volume of 100 mL may be entrained through a 14-G catheter in 1 second. With increased venous pressures, air embolism becomes less likely. In the Trendelenburg position, if air embolism does occur, the likelihood of the air migrating to the brain is reduced when compared to 0° or greater elevation.

Rosen M, Latto P, Ng WS, et al., eds. Practical aspects of technique. In: *Handbook of Percutaneous Central Venous Catheterisation*. 2nd ed. Philadelphia, PA: W.B. Saunders Company; 1992: chap 3, 45-52.

10. **The answer is C.** This question is actually asking about the distribution of the patient's West zones. These theoretical zones are distributed based on gravity and determine the pressure relationships among the pulmonary arteries, pulmonary veins, and alveoli. In West zone 1, alveolar pressure exceeds pulmonary artery and pulmonary venous pressure. In West zone 2, pulmonary arterial pressure exceeds alveolar pressure, which exceeds pulmonary venous pressure. A PAC positioned in either West zone 1 or 2 will be susceptible to alveolar pressure, and measurements can be expected to reflect alveolar or airway pressure rather than left atrial pressure. In West zone 3, pulmonary arterial pressure exceeds pulmonary venous pressure, which exceeds alveolar pressure; the tip of the PAC must lie in zone 3 for PAWP to accurately reflect left atrial pressure. The CXR demonstrates a patient in the upright position; line C would most closely reflect West zone 3 (because it is pointing downward) and is

therefore the most accurate waveform. A small pneumothorax or lobar pneumonia should not significantly derange PAC pressure waveforms.

Schroeder R, Barbeito A, Bar-Yosef S. Cardiovascular Monitoring. In: Miller RD, Erikson LI, Fleisher LA, et al., eds. Miller's Anesthesia. 8th ed. Philadelphia, PA: Churchill Livingstone; chap 45, 1345-1395.

11. **The answer is B.** Positive pressure ventilation has many effects on the cardiovascular system, with the commonly cited effect being reductions in preload secondary to increased intrathoracic pressures. It is important to remember that elevations in intrathoracic pressure, in effect, squeeze the ventricle and result in reductions in afterload. These combined effects result in the sometimes-observed flash pulmonary edema from ventilator disconnection (secondary to the sudden increase in left ventricular afterload and right ventricular preload). Dead space generally increases with positive pressure ventilation because of the increase in the proportion of West zone 1 associated with alveolar distention (alveolar pressure > pulmonary arterial pressure > pulmonary venous pressure). Adequate ventilation should not be associated with tachycardia, which can be caused by feelings of dyspnea, anxiety, or a stress response from inadequate oxygen delivery to the myocardium.

MacIntyre NR. Mechanical ventilation—adverse effects of positive-pressure ventilation. In: Vincent JL, Abraham E, Moore FA, Kochanek PM, Fink MP, eds. Textbook of Critical Care. 7th ed. Philadelphia, PA: Elsevier; 2017: chap 39, 184-188.

12. **The answer is A.** Thermometer filaments are metal and are appreciable on x-ray; this allows one to determine if a Foley catheter in place has a thermometer function available. The resistance of the metal increases with decreasing temperature, and vice versa in a predictable fashion; this allows calculation of temperature. This technology and the materials used to make them are inexpensive. There is no magnetic or compliance component to commonly used temperature technology. Photon absorption, specifically in the infrared bandwidth, is commonly used by bedside nurses in the auricular cavity. However, these devices are not typically indwelling.

Dorsch JA, Dorsch SE, eds. Temperature monitoring. In: Understanding Anesthesia Equipment. 5th ed. Philadelphia, PA: Lippincott Williams & Wilkins; 2008: chap 29, 858-870.

13. **The answer is D.** Dopamine is widely used as an inotrope in patients presenting in septic shock, but its inotropic effects (e.g., increase in cardiac output) do not necessarily result in increased MAP. There is heterogeneity with the hemodynamic response to dopamine depending on the underlying condition of the patient, including variable increases in systemic vascular resistance (SVR). Most of the increased blood pressure (BP) generally appreciated from dopamine results from increased cardiac stroke volume (SV). Norepinephrine has been demonstrated to increase CO to the same extent as dopamine while yielding an increase in MAPs; this is secondary to strong α-1 and β-1 adrenergic properties. Epinephrine is a potent inotrope (β-1 properties) but does not necessarily augment BP to the same degree as norepinephrine in a consistent fashion across all dosing ranges. Phenylephrine is purely a sympathomimetic α-1 acting agent and therefore does not augment CO.

Teboul J-L, Monnet X, Jozwiak M. Inotropic therapy—hemodynamic effects of inotropic agents in critically ill patients, effects on cardiac output. In: Textbook of Critical Care. 7th ed. Philadelphia, PA: Elsevier; 2017: chap 90, 628-636.

14. **The answer is B.** SVR is a calculated number, and therefore is not directly measured. The formula for SVR is:

$$SVR = [(MAP - CVP)/CO] \times 80$$

As demonstrated, there is no factor included for ventricular volume.

Schroeder R, Barbeito A, Bar-Yosef S. Cardiovascular monitoring. In: Miller RD, Erikson LI, Fleisher LA, eds. Miller's Anesthesia. 8th ed. Philadelphia, PA: Churchill Livingstone; chap 45, 1345-1395.

15. **The answer is A.** To minimize interference during EEG recording, the electrodes are designed to fixate to the scalp and provide minimal motion at both the skin–electrolyte and electrolyte–metal junctions. This is achieved by maximizing the amount of gel used; the gel creates an electrode–gel bridge through which maximal conduction occurs. As such, the electrodes are not ideally closer to the skin, but have more consistent contact. To maximize mechanical stability of the electrode and the skin in its vicinity, the physical load on the electrode should be kept as small as possible, and lightweight and flexible electrode leads are applied.

Schomer DL, Epstein CM, Herman ST, et al. Recording principles. In: Schomer DL, Lopes de Silva FH, eds. *Electroencephalography: Basic Principles, Clinical Applications, and Related Fields.* 7th ed. Philadelphia, PA: Lippincott Williams & Wilkins; 2018: chap 5, 104-153.

16. **The answer is A.** The waveform shown here on the right demonstrates urgent intracranial hypertension. This is demonstrated by P wave reversal. Normally, the P1 wave is the highest pressure point (reflecting cardiac pulsation), followed by P2, which is cerebral arterial recoil, followed by P3, which reflects cerebral venous engorgement. A P2 wave exceeding the P1 wave is reflective of decreased cerebral compliance and urgent intracranial hypertension. Aggressive management must be pursued, which in this case would involve administration of mannitol. The patient's BP is low, but upon calculating the mean arterial pressure (MAP, which is 85), a cerebral perfusion pressure (CPP) of 65 mmHg is confirmed. Considering that all of the other measures would be inadequate to treat this urgent ICP elevation, mannitol should be given now, and a reduced BP from the diuresis can be treated later if appropriate (see accompanying waveforms).

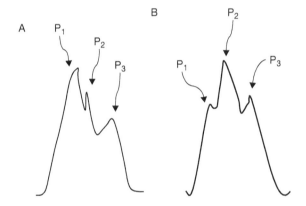

A: Normal ICP Waveform;
B: Urgent Intracranial Hypertension Waveform.
Images created by George Williams, MD.

Chesnut RM. Intracranial pressure. In: Le Roux PD, Levine JM, Kofke WA, eds. *Monitoring in Neurocritical Care.* 1st ed. Philadelphia, PA: Elsevier; 2013: chap 34, 338-347.

17. **The answer is C.** The patient's ABG demonstrates adequate ventilation but inadequate oxygenation. The treatment of choice to maximize alveolar recruitment is CPAP, which in turn will improve oxygenation. While BiPAP could be used for the positive end-expiratory pressure (PEEP) component, it is not indicated since the patient is maintaining a normal $PaCO_2$ and has no respiratory acidosis. Amantadine may improve the mental status of a patient following a basal ganglia stroke over hours to days, but would not be an appropriate intervention for a patient in respiratory distress.

Yu F, Hill NS. Non-invasive positive pressure ventilation. In: Vincent JL, Abraham E, Moore FA, Kochanek PM, Fink MP, eds. *Textbook of Critical Care.* 7th ed. Philadelphia, PA: Elsevier; 2017: chap 62, 373-379.

18. **The answer is C.** Every 20 cm change in height of a transducer from the level plane of what one is attempting to measure results in a change of 15 mmHg in the pressure measured. If the transducer is above the circle of Willis, then the pressure would appear lower than it actually due to the effect of gravity in our atmosphere. Similarly, if the transducer is below the circle of Willis, then the pressure would appear higher than it actually is, again, secondary to the effect of gravity in our atmosphere. This allows us to accurately correct for the error in the monitor and determine that the ICP is actually 39 mmHg. Since this patient's mean arterial pressure (MAP) is 77 mmHg, the CPP is actually 38 mmHg.

   Chesnut RM. Intracranial pressure. In: Le Roux PD, Levine JM, Kofke WA, eds. *Monitoring in Neurocritical Care.* 1st ed. Philadelphia, PA: Elsevier; 2013: chap 34, 338-347.

19. **The answer is C.** Preoxygenation is one of the single most efficacious techniques that can be used to prevent desaturation following induction for intubation. Preoxygenation for 5 minutes with 100% FiO_2 has been demonstrated to achieve a sustained saturation of greater than 90% for approximately 6 minutes. NGT insertion would not be indicated in this case and may actually be harmful given the unstable condition of this patient. No indications for an RSI are provided in this case. These indications include trauma, recent oral intake, bowel perforation, ileus, or pregnancy.

   Hagberg CA, Artime CA. Airway management in the adult. In: Miller RD, Erikson LI, Fleisher LA, et al., eds. *Miller's Anesthesia.* 8th ed. Philadelphia, PA: Churchill Livingstone: chap 55, 1647-1683.

20. **The answer is D.** Whenever a patient is difficult to intubate, one should call for help following two or more failed attempts at direct laryngoscopy, regardless of potential improvement in visualization. Attempting to use adjunct techniques is maybe appropriate, but only after calling for help so that further resources are available. In this case, awakening the patient or returning to spontaneous ventilation is not a feasible option. Please review the American Society of Anesthesiologists difficult airway algorithms, (see the two following algorithms).

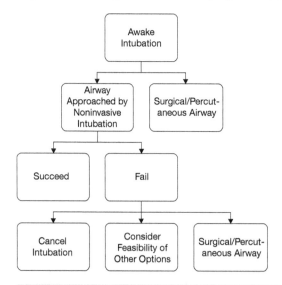

Difficult Airway Algorithm for Awake Intubation [Image created by George Williams, MD; Adapted from American Society of Anesthesiologists Task Force on Management of the Difficult Airway. Practice guidelines for management of the difficult airway: an updated report by the American Society of Anesthesiologists Task Force on Management of the Difficult Airway. Anesthesiology. May 2003;98(5):1269-1277.]

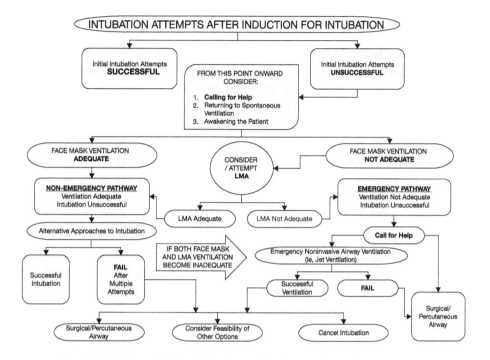

Difficult Airway Algorithm for Intubation After Induction [Image created by George Williams, MD; Adapted from American Society of Anesthesiologists Task Force on Management of the Difficult Airway. Practice guidelines for management of the difficult airway: an updated report by the American Society of Anesthesiologists Task Force on Management of the Difficult Airway. Anesthesiology. May 2003;98(5):1269-1277.]

American Society of Anesthesiologists Task Force on Management of the Difficult Airway. Practice guidelines for management of the difficult airway: an updated report by the American Society of Anesthesiologists Task Force on Management of the Difficult Airway. *Anesthesiology*. May 2003;98(5):1269-1277. doi:10.1097/00000542-200305000-00032

21. **The answer is A.** $ETCO_2$ is a highly useful tool, more commonly applied to patients who are intubated; however, it can be used in patients who are receiving oxygen via nasal cannula or face mask. The capnograph is frequently an infrared absorption device, readily available for bedside use. There is normally a gradient of 3 to 4 mmHg between partial pressure of carbon dioxide in arterial blood ($PaCO_2$) and $ETCO_2$, unless an open system such as a nasal cannula, face mask, and so on is being used. As such, it is normal to have a low value for $ETCO_2$ when used in this fashion. The normal RR indicates that the patient is not overly sedated (reflected by a RR of less than 10) or anxious (tachypnea), and therefore no further intervention without a clinical cause would be warranted. If the patient was intubated and suddenly had a drop in $ETCO_2$, a pulmonary embolism workup would be appropriate.

Marino PL, Sutin KM, eds. Cardiac arrest. In: *ICU Book*. 3rd ed. Philadelphia, PA: Lippincott Williams & Wilkins; 2007: chap 15, 277-296.

22. **The answer is D.** $SjvO_2$ is useful in determining outcomes in neurologically ill patients in whom there is a question about mismatch in oxygen supply and demand. Stocchetti et al. demonstrated a ±5% variance in values between the right and left sides, although no one side was determined to be more accurate than the other in patients with bilateral, predominantly unilateral, cortical, or deeply located lesions. The authors used fiber-optic catheters for continuous $SjvO_2$ saturation data, although this is not a prerequisite for accurate measurement.

Prakash A, Matta BF. Jugular bulb oximetry. In: Le Roux PD, Levine JM, Kofke WA. *Monitoring in Neurocritical Care*. 1st ed. Philadelphia, PA: Elsevier; 2013: chap 32, 320-326.

Stocchetti N, Paparella A, Bridelli F, et al. Cerebral venous oxygen saturation studied with bilateral samples in the internal jugular veins. *Neurosurgery*. January 1994;34(1):38-43. doi: 10.1097/00006123-199401000-00007

23. **The answer is B.** Jugular venous bulb saturation ($SjvO_2$) is a reflection of cerebral oxygen supply and demand. While a low $SjvO_2$ may be clearly indicative of a global mismatch of the supply to demand ratio, an elevated $SjvO_2$ is more difficult to isolate in terms of causative derangements. Potential causes include:

    a. Focal cerebral ischemia, if the reduced oxygen saturation from the ischemic brain is offset by a high oxygen saturation from surrounding hyperemic brain

    b. Oxygen-limited cytochrome turnover

    c. Restrictive oxygen diffusion

    d. Extracerebral contamination of blood in the jugular bulb when cerebral blood flow is low

    e. Rapid drawing of the blood sample through the catheter at rates greater than 2 mL/minute (or 30 μL/second).

    Knowledge of the patient's cerebral blood flow and/or cerebral metabolic rate is needed to further delineate a cause of elevated $SjvO_2$. Cormio et al. demonstrated that higher $SjvO_2$ is associated with poorer outcomes when compared to severely head-injured patients who had a normal $SjvO_2$.

    Cormio M, Valadka AB, Robertson CS, et al. Elevated jugular venous oxygen saturation after severe head injury. *J Neurosurg*. January 1999;90(1):9-15. doi:10.3171/jns.1999.90.1.0009

    Prakash A, Matta BF. Jugular bulb oximetry. In: Le Roux PD, Levine JM, Kofke WA, eds. *Monitoring in Neurocritical Care*. 1st ed. Philadelphia, PA: Elsevier; 2013: chap 32, 320-326.

24. **The answer is B.** The Lindegaard index was developed to determine the likelihood of vasospasm with greater accuracy. It is defined as the ratio between the mean flow velocity in the middle cerebral artery (MCA) and the mean flow velocity in the extracranial internal carotid artery (ICA); the MCA was chosen because it is the only artery in which threshold velocities have been clearly defined above which vasospasm is suspected. There is no firm consensus for other vessels. Lower frequencies (1–2 Hz) are used to maximize bone penetration. Four acoustic windows (transtemporal, transorbital, suboccipital, and retromandibular) are used, corresponding to the points at which sound can most easily penetrate the skull to allow assessment of the vessels. A description of a brain-death pattern found on TCD has been published; However, it is not universally accepted as defining brain death.

    Rasulo FA, De Peri E, Lavinio A, et al. Transcranial Doppler ultrasonography in intensive care. *Eur J Anaesthesiol Suppl*. 2008;42:167-173. doi:10.1017/S0265021507003341

25. **The answer is A.** EVD weaning is a source of significant debate and variation in practice. Choices A, B, and D are employed by different surgeons; however, only A has been demonstrated by a randomized control trial to be superior to choice B in terms of length of stay. Klopfenstein et al. demonstrated that rapid weaning results in shorter lengths of stay and no increase in shunt insertion rates.

    Klopfenstein JD, Kim LJ, Feiz-Erfan I, et al. Comparison of rapid and gradual weaning from external ventricular drainage in patients with aneurysmal subarachnoid hemorrhage: a prospective randomized trial. *J Neurosurg*. February 2004;100(2):225-229. doi:10.3171/jns.2004.100.2.0225

26. **The answer is D.** Catheter tunneling has been shown to reduce infection rates at the time of insertion; however, it still resulted in long-term infection rates of 17% (compared to 0%–22% for traditional EVDs). A correlation between irrigations and infection rates has been demonstrated and as such has led to the development of highly effective protocols (that restrict EVD manipulation and reduce infection rates). Prophylactic catheter changes every 5 days have not demonstrated reduced infection rates compared to allowing a catheter to remain.

Dasic D, Hanna SJ, Bojanic S, et al. External ventricular drain infection: the effect of a strict protocol on infection rates and a review of the literature. *Br J Neurosurg.* October 2006;20(5):296-300. doi:10.1080/02688690600999901

27. **The answer is A.** Hypermagnesemia may potentiate neuromuscular blockade by inhibiting acetylcholine release from the motor terminal as well as reducing end plate sensitivity to acetylcholine. Hypothermia reduces the metabolism of anesthetic drugs and therefore should be considered a sedative in its own right. Renal insufficiency impairs clearance of most muscle relaxants. Gentamycin, hypernatremia, hyperlithiumemia, hypokalemia, and hypocalcemia potentiate the effect of neuromuscular blocking agents.

Nacuib M, Len CA, Meistelman C. Pharmacology of neuromuscular blocking drugs. In: Miller RD, Erikson LI, Fleisher LA, et al., eds. *Miller's Anesthesia.* 8th ed. Philadelphia, PA: Churchill Livingstone: chap 34, 958-994.

28. **The answer is D.** The respiratory quotient is defined as the production of carbon dioxide divided by consumption of oxygen. FiO_2, partial pressure of water, and $PaCO_2$ are all components of the alveolar gas equation, along with the respiratory quotient. Type and status of nutrition are key factors in determining the respiratory quotient, but the consumption of oxygen must be measured and therefore most affects the respiratory quotient of all of the variables listed.

Gentile MM, Davies JD. Bedside monitoring of pulmonary function. In: Vincent JL, Abraham E, Moore FA, Kochanek PM, Fink MP, eds. *Textbook of Critical Care.* 7th ed. Philadelphia, PA: Elsevier; 2017: chap 35, 158-166.

29. **The answer is C.** A brain tissue oxygen ($PbtO_2$) monitor is inserted in the white matter, placed on the side of the injury and near, but not within, the infarct or hemorrhage. Low $PbtO_2$ (less than 20 mmHg) in patients with poor neurological exam may be indicative of ischemia, catheter malposition (within infarcted tissue) or malfunction. By briefly raising the FiO_2 to 100%, the adequacy of placement and catheter function can be assessed—an increase in $PbtO_2$ suggests a functioning probe and likely hypoxic brain tissue; while a lack of increase suggests malposition or nonfunctioning probe, and a CT brain should be obtained. If the FiO_2 challenge is suggestive of ischemic brain, then treatment should be aimed at improving cerebral blood flow (e.g. by increasing MAP or decreasing ICP) and oxygen content (e.g. transfusing pRBC, or increasing FIO_2 or PEEP), as well as reducing cerebral metabolic demand (e.g. treating fever, seizures, pain, or agitation). For this patient, all the aforementioned variables are optimized.

Kurtz P, Schmidt JM, Claassen J, et al. Anemia is associated with metabolic distress and brain tissue hypoxia after subarachnoid hemorrhage. *Neurocrit Care.* 2010;13(1):10-16. doi:10.1007/s12028-010-9357-y

Le Roux P, Menon DK, Citerio G, et al. The International Multidisciplinary Consensus Conference on Multimodality Monitoring in Neurocritical Care: a list of recommendations and additional conclusions: a statement for healthcare professionals from the Neurocritical Care Society and the European Society of Intensive Care Medicine. *Neurocrit Care.* 2014;21(suppl 2):S282-S296. doi: 10.1007/s12028-014-0077-6

Oddo M, Bösel J. Monitoring of brain and systemic oxygenation in neurocritical care patients. *Neurocrit Care.* 2014;21(suppl 2):S103-S120. doi:10.1007/s12028-014-0024-6

30. **The correct answer is B.** The optic nerve is contiguous with the subarachnoid space, making it sensitive to changes in ICP, with an increase in ICP resulting in an enlargement of the ONSD. Utilizing ultrasound B-mode, the ONSD is measured 3 mm posterior to the retina, and a diameter of greater than 5 mm is highly sensitive and specific for ICP >20 mmHg. Since the patient has a moderately sized hemorrhage with low GCS, an ONSD of 5.5 mm is highly suggestive of acutely raised ICP of >20 mmHg, and would warrant treatment with hyperosmolar therapy until an ICP monitor can be placed; which cannot be done until the International Normalized Ratio (INR) is checked and corrected. Hemicraniectomy is not yet indicated. The other answers are distractors.

Dubourg J, Javouhey E, Geeraerts T, et al. Ultrasonography of optic nerve sheath diameter for detection of raised intracranial pressure: a systematic review and meta-analysis. *Intensive Care Med.* 2011;37(7):1059-1068. doi:10.1007/s00134-011-2224-2

Maissan IM, Dirven PJAC, Haitsma IK, et al. Ultrasonographic measured optic nerve sheath diameter as an accurate and quick monitor for changes in intracranial pressure. *J Neurosurg.* 2015;123(3):743-747. doi:10.3171/2014.10.JNS141197

Rajajee V, Vanaman M, Fletcher JJ, et al. Optic nerve ultrasound for the detection of raised intracranial pressure. *Neurocrit Care.* 2011;15(3):506-515. doi:10.1007/s12028-011-9606-8

31. **The correct answer is B.** This patient has a left sided moderate pneumothorax while on positive pressure ventilation. Ultrasound was initially used to identify the pneumothorax based on three features: (1) loss of the normal lung sliding, a very sensitive but nonspecific sign of pneumothorax; (2) absence of "B-lines," and (3) the identification of a lung point, or transition point between normal and collapsed lung. These three findings are needed to diagnose pneumothorax on ultrasound. Since the patient was hemodynamically stable, a chest x-ray was obtained and confirmed the pneumothorax; had there been hemodynamic instability (i.e., tension pneumothorax), then immediate needle decompression (by placing a large gauge needle in the mid-clavicular line, 2nd intercostal space) would have been appropriate. Guidelines recommend placement of a thoracostomy tube in any mechanically ventilated patients with a pneumothorax; although a retrospective study suggests that observation may be appropriate in those without tension pneumothorax. A thoracostomy tube can be placed above the rib in the "triangle of safety" of the axilla. Alternatively, a small-bore catheter can be placed anteriorly along the 2nd intercostal space, mid-clavicular line, using the seldinger technique. Lowering the PEEP may lower the risk for progression to tension pneumothorax, but the risk persists nonetheless. Extubation is not possible given the acute SAH and low GCS. Sending the patient for clipping or coiling is risky without first treating the pneumothorax.

Havelock T, Teoh R, Laws D, et al. Pleural procedures and thoracic ultrasound: British Thoracic Society Pleural Disease Guideline 2010. *Thorax.* 2010;65(suppl 2):ii61-ii76. doi:10.1136/thx.2010.137026

Hsu C-W, Sun S-F. Iatrogenic pneumothorax related to mechanical ventilation. *World J Crit Care Med.* 2014;3(1):8-14. doi:10.5492/wjccm.v3.i1.8

Lichtenstein DA. BLUE-protocol and FALLS-protocol: two applications of lung ultrasound in the critically ill. *Chest.* 2015;147(6):1659-1670. doi:10.1378/chest.14-1313

Moore FO, Goslar PW, Coimbra R, et al. Blunt traumatic occult pneumothorax: is observation safe?—results of a prospective, AAST multicenter study. *J Trauma.* 2011;70(5):1019-1023; discussion 1023-1025. doi:10.1097/TA.0b013e318213f727

32. **The correct answer is C.** Microdialysis measures the chemistry of the extracellular space within a small area in brain, as a means of detecting secondary brain injury, and typically in conjunction with ICP monitoring. A microdialysis catheter is typically inserted into the white matter via burr hole or under visualization during craniotomy. Perfusion fluid is passed through the catheter at a set rate, which creates a gradient for bidirectional flow (between the perfusion fluid and interstitial fluid compartments) through a porous membrane at the tip of the catheter. The perfusion fluid returning from the catheter typically contains molecules such as glucose, lactate, and pyruvate - components of the tricarboxylic acid cycle, dependent on mitochondrial function. Under normal physiologic conditions, adenosine triphosphate (ATP) production occurs by glycolysis of glucose to pyruvate for utilization in the tricarboxylic acid cycle. During hypoxic (partial brain oxygen, or $PbtO_2$, less than 20 mmHg), or anaerobic conditions (e.g., due to raised ICP or reduced cerebral blood flow) pyruvate levels are reduced by metabolism to lactate, resulting in a high LPR (LPR >25–40). LPR can also be elevated during nonischemic metabolic distress, or mitochondrial dysfunction, however, pyruvate levels will be normal or high, and $PbtO_2$ will be $\geq$20 mmHg. Our patient had normal $PbtO_2$, normal pyruvate level and high LPR, suggestive of mitochondrial dysfunction. All the other choices would be expected to result in an ischemic profile (low $PbtO_2$ and pyruvate and high LPR).

Hutchinson P, O'Phelan K. International multidisciplinary consensus conference on multimodality monitoring: cerebral metabolism. *Neurocrit Care.* 2014;21(suppl 2):S148-S158. doi:10.1007/s12028-014-0035-3

33. **The correct answer is B.** Our patient is in septic shock, which requires timely acquisition of cultures, lactic acid, initiating antibiotics, and fluid resuscitation. This question is focused on how to best determine whether a patient in shock has been adequately resuscitated—a critical

question, since too little fluid leads to inadequate preload, reduced cardiac output (CO) and oxygen delivery, and consequently tissue hypoperfusion. Conversely, excessive volume loading, without further increase in CO, would lead to hemodilution and tissue edema. Fluid overload has been associated with worse outcomes in critically ill patients, and current guidelines recommend frequent assessment for ongoing need for resuscitation prior to fluid administration. Fluid responsiveness can be assessed by several methods. Traditional static measures of cardiac preload, such as central venous pressure (CVP) and pulmonary capillary wedge pressure (PCWP) are unreliable for predicting fluid responsiveness. Dynamic measures of cardiac preload, such as stroke volume variation (SVV) and pulse pressure variability (PPV) require an arterial line, and are excellent measures of volume responsiveness in shock patients - with some notable exceptions: spontaneous respiration; tidal volume (TV) <8 mL/kg; PEEP >5; low lung compliance (i.e., ARDS); and when arrhythmias are present. Our patient was spontaneously breathing, limiting the diagnostic accuracy of SVV/PPV. Variation in inferior vena caval size during mechanical ventilation, as measured by echocardiography, is another means of assessing fluid responsiveness, but seems to be less sensitive and specific than SVV/PPV, with similar limitations. A third technique involves an "autotransfusion," by passively raising the legs to 40 degrees in a supine patient, which has been shown to be a sensitive and specific assessment for volume responsiveness, potentially even in spontaneously breathing patients, during low-tidal ventilation, and with cardiac arrhythmia.

Charbonneau H, Riu B, Faron M, et al. Predicting preload responsiveness using simultaneous recordings of inferior and superior vena cava diameters. *Crit Care.* 2014;18(5):473. doi:10.1186/s13054-014-0473-5

Cherpanath TGV, Hirsch A, Geerts BF, et al. Predicting fluid responsiveness by passive leg raising: a systematic review and meta-analysis of 23 clinical trials. *Crit Care Med.* 2016;44(5):981-991. doi:10.1097/CCM.0000000000001556

Micek ST, McEvoy C, McKenzie M, et al. Fluid balance and cardiac function in septic shock as predictors of hospital mortality. *Crit Care.* 2013;17(5):R246. doi:10.1186/cc13072

Monnet X, Marik PE, Teboul J-L. Prediction of fluid responsiveness: an update. *Ann Intensive Care.* 2016;6(1):111. doi:10.1186/s13613-016-0216-7

Zhang Z, Xu X, Ye S, et al. Ultrasonographic measurement of the respiratory variation in the inferior vena cava diameter is predictive of fluid responsiveness in critically ill patients: systematic review and meta-analysis. *Ultrasound Med Biol.* 2014;40(5):845-853. doi:10.1016/j.ultrasmedbio.2013.12.010

28

Clinical Cases

ASMA ZAKARIA, BÜLENT YAPICILAR, AND POUYA TAHSILI-FAHADAN

■ QUESTIONS

1. An 18-year-old man admitted to the hospital with a gunshot wound to the head and intractable intracranial hypertension is being de-escalated from hyperosmolar therapy with hypertonic saline and slowly rewarmed at 0.25°C/hour to target temperature of 37°C. His current temperature is 35.5°C. The nurse informs you that his serum potassium is 2.0 mEq/L, despite having received approximately 120 mEq of potassium chloride in replacement that day, and the urine output has been consistently greater than 200 mL/hour. Additional pertinent labs include Na 153 mEq/L, Mg 1.5 mEq/L, and HCO$_3$ 20 mEq/L. You notice a change on the telemetry monitor and order a stat ECG (see following image). What is the likely cause of this abnormality?

   A. Acute myocardial infarction (MI)
   B. Acute pulmonary embolism
   C. Hypokalemia
   D. Acidosis
   E. Hypothermia

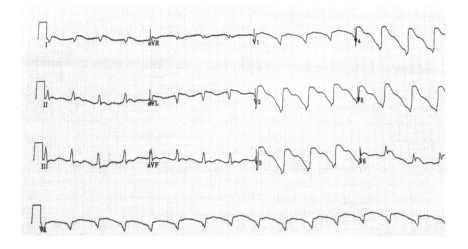

2. A 44-year-old morbidly obese woman with hypertension and diabetes is found slumped over in a bathroom stall. At the scene, her blood pressure (BP) is documented at 180/90 with a pulse of 78; her blood sugar is 180 mmol/L. CT scan of the head is shown. What is the likely cause of this patient's findings?

A. Hypertensive intracerebral hemorrhage (ICH)
B. Embolic stroke with hemorrhagic conversion
C. Venous sinus thrombosis
D. Aneurysmal subarachnoid hemorrhage (SAH)
E. Hemorrhagic encephalitis

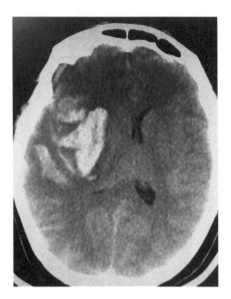

3. A 29-year-old C5–C6 quadriplegic patient is being prepared for transfer to a rehabilitation facility when you are paged for with the following finding. What is an appropriate long-term therapy for this condition?

A. Permanent pacemaker
B. PRN intravenous (IV) atropine
C. PO albuterol
D. PO theophylline
E. All of the above

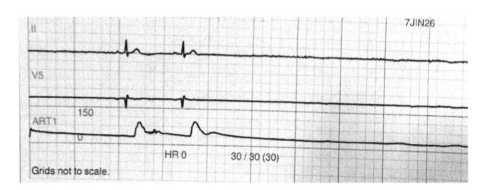

4. A 67-year-old woman was transferred from an outside facility with a diagnosis of viral meningitis and coma. She had presented to the outside hospital with complaints of nausea, vomiting, ataxia, and progressive lethargy. The patient had a history of ovarian cancer in remission for 3 years and was otherwise healthy. CT scan and MRI brain were unremarkable. Lumbar puncture (LP) revealed a white blood cell (WBC) count of 15 (40% N, 20% L, and 40% M), red blood cell (RBC) count 250, glucose 40, and protein 100. All bacterial and viral cultures and polymerase chain reactions (PCRs) were negative, and she was empirically treated with acyclovir. Upon your evaluation, the patient was comatose with sluggish pupillary response, dysconjugate gaze, absent oculocephalic reflexes, extensor posturing bilaterally, and brisk reflexes. She was breathing over the ventilator and was hemodynamically stable. LP was repeated and showed WBC 18 (100% M), RBC 50, glucose 28, and protein 150. Serum glucose was

150 mg/dL. EEG revealed generalized delta and theta activity without rhythmicity. Brain MRI with contrast is shown on the right. What is the most likely cause of the patient's condition?

A. Miller–Fisher syndrome
B. Bickerstaff brainstem encephalitis
C. Meningeal carcinomatosis
D. Pontine infarction
E. Nonconvulsive status epilepticus (NCSE)

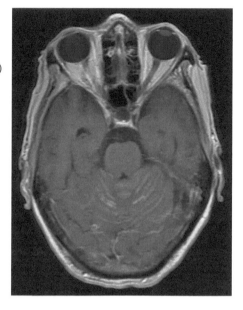

5. A 60-year-old patient with diabetes and hypertension is transferred to your ICU from another facility, where he was being treated for urosepsis. The patient has been on stable, low-dose vasopressors for 4 days, is on antibiotics, and appears adequately volume resuscitated. On reviewing the chart, you realize that the patient has not received nutrition since his admission to the hospital 5 days ago because he was on vasopressors. You would:

A. Insert a feeding tube and advance to full dose tube feeds despite vasopressors
B. Order total parenteral nutrition (TPN)
C. Order peripheral parenteral nutrition (PPN)
D. Start a dextrose solution—it should provide enough calories!
E. Start trophic feeds through the gut at 10 to 20 mL/hour while he is on vasopressors and supplement with TPN or PPN

6. A 40-year-old woman is admitted to the hospital after witnessed cardiac arrest for 20 minutes. Bystanders performed CPR until emergency medical services (EMS) arrived. Hypothermia protocol was initiated after admission to the hospital, and the patient was noted to have frequent myoclonic jerks during rewarming. Brainstem reflexes were intact and the patient had flexor posturing to painful stimulation. MRI brain revealed scattered diffusion-weighted imaging changes in the cortex but no damage to the deep structures. EEG was performed and is shown in the following image. What is the next step in management?

A. Have a family discussion regarding irreversible brain damage and comfort care
B. Load with an antiepileptic agent until myoclonic jerks stop since they are difficult for the family to watch; then proceed with comfort care
C. Continue EEG monitoring and titrate antiepileptic agents until the seizures stop or burst suppression (BS) is achieved
D. Load with antiepileptic drugs until clinical myoclonus stops and then wait for the patient to wake up for 2 more days
E. Recool the patient and rewarm more slowly next time

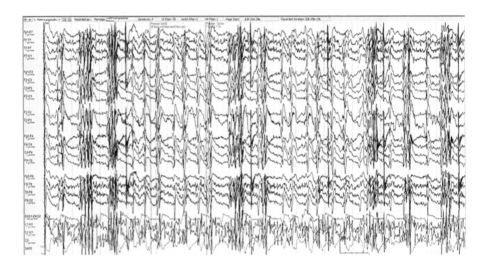

7. A 60-year-old woman with a history of hypertension presented with a cerebellar intraparenchymal hemorrhage (IPH), fourth ventricle intraventricular hemorrhage (IVH), hydrocephalus with partial brainstem dysfunction, and somnolence on examination. She was emergently taken for surgical decompression and did well. A conventional angiogram was subsequently performed and is shown in the following images. Your next steps in management include all of the following, **except**:

A. Wean external ventricular drain (EVD) and tightly control blood pressure (BP)
B. Use intrathecal tissue plasminogen activator (tPA) to allow quick dissolution of the IVH to facilitate EVD wean
C. Take a detailed family history
D. Send genetic testing
E. Continue outpatient, staged management of this condition

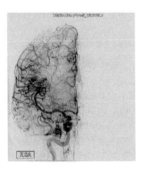 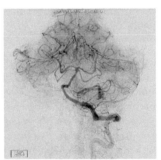

8. A 35-year-old, 2 days postpartum woman had sudden onset of the worst headache of her life. Her blood pressure (BP) upon arrival to the ED was 180/90, and she was somnolent but had a nonfocal neurologic examination. Opening pressure was normal on lumbar puncture (LP), and cerebrospinal fluid (CSF) was clear with normal chemistries and cell count. Imaging studies are shown in the following images. What is the most likely diagnosis?

A. Eclampsia/preeclampsia
B. Posterior reversible encephalopathy syndrome (PRES)
C. Venous sinus thrombosis
D. Reversible cerebral vasoconstriction syndrome (RCVS)
E. Sheehan's syndrome

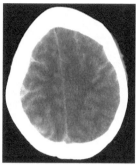 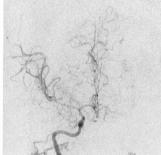 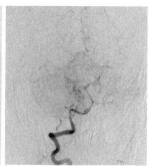

9. An 18-year-old G1P0 woman presented with a severe headache behind her right ear, followed by a left-sided tingling sensation and a complex partial seizure. She is admitted to your ICU for close monitoring and treatment while she continues to have frequent complex partial seizures. On examination, she is awake, but somnolent with left-sided hemiparesis. Imaging studies are shown here. What is the most likely diagnosis?

   A. Eclampsia/preeclampsia
   B. Posterior reversible encephalopathy syndrome (PRES)
   C. Cerebral venous sinus thrombosis (CVST)
   D. Reversible cerebral vasoconstriction syndrome (RCVS)
   E. Sheehan's syndrome

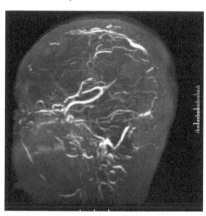 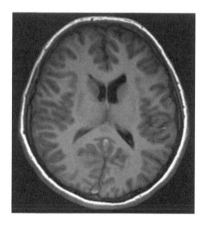

10. A 65-year-old alcoholic with traumatic brain injury (TBI), bifrontal contusions, and right-sided epidural hematoma with midline shift and uncal herniation is admitted to your ICU. After initial decompression, intracranial pressure (ICP) remained within normal limits. Four days postoperatively, the patient is now off all sedation and is still poorly responsive. He has intact brainstem reflexes, withdraws on the right, and flexes on the left. Imaging studies and EEG are shown in the following images. What is the cause of his poor mental status?

   A. Bifrontal injury
   B. Diffuse axonal injury
   C. Persistent effects of midline shift after initial injury
   D. Nonconvulsive status epilepticus (NCSE)
   E. All of the above

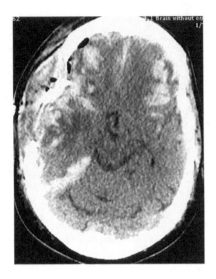

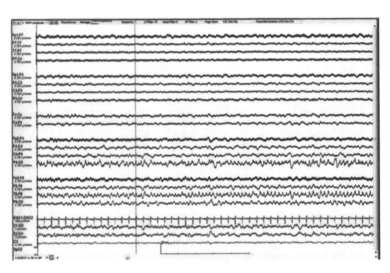

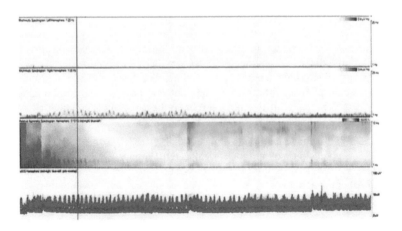

11. An 80-year-old woman is admitted to your ICU with mild traumatic brain injury (TBI) after a fall in her dialysis center. The dialysis had been discontinued due to hypotension and frequent runs of nonsustained ventricular tachycardia (VT). Upon admission, the patient was initially hemodynamically stable but developed acute hypotension requiring pressors, abdominal distension, and diffuse peritoneal signs the next day. Kidney-ureter-bladder (KUB) x-ray was performed and is shown in the image on the right. What is the next step in management?

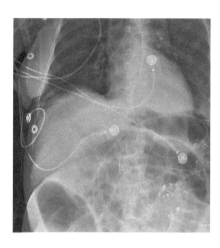

A. Right upper quadrant (RUQ) ultrasound
B. Stat gastroenterology medicine consult for endoscopic retrograde cholangiopancreatography (ERCP)
C. Nasogastric tube (NGT) to low intermittent wall suction to decompress the gaseous distension
D. Rectal tube to decompress the gaseous distention
E. Intravenous (IV) antibiotics and stat general surgery consult

12. A 46-year-old man is admitted to your ICU after facial assault with a penetrating object through his orbit. You are called to the bedside on postop day 1 after removal of the object because the patient is in severe pain. Upon your examination, the eye is swollen, injected, and pulsating. The pupil is minimally reactive and extraocular movements are difficult to assess because of pain. He has light perception on visual acuity, which is unchanged from the time of presentation. What is the most likely diagnosis?

A. Orbital cellulitis
B. Orbital hematoma
C. Cavernous sinus thrombosis
D. Carotid-cavernous fistula (CCF)
E. Orbital compartment syndrome

13. A 78-year-old man with a history of hypertension, hyperlipidemia, and mild hearing loss is brought to the hospital by ambulance after a motor vehicle accident. He is intubated in the ED for airway protection and undergoes massive blood transfusion for hemorrhagic shock. He is admitted to the ICU. Which of the following reduces the risk of delirium in the ICU?

A. Benzodiazepine-induced coma
B. Mechanical ventilation
C. Polytrauma
D. Metabolic acidosis
E. Sedation with dexmedetomidine

14. A 65-year-old man with a history of hypertension and hyperlipidemia is found down at home by his son at 6 p.m. after he does not show up at his granddaughter's birthday. He was last seen normal the day before at 9 p.m. He is taken to the ED. His initial vital signs are blood pressure (BP) 178/92 mmHg, heart rate (HR) 109/min, respiratory rate (RR) 22/min, and is afebrile. On examination, the HR is irregularly irregular. He is awake but aphasic with right lower facial droop and flaccid right arm. His initial National Institutes of Health Stroke Scale

(NIHSS) score is 18. A noncontrast CT scan of the brain shows loss of grey-white matter differentiation in the left frontal lobe and hypoattenuation of the left caudate without any evidence of intracranial hemorrhage. A CT angiogram of the head shows an occlusion of the first segment of the middle cerebral artery (MCA); and perfusion CT estimates an infarct size of 28 mL. At baseline, the patient is independent with activities of daily living and enjoys an active lifestyle. What is the next step in management?

A. Start aspirin 325 mg. Patient is not eligible for either intravenous (IV) thrombolysis or endovascular thrombectomy

B. Initiate IV thrombolysis with alteplase based on neuroimaging evidence of salvageable tissue

C. Proceed with endovascular thrombectomy based on mismatch between severity of the neurological deficit and infarct volume

D. Initiate IV thrombolysis with alteplase followed by endovascular thrombectomy

E. Need to calculate the ratio of the volume of ischemic tissues on perfusion CT to infarct volume to decide on acute treatment

15. A 72-year-old woman with a past medical history of diabetes, hypertension, hyperlipidemia, and atrial fibrillation on warfarin presents to the ED with a new severe dysarthria, left-sided weakness, and neglect (National Institutes of Health Stroke Scale [NIHSS] score 17). Her vital signs are blood pressure (BP) 169/83 mmHg, heart rate (HR) 87/min, respiratory rate (RR) 18/min, and temperature 37.4°C. Her International Normalized Ratio (INR) is 1.3. She was last seen 12 hours prior to presentation. MRI of the brain shows an acute stroke in the territory of the right middle cerebral artery (MCA) without evidence of intracranial hemorrhage. Infarct volume on diffusion-weighted imaging (DWI) is measured 48 mL; and volume of ischemic tissue on MRI perfusion scan is calculated as 110 mL. Magnetic resonance angiography (MRA) shows an occlusion of the right proximal MCA. What is the best treatment for her stroke?

A. Start intravenous (IV) alteplase infusion based on clear evidence of salvageable brain tissue and absence of intracranial hemorrhage

B. Start heparin drip with a goal partial thromboplastin time (PTT) 1.5 to 2 times the normal

C. Start warfarin for secondary stroke prevention

D. Immediate endovascular thrombectomy

E. Start aspirin 325 mg

16. A 70-year-old man is admitted to the neurointensive care unit for aneurysmal subarachnoid hemorrhage (SAH). He is intubated on mechanical ventilation. On day 3 of admission, he develops septic shock. He is fluid resuscitated and broad-spectrum antibiotics with vancomycin plus piperacillin/tazobactam are administered. Despite early and aggressive treatment, 12 hours later, he remains hemodynamically unstable necessitating escalating doses of norepinephrine (>1 mg per hour) to maintain a systolic blood pressure (SBP) >90 mmHg. Which intervention has been shown to decrease vasopressor requirement and mortality in septic shock?

A. Switch antibiotics to linezolid plus meropenem

B. Add vasopressin infusion

C. Add intravenous (IV) infusion of hydrocortisone 200 mg per day

D. Add oral fludrocortisone 50 mcg daily

E. Add IV hydrocortisone 50 mg 4 times a day plus fludrocortisone 50 mcg daily

■ ANSWERS

1. **The answer is C.** These ECG changes are typically seen with severe refractory hypokalemia. The earliest ECG changes associated with hypokalemia are a decrease in T-wave amplitude followed by a ST segment depression and T-wave inversions. Subsequently, the PR interval may be prolonged with an increase in amplitude of the P wave. U waves (a positive deflection after the T wave) may be seen and in severe hypokalemia may fuse with the T wave to form giant U waves as seen in the ECG. A pseudo-prolonged QT interval may be seen, which is actually a QU interval in the absence of a T wave. The most common cause of hypokalemia is renal losses after diuretic use (more commonly thiazide than loop or osmotic diuretics), especially if two diuretics acting on different parts of the tubular system are used. Patients who develop secondary hypoaldosteronism from liver disease, congestive heart failure (CHF), or nephrotic syndrome are also at risk. Antibiotics such as penicillins and aminoglycosides can promote potassium loss. In the neurocritical care setting, patients receiving mannitol or hypertonic saline infusions have been noted to develop hypokalemia because of the diuretic effect and as a consequence of the high-sodium load reaching the collecting ducts. For this reason some centers use potassium-sparing diuretics in conjunction with mannitol to avoid symptomatic hypokalemia in the setting of intracranial pressure (ICP) management. Hypokalemia can be refractory if concomitant hypomagnesaemia is not corrected. The exact etiology of this is not known, but it may be multifactorial. Low intracellular magnesium levels may increase potassium wasting from the collecting tubules, especially in the setting of additional factors such as an increase in distal sodium delivery. ECG changes in hypomagnesemia include an increased PR and QT interval, widened QRS complex, and flattened T wave. The findings can be identical to those seen in hypokalemia; however, in this case, the patient's potassium level is much lower than his magnesium level and, given the refractory nature of his disease, hypokalemia is the more likely cause. Hypothermia at 35°C (95°F) is associated with sinus tachycardia. As the core body temperature drops further (<90°F or 32°C), sinus bradycardia with prolongation of PR interval, QRS widening, and QT interval are seen. Osborn waves (an upward deflection after the QRS complex) are seen below 86°F or 30°C.

Ashurst J, Sergent SR, Sergent BR. Evidence-based management of potassium disorders in the emergency department. *Emerg Med Pract*. 2016;18(11):1-24.

Bilotta F, Giovannini F, Aghilone F, et al. Potassium sparing diuretics as adjunct to mannitol therapy in neurocritical care patients with cerebral edema: effects on potassium homeostasis and cardiac arrhythmias. *Neurocrit Care*. 2012;16(2):280-285. doi:10.1007/s12028-011-9652-2

El-Sherif N, Turitto G. Electrolyte disorders and arrhythmogenesis. *Cardiol J*. 2011;18(3):233-245.

2. **The answer is D.** This axial CT scan of the head shows an intraparenchymal hemorrhage (IPH) with a sylvian SAH and a small subdural hematoma (SDH), with the outline of an aneurysm visible lateral to the IPH. Approximately 20% of patients with aneurysmal rupture have associated IPH, occurring more commonly in patients with anterior communicating artery (AComm), distal anterior cerebral artery, and distal middle cerebral artery (MCA) aneurysms. These patients present with callosal, interhemispheric, and sylvian/temporal hematomas. In addition, patients may have concurrent intraventricular hemorrhage (IVH) and SDH. Rarely, patients may present with IPH, IVH, or SDH without any evidence of SAH. In these cases, a history of thunderclap headache, absence of risk factors for IPH or IVH, and absence of a history of trauma should raise the suspicion of a saccular aneurysm. Likely causes of the absence of SAH are the location of the dome of the aneurysm close to the ventricular system or brain parenchyma and delayed presentation after the hemorrhage, with radiographic resolution of subarachnoid blood. Another theory is that the IPH/IVH may represent a rebleed after the subarachnoid space has been scarred down by a sentinel hemorrhage.

Shigematsu H, Sorimachi T, Aoki R, et al. Acute subdural hematoma caused by a ruptured cavernous internal carotid artery giant aneurysm following abducens nerve palsy: case report and review of the literature. *Acta Neurochir (Wien)*. 2015;157(7):1113-1116. doi: 10.1007/s00701-015-2428-2

Thai QA, Raza SM, Pradilla G, et al. Aneurysmal rupture without subarachnoid hemorrhage: case series and literature review. *Neurosurgery*. 2005;57(2):225-229. doi:10.1227/01.NEU.0000166535.59056.FA

Thapa A, Kc B, Shkya B. Pure acute on chronic subdural hematoma due to ruptured posterior communicating artery aneurysm: unsuspecting entity. *World Neurosurg*. 2018;114:335-338. doi:10.1016/j.wneu.2018.03.211

3. **The answer is E.** Patients with acute spinal cord injury suffer a myriad of complications of which pulmonary and cardiac are the most common. Among the cardiac complications, shock and hypotension occur early and are usually the reason for ICU admission in the first week after injury. Sinus bradycardia, dysrhythmia, and cardiac arrest can occur subsequently, usually within the first 14 days after injury. Acute spinal cord injury above T6 can disrupt the descending sympathetic pathways to the intermediolateral cell column in the T1-L2 spinal cord. This results in loss of supraspinal sympathetic control and unopposed parasympathetic activity in the respiratory and cardiac systems in quadriplegic patients, making them prone to prolonged episodes of bradycardia, pauses, and intermittent heart blocks, especially when suctioned or turned. Atropine should be readily available for patients with bradycardia, and 0.5 to 1 mg should be administered when symptomatic or prophylactically before suctioning. Oral albuterol and theophylline can be used to increase resting heart rate, although there are no randomized trials to support this. Some patients with significant heart block or recurrent cardiac arrests may require a permanent pacemaker.

Casha S, Christie S. A systematic review of intensive cardiopulmonary management after spinal cord injury. *J Neurotrauma*. 2011;28(8):1479-1495. doi:10.1089/neu.2009.1156

Evans CH, Duby JJ, Berry AJ, et al. Enteral albuterol decreases the need for chronotropic agents in patients with cervical spinal cord injury-induced bradycardia. *J Trauma Acute Care Surg*. 2014;76:297-302. doi:10.1097/TA.0000000000000118

Hagen EM, Faerestrand S, Hoff JM, et al. Cardiovascular and urological dysfunction in spinal cord injury. *Acta Neurol Scand Suppl*. 2011;191:71-78. doi:10.1111/j.1600-0404.2011.01547.x

Moerman JR, Christie B 3rd , Sykes LN, et al. Early cardiac pacemaker placement for life-threatening bradycardia in traumatic spinal cord injury. *J Trauma Acute Care Surg*. 2011;70(6):1485-1488. doi:10.1097/TA.0b013e3182185509

4. **The answer is C.** The history of ovarian cancer and the diffuse leptomeningeal enhancement are suggestive of meningeal carcinomatosis. Meningeal carcinomatosis is seen in 1% to 5% of patients with solid tumors (commonly breast, nonsmall-cell lung cancer, and melanoma), 5% to 15% of patients with leukemia/lymphoma (leukemic/lymphomatous meningitis), and 1% to 2% of patients with primary brain tumors. Neurologic symptoms usually localize to several regions of the neuraxis, with those involving the spinal cord and cauda equina being most common, followed by cranial neuropathies and hemispheric dysfunction. Patients often present with signs of hydrocephalus and elevated intracranial pressures (ICP). Diagnosis is made by having a high index of suspicion, meningeal enhancement (often most prominent in the basal meninges, dorsal spinal column, and cauda equina), cerebrospinal fluid (CSF) monocytosis, and isolating tumor cells in CSF on cytology. Although the latter is the gold standard, tumor cells are isolated in only 50% of samples on the first LP, with the yield increasing to 80% on the second puncture. There is no added benefit of subsequent LPs. Treatment is mostly palliative, with median survival of 2 to 3 months. Whole brain radiation therapy and intrathecal chemotherapy are the mainstays of treatment and may prevent further neurologic deterioration and improvement in quality of life. Supportive treatments such as antiepileptic medications, pain medications, and occasionally corticosteroids in patients with concomitant parenchymal disease should be prescribed. Miller–Fisher syndrome is a demyelinating cranial and peripheral neuropathy, which is a variant of Guillain–Barré syndrome (GBS) and is defined by a triad of areflexia, ophthalmoplegia, and ataxia. Patients classically do not have signs of encephalitis or encephalopathy. Anti-GQ1b antibodies are present in 90% of patients. Bickerstaff brainstem encephalitis presents with ataxia, ophthalmoplegia, hyperreflexia, and alteration of consciousness. Hyperintense lesions are seen in the midbrain, pons, and medulla on MRI. A significant number of patients have evidence of concurrent axonal GBS, suggesting

that this may be another variant of the disease. The progression of symptoms and MRI findings preclude pontine infarction, and the EEG does not support a diagnosis of NCSE.

Clarke JL. Leptomeningeal metastasis from systemic cancer. *Continuum.* 2012;18(2):328-342. doi: 10.1212/01.CON.0000413661.58045.e7

Cui J-Z, He J-Y, Li Q, et al. Advancements in diagnosis and treatment of meningeal carcinomatosis in solid cancer. *Neuroimmunol Neuroinflamm.* 2017;4:167-178. doi:10.20517/2347-8659.2017.26

Miller E, Dy I, Herzog T. Leptomeningeal carcinomatosis from ovarian cancer. *Med Oncol.* 2012; 29(3):2010-2015. doi:10.1007/s12032-011-0076-9

5. **The answer is A.** Initiation of enteral nutrition (EN) in critically ill patients is not always clear cut. It is preferable to use EN in critically ill patients as it reduces infectious complications, promotes enterocyte health while maintaining a strong mucosal barrier, and has a lesser stress response than parenteral nutrition (PN). However, there is concern that initiating EN in a patient with hemodynamic compromise and possible splanchnic vasoconstriction may promote nonocclusive mucosal ischemia (NOMI) due to increased oxygen demand. Turza et al. recommend a four-stage approach to initiating EN in patients requiring vasopressors:

   a. Evaluate the patient's medical and nutritional history. Patients with multiple vascular risk factors may be predisposed to NOMI, while those with poor nutritional response or high metabolic demand will benefit from early nutrition.

   b. Evaluate the current physiologic state. Low-dose, nonescalating vasopressors in patients who are volume resuscitated and able to maintain a mean arterial pressure (MAP) greater than 60 should not deter the initiation of EN. Alternately, patients with dropping urine output, worsening lactate levels, and base deficit and those requiring frequent transfusions may not be able to tolerate EN.

   c. Establish gastrointestinal (GI) access and pick appropriate tube feeds. The use of formulas with lower osmolarity (<700 mOsm) and fiber content and simpler sugars will reduce metabolic demands, improve transit time, and reduce dysmotility, thereby alleviating factors which may result in the bacterial overgrowth that worsens NOMI.

   d. Postinitiation monitoring includes serial abdominal examinations and gastric residual checks. Laboratory monitoring of lactate, white blood cell counts, and hemoglobin levels or radiologic testing may be performed if there is concern for ileus.

   At times, a combination of trophic EN and supplemental PN is adopted as an intuitive compromise. This has been shown to increase the risk of nosocomial infections in a retrospective review of trauma patients.

   Elke G, van Zanten AR, Lemeirux M, et al. Enteral versus parenteral nutrition in critically ill patients: an updated systematic review and meta-analysis of randomized clinical trials. *Crit Care.* 2016;20(1):117. doi: 10.1186/s13054-016-1298-1

   Lewis SR, Schofield-Robinson OJ, Alderson P, et al. Enteral versus parenteral nutrition and enteral versus a combination of enteral and parenteral nutrition for adults in the intensive care unit. *Cochrane Database Syst Rev.* 2018;6:CD012276. doi:10.1002/14651858.CD012276.pub2

6. **The answer is C.** The EEG is consistent with postanoxic status epilepticus (PSE). Although this diagnosis usually portends a poor prognosis, the administration of therapeutic hypothermia (TH) to postcardiac arrest patients has made the prediction of outcomes based on American Academy of Neurology (AAN) criteria more difficult. In a prospective study by Rossetti et al., three clinical variables were demonstrated to have higher false-positive rates compared to the AAN guidelines: incomplete brainstem reflexes, myoclonus, and absent motor responses to pain. Early lack of reactivity on continuous EEG, prolonged periods of discontinuity, epileptiform discharges or seizures, and absent cortical responses on somatosensory evoked potentials (SSEP) were strongly associated with mortality. PSE is independently associated with a poor outcome after anoxic injury. However, in the presence of brainstem reflexes, SSEP responses, and EEG reactivity can have a favorable outcome if the condition is treated as status epilepticus (SE).

Rossetti AO, Oddo M, Logroscino G, et al. Prognostication after cardiac arrest and hypothermia: a prospective study. *Ann Neurol*. 2010;67(3):301-307. doi:10.1002/ana.21984

Sandroni C, Geocadin RG. Neurological prognostication after cardiac arrest. *Curr Opin Crit Care*. 2015;21(3):209-214. doi:10.1097/MCC.0000000000000202

Taccone F, Cronberg T, Friberg H, et al. How to assess prognosis after cardiac arrest and therapeutic hypothermia. *Crit Care*. 2014;18(1):202. doi:10.1186/cc13696

7. **The answer is B.** The patient has multiple arteriovenous malformations (AVMs) warranting a detailed family history and genetic workup. Intrathecal tPA is contraindicated in this setting. Intracranial vascular malformations include developmental venous anomalies (DVA), capillary telangiectasias, AVM, and cavernous malformations, each of which have different natural histories and treatment options.

   • Capillary telangiectasias are usually angiographically occult lesions, detected incidentally on contrast-enhanced MRI or CT scans, and are rarely symptomatic. They are benign, thin-walled capillaries surrounded by normal brain parenchyma, do not need treatment or follow-up, and account for 4% to 12% of all vascular malformations. De novo development has been reported.

   • DVA also known as venous angiomas are congenitally enlarged, thickened, hyalinized venous vessels draining normal brain tissue. They are the most common intracranial vascular malformation, with a prevalence of 2.5%, discovered mostly incidentally and often associated with cavernous malformations. A causative link between the two has been suggested, with DVAs being a precursor to cavernous malformations. DVAs can be detected on MRI, CT scan, and angiogram as a single dilated vein or caput medusa. They usually have a benign clinical course with low morbidity and mortality and do not warrant treatment.

   • AVMs are a collection of abnormal blood vessels, comprising arteries, veins, and an intervening collection of abnormal vessels called the nidus. They are congenital lesions with an incidence of 1 per 100,000, often presenting as an intracerebral hemorrhage (ICH) in the third to fourth decade. The bleeding risk varies according to size, location, draining pattern, and so on. Magnetic resonance angiography (MRA) and CT angiography (CTA) can both visualize AVMs; however, conventional angiography remains the gold standard for diagnoses, formulation, and implementation of a treatment plan which may include a combination of surgery, embolization, and radiation therapy.

   • Cavernous malformations are acquired or congenital lesions formed by endothelium-lined vascular spaces without intervening brain parenchyma. They can be seen on CT and MRI as "popcorn"-shaped dystrophic calcifications or hemosiderin deposits from prior hemorrhages. They are angiographically occult and most commonly present with seizures. Treatment is not always warranted, but surgical resection is often necessary if associated with recurrent hemorrhages or intractable epilepsy.

   • Dural arteriovenous fistulas are malformations located in the meninges fed by dural arteries and drained by dural or leptomeningeal venous channels. The most common location is the transverse sinus. They can develop after trauma, venous thrombosis, or spontaneously, and account for 10% to 15% of all cranial malformations. Clinical presentation includes headache, neurologic deficits, bruits, and hemorrhage, with a cortical drainage pattern consistent with more aggressive behavior. Six-vessel cerebral angiogram remains the gold standard in diagnosing a fistula. Treatment includes endovascular or surgical interventions, with surgery being the more definitive approach.

Chalouhi N, Dumont AS, Randazzo C, et al. Management of incidentally discovered intracranial vascular abnormalities. *Neurosurg Focus*. 2011;31(6):E1. doi:10.3171/2011.9.FOCUS11200

Ene C, Kaul A, Kim L. Natural history of cerebral cavernous malformations. *Handb Clin Neurol*. 2017;143:227-232. doi:10.1016/B978-0-444-63640-9.00021-7

Flemming KD, Lanzino G. Management of unruptured intracranial aneurysms and cerebrovascular malformations. *Continuum*. 2017;23(1):181-210. doi:10.1212/CON.0000000000000418

8. **The answer is D.** RCVS unifies a group of disorders with similar clinical and radiographic characteristics, such as Call–Fleming syndrome, benign angiopathy of the central nervous system (CNS), migrainous angiitis, drug-induced cerebral angiopathy (selective serotonin reuptake inhibitors [SSRIs], marijuana), and postpartum angiopathy (hormonal changes, serotonergic surge). Typically, patients present with a thunderclap headache with or without focal neurologic signs, normal CSF analysis without evidence of CNS inflammation, exclusion of other causes of sudden severe headache (aneurysm or vascular abnormalities), and presence of segmental cerebral arterial vasoconstriction on catheter, CT, or magnetic resonance angiography (MRA), which resolves within 12 weeks. Cortical (nonaneurysmal) subarachnoid hemorrhage (SAH) is the most common radiographic finding. The gold standard for diagnosis is detecting the presence and subsequent resolution of segmental vasoconstriction on conventional angiography. In most cases the vascular changes resolve without treatment. Calcium channel blockers (nimodipine, verapamil), glucocorticoids, and intravenous (IV) magnesium have been tried with limited success. Although the course is usually benign, severe vasospasm has been reported resulting in transient ischemic attacks (TIAs), seizures, and ischemic and hemorrhagic infarctions. Intraarterial milrinone and verapamil as well as angioplasty have been attempted with some success in severe or refractory cases. Preeclampsia is defined as pregnancy-induced hypertension with proteinuria, but there is no information about urine studies in this case and the condition is not associated with the imaging findings of cerebral vasoconstriction. Eclampsia, a life-threatening condition occurring in pregnancy or early puerperium, is the occurrence of a tonic–clonic seizure in the setting of preeclampsia. Treatment includes IV magnesium to a goal of 4 to 7 mEq/L (4–6 g IV loading dose, then 1–2 g/hour), BP control with IV hydralazine or labetalol, and emergent termination of pregnancy. If the patient continues to have seizures, the dose of magnesium may be increased (with close observation for respiratory failure or heart block). IV anticonvulsants and mechanical ventilation can be initiated in refractory cases. PRES is characterized by headache, confusion, seizures, and visual loss with acute subcortical and cortical edema on MRI. Although classically seen in the parietooccipital lobes, brainstem, and cerebellum, the edema can extend as far anteriorly as the temporal and frontal lobes. PRES can be seen in the setting of malignant hypertension, eclampsia, hypercalcemia, and due to drugs such as tacrolimus and cyclosporine. Sheehan's syndrome, or postpartum pituitary necrosis, is a complication of postpartum hypovolemic shock resulting in panhypopituitarism. The most common presenting symptom is agalactorrhea.

Albano B, Del Sette M, Roccatagliata L, et al. Cortical subarachnoid hemorrhage associated with reversible cerebral vasoconstriction syndrome after elective triplet cesarean delivery. *Neurol Sci.* 2011;32(3):497-501. doi:10.1007/s10072-011-0505-8

Lamy C, Oppenheim C, Mas JL. Posterior reversible encephalopathy syndrome. *Handb Clin Neurol.* 2014;121:1687-1701. doi:10.1016/B978-0-7020-4088-7.00109-7

Velez A, McKinney JS. Reversible cerebral vasoconstriction syndrome: a review of recent research. *Curr Neurol Neurosci Rep.* 2013;13(1):319. doi:10.1007/s11910-012-0319-y

9. **The answer is C.** CVST is a rare disorder affecting 3 to 4 adults per million annually. With the increasing use of oral contraceptives (OCP) in the past few decades, the disease has become more prevalent in adult women of child-bearing age with an almost six-fold increase in the risk of CVST among OCP users. This is followed by patients with inherited thrombophilia, hypercoagulability associated with pregnancy and puerperium, and head and neck infections. Presentation is varied and dependent on the location and extent of venous involvement. Headache is a ubiquitous presenting complaint, accompanied by seizures in 47% and paresis in 43% of patients. The majority of patients have an indolent course with symptoms developing over days to months. Rarely, they may resemble an arterial infarction but with a waxing and waning course. Focal edema and infarctions are often seen when cortical veins are involved. Larger infarctions and hemorrhages are associated with worsening mental status and coma. Abnormal signal change in the venous sinus on MRI with concomitant loss of flow on magnetic resonance venography (MRV) is diagnostic. Treatment includes systemic anticoagulation with weight-based low molecular weight heparin or unfractionated

heparin with transition to vitamin K antagonists to a goal International Normalized Ratio (INR) of 2 to 3 for 3 to 6 months. Patients with a history of deep vein thrombosis (DVT) or recurrent CVST will need indefinite treatment. Intraparenchymal hemorrhage (IPH) is not a contraindication to anticoagulation in this population. Local administration of endovascular thrombolysis has been reported, but there is insufficient efficacy or safety data available to justify its utility in patients who are not refractory to systemic anticoagulation. Decompressive hemicraniectomy can be performed in the setting of malignant cerebral edema with reasonable outcomes. Over 80% of the patients have favorable recovery. Mortality of 7% to 13% is seen within the first month, usually due to cerebral edema in the acute phase or due to underlying cause on subsequent follow-up.

Bhogal P, AlMatter M, Aguilar M, et al. Cerebral venous sinus thrombosis. *Clin Neuroradiol.* 2017;27(2):235-240. doi:10.1007/s00062-016-0540-1

Ferro JM, Crassard I, Coutinho JM, et al. Second International Study on Cerebral Vein and Dural Sinus Thrombosis (ISCVT 2) Investigators. Decompressive surgery in cerebrovenous thrombosis: a multicenter registry and a systematic review of individual patient data. *Stroke.* 2011;42(10):2825-2831. doi 10.1161/STROKEAHA.111.615393

Martinelli I, Passamonti SM, Rossi E, et al. Cerebral sinus-venous thrombosis. *Intern Emerg Med.* 2012;7(suppl 3):S221-S225. doi 10.1007/s11739-012-0806-9

10. **The answer is E.** The patient has suffered a severe head injury with multiple contusions, cerebral edema, and herniation. Individually, each of these conditions can result in a persistent comatose state. In addition, the patient is having nonconvulsive focal seizures, which may be contributing to the encephalopathy. The growing recognition of nonconvulsive seizures (NCS) in the critically ill population and the need for treatment has been a topic of debate in recent years. Are these seizures a cause of the encephalopathy or simply a manifestation of the dying brain? Similarly, should they be aggressively treated with the hope of resolution of coma or are they a hallmark of irreversible brain injury and a poor prognostic sign? Although case reports supporting both arguments exist, these questions are yet to be answered in a randomized controlled trial. Additionally, many reports of NCSE lump together patients who are delirious with patients who are deeply comatose in the setting of NCS, making it all the more difficult to establish prognosis. Until the availability of further evidence, the best way to approach these situations is to look at the entire clinical picture. Aggressive treatment, with its risks, may be warranted if the clinical picture looks worse than can be explained by the level of injury. Similarly, in the setting of a devastating injury, administration of further sedatives to treat focal NCSE may not be worthwhile.

Al-Mufti F, Claassen J. Neurocritical care: status epilepticus review. *Crit Care Clin.* 2014;30(4): 751-764. doi:10.1016/j.ccc.2014.06.006

Bermeo-Ovalle A, Bleck T. Status epilepticus in the intensive care unit. *Semin Neurol.* 2016;36(6): 492-501. doi:10.1055/s-0036-1592357

11. **The answer is E.** Pneumobilia, defined as air within the hepatic portion of the biliary tree, suggests an abnormal communication between the intestine and biliary tree or the presence of gas-forming bacteria within the biliary tree. It can be differentiated and is managed differently, from air within the portal venous system by its appearance on abdominal CT scan (see image on following page). The flow of bile toward the hilum of the liver directs the air more centrally in pneumobilia as opposed to air in the portal system, which follows an extensive branching pattern approaching the capsule. Causes of pneumobilia include surgical or spontaneous (gallstones, peptic ulcer disease) biliary-enteric anastomoses, incompetent sphincter of Oddi, and, less commonly, infections such as emphysematous cholecystitis, acute cholangitis, and liver abscesses. Portal venous gas is associated with mesenteric ischemia in 50% of the patients and can be seen postoperatively or secondary to gastric ulcers, diverticulitis, small

bowel obstruction (SBO), or septicemia. Fifteen percent of cases are idiopathic. Our patient had mesenteric ischemia likely secondary to embolism and hypoperfusion.

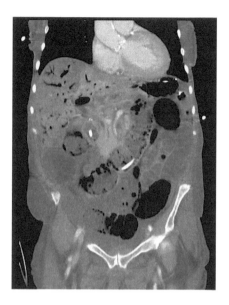

Rajkovic Z, Papes D, Altarac S, et al. Differntial diagnosis and clinical relevance of pneumobilia or portal vein gas on abdominal x-ray. *Acta Clin Coat.* 2013;52(3):369-373.

Sherman SC, Tran H. Pneumobilia: benign or life-threatening. *J Emerg Med.* 2006;30(2):147-153. doi: 10.1016/j.jemermed.2005.05.016

12. **The answer is D.** The patient has a CCF, which is an abnormal communication between the arterial and venous blood within the cavernous sinus and is characterized by pain, chemosis, pulsatile proptosis, ocular bruit, and progressive vision loss. The most common form of CCF is a direct communication between the internal carotid artery (ICA) and cavernous sinus (type A) usually as a result of trauma (young males) or aneurysm rupture (older women). Traumatic CCFs are the most common type, accounting for 75% of all CCFs, and occur in 0.2% of all head trauma and 4% of basilar skull fractures. Conventional angiogram is the gold standard for diagnosis. Endovascular transvenous embolization of the fistula while maintaining patency of the ICA is the mainstay of treatment, with greater than 80% cure rates at 1 year. Symptoms of chemosis and proptosis usually resolve within hours to days of intervention, while cranial nerve (CN) palsies may persist for a few weeks. Visual loss may or may not be reversed depending on the degree of blindness at presentation and the underlying cause. Cavernous sinus thrombosis is a close differential diagnosis and usually presents with ptosis, chemosis, proptosis, CN palsies, vision loss, and a dilated, sluggishly reactive pupil. The most common etiology is infectious with direct spread from the nose, sinuses, or teeth. Diagnosis is made by clinical findings, MRI, and magnetic resonance venography (MRV), and treatment includes intravenous (IV) antibiotics and close monitoring for complications such as meningitis, vision loss, sepsis, or septic emboli. Orbital cellulitis is a bacterial infection of the tissues surrounding the eye, including eyelids, eyebrows, and cheeks, resulting in swelling of the eyelids, pain with eye movements, fever, and decreased vision if not treated promptly. Orbital hematomas can be preseptal or postseptal. Preseptal hemorrhages are usually posttraumatic and benign, resulting in extensive ecchymoses of the eyelids. Postseptal hemorrhages may occur due to trauma, surgical intervention, arteriovenous malformations, or bleeding diathesis, among other causes, and can lead to orbital compartment syndrome with increase in intraocular pressures and vision loss from orbital nerve compression.

Chi CT, Nguyen D, Duc VT, et al. Direct traumatic carotid cavernous fistula: angiographic classification and treatment strategies. Study of 172 cases. *Interv Neuroradiol.* 2014;20(4):461-475. doi:10.15274/NRJ-2014-10020

Sobin L, Jones K, Tatum S. Spontaneous carotid-cavernous fistula: challenges in clinical and radiologic diagnosis. *Am J Emerg Med.* 2014;32(6):691. doi:10.1016/j.ajem.2013.12.008

13. **The answer is E.** A systematic review identified eleven risk factors for developing delirium in the ICU. These included age, dementia, hypertension, poly-trauma, emergency surgery prior to ICU admission, sedative-induced coma, delirium on the day prior, use of mechanical ventilation, metabolic acidosis, multi-organ failure and APACHE II score. Factors that were clearly associated with reduction in delirium were dexmedetomidine. It is unclear if this was a physiological effect of the drugs itself or because dexmedetomidine use was associated with less benzodiazepine use.

    Zaal IJ, Devlin JW, Peelen LM, et al. A systematic review of risk factors for delirium in the ICU. *Crit Care Med.* 2015;43(1):40-47. doi:10.1097/CCM.0000000000000625

14. **The answer is C.** The patient is out of 4.5-hour time window for IV thrombolysis. However, he is a candidate for endovascular thrombectomy based on the recent DWI or CTP Assessment with Clinical Mismatch in the Triage of Wake-Up and Late Presenting Strokes Undergoing Neurointervention with Trevo (DAWN) trial. In this trial, patients with occlusion of the intracranial internal carotid artery (ICA) or proximal middle cerebral artery (MCA) who had last been known to be well 6 to 24 hours earlier and showed evidence of salvageable brain tissue were randomly assigned to thrombectomy plus standard care (the thrombectomy group) or to standard care alone (the control group). Enrolled patients had good premorbid baseline defined as modified Rankin scale (mRS), 0 to 1. Infarct volume was assessed on diffusion-weighted imaging (DWI) sequence of brain MRI or perfusion CT scan using the automated RAPID software. Presence of salvageable brain tissue was based on a mismatch between severity of their neurological deficits and the volume of infarcted brain, and not the ratio of the volume of ischemic tissue at risk to infarct volume:

Group	Age (years)	NIHSS	Infarct Size (mL)
A	≥80	≥10	<21
B	18–80	≥10	<31
C	18–80	≥20	31–51

    DAWN trial measured "utility-weighted mRS" at 90 days as the primary outcome. In contrast to mRS, a lower score in "utility-weighted mRS" indicates a better outcome (ranges from 0 = death to 10 = no deficits). At 90 days, the "utility-weighted mRS" was 5.5 for the thrombectomy group compared to 3.4 in the control group, and 49% of patients in the thrombectomy group achieved functional independence versus only 13% in the control group. These translate to number-to-treat (NTT) of 2 and 2.8 for less disability and functional independence at 90 days, respectively. Rate of procedure-related complications was very low. Serious adverse events including mortality and stroke-related death at 90 days as well as and symptomatic intracerebral hemorrhage (ICH) were similar between the two groups.

    Nogueira RG, Jadhav AP, Haussen DC, et al. Thrombectomy 6 to 24 hours after stroke with a mismatch between deficit and infarct. *N Engl J Med.* 2018;378(1):11-21. doi:10.1056/NEJMoa1706442

15. **The answer is D.** The patient is not a candidate for IV alteplase as she presents out of 4.5-hour treatment time window. However, she is a candidate for endovascular thrombectomy. In DEFUSE 3 trial, patients 6 to 16 hours after they were last known to be well who had a proximal MCA or internal carotid artery (ICA) occlusion, an initial infarct size of less

than 70 mL, and a ratio of the volume of ischemic tissue on perfusion imaging to infarct volume of 1.8 or more were randomly assigned to thrombectomy plus standard medical therapy (thrombectomy group) or standard medical therapy alone (control group). Thrombectomy was associated with better functional outcomes (odds ratio, 2.77) and lower mortality (14% vs. 26% in the control group) without a difference in symptomatic intracranial hemorrhage or serious adverse events.

Albers GW, Marks MP, Kemp S, et al. Thrombectomy for stroke at 6 to 16 hours with selection by perfusion imaging. *N Engl J Med.* 2018;378:708-711. doi:10.1056/NEJMoa1713973

16. **The answer is E.** Two recent trials (ADRENAL and APROCCHSS) studied the effects of adjunctive glucocorticoid therapy and glucocorticoid + mineralocorticoid therapy in patients with septic shock. In the former study, 3,800 patients with septic shock who were undergoing mechanical ventilation were randomized to receive hydrocortisone (at a dose of 200 mg per day) or placebo for 7 days (or until death or discharge from the ICU). Although patients in the hydrocortisone group had faster resolution of shock (3 days vs. 4 days in the control group), no significant between-group difference was found in mortality. In APROCCHSS, the effect of hydrocortisone plus fludrocortisone in patients with septic shock was compared to the placebo. Mortality was significantly lower in the hydrocortisone-plus-fludrocortisone group than in the placebo group at ICU and hospital discharge, and at 90 and 180 days. In addition, hydrocortisone plus fludrocortisone therapy increased the number of vasopressor-free and organ-failure-free days without increasing the rate of serious adverse events except for hyperglycemia.

Annane D, Renault A, Brun-Buisson C, et al. Hydrocortisone plus fludrocortisone for adults with septic shock. *N Engl J Med.* 2018;378:809-818. doi:10.1056/NEJMoa1705716

Venkatesh B, Finfer S, Cohen J, et al. Adjunctive glucocorticoid therapy in patients with septic shock. *N Engl J Med.* 2018;378:798-808. doi:10.1056/NEJMoa1705835

Index

Italic page numbers indicate Answer rationales for the respective Question.